Acupuncture

A COMPREHENSIVE TEXT

Shanghai College of Traditional Medicine

TRANSLATED AND EDITED BY JOHN O'CONNOR AND DAN BENSKY

Eastland Press
SEATTLE

Eastland Press, Inc.
P.O. Box 99749
Seattle, WA 98139, USA
www.eastlandpress.com

Library of Congress Catalog Card Number: 81-65416
ISBN: 978-0-939616-00-8
Printed in the United States of America

Section III. chapter 10, "A Summary of Research Concerning the
Effects of Acupuncture," was initially published in the *American
Journal of Chinese Medicine* Vol. 3, No. 4, pp. 377-394, 1975, and
is reprinted here in revised form by permission of the American
Journal of Chinese Medicine, Inc., P.O. Box 555, Garden City,
New York 11530.

26   25   24   23

Calligraphy by James Wang and Lilian Bensky.
Cover design by Patricia O'Connor.

To Our Parents

Erma Jean and John   and   Judith and Leonard
O'Connor   Bensky

we gratefully dedicate
this translation.

Table of Contents

Editors' Foreword*

This book was written in 1974 by the Shanghai College of Traditional Medicine as a completely revised and expanded, one-volume edition of a four-volume work authored by the same school in 1962. It is unquestionably the most comprehensive book written about the modern practice of acupuncture in China, describing in detail the characteristics of some 1,000 points, more than 20 therapeutic methods ranging from body, ear, head and foot acupuncture to moxibustion, ultra-violet radiation and surgical techniques, and a wide assortment of prescriptions for the treatment of more than 100 diseases. Although one focus of the book is upon modern research, its strength lies as much in the extensive discussion and interpretation of ancient concepts and techniques. For, in addition to journals of modern research, the authors of this book have drawn their material from scores of ancient works whose theories, techniques and prescriptions are cited throughout the text.

We had two main objectives in translating this book: first, to produce a reference text for English-speaking students and practitioners of acupuncture; and second, to present an overview of the practice of acupuncture in modern China.

In pursuing the first objective, the guiding principle of our work has been to translate the book into clear, understandable English, not pidgin Chinese, nor Latin or Greek. While this approach is by no means universally followed, we believe that it permits the transmission of knowledge about Chinese medicine into English in a way which best accommodates the need for both clarity and fidelity. Therefore, only three words—Yin, Yang, and Qi—are left in their transliterated form. All other words have been translated into their common English equivalencies.

On the other hand, we have chosen to capitalize many words in translation which, were we not to do so, might confuse the reader. For example, the term Miscellaneous channels refers to eight specific vessels in traditional Chinese medicine. Had we used the lower case (miscellaneous), the reader might mistakenly think that the reference is to no particular channels, just *miscellaneous* ones. Similarly, the words Excess and Deficiency describe specific pathological conditions in Chinese medicine which are similar to, yet quite distinct from the ordinary connotations which attach to the words excess and deficiency. While capitalization of these and other key words may occasionally distract the reader, we believe this to be a lesser evil than either transliteration or Latinization.

Most of the political language (obligatory in the mid-1970's) has been deleted from this translation; some has been retained. Redundancy and textual surplusage has been pared to a minimum in the interests of economy. Nor have we hesitated to paraphrase where to do so would, in our opinion, facilitate the expression of ideas in the original text.

Still, we have omitted little of substance from the original. Discussion of the Western etiology of diseases set forth in Section IV of the Chinese text has been eliminated here. Students of medicine in

*Throughout this book, 'Editors' refers to the translators and editors of this English translation, and not to the editors of the original Chinese text.

China today are exposed to both traditional Chinese as well as modern Western descriptions of physiology and pathology in a continuing effort to forge a 'combined medicine'. It is assumed, however, that the reader of this translation is either already familiar with Western pathology, or has ready access to other English language sources for this information.

We also chose to omit from this translation the descriptions of the ceramic needle acupuncture method used by certain minority nationalities in southwestern China, and electric shock therapy (not to be confused with electro-acupuncture), with which students of Western medicine are probably familiar.

Finally, certain portions of the brief description of traditional Chinese pathology provided in Section I of the original text have been replaced with what we believe is a more thorough discussion in the Editors' Introduction.

With respect to our second objective, the original text presumes that its readers already have at least a rudimentary understanding of Chinese medical theory. We have therefore added our own introduction to the theoretical basis of Chinese medicine so as to provide even beginners with a knowledge of the fundamentals. We have also elected to retain discussion of certain diseases regularly encountered by the Chinese, but rarely seen by Western acupuncturists (e.g., malaria, schistosomiasis).

In this translation, we have used a modified version of the widely accepted acupuncture point numbering system* devised by the American Society of Chinese Medicine, which is based on that of Soulie de Morant. We have added quite a few new listings to the number of miscellaneous and new points in that system. Furthermore, many teachers of acupuncture from Asia are unfamiliar with any Western system of numbering and for them, as well as other interested Westerners, we have supplied a transliteration of the Chinese name for each point every time it is mentioned in the text. For this and all other purposes (names, places, book titles, etc.), the official *Pinyin* transliteration system of the People's Republic of China has been utilized. For those who are unfamiliar with this system, an abbreviated conversion table has been provided in Appendix II.

This book can be used in two different ways. First, it can be used as a reference text. For this purpose, we have prepared an extensive general index to complement the table of contents. There is also a bibliography of ancient and modern medical sources upon which this book is based, and a table of abbreviated titles which are used throughout the translation (Appendix I). In addition to the general index, there is an index of acupuncture points which identifies those prescriptions throughout the book wherein each point appears, and a cross index of transliterated point names to numbers (Appendix IV). Finally, some readers may find the table of Chinese dynasties helpful (Appendix III).

Second, this book can also be used as an educational text. We suggest that a student read the Editors' Introduction while simultaneously studying the introductory parts of Sections I and II (Channels and Points). After assimilating this material, a student should finish those Sections and then proceed to Sections III and IV (Techniques and Therapy).

Many friends have helped us over the long course of this project, but space limits those who we can thank by name.

Our wives, Pat and Lilian, brought this book to fruition. Without their talent, hard work and support we would still be discussing what to do. With their help, we have done it.

Peggy Welker, Cathy Nelson and Sherry Flack performed a multitude of tasks preparing this book for publication. We would also thank Lee Hiller, Jackie Ann Knapman and Alan Fonorow. Many colleagues have given us the benefit of their expert advice on technical and philosophical points, especially Chen Daquan, Kenneth Dewoskin, Ted Kaptchuk, Lin Shuenfu, Charles Lincoln, Richard Roppel and Howard Schubiner.

All mistakes are ours alone. We would appreciate comments from our readers.

* See note regarding Bladder channel points B-36 to B-54 opposite page 119.

Chicago
August, 1981

Editors' Introduction to Chinese Medicine

by Dan Bensky

Traditional Chinese medicine has developed over a period of at least 3,000 years. To attempt to practice even but a single aspect of this medicine, acupuncture, without some understanding of its philosophical and theoretical underpinnings will lead the practitioner to less than optimal results.

Acupuncture performs certain functions in traditional Chinese medicine. It regulates the flow of Qi through the channels and Organs, removes blockages, strengthens the body's Protective Qi and lessens the virulence of Excesses. To be able to use acupuncture effectively against the full panoply of illnesses it is capable of treating, one must understand the meaning of Qi, channels, Organs and Excesses, how blockages manifest themselves, and how traditional Chinese medicine conceptualizes disease. Using acupuncture without understanding its philosophical and theoretical basis is like using antibiotics with no knowledge of Western physiology, anatomy, and pharmacology: the results will be unpredictable at best.

The following introduction to traditional medical theory, although by necessity brief, will provide a foundation for understanding the practices described in the main text. The first section briefly describes the history of traditional medicine in China, followed by a discussion of its philosophical context. The major portion of the introduction explores traditional physiology, pathology, and diagnosis.

HISTORY OF CHINESE MEDICINE

Archeological finds of the late Shang Dynasty (c. 1000 B.C.) include both acupuncture needles and divination bones on which were inscribed discussions of medical problems. In the Han Dynasty (206 B.C.-220 A.D.), the basics of Chinese medical theory and practice were firmly in place. Prominent among them were the concepts of Yin and Yang, the Five Phases, channel theory, various needling methods, a pharmacopeia and a relatively sophisticated approach to therapy. By the 4th century A.D., the medical classics that laid the foundations of Chinese medicine had been written.

The most important of these is the *Yellow Emperor's Inner Classic*. This work is written in the form of a dialog between the legendary ruler, the Yellow Emperor, and his minister, Qi Bo, on the subject of medicine. The two parts of this work are quite different in scope. The first, *Simple Questions,* discourses upon general theoretical questions, while the second, *Spiritual Axis,* focuses more closely upon acupuncture. These are the oldest extant books on Chinese medicine and are frequently cited in this text.

Many other medical classics were also produced at this time. *Discussion of Cold-Induced Disorders* is the most important clinical text of this era. Its principal focus is herbal prescriptions, although it was heavily influenced by channel theory. The *Classic of the Pulse* describes this

1

important facet of diagnosis. Two other works expanded upon the contents of the *Inner Classic*. The *Classic of Difficulties* discusses some of the less penetrable concepts of the *Inner Classic*. The *Systematic Classic of Acupuncture and Moxibustion* arranges in a convenient order the references to acupuncture found in the *Inner Classic*, together with those of certain other works, since lost.

Chinese medicine continued to develop in later dynasties as the fundamental concepts set forth in the early classics were refined and expanded. This later history, described in Section I, chapter 2 of the main text, demonstrates that traditional medicine is a constantly evolving art.

PHILOSOPHICAL BACKGROUND OF CHINESE MEDICINE

Patterns

In the West we are accustomed to viewing events in a linear fashion, that is, A causes B which with C causes D. Classical Chinese thought moves in an entirely different dimension, one in which various phenomena are interrelated as part of a pattern. According to the mythology surrounding the birth of the Chinese language, the legendary sage-ruler Fu Xi (also credited with discovering the trigrams of the *Book of Change*) discerned the patterns in heaven and earth, and from them fashioned the characters of the Chinese language. This sense of phenomena as intertwined patterns has important ramifications. There is an overwhelming sense of context: events or objects by themselves have no meaning. Meaning is derived from participation in the patterns. From this grows the feeling that all things are closely interrelated to each other.

In medicine these differences in philosophy appear in many ways. While the primary mode of thought in Western medicine is analytical, dissecting things until the causal links shine through, in Chinese medicine exactly the opposite occurs. Signs and symptoms are pieced together and synthesized, until a picture of the whole person appears. This piecing together is the very heart of the Chinese diagnostic process, as we will show in our discussion of Organs further on. Based on this perspective, disease in Chinese medicine can only meaningfully be presented in terms of a particular patient at a particular time. Treatment in Chinese medicine is centered on the person rather than the disease.

Continuum

The West has tended to place different qualities in discrete, non-interchangeable categories. For example, mainstream Western thought posits a Mind/Body dichotomy. To this way of thinking, the Mind and Body are separate entities which sometimes interact with each other. Traditional Chinese thought, on the other hand, tends to view all phenomena as existing along a continuum with two poles. Thus, there are differences of shade but not of kind. Returning to our example, the Chinese would devise a continuum between the two poles, "Mind" and "Body", placing various aspects of being human along the line: one aspect may tend more to the "Mind-side" than another, and yet more to the "Body-side" when compared to still others. In traditional Chinese medicine mental, emotional, and physical illness are closely related, not absolutely different in kind. Traditional medicine takes the entire person into account, both in diagnosis and treatment.

Another facet of this perspective is that vital substances in the body are regarded as amalgams of what we would call "matter" and "energy." Certain concepts such as Qi, Blood, Spirit, Essence, etc., have attributes of both. If one remembers that some of these tend more to the energy side of a continuum, and others more to the matter side, their meaning is easier to assimilate.

Harmony

The lifestyle of the modern West emphasizes competition and confrontation. This culture-bound view of the universe was very strong during the formative years of modern Western medicine, and has influenced it greatly. Disease is primarily due to causes that can be killed, cut-out, or contained. When this is impossible, treatment is usually unsuccessful. This is still the predominant paradigm of Western medicine.

In social and natural relationships the Chinese traditionally prized harmony above all. A positive, harmonious feeling of wellness is the Chinese ideal of health. Disease is viewed as disorder in the body, and treatment is directed toward properly ordering or "harmonizing" the body. (Again, notice how disease and treatment are conceptualized in terms of the body.) This perspective has given Chinese medicine a handle on many chronic, debilitating conditions. Moreover, when reading about the functions of the points in the text, there are many which are said to "harmonize," "regulate," "adjust," "facilitate," "benefit," "calm," and so on, further illustrating the importance of harmony in Chinese medicine.

Function

Modern science places a great deal of emphasis on a correct understanding of the body's structure, and how it changes during the course of disease. Physiology and pathology are linked with structure; function is a result of structure. Whenever possible, a disease is described by what it does to the tissues involved.

Chinese medicine places the emphasis almost totally on function. What happens is considered more important than what something has come to look like. For example, the exact physical substrate of the Organs was rarely subjected to intensive investigation in traditional China for many reasons, one of which being that it was not considered important. This is a major obstacle for beginning students, who find it difficult to understand how the Organs perform their functions (i.e., what is the mechanism). In Chinese medicine the Organs *are* the functions and no mechanism, explicable on a structural or morphological level, is necessary. There has been much research in recent years as to the "scientific" or "physiological" bases for traditional concepts and treatments. These are important as translations of traditional Chinese natural philosophy into modern science, but they cannot be substituted for an understanding of the tradition itself. For example, while patients with Deficient Kidney Yin may have increased levels of certain steroid metabolites in their urine, diagnosis and treatment of Deficient Kidney Yin does not proceed on that level.

Correspondence

Traditional Chinese thought made extensive use of long chains of correspondences so as to rationalize the cosmos. This type of thinking was also prominent in medieval and Renaissance Europe, but is no longer a part of mainstream scientific thought. The correspondences, which in medicine linked aspects of the microcosm of man with the macrocosm of the cosmos, were one manifestation of the Chinese feeling for patterns and interrelationships. In some cases, however, these correspondences were based on superficial appearances and hindered the search for truth. In other cases they were empirical lists whose underlying philosophical unity was contrived by metaphysical manipulation. Further discussion of the correspondences is presented in connection with the Five Phases below.

Ambiguity

In modern science, precision of measurement and conceptualization is the ideal. Traditional Chinese thought, however, has an affinity for vagueness. This is due to an appreciation that in nature things are rarely cut and dried, but instead are rather blurred. This is also true of traditional medicine. The definitions, diagnostic entities, and therapeutic guidelines presented in the introduction and main text will often seem maddeningly amorphous. This may hinder the student from feeling comfortable with the ideas. It is also a frustrating aspect of translation, where vague concepts in Chinese are often unavoidably translated into concepts which have very definite meanings in English. It is a paradox that although a traditional medical concept may be presented in a few sentences with clarity, a more faithful expression of the idea would be less precise.

All of the above characteristics are embedded in the very fiber of Chinese medicine. They are the reasons Chinese medicine views the body in such a different way than Western science. Because of these differences, translation of terms is a major problem. Words in Chinese that mean 'blood', 'liver', 'wind', etc., have very different connotations than the English words, yet also share a degree of common meaning. In this text, when such terms are used in the traditional sense they are capitalized. For example, Congealed Blood is a traditional term and does not imply the presence of a hematoma, nor does Deficient Kidney Yin mean that the kidneys are diseased. What it is that distinguishes a Chinese term from its English counterpart will be discussed in the following sections. As each of the terms is described, the problems inherant to translation will become clearer.

Chinese medicine is an empirical science. Theory can never be divorced from practice. All aspects of its conceptual framework are closely interrelated. This makes it difficult to study, as one is caught in a circle of terms with no well-defined point of entry. So far as possible, this introduction follows a step-by-step approach. Inevitably, however, some terms will appear in context before they are separately explained.

We begin with an explanation of the fundamental properties and functions of the body.

FUNDAMENTAL PRINCIPLES

Yin and Yang

The root of many of the ideas to be discussed in the following pages, and in fact much of the Chinese world view itself, lies in the concept of Yin and Yang. These terms have been used in a somewhat technical sense for over 2000 years, having expanded beyond their original meanings of the shady and sunny sides of a mountain, respectively. Yin and Yang are emblems of the fundamental duality in the universe, a duality which is ultimately unified. The symbol of *Taiji* or the Great Polarity (below) demonstrates the Yin/Yang concept in a graphic form. Herein, black signifies Yin and white signifies Yang. The two colors coil around, fade into, and penetrate each other. Both are necessary for the whole to exist. An appreciation of this close relationship is vital if one wishes to look at the processes of health and disease through traditional Chinese eyes.

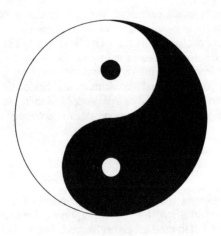

Taiji
Great Polarity

4

The qualities of Yin and Yang are projected to all levels of the cosmos through a system of correspondences. Some of the more general correspondences are listed below:

YIN	YANG
Earth	Heaven
Female	Male
Night	Day
Moon	Sun
Low	High
Heaviness	Lightness
Falling tendency	Rising tendency
Movement inward	Movement outward
Relative stasis	Clear action

It must be remembered that Yin and Yang are complementary and not contradictory. Nor is one regarded as "good," and the other "bad." Rather, a harmony is sought between them and any imbalance avoided. Because the Yin/Yang concept is all pervasive in Chinese thought, it was naturally adopted by the founders of Chinese medicine. Distinguishing between the Yin and Yang qualities of a person's constitution, or the character of one's illness is an important step in the process of synthesis necessary to making a traditional diagnosis. Many examples of the application of the Yin/Yang concept in medicine will be encountered later. Some general medical correspondences are listed below:

YIN	YANG
Interior	Exterior
Front	Back
Lower section	Upper section
Bones	Skin
Inner Organs	Outer Organs
Blood	Qi
Inhibition	Stimulation
Deficiency	Excess

All of these applications of Yin and Yang are relative. What is Yin in relation to one thing may be Yang in relation to another. For example, the front of the body is Yin compared to the back. Yet on the front of the body itself, the chest is Yang in relation to the abdomen. In traditional physiology, pathology, diagnostics, and treatment, Yin and Yang provide the broad parameters within which all other observations and conceptualizations are gathered.

Five Phases

Since approximately 400 B.C. the Chinese used another set of concepts in their attempt to understand the world. These were the Five Phases—Wood, Fire, Earth, Metal, and Water. The Five Phases were regarded as five properties inherent in all things. It is important that these phases be understood as processes or tendencies, and not as elemental building blocks. The Chinese word that we translate as phase *(xing)* means to walk, to move, and perhaps most pertinent, a process. We therefore refer to the Five Phases, rather than to the Five Elements. The phases provide a system of correspondences and patterns within which numerous phenomena are arranged, especially in ways that relate to the process of change.

More specifically, each phase is a symbol that represents a category of related functions and qualities. For example, Wood is associated with active functions that are in a phase of growing or

5

increasing. Fire represents functions that have reached a maximal state, and are about to begin to decline. Metal symbolizes functions that are declining, and Water represents those functions that have actually reached a maximal state of decline, and are about to change in the direction of growth. Finally, Earth designates balance or neutrality. In a sense, Earth is a "buffer" between the other phases.

The application of the Five Phases to seasonal growth is but one example of how the system was used. In time, the five generic categories were used for the classification of virtually all phenomena from colors and sounds to odors, tastes, emotions, animals, dynasties, planets, and ultimately all known things in the cosmos. (Originally, political and astronomical correlations were the most important.) Correspondences were also found between the phases and the Organs and anatomical regions; hence, the relationship of the Five Phases to medicine. (See the table of correspondences below.)

There are thirty-six possible sequences in which to order the phases, and although many have appeared in China over the ages, the most important two in Chinese medicine are the production and conquest sequences. These are often applied to physiology, pathology, diagnosis, and the classification and selection of acupuncture points for treatment. (See Section II, chapter 1 of the text.) The following diagram illustrates these sequences. Wood produces Fire which produces Earth which produces Metal which produces Water which produces Wood. Thus, the cycle repeats itself. In the conquest sequence, Wood conquers Earth which conquers Water, etc.

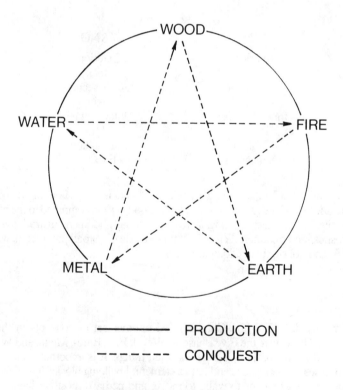

Five Phases

TABLE OF CORRESPONDENCES ASSOCIATED WITH THE FIVE PHASES

	WOOD	FIRE	EARTH	METAL	WATER
Direction	East	South	Center	West	North
Season	Spring	Summer	Long Summer	Autumn	Winter
Climatic Condition	Wind	Summer Heat	Dampness	Dryness	Cold
Process	Birth	Growth	Transformation	Harvest	Storage
Color	Green	Red	Yellow	White	Black
Taste	Sour	Bitter	Sweet	Pungent	Salty
Smell	Goatish	Burning	Fragrant	Rank	Rotten
Yin Organ	Liver	Heart	Spleen	Lungs	Kidneys
Yang Organ	Gall Bladder	Small Intestine	Stomach	Large Intestine	Bladder
Opening	Eyes	Tongue	Mouth	Nose	Ears
Tissue	Sinews	Blood Vessels	Flesh	Skin/Hair	Bones
Emotion	Anger	Happiness	Pensiveness	Sadness	Fear
Human Sound	Shout	Laughter	Song	Weeping	Groan

Application of the Five Phases to Medicine

There are innumerable correspondences associated with the Five Phases. Those which have medical significance are set out in the previous table. Where to draw the line between those which are clinically useful and those which are not can be quite difficult, and in the end will depend on one's experience and philosophy. Some practitioners may take a dim view of omitting such correspondences as planets and grains. On the other hand, odors are not included on many lists, although some practitioners feel that they are clinically important.

The correspondences used in medicine are of two kinds: those which in the Chinese mode of thought make sense metaphysically, or arise from associations independent of the body (often forced), and those which are based on the actual functions of the Organs, or appear as empirical phenomena in nature. The color correspondences, for example, are of natural origin: green for Wood (trees), red for Fire, yellow for Earth (the soil of Northern China, where these correspondences originated, is yellow), white for Metal (silvery luster), black for Water (the inky depths of the ocean). Other correlations, however, often strained, are posited for the seasons, climatic conditions, directions, tastes and odors. The nose, for example, as far as we can tell, has no relationship with Metal and was not thought to have one by the ancient Chinese. On the other hand, as the opening most often affected by diseases of the Lungs, it shares a natural correspondence with that Organ, and the nasal tract is regarded as an extension of the Lungs in Chinese physiology. In a similar way, the association of anger and the Liver is most probably due to careful observation of people, rather than to any perception of the 'wood-ness' in the process of getting angry. (Anger is associated with the Wood phase.) These distinctions are important not only in enabling one to better understand the dynamics behind the use of the Five Phase theory in diagnosis, but also in viewing the whole system in proper perspective.

The world view underlying the Five Phase theory, that of a system of correspondences, is at the foundation of Chinese medical philosophy. However, in modern Chinese texts on traditional medicine (such as the present work), the importance of specific constituents among the correspondences is de-emphasized and there are relatively few references to them. Rather, the Five Phases are generally used only as a shorthand method to remember the relationships among the Organs (when convenient), or as the theoretical context from which certain methods of selecting points is derived. A mechanical application of the theory, however, such as basing the selection of points solely on the Five Phases, is never encountered in this text and is actively discouraged.

FUNDAMENTAL PROPERTIES

Qi

Qi (pronounced "chee," as in cheese) is an untranslatable word in the Chinese medical lexicon. It signifies a tendency, a movement, something on the order of energy. There are two main aspects of Qi. On the one hand, Qi is thought of as matter without form. When this substance is diseased certain symptoms appear. Qi is also a term for the functional, active aspect of the body. When Chinese doctors do the work of diagnosis (taking a history, feeling the pulse, etc.) they are measuring different types of Qi. When acupuncture is used, the Qi is said to be 'obtained' and then manipulated. Qi is thus an example of the absence of the matter/energy dichotomy in Chinese medicine. In Section I, chapter 1 of the main text the various forms of Qi are discussed at greater length. Nonetheless, a brief description is warranted here.

Source Qi is the basal energy of the body formed from the Essence of the Kidneys, the nutrients absorbed from food, and the energy absorbed by the Lungs from the air. It flows through the entire body and is the basis for all movement and action. While it is impossible to define precisely, there exist diagnostic means to measure its strength, and treatments to reinforce it. Source Qi manifests itself in the following ways:

Organ Qi: the physiological activity and functions of each Organ.
Channel Qi: the transportive and moving functions of the channels.

Nourishing Qi: the Qi that moves with the Blood. Its main physiological functions are transforming and creating Blood, moving with the Blood, and helping the Blood to nourish the tissues of the body.

Protective Qi: the Qi that travels outside the channels and Organs. It warms the Organs, travels between the skin and the flesh to regulate the opening and closing of the pores (thereby providing for the body's defense against external diseases), and protects and moistens the skin and hair.

Ancestral Qi: the Qi that collects in the chest, with its center at point Co-17 *(Shanzhong)*. It travels up to the throat and down into the abdomen. This Qi underlies breathing and speaking, regulates the beating of the Heart, and is important in strengthening the body when cultivated through meditation.

Blood

Although the red liquid which circulates throughout the body is called blood in Western medicine, that is only part of the Chinese conception of Blood. In addition to being a substance, Blood is also regarded as a force, a level of activity in the body which is involved with the sensitivity of the sense organs, as well as a deep level of the body in the progression of febrile diseases. Traditionally, it is said that Blood is manufactured in the Middle Burner, using the Qi derived from the air in the Lungs and food digested by the Spleen. The major function of Blood is to carry nourishment to all parts of the body. It is therefore closely related to Nourishing Qi.

Qi and Blood

The relationship between Qi and Blood is a good illustration of Yin/Yang theory. Qi is Yang and Blood is Yin. Qi is the "commander" of Blood because Blood depends on Qi for its formation from air and food, and for power to move through and remain in the channels. Blood is the "mother" of Qi, because the strength of the Qi depends on the nutrition and moisture carried in Blood. The two qualities thus complement each other.

As previously mentioned, Qi and Blood are intimately related. In the section on diagnostics, many of the symptoms of Qi or Blood will be discussed. Although the identification of a Qi or Blood problem is usually only part of the winnowing process which culminates in a description of the health of the body centered on the Organs, Qi and Blood are often the focus of treatment themselves.

Disturbances in the function of Qi fall under two general headings: Deficient Qi and Stagnant Qi. Although the specific symptoms reflecting Deficient Qi in a particular Organ vary according to the affected Organ, certain factors such as heredity, age, improper living habits, or chronic long-term disease may result in Deficient Source Qi, which is manifested in general lassitude, depression, pallid complexion, pale swollen tongue, and an empty and/or fine pulse.

Stagnant Qi occurs when the Qi does not flow smoothly through the channels. This stagnation in the channels is regarded as the origin of pain, and can be dispersed by using acupuncture to stimulate the flow of Qi. In addition to pain, Stagnant Qi may result in a full or bloated feeling in the chest or abdomen. A common consequence of Stagnant Qi is that the Qi in the Lungs or Stomach, which normally flows downward, rebels upward and results in coughing or vomiting, respectively. This condition is called Rebellious Qi, a subgroup of Stagnant Qi.

In certain respects, the diseases of Blood parallel those of Qi. Qi is the commander of Blood, and Stagnant Qi can often lead to Congealed Blood. Blood nourishes Qi and Deficient Blood can predispose one to Deficient Qi. This is a consequence of the nutritive (Blood-Yin) and functional (Qi-Yang) reciprocal relationship between the two.

Deficient Blood has numerous origins. Among the most common are loss of blood, malnutrition, Deficient Spleen (the Organ that produces and controls Blood), and Congealed Blood. The most common symptoms include dizziness, pallid complexion, dry skin, loss of hair (which is considered to be an extension of Blood), pale lips and tongue, and a fine pulse.

Congealed Blood results from two distinct injuries to the body. One is direct damage to the body's tissues which stops the flow of Blood. The other is chronic Stagnant Qi, wherein the Blood is not being pushed through the vessels smoothly enough, and congealing results. The primary symptoms of Congealed Blood include local, steady, fixed pain (often stabbing), congealed spots on the side of the

9

tongue, hard swellings, and a rough pulse.

The major differences between the pain of Stagnant Qi and that of Congealed Blood include the following: pain from Stagnant Qi is characterized by dullness, episodic nature, lack of a specific location, and the absence of anything palpable at the site of pain; pain from Congealed Blood is usually stabbing, fixed at the site of a swelling, and of long duration.

Another problem associated with Blood is bleeding. This can result from Organ dysfunction or Hot Blood. When Hot Blood is the cause, the hemorrhaged blood is bright red. If other factors are responsible (e.g., Deficient Spleen in some cases of uterine hemorrhage), the blood may be pale or dark in hue. Hot Blood is also the cause of rashes and other skin disorders. Symptoms of Hot Blood include fever, restlessness or delirium, a dark purplish tongue, and a quick pulse accompanying the appearance of a rash.

Essence and Spirit

Essence (a Yin characteristic) is that aspect of the body which is the basis for all growth, development and sexuality. Congenital Essence is that part of the body's Essence which is inherited from the parents. After birth this Essence, which is akin to an inborn constitution, determines each of our growth patterns. Congenital Essence can never be replaced if lost, but can be supplemented by acquired Essence, which is derived from food. Essence also has the narrow meaning of semen.

Spirit (a Yang characteristic) is the force behind one's mental state and actions. All forms of consciousness and thought are manifestations of Spirit.

Fluids

The fluids of the body include sweat, urine, saliva, tears and the various secretions. Fluids are either thin (Yang) or thick (Yin). The thin fluids moisten the muscles, skin, flesh, and the membranes of the sensory and excretory openings. The thick fluids moisten and nourish the inner Organs and Brain, and facilitate the movement of the bones and joints.

THE ORGANS

The concept of the Organs (also called Viscera) in Chinese medicine is radically different from that of contemporary Western medicine. Understanding this difference is very important because the physiology and pathology of the Organs is fundamental to the understanding and treatment of disease. If the Chinese conception of the Organs is not understood, any attempt to use acupuncture or any other mode of traditional Chinese therapy will be muddled, especially if one tries to freely transfer ideas which are tied together only by the most tenuous of connections.* As will soon become apparent, anyone assuming that treatments which are regarded by the Chinese as beneficial to the Liver will automatically be useful against Western-defined hepatic disorders, will become confused and probably upset at the lack of success.

Perhaps the salient characteristic of the Chinese conception of the Organs (to a modern Westerner) is the lack of emphasis on the physical structure. Although many of the terms for the Organs are similar to Western appellations, they do not refer to the specific tissue, but rather to semi-abstract concepts which are complexes of closely interrelated functions. These functions, which are fully described in traditional texts, are not based on surgical discoveries, but on clinical observation of patients over many hundreds of years. This lack of concreteness has many explanations, the principal one being the relative lack of emphasis placed on the physical structure. Although a Chinese doctor

---

*As stated earlier, because the meanings of the terms Organ, Liver, Heart, etc., in Chinese medicine are so different from their Western counterparts, we have capitalized them throughout the text. The same holds true for the basic qualities (e.g. Essence), and Excesses (e.g. Wind).

believes most Organs have some kind of physical presence in the body, one Organ, the Triple Burner, has no anatomical substrate. Instead, it is rather the outward manifestations of the complexes that are focused upon. This is reflected in the traditional name for the physiology of the Organs, *zang xiang,* the phenomena (signs) of the Organs.

The Organs are divided into two principal groups: the Yin (Inner) and Yang (Outer) Organs. The five Yin Organs, which are the core of the entire system, are the Liver, Heart, Spleen, Lungs and Kidneys. (In discussions of the channels a sixth Organ, the Pericardium, is added, but otherwise it is an adjunct of the Heart.) The six Yang Organs are the Gall Bladder, Small Intestine, Large Intestine, Stomach, Bladder, and Triple Burner. Within the description of these Organs almost all the body's functions are defined and explained. Some students of Chinese medicine, not understanding that the Organs are functional complexes rather than anatomical structures, wonder about the absence of a pancreas, thyroid, adrenals, and so on from Chinese "anatomy." They either put this down to the primitive nature of Chinese medicine, or try to explain the absence on the basis of one to one correspondences (the thyroid is part of the Heart, the adrenals belong to the Kidneys, and so on). Actually, the gestalt of Chinese medicine is more complex than either of these simplifications, and although both contain elements of truth, it is best to come to grips with the Chinese concept of the Organs on its own terms. The description of problems in or among the Organs is the basis for understanding disease.

The Yin Organs are described in the literature more fully than the Yang Organs. The Yin Organs are said to "store and not drain," meaning that their functions are directed toward sustaining homeostasis, both physically and mentally. The Yang Organs are said to "drain and not store," referring to their role in the transformation and disposal of food and waste. All the Yang Organs receive food or a product of food and pass it along. Each Yang Organ is associated with a Yin Organ by a special Yin/Yang relationship.* Pairs of Yin and Yang Organs so linked belong to the same Phase, their channels are sequential to each other in the circulation of Qi, their functions are closely linked, and disease in one usually affects the other. In acupuncture, the channel corresponding to the Yang Organ is often used to treat disorders of its related Yin Organ.

Section I, chapter 3 of the main text lists some of the disorders associated with the various Organs in the context of the channel system.

With this we come to the very heart of traditional Chinese medicine—the patterns of disease. The classification of disorders and the aim of treatment in Chinese medicine is based on pathological patterns of the various Organs. The word that the Chinese use for notating the problems of the Organs is *zheng,* which means 'emblem.' This is an example of the abstract in Chinese medicine, in that the signs and symptoms of disease are grouped into 'emblems' which represent the state of health of the patient as a whole. Hans Agren calls these 'manifestation types', while Ted. J. Kaptchuk translates this term as 'pattern', a translation which we have adopted in this introduction and throughout the text.

The active purpose of Chinese medicine is to "discern patterns and institute treatment." Therefore, without a diagnosis of a pattern there can be no treatment of the underlying problem. In order to facilitate understanding of the various prescriptions set forth in Section IV of the text, common patterns associated with the Organs will be discussed below, after a brief description of the functions of each Organ. The mechanisms of disease are dealt with further on.

Because the focus of diagnosis and the conceptualization of the body in Chinese medicine differ so much from Western medicine, the fact that a Western-defined disease may have more than one corresponding Chinese pattern, or one Chinese pattern may appear under different Western-defined disease headings should come as no surprise. To orthodox practitioners of Western medicine, the patterns described below will be regarded merely as syndromes or groups of symptoms. In the context of Western medicine this would be true. There, most cases are diagnosed with confidence from the inside out, i.e., with a blood test, scan, x-ray, etc., so that some kind of information from inside the body is necessary to name a disease with confidence. But Chinese medicine approaches patients from the outside in. The senses of the doctor and patient are used to garner information which the doctor can synthesize into a total picture of how the patient is operating at that time. To doctors of Chinese medicine, this is the only way to get at the root of the problem. They view Western doctors as

*Also called the Inner/Outer relationship. The channels to which the Organs pertain share the same Yin/Yang relationship.

ordinarily providing only symptomatic treatment. . . exactly how Western doctors view their Chinese counterparts.

It should be noted here that each of the vital Organs is responsible as well for a variety of disorders that appear along the path of its associated channel. The paths of the channels are described in Section I of the text. It should also be mentioned that in discussing the patterns of disease, it is necessary to use terminology that will not be properly explained until we reach the Mechanisms of Disease and the Eight Parameters later in this introduction.

Liver and Gall Bladder

These Organs correspond to the Wood phase, the direction east, the spring season, the climatic condition of wind , the color of green, the emotion of anger, the taste of sour, the odor goatish, and the sound of shouting. Their point of entry is the eyes. They control the sinews (muscles, joints), and their health is reflected in the nails.

The Liver is the Organ that is responsible for spreading and regulating the Qi throughout the body. Its character is flowing and free. Thus, depression or frustration can disturb its function. It is also responsible for storing Blood when the body is at rest. This characteristic, combined with its control over the lower abdomen, makes it the most important Organ with regard to women's menstrual cycle and sexuality. The Gall Bladder stores and excretes gall, which is produced by the Liver. Together with the Heart, the Gall Bladder is responsible for decision-making.

Depression or long-term frustration can upset the Liver's spreading function and result in continuing depression, a bad temper and a painful, swollen feeling in the chest and sides. If it worsens, it may lead to disharmony between the Liver and the Stomach and/or Spleen. This disorder is marked by the "rebellion" of Qi in the latter two Organs, whereby the Qi moves in the opposite direction than is normally proper. In the case of the Stomach, whose Qi normally descends, rebellious Qi means hiccoughing, vomiting, etc. The Qi of the Spleen, on the other hand, is ordinarily directed upward; rebellious Qi in this Organ means diarrhea.

Depression of the Liver Qi is often the root cause of many women's disorders, including menstrual irregularities, swollen and painful breasts, etc.

One of the Liver's most important functions is storage of Blood, with the attendant emphasis upon nourishing and moistening. When the Liver Blood is deficient (more severe cases are called Deficient Liver Yin), the Liver is incapable of moistening. This is manifested in dry, painful eyes with blurred or weak vision, lack of suppleness or pain in moving the joints, dry skin, dizziness (lack of Blood in the head), and infrequent or spotty menstruation. When the Deficient Liver Yin reaches a certain degree of severity, the conditions Rising Liver Fire or Hyper Liver Yang Ascending occur. These conditions are evidenced in ill-temper, restlessness, headache, vertigo, red face and eyes, and a parched mouth. They result when the Liver Yin is so deficient as to be incapable of securing the Liver Yang, which rises uncontrollably to the head. While many of the symptoms appear as disorders of the head, a weakness in the lower joints may also be observed.

The various meanings conveyed by the word Wind are described more fully under the topic of the Six Excesses which is set out in Mechanisms of Disease, below. However, it is necessary here to discuss Liver Wind, or the pattern, Interior Movement of the Liver Wind. This pattern often appears as a progression in the development of the condition Liver Fire, or Liver Yang Rising in Excess. Movement of the Interior Wind is evidenced by sudden onset of the following symptoms: dizziness while moving about, spasms, paralysis, difficulty in movement, severe vertigo, etc. These symptoms represent the transitory, disorienting, and ultimately disassociative function of Wind.

The principal disease associated with the Gall Bladder is a disorder affecting the flow of gall, caused by Dampness and Heat. This is manifested by pain in the region of the Liver, an oppressive sensation of fullness in the abdomen, and yellowish eyes, skin, urine and tongue.

Heart and Small Intestine

These Organs correspond to the Fire phase, the southerly direction, the summer season, the climatic condition of heat, the color red, the emotion of happiness, the sound of laughter, the taste of bitterness, the odor of burning. Their point of entry is the tongue. They control the blood vessels and are reflected in the face.

The Heart controls the blood vessels and is responsible for moving the Blood through them. It also stores the Spirit, and is therefore the Organ most frequently associated with mental processes. The Small Intestine separates the waste material from the nutritious elements in food. The nutritious elements are distributed throughout the body, while the waste is sent on to the Large Intestine.

Almost all the disorders of the Heart are those of weakness. The four categories of Heart weakness are Deficient Heart Qi, Deficient Heart Yang, Deficient Heart Blood, and Deficient Heart Yin.

The principal functions of the Heart are associated with the Spirit and Blood vessels. Thus, certain symptoms, among them some forms of emotional distress, dizziness, palpitations, shortness of breath, and lack of vitality in the face, are common to all the Heart's disease patterns. Deficient Qi in this Organ is marked by general lassitude, panting and shallow breathing, and frequent sweating. When the face is swollen and ashen gray or bluish-green, and the limbs cold, the condition is called Deficient Heart Yang. Restlessness, irritability, dizziness, absentmindedness, and insomnia are typical symptoms of Deficient Heart Blood. In more advanced cases, Deficient Heart Yin develops with a flushed feeling in the palms and face, low grade fever, and night sweating.

The pattern Heart Excess arises from an excess of Heart Fire. This is marked by fever, sometimes accompanied by delirium, a racking pulse, intense restlessness, insomnia or frequent nightmares, a bright red face, a red or blistered and painful tongue, and often a burning sensation during urination. The latter symptom is considered to be the result of Heat being transferred from the Heart to the Small Intestine, interfering with the Small Intestine's role in metabolism and the body's management of water.

Spleen and Stomach

These Organs correspond to the Earth phase, the central direction, the season of long summer (the end of summer), the climatic condition of dampness, the color yellow, the emotion of pensiveness, the taste of sweetness, fragrant odor and the sound of singing. Their opening is the mouth. They control the flesh and the limbs.

The Spleen is the principal Organ of digestion. It transports nutrients and produces and regulates the Blood (regulates in the sense of keeping it within the channels). It is responsible for the transformation of food into nourishment. The relationship between the Spleen and the Stomach is a particularly strong example of the Yin/Yang relationship between Organs. The Stomach receives food; the Spleen transports nutrients. The Stomach moves things downward; the Spleen upward. The Stomach likes dampness; the Spleen dryness (i.e., the Stomach, being Yang, easily copes with Dampness (Yin) but has trouble with Dryness (Yang)).

When the Spleen is weak, the body is unable to use the nourishment in food. This leads to general lassitude and fatigue, and a pasty complexion. The upper abdomen is the province of the Spleen, and Deficient Spleen Qi is marked by a sense of malaise or fullness in that area. Because the transportive function requires that the Spleen distribute its Qi upward, weakness in the Spleen is usually accompanied by diarrhea. The Spleen Qi is also referred to as the Middle Qi, responsible for holding the Viscera in place. Insufficiency of the Middle Qi presages prolapsed stomach, kidneys, etc. In more severe cases, the Spleen Yang Qi is Deficient. This pattern is manifested in diarrhea, cold limbs, and abdominal pain that can be soothed by the warmth of frequent hot drinks, application of the hands, or moxibustion.

When many of the above symptoms are accompanied by bleeding, especially from the digestive tract or uterus, the condition is called Spleen Not Controlling the Blood.

Cold and Dampness Harassing the Spleen is a manifestation type characterized by a pent-up feeling in the chest and a bloated sensation in the abdomen, lassitude, lack of appetite and taste, a feeling of cold in the limbs, a dark yellowish hue to the skin, some edema and diarrhea or watery stool. The Cold and Dampness prevent the Spleen from performing its transforming and transporting functions. This leads to a great disturbance in water metabolism and is one of the origins of Phlegm.

While there are some patterns describing Deficiency of the Stomach (many of these originate in the

Spleen), most Stomach disorders stem from Excess. Stomach Fire is a painful, burning sensation in the Stomach, unusual hunger, bleeding from the gums, constipation, and halitosis. Rebellious Stomach Qi was described earlier.

Lungs and Large Intestine

These Organs correspond to the Metal phase, the westerly direction, the season of autumn, the dry climatic condition, the color white, the emotion of melancholy, the pungent taste, the rank odor, and the sound of crying. Their opening is the nose. They govern the skin.

The Lungs are responsible for taking Qi from the air, and for the energy state of the Qi in the body. They also control that part of the liquid metabolism which distributes the liquids to the skin.

The Lungs are called the delicate Organ because they are the first to be attacked by exogenous disease. Such disease also causes what is called the Non-Spreading of the Lung Qi. The primary symptom associated with the Lungs is coughing. This is a form of Rebellious Qi, since the Lung Qi normally flows downward. When coughing is accompanied by lassitude, shortness of breath, light foamy phlegm, and weakness in the voice, it is called Deficient Lung Qi. When the cough is a dry one, with little phlegm, parched throat and mouth, and Deficient Yin symptoms such as night sweating, low grade fever, red cheeks, etc., the condition is referred to as Deficient Lung Yin.

The Large Intestine is considered important in the metabolism of water and the passing of water. The Large Intestine extracts water from the waste material it receives from the Small Intestine and sends it on to the Bladder, excreting the solid material as stool. However, many disorders affecting this Organ are categorized as Spleen and Stomach patterns. Certain kinds of abdominal pain are regarded as manifestations of a blockage of Qi or Blood in the Large Intestine.

Kidneys and Bladder

These Organs correspond to the Water phase, the winter season, the cold climatic condition, the southerly direction, the color black, the emotion of fear, the taste of salt, a rotten smell, and the sound of groaning. Their sensory organ is the ear. Their openings are the urethra and anus. They control the bones, marrow, and brain and their health is reflected in the hair of the head.

The Kidneys store Essence and are thus responsible for growth, development, and the reproductive functions. They assume the primary role in water metabolism and control the body's liquids. They also hold the body's most fundamental Yin and Yang. The Bladder transforms fluids into urine and excretes it from the body.

The Kidneys are the repositories of the basal Yin and Yang of the body. Therefore, any disorder, if sufficiently chronic, will involve the Kidneys. Furthermore, a disease of the Kidneys will usually lead to problems in another Organ. Methods of strengthening the Kidneys are therefore used by the Chinese to increase or maintain vitality and health. The symptoms of Deficient Kidney Yang or Yin are the classic symptoms of that type and will appear, to a certain extent, in Deficient Yang or Yin patterns of any Organ.

The symptoms of Deficient Kidney Yin are easy to understand and memorize if one learns the correspondences of the Kidneys, and remembers that Yin represents the structive, nourishing, and fluid aspects of the body. The lower back is weak and sore, there is ringing in the ears and loss of hearing acuity, the face is ashen or dark, especially under the eyes. Dizziness, thirst, night sweats and low grade fevers are common. Men have little semen and tend toward premature ejaculation, while women have little or no menstruation.

Deficient Kidney Yang symptoms are by and large associated with loss of energy or warmth. As with Deficient Kidney Yin, there is ringing in the ears, dizziness, and soreness in the lower back. However, the soreness is characterized by a sensitivity to cold. There is lassitude, fatigue and a feeling of coldness. There is a notable weakness in the legs. In men, there is a tendency towards impotence, and in both sexes, clear and voluminous urine or incontinence.

Most commonly, Deficient Kidney Yin produces similar disorders in the Heart and Liver, while Deficient Kidney Yang disturbs the functions of the Spleen and Lungs. (Of course, the disease progression could be in the opposite direction.) All of these conditions, except for that affecting the Lungs, have been previously described. The pattern associated with the Lungs is called Kidney Not Receiving Qi, which is a type of wheezing characterized by difficult breathing, primarily during inhalation. In addition to the Deficient Kidney Yang symptoms, this condition is also evidenced in a faint voice, coughing, puffiness in the face, and spontaneous sweating.

The Kidneys perform important functions in the metabolism of water. When these functions are disrupted, the condition Deficient Kidneys (leading to) Spreading Water occurs.

Pericardium and Triple Burner

These two Organs are said to correspond to the "Ministerial Fire," as distinguished from the "Sovereign Fire" of the Heart and Small Intestine. As mentioned previously, the Pericardium has no separate physiological functions, although it is mentioned with regard to the delirium induced by high fevers. At least as far back as the 3rd century *Classic of Difficulties,* the Triple Burner was described as "having a name but no form." In the *Inner Classic,* the Triple Burner was regarded as an Organ that coordinated all the functions of water metabolism. In other traditions, the Burners were but three regions of the body that were used to group the Organs. The Upper Burner includes the chest, neck, head and the functions of the Heart and Lungs. The Middle Burner spans the region between the chest and the navel, and includes the functions of the Stomach and Spleen. The Lower Burner contains the lower abdomen and the functions of the Kidneys and Bladder (and usually the Liver which, however, is sometimes placed in the Middle Burner). As such, the Upper Burner has been compared to a mist which spreads the Blood and Qi, the Middle Burner is like a foam which churns up food in the process of digestion, and the Lower Burner is likened to a swamp where all the impure substances are excreted. This description is commonly used in diagnosis. Later in the text, the reader will discover that as a channel, the meaning and use of the Triple Burner is different again. This is a puzzle even to the Chinese, and journals of traditional medicine are full of articles addressing the problem of this Organ.

Functional Inter-relationships Among the Organs

By way of summary, some examples of the functional inter-relationships among the Organs are provided below.

The Spleen, Liver and Heart are the three Organs that have the most direct relationship with the Blood. The Spleen creates it, the Liver stores it, and the Heart moves it. Any problem associated with the Blood will involve at least one of these Organs.

The Liver and the Kidneys are closely related. Their channels cross in many places. The Liver stores Blood; the Kidneys store Essence. These substances, both of which are Yin, have a considerable influence on the reproductive functions.

The Heart (Upper Burner, Fire) and the Kidneys (Lower Burner, Water) keep each other in check and are dependent upon one another. The Spirit of the Heart and the Essence of the Kidneys cooperate in establishing and maintaining consciousness.

The Spleen's digestive function is associated with the distributive function of the Liver. Disharmony between these two entities results in various digestive troubles. The transportive and digestive functions of the Spleen (also called the Middle Qi) depend upon the strength of the Kidney Yang.

Although the Lungs govern the Qi, the Qi from the Lungs must mix with the Essence from the Kidneys before Source Qi is produced. The Lungs govern the Qi, the Liver spreads it, and the Kidneys provide its basis.

THE CHANNELS

The channels are one of the most important and unique concepts in Chinese medicine. Although they are described in great detail in the main body of the text (all of Section I), it is necessary to touch on some of the more important aspects here. The channels are regarded as three-dimensional passageways through which the Qi and Blood flow at different levels of the body. Therefore, it is inappropriate to refer to the channels by using the two-dimensional term "meridian," as is common in English translations.

The channels are important to every facet of Chinese medicine, particularly acupuncture. Their graphic ordering illustrates many of the linkages among the Organs and their respective openings and sense organs. In some ways, the channels also delineate the Organs' spheres of influence in the body. This is particularly important in the selection of points to treat certain localized problems, discussed more fully in the main text.

Most prominent among the channels are the Fourteen channels, twelve of which are bilaterally oriented in the body and are extensions of the twelve Yin and Yang Organs. The name of each is derived from the extremity which it traverses, the particular aspect of the limb through which it passes, and the Organ with which it is associated. By way of overview and as a preface to the text, we list them here in order of the sequential circulation of Qi. Abbreviations for each of the Fourteen channels is placed in parenthesis after the full name.

1. Arm Greater Yin Lung channel (L)
2. Arm Yang Brightness Large Intestine channel (LI)
3. Leg Yang Brightness Stomach channel (S)
4. Leg Greater Yin Spleen channel (Sp)
5. Arm Lesser Yin Heart channel (H)
6. Arm Greater Yang Small Intestine channel (SI)
7. Leg Greater Yang Bladder channel (B)
8. Leg Lesser Yin Kidney channel (K)
9. Arm Absolute Yin Pericardium channel (P)
10. Arm Lesser Yang Triple Burner channel (TB)
11. Leg Lesser Yang Gall Bladder channel (GB)
12. Leg Absolute Yin Liver channel (Li)

The remaining two channels are situated on the midline of the body, one principally on the back—the Governing channel (Gv), and the other on the front—the Conception channel (Co). Only these fourteen channels have their own acupuncture points.

With Pulse (also translated as Blood Vessels), we again encounter that degree of vagueness and overlapping that exists in Chinese medicine. Pulse is defined as the Vessels through which Blood and Qi flow. As such it seems to mean the same as the channels. The term Pulse Qi, in fact, is taken to be synonymous with Channel Qi. However, as the Pulse is associated with the Heart, the emphasis is placed on the movement of Blood.

THE MECHANISMS OF DISEASE

As we noted earlier, when the various entities and forces in the body are in harmonious balance, there is health. When this balance is disturbed, there is illness. The development of disease depends on two factors: the strength of the body itself, and the strength of the disease-causing quality. If the body is truly strong there is no way for disease to gain a foothold. Also, many disorders arise from internal disharmonies with little or no effect from exogenous influences. In Chinese medicine much emphasis is placed on the prevention of disease by the promotion of general health and the early treatment of disharmonies. In the *Yellow Emperor's Inner Classic,* written approximately 200 B.C., it is said that treating disease after it has manifested itself is like waiting to dig a well until after one is thirsty.

In Chinese medical terminology, the physiological activities of the Organs, the Qi, the Blood, etc., all of which have the power to resist disease, are called the Normal Qi. The course of disease is seen as a struggle between the Normal Qi and the disease-causing quality. Treatment of the disease at any particular time depends on the relationship between these two forces. Disorders which are primarily caused by internal disharmony require careful treatment so as to properly regulate the Organs.

The causes of disease are divided into three categories: those coming from outside the body, those arising inside the body, and those whose origins are neither outside nor inside. In addition, there is another concept, that of Phlegm, which is pertinent here but will be discussed last.

The Six Excesses

The Six Excesses are Wind, Cold, Heat, Dampness, Dryness and Summer Heat. They conform to the Five Phase correspondences (both Heat and Summer Heat correspond to Fire). The term Excess might also be translated as Abnormality, Evil, or Pernicious Influence. When normal environmental forces become excessive (e.g., a particularly cold spell in winter), or occur unseasonably (e.g., a warm spell in the middle of winter), they may cause disease. However, because of individual physical make-up and a latency period in some diseases, people may have a different disease at the same time and the same disease at different times. Clinical differentiation of the Excesses is made on the basis of symptoms, not tests aimed at discovering a precisely defined disease-causing agent. That is to say, the disease is described in terms of the body's response, rather than in terms of an autonomous disease. Therefore two people may catch the same "disease" (in the Western sense) at the same time yet because of differences in their environment and constitution they may exhibit different patterns. Thus, the Excess "responsible" for the disease may be different.

Sometimes an imbalance among the Organs internally will lead to symptoms similar to those of an externally caused illness. Using tools of diagnosis (discussed below), it is possible to differentiate between symptoms caused by external Excess and those caused by an imbalance within the body itself.

The Excesses (with the exception of Heat) are each related to a particular season and associated with either Yin (which injures Yang forces), or Yang (which injures Yin substances). The symptomatic manifestations of each Excess resemble the characteristics of their seasonal counterparts in nature. The original relationships between the Excesses and the seasons were based on the weather patterns in ancient northern China, and do not necessarily hold true for other parts of the world.

Wind (Spring/Yang)

Diseases caused by Wind arise suddenly and change quickly. They may be accompanied by symptoms such as spasms, vertigo, itching, or a pain which often changes location. Wind diseases of an exogenous origin usually affect the skin, head, throat, and Lungs first. Wind is the Excess which carries other Excesses into the body.

Internally, when the Liver (Wood-Wind) Yang is hyperactive, dizziness, convulsions, etc., ensue. Similar symptoms accompany high fevers. Both are called Interior Wind.

Cold (Winter/Yin)

The principal symptom of this Excess is that the body, or a part of the body, feels cold. Cold causes things to congeal; in the body this causes pain. (Pain is caused by obstruction in the flow of Qi or Blood.) Cold causes things to contract; in the channels this causes cramps and spasms. When Cold diseases are present, the body excretions (mucus, phlegm, urine, stool, etc.) are white or clear and watery.

When the Yang Qi is weak, symptoms similar to those caused by Cold appear.

Heat (Yang)

The main characteristic of Heat is that the body or a part thereof feels hot. Heat easily injures the body fluids. Thus, the tongue and stool become dry, and the patient is thirsty. Heat can cause the Blood to travel outside the channels, leading to hemorrhage or rashes. In the presence of Heat-caused diseases, body excretions are dark or yellow, sticky and/or foul smelling. Sometimes, the act of expulsion causes Heat in the part of the body involved. Often, disease caused by one of the other Excesses transforms into Heat within the body. Heat is sometimes called Fire.

Dampness (Long Summer/Yin)

This Excess often appears during damp weather or when a person comes into contact with moisture for a prolonged period of time. Dampness is sluggish and stagnating. Diseases caused by this Excess take a long time to cure. When Dampness is on the external portions of the body, the patient feels pent-up, the limbs heavy, and the head swollen. When Dampness invades the channels and joints, movement is difficult, numbness may appear, and if there is pain, it is fixed in one place. The entire body or a part thereof is affected by swelling or edema. Dampness tends to attack the Spleen. When the Spleen's transforming and transporting functions are weak, Interior Dampness may result.

Dryness (Fall/Yang)

Dryness attacks the liquids of the body and may result in dry skin, chapped lips, hacking cough, constipation, etc. When the body's Yin substances are seriously depleted (as in the latter stages of a long febrile disease), similar symptoms appear.

Summer Heat (Summer/Yang)

The primary characteristic of Summer Heat is fever with pronounced sweating. This injures the Yin and the Qi. Dampness almost always accompanies this Excess.

The Seven Emotions

The Seven Emotions are happiness, anger, worry, pensiveness, sadness, fear, and terror. They are linked with the Five Phase system of correspondences, with a couple of additions (both worry and sadness correspond to Metal; both fear and terror correspond to Water). In addition to the Seven Emotions, frustration upsets the free-flowing nature of the Liver and, not surprisingly, often leads to anger. These are normal emotions which can lead to illness if sustained for a long period of time. These emotions either adversely affect those Organs associated with the same Phase, or upset the Yin/Yang balance in the body. Emotion-related diseases, which might be labelled psychosomatic in Western medicine, are treated like any other disease in Chinese medicine.

Causes Which Are Neither Outside Nor Inside

These refer to parts of patterns (not really causes) that are neither Excesses nor emotions. Inconsistency in the quantity, quality, or time of eating causes indigestion and related diseases. Quality here refers both to the sanitary level of food and to the traditional classification of foodstuffs as either Cold or Hot. Each Organ is associated with a corresponding taste in the Five Phase system. Too much of one taste will injure the corresponding Organ.

Sexual activity and the reproductive functions are linked with the Kidneys in men, and with both the Kidneys and the Liver in women. When excessive sexual activity occurs, the Yin and Yang of these Organs may be damaged. If a woman gives birth too many times, the Conception and Penetrating channels (discussed in the main text) may be injured, resulting in menstrual problems. The same is true of manual labor: when performed in suitable amounts it benefits the body; when done to excess, the body is injured.

Phlegm

In Chinese medicine the word Phlegm does not refer exclusively to the secretions that are coughed up from the Lungs, but rather to stagnant water in the body. Traditionally, its formation is due to dysfunction in the water metabolism, especially in the transforming/transporting functions of the Spleen. Therefore, the Spleen is called the source of Phlegm. When the water in the body becomes stagnant, it transforms into Phlegm. There are many possible reasons for this stagnation, but the most common are Deficient Qi and Heat. Phlegm is both the result of dysfunction and the cause of further dysfunction. When Phlegm collects in the Lungs there is coughing and wheezing with profuse Phlegm. When it enters the Stomach there is nausea and vomiting. When it invades the channels hard swellings occur. And when it surrounds the Heart delirium ensues.

In actuality, the various causes of disease overlap and occur together. Diagnosis is directed toward determining the relationships which exist at a particular time between the different disease-causing qualities and the Organs.

THE EIGHT PARAMETERS

The ideal diagnosis in traditional Chinese medicine gives a conceptual picture of the root dysfunction of the body and suggests a structure for possible treatment. The first stage in the winnowing process utilizes the Eight Parameters. These are four pair of broad polarities that provide a preliminary description of the nature and strength of the disease. The Eight Parameters (also known as the Eight Principles) are Exterior/Interior (depth of disease), Hot/Cold (nature of disease), Excessive/Deficient (strength of disease versus that of body), and Yin/Yang (overall quality of condition). When used as the first step in diagnosis, these parameters enable the doctor to establish in general terms the location, quality and strength of a disease. After this is done, other diagnostic methods are applied to pinpoint the disease and identify the requisite treatment. It must be remembered that disease are complex and everchanging. Sometimes two different or even contradictory parameters will appear simultaneously. As the disease progresses, it may move from one parameter to another. It is therefore important to monitor the changes and tailor each treatment to fit the particular person at that particular time. Consequently, Chinese doctors continuously adjust the treatment as the disease progresses.

Exterior/Interior

These parameters delineate the location of disease. The disease process is understood to evolve in primarily one of two ways. In the first, the body's balance betwen Yin and Yang is upset. These are always Interior diseases. In the second, an Excess enters from outside the body and the body struggles with it. Such diseases usually begin as Exterior conditions and may progress to become Interior ones. These two processes are not mutually exclusive. In fact, if there is no weakness in the body's Exterior armour, no Excess can get in. Here the skin, flesh, and channels are defined as Exterior, while the Organs and deeper body tissues, like the bones, are Interior.

Exterior symptoms include chills, fever, headache, sore limbs, runny nose, coughing, sore throat, and a floating pulse. Ordinarily, Excesses first encroach upon the body through the skin or nose, which are both related to the Lungs. If the Excess succeeds in penetrating these outer defenses there must be a weakness in the Protective Qi. Chills may result, which is the definitive symptom of Exterior conditions. The presence of perspiration is an important indicator of the strength of the Protective Qi. If the Excess is in the outer and higher parts of the channels, headaches and soreness result. This is also reflected in a floating pulse. Below are some of the relationships of the Exterior condition with the other parameters.

Exterior Cold
The chills are stronger than the fever, the fur on the tongue is white and moist, head and body pains are severe, mucus is clear or white, the throat may be itchy and the voice raspy, the pulse is floating and tight.

Exterior Hot
The fever is high, the fur on the tongue is dry and yellow, the throat is very painful and inflamed, mucus from the nose or lungs is yellow and congealed, and the pulse is floating and rapid.

Exterior Excess
There is no perspiration. This usually occurs in a Wind Cold disease when the Cold Excess is so strong that the pores are blocked.

Exterior Deficiency

There is perspiration without the usual corresponding break in the fever. This is due to a weakness in the Protective Qi, which is unable to properly regulate the pores.

Interior symptoms, as distinct from Exterior symptoms, are those involving the Organs and deeper tissues of the body. They may arise from Excesses lodged in Exterior portions of the body which penetrate the external defenses and enter the Organs, or from Excesses which directly attack the Organs themselves. Other causes include emotional imbalance, improper living habits, etc., which disturb the harmony among the functions of the Organs. The many varieties of Interior patterns have been discussed in the preceding section on the Organs.

There are some symptoms that commonly indicate the presence of Interior diseases, rather than Exterior ones. These include fever without chills, a feeling of coldness in the body, irritability, pain in the trunk, vomiting, and changes in the body of the tongue. The condition of the stool and urine, and the existence and type of thirst (usually normal in Exterior conditions), are important signs in determining the nature of an Interior disease. A comparison between Interior Cold and Interior Hot diseases will serve to give a general idea how these symptoms are actually used in diagnosis.

Interior Cold

Typical symptoms include a pale complexion, sensitivity to cold, cold in the extremities, no thirst or a desire to drink hot liquids, pain in the abdomen which diminishes upon the application of heat, copious and clear urine, watery stool, pale tongue with white fur, and a deep, slow pulse.

Interior Hot

Common symptoms include a flushed complexion, fever, irritability, thirst for cold beverages, sweating, scanty dark urine, constipation or diarrhea containing pus or blood, a dark red tongue with yellow fur, and a quick pulse.

Under certain conditions, and in diseases due to external factors, there is a period when the symptoms are half Exterior and half Interior. This occurs when there are alternating chills and fever, a pent-up feeling in the sides and chest, irritability and restlessness, nausea, lack of appetite, a bitter taste in the mouth, a dry parched mouth, vertigo, and a wiry pulse. A carefully balanced plan of treatment, focusing upon the channels which traverse the middle of the extremities, is required. These channels (Liver, Gall Bladder, Triple Burner and Pericardium) correspond to the half Exterior/half Interior level of the body.

If an Excess attacks both the Exterior and Interior portions of the body simultaneously, or if an Exterior disease compounds a pre-existing Interior condition, these two parameters come into play at the same time. In such instances the selection of points will depend on a careful evaluation of the circumstances and a decision as to the relative importance of each parameter.

Hot/Cold

These parameters delineate the activity of the body and the quality of the disease. When the body is attacked by a Yang Excess, or when the Yin substances are depleted, then Hot symptoms develop. When the body is attacked by a Yin Excess, or the Yang activities are weak, Cold symptoms develop. Because the difference between these groups of symptoms has already been discussed under the description of Cold and Heat Excesses, they will only be summarized here.

Hot

A flushed face, red eyes, heat in any part of the body, fever, irritability, thirst for cold liquids, constipation, scanty dark urine, dark red tongue, rapid pulse, dark, putrid and/or thick secretions.

Cold

A pale complexion, quiet attitude, tendency to curl up, cold in any part of the body, general feeling of cold, lack of thirst or thirst for only hot liquids, severe, localized pain, diarrhea, long clear urine, slow pulse, thin, clear and/or white secretions.

When various parts of the body are in different states of health, the Hot and Cold parameters may appear simultaneously. When either Hot or Cold is severe, 'false' symptoms may appear. In a Hot disease this usually takes the form of cold in the limbs because the Yang energy is locked inside the trunk and cannot spread to the limbs. In Cold diseases a flushed face, sore throat, and irritability may appear due to the rising of the weak Yang. In such cases as these, the majority of the symptoms, and particularly the tongue, pulse, and thirst factors, will accurately reflect the state of the body.

Excessive/Deficient

These parameters concern the quality of the body's resistance (the Normal Qi) versus the strength of the disease. If the disease occurs less because of a weakness in the body than because of the strength of the Excess, the disease is called an Excessive disease. If the condition of the body is very weak and that of the disease not necessarily strong, or if the disease is caused primarily by internal disharmony or weakness, it is called Deficient. At the risk of oversimplification, acute diseases tend to be Excessive, and chronic ones Deficient.

Excessive*
Symptoms of Excess vary widely depending on the quality and location of the disease. However, when contrasted to Deficient diseases, the following symptoms are important: the voice is normal or louder than normal, breathing is heavy, if there are pains in the chest or abdomen they are felt as hard or elastic lumps which react painfully to pressure, the fur on the tongue is thick, and the pulse has strength.

Deficient
Deficient symptoms vary depending on whether it is the Qi, Blood, Yang, Yin or a particular Organ that is affected. However, when contrasted with symptoms of Excess, symptoms of Deficiency may be summarized as follows: the patient is quiet and withdrawn, the voice is soft and low, the complexion varies from sickly yellow to ghastly pale, breathing is light, pain is diminished upon massage or pressure, swellings are soft, there is little or no fur on the tongue and the pulse is weak.

As a disease progresses, changes occur with respect to these two parameters and, if conditions are appropriate, they can both appear simultaneously. In such cases, judicious diagnosis is essential to proper treatment.

Yang/Yin

Yang and Yin are the larger parameters within which the others are subsumed. Exterior, Hot, and Excessive symptoms are Yang; Interior, Cold, and Deficient symptoms are Yin. The classic Yang symptoms correspond to Excessive/Hot conditions, while classic Yin symptoms correspond to Deficient/Cold conditions. Of course, almost all diseases include both Yang and Yin elements.

DIAGNOSTICS

In any form of medicine, diagnostics acts as a bridge between theory and treatment. Since both theory and treatment in Chinese medicine are very different from their Western counterparts, it is

*The word which we translate as Excessive is entirely different from that which we previously translated as Excess. It is important to keep them straight. An Excess does not invariably lead to an Excessive condition, nor are all Excessive conditions caused by Excesses. We apologize for the confusion, but other translations are either less accurate or more awkward.

An Excess (the noun) refers to certain disease-causing factors. Excessive (the adjective), or a symptom of Excess, refers to the quality of the body's resistance in relation to the strength of a disease.

natural that the direction and technique of diagnosis also differ. As we discussed earlier, the Chinese doctor aims at constructing a description of the patient's body as a whole, using patterns or manifestation types. The patterns emerge from observing the interplay of the causes of disease with the functional groups of the Organs. In the context of Western medicine, however, these patterns are merely regarded as groups of symptoms. Therefore, what in Chinese medicine is viewed as treatment that gets to the root of a problem, Western medicine regards as only symptomatic therapy, and vice versa.

This paradox is reflected in Chinese diagnostic techniques. Chinese diagnosis works from the outside in. The doctor uses his or her senses directly to monitor the condition. Many of the things examined on the body are similar to those examined by Western physicians, but some of the examinations (e.g., the tongue and pulse) are performed differently and from an entirely different perspective than are similar techniques employed by Western physicians. Several of the diagnostic techniques of Chinese medicine, such as palpation of certain groups of acupuncture points or diagnosis by sensitivity at points on the ear, are totally unknown to orthodox Western medicine. In Western medicine, as we pointed out earlier, most definitive diagnoses are made from the inside out, through the use of various laboratory tests, to examine parts of the body that are usually inaccessible by other means. The results of these tests are then reconciled with the clinical presentation of the patient.

The four principal categories of Chinese diagnostic technique are 1) looking, 2) listening/smelling (the same word in Chinese), 3) asking, and 4) palpating. All the information needed by a Chinese doctor in diagnosing disease and determining treatment is encompassed by these four areas of inquiry. The formulation of a diagnosis itself points to the strategy of treatment. In fact, without a proper understanding of the four methods of diagnosis, optimal use of any Chinese therapeutic technique, including acupuncture, is impossible.

Looking

The first thing a doctor does when a patient walks into his office is to "look the Spirit over." Spirit here means the combination of the patient's facial expression, muscle tone, posture, mode of speech, and general appearance. If the disease is not serious the patient will be spirited, have good complexion, clear eyes and speech, normal posture, and be quick in replying to questions. When some diseases reach a certain point of seriousness, the patient's face becomes dark, she shows little interest in what goes on around her, loses normal posture, talks slowly with frequent pauses, and, in short, becomes dispirited. Sometimes one facet (e.g., speech or posture) of a dispirited patient will suddenly seem to change for the better with no corresponding improvement in other aspects. This is a sign that the disease has entered a very serious stage, because it represents a serious imbalance.

Certain physical types are prone to certain disorders. Fat people are likely to come down with diseases having as their source Phlegm and Dampness, while thin people more easily suffer from Deficient Yin.

Changes in skin color, especially of the face, are important. Often, the appearance of a color indicates some problem with the Organ to which it corresponds. A pale complexion reflects a Deficient or Cold condition. If the face is chalky and bloated, this signifies Deficient Qi. If the face is pale and lusterless there is insufficient Blood. A patient with roundworm has small white spots on the cheeks and black areas above the pupils on the eyeballs. A dark, bluish-green hue to the face reflects a blockage of the energy flow in the body usually accompanied by pain. The blockage may have been caused by either Wind/Cold, Congealed Blood, or stagnant Qi.

Red signifies Heat. If it appears as a light tinge that comes primarily to the cheeks in the afternoon, it is Deficient Heat. If the face is flushed and the eyes red, it is Excessive Heat. A yellow color comes from Dampness and Deficiency. In Chinese medicine, there are two kinds of jaundice: Yang jaundice caused by Damp Heat where the skin is a bright orange-yellow, and Yin jaundice caused by Damp Cold where the skin is a pale yellow. Black, which is most commonly observed under the eyes, signifies Deficient Kidneys and Congealed Blood.

One interesting method used in diagnosing infants and small children is to examine the veins on the radial side of the index finger to determine the nature and seriousness of the disease. In normal children, when this vein is rubbed it turns faintly red and is indistinct. Bright red signifies that the child has contracted a Hot disease. If it is purple, the Heat is very strong. If it is green or dark blue, there is Wind in the body. The first segment of the finger is called the Wind segment, the second the Qi segment, and the tip is called the Life segment. When the vein is only visible in the Wind segment, the disease is mild. When it reaches the Qi segment it is more severe. When the vein is visible in the Life segment, the disease is in a very dangerous stage. This technique is useful because it gives information about the condition of a patient with common childhood diseases, at an age when it is most difficult to take the pulse.

Inspection of the tongue occupies a prominent place in Chinese diagnostics. The tongue is closely connected (through the channels) with the Heart and Spleen, and therefore reflects the condition of the Blood. For diagnostic purposes, the body of the tongue is divided into areas representing various Organs, as shown in the following illustration.

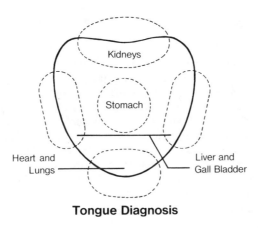

Tongue Diagnosis

Localization of any of the following conditions usually signifies a disorder in the corresponding Organ.

In diagnosis, changes in the shape, fur, and body of the tongue are all important. The meaning of these changes is expressed in terms of the Six Excesses and Eight Parameters, discussed above. When the tongue is examined, it must be done under light that is as close to natural light as possible. Otherwise, there may be incorrect observation of the color of the body or fur. It is also necessary to ascertain if the patient has eaten or drank anything (e.g., cherries, coffee) that would affect the color of the fur.

The healthy tongue is moderately red, neither too fat nor too pointed, slightly moist with no fur or a thin white fur, and usually without crevices. If a person has a tongue like this it signifies that any disease he might have is mild at the time.

The shape and physical alteration of the body of the tongue are the first things to look for. A fat tongue with indentations of teeth along the edges indicates either Deficient Qi or a surfeit of Dampness in the body. Differentiation depends on the condition of the fur. A white, moist fur reflects Deficient Qi, a greasy fur Dampness. A tongue that is thin and narrow indicates either insufficiency of Yin liquids, or both Deficient Qi and Yin. If the body of the tongue is red, then the problem is that of Deficient Yin alone. If it is pale, both the Qi and Yin are weak.

Red eruptions on the tip or the edges of the tongue indicate intense Heat. Red or purplish eruptions on the sides of the tongue (in the Liver area) indicate Congealed Blood, pain, or tension due to disturbances of the Liver's spreading function. They are often observed among women with menstrual problems.

Cleavages in the tongue, either superficial or deep, indicate the presence of Heat or dryness in the body. In a small minority of cases it is congenital and has no particular meaning.

The color of the tongue changes depending upon the degree of Heat in the body, and upon the condition of the Qi and Blood. A normal tongue is light red. If the color is lighter it is called pale, if darker it is called red, and if still darker it is called deep-red. Sometimes the tongue contains areas that are dark blue or purple.

A pale tongue signifies Deficient Blood and Qi. If it is very pale, it may be a symptom of Interior Cold. A red tongue indicates the presence of Interior (Deficient) Heat. In conditions of Excessive Heat the entire tongue is red, whereas with Deficient Heat only the tip is so colored. If the tongue is dark red, the Heat is correspondingly deeper in the body. A deep-red tongue with sores is symptomatic of Fire in the Heart.

When the tongue manifests purple or dark blue patches, there is an impediment to the flow of Qi and Blood. If these patches are localized then the problem is limited to that area of correspondence in the body.

Healthy people have a thin layer of fur on the tongue. Changes in the appearance and color of this fur are helpful in diagnosis. A normal tongue has a slightly moist fur. If there is too much moisture, such that there is a semi-transparent film over the tongue, the fur is called wet. This indicates the presence of Dampness in the body. Excessive dryness of the fur indicates an insufficiency of fluids (this is one of the first symptoms of this condition). If one can see the tongue through the fur, the fur is called thin. This signifies that the Excess indicated by the fur (usually Dampness, Heat, or Cold) is weak. If the fur is very thick and appears to have some kind of greasy matter upon it, it is called greasy. This characteristic indicates serious Dampness, Phlegm, or indigestion. If the Yin liquids are seriously depleted or the Stomach Qi is weak, the tongue will have no fur at all. This is called a stripped tongue.

The color of the fur is one of the most important indicators in determining the nature of a disease in the body. The fur is usually thin and white on a healthy person. If a patient has this kind of fur, the disease is not serious, or is still at the Exterior stage. A white, wet fur indicates Cold. A white, dry fur indicates that the Cold Excess is in the process of transforming into Heat. A thick, greasy white fur indicates the presence of Phlegm and Dampness. A yellow fur signifies Heat.

In the course of diagnosis, many other parts of the body come under the scrutiny of the doctor. Here, we will mention a few of the more common manifestations that a Chinese doctor would look for. Most of these are related to the series of correspondences revolving around the Five Phases, but some are based only on experience.

The hair reflects the health of the Kidneys and of the Blood. Thus, thinning, dry hair indicates Deficient Kidney Qi or weak Blood. The differences in color and moisture of the lips are similar to those of the body of the tongue. If the corners of the lips do not close firmly and the groove between the nose and the upper lip is shrunken, then the Qi is close to exhaustion and the disease is probably terminal. Drooling saliva is due to either a Deficient Spleen or Heat in the Stomach. Red, swollen, or bleeding gums are caused by Stomach Fire. Pale, swollen gums and loose teeth can be traced to Deficient Kidneys.

More recently, inspection of skin eruptions on the ears has been used in diagnosis. (See Section III, chapter 7 of text on ear acupuncture.)

Listening and Smelling

A doctor must pay attention to the patient's breathing, mode of speech, and cough, as these are important indicators of the body's health. In Deficient diseases, the breathing is shallow and soft; rough, heavy breathing occurs in diseases of Excess. Asthmatic wheezing is divided into two categories. Excessive wheezing (the Lungs are the main problem) is characterized by a high and rough sound to the breathing, with the exhalations being particularly forced. In cases of Deficient wheezing (the Kidneys not grasping the Qi is the main problem), the sound is low and there is more trouble inhaling. Speech and coughs are differentiated as Excessive or Deficient in the same manner. A cough that produces gurgling sounds in the throat is due to Phlegm and/or Dampness. A dry, hacking cough is caused by Dry Heat in the Lungs.

The nose is also an important diagnostic tool. In Excessive Hot diseases the various secretions and excretions of the body have a very foul odor, while in Excessive Cold diseases they may smell like rotten fish. Congestion of food may cause the patient to have rotten, sour breath.

The odors which correspond to the various Organs have two principal diagnostic functions. First, the doctor may smell them and distinguish which Organ is affected. Secondly, patients themselves may smell them and be able to tell if the particular Organ in question is making improvement.

Asking

Asking the patient about his or her past medical history, present condition, and life-style provides doctors, both Chinese and Western, with one of the most important sources of diagnosis. It must, however, be combined with the other methods of diagnosis to correct for the patient's subjective bias, and to fill in information the patient cannot give. Traditionally, there are ten areas on which Chinese doctors concentrate when interviewing patients. These are discussed below.

Chills and Fever

Chills and fever appearing simultaneously indicate Exterior conditions. If the chills are stronger, it is a Wind/Cold disease; if the opposite is true, it is Wind/Hot condition. Alternating chills and fever is the primary symptom of half Exterior/half Interior conditions. Continuing fever without chills indicates that the disease has moved inward. When the Heat has entered the Stomach and Intestines there is a constant fever that rises in the evening. Generally, if the fever rises during the night the condition is serious. A patient with a severe Deficient Yin condition develops a low fever daily, or a feeling of heat in the soles and palms in the afternoon or evening, which breaks late at night when the patient sweats heavily. Irregular periods of low fever accompanied by lassitude indicate Deficient Qi. Chills or coldness in the limbs are symptoms of Deficient Yang of either the Spleen or Kidneys.

Perspiration

If, during Exterior conditions, there is no perspiration, this shows that the Excess has bottled up the Protective Qi preventing the body from expelling the Excess. If there is sweating but no corresponding break in the fever, this indicates that the Protective Qi is too weak to expel the disease. If there is an excess of perspiration during the day, this is called spontaneous sweating and indicates Deficient Qi. Heavy sweating at night signifies Deficient Yin.

Head and Body

New headaches are usually caused by exogenous Excesses, while old or recurring headaches are usually due to internal factors. Violent headaches indicate Excessive conditions, and dull ones indicate Deficient conditions. Headaches that increase in intensity after encountering cold are caused by Wind and Cold. Those that worsen in hot environments are usually caused by hyperactive Liver Yang. When the head feels under a lot of pressure, as if it is encased in a bag, the cause is Dampness. Frontal headaches are associated with Yang Brightness (Stomach and Large Intestine), and those concentrated behind the hairline with Greater Yang (Small Intestine and Bladder). These names refer to the channels which traverse that particular area of the head. (See Section I, chapter 3 of the text.) Headaches at the vertex are caused by Liver dysfunction.

In Chinese medicine there are three kinds of vertigo. The first, related to hyperactive Liver Yang, feels as if one is on a ship, walking unsteadily. In the second, associated with Wind and Phlegm, everything seems to be spinning around. The third, vertigo caused by insufficient Blood and Qi, is characterized by dizziness, unclear vision, and a ringing in the ears.

It is most important to ask the patient to identify any place on or in the body that feels strange or painful. These pains can be significant in themselves as identifying a local disorder, or they can reflect disease elsewhere in the channel along which they are located. Pain that moves around is due to Wind or Stagnant Qi. Pain which remains in one place is caused by Cold, Dampness or Coagulated Blood. Pain which lessens upon pressure of massage is Deficient. Conversely, pain which intensifies upon pressure is Excessive. Insufficiency of Blood and Qi can cause soreness and/or numbness in the muscles and sinews. Dampness may cause the body to feel heavy.

Urine and Stool

An excess of urine, especially at night, is due to Deficient Kidney Yang which, if severe, can lead to incontinence. Sparse urine can be caused by Heat drying up the liquids in the body, or by Qi of the Bladder being too weak to pass urine. Deficiency in general can result in urine that is passed weakly or in a dripping manner.

When Heat enters the body from outside and penetrates into the Stomach and Intestines, the abdomen feels bloated and painful and there is constipation. In Deficient Yin conditions where there is an absence of fluids, constipation occurs without a feeling of bloatedness. In old age, the body loses the energy to expel stool; this is called Cold constipation.

Massive and sudden diarrhea is a condition of Excess. Long-term diarrhea results from Deficient Spleen. Frequent diarrhea with small amounts each time and a feeling immediately afterward that one has to go again (as in dysentery) is caused by Damp Heat in the Intestines. If diarrhea is accompanied by pain in the abdomen which diminishes after the diarrhea, the cause is usually congestion of food. This arises from a disorder affecting the Spleen/Stomach's function of transformation and transportation of food. If the pain occurs under some kind of emotional stress and is not relieved by the diarrhea, the cause is probably an imbalance between the Spleen and the Liver. Diarrhea every morning at dawn (called five o'clock or cock-crow diarrhea) is caused by Deficient Spleen and Kidney Qi, and is most common among the elderly.

Diet and Appetite

Different kinds of thirst indicate disorders related to different Excesses. Not being thirsty, or desiring warm drinks, indicates Cold. A strong desire for cold drinks indicates Heat. The absence of thirst, or only slight thirst, or spitting up liquid immediately after drinking indicates Dampness.

Usually, a good appetite shows that a disease is not too serious. Lack of appetite with a bloated feeling after eating is caused by either a weak Spleen or Damp Heat in the Middle Burner. Heat in the Stomach may cause one to eat a lot, be constantly hungry, and have a noisy stomach. The presence of certain tastes in the mouth has diagnostic significance (as determined by the correspondences of the Five Phases). Bitterness is associated with Heat; sweetness or blandness with Dampness or a weak Spleen; rotten tastes accompany congestion of food; sour tastes are associated with dysfunction of the Liver.

Chest and Abdomen

The basic rules governing pain in these areas are the same as those previously described for the head and body. A feeling of depression in the chest accompanied by shortness of breath is due to Deficient Qi. Swollen and painful chest and sides indicates dysfunction of the Liver or Gall Bladder. A feeling of bloatedness in the abdomen that is relieved by belching or passing gas is caused by stagnation of either Qi or Food.

Eyes and Ears

The eyes are the sensory organs associated with the Liver. Red, irritated eyes are caused by hyperactive Liver Yang. Loss of vision accompanied by dry, dull eyes is usually symptomatic of Deficient Liver and Kidney Yin. The ears are the sensory organs of the Kidneys, and progressive loss of hearing or tinnitus is usually caused by a weakness of the Kidneys. The paths of the Lesser Yang channels (those associated with the Triple Burner and Gall Bladder) travel around and into the ears. Hot diseases of exogenous origin often enter the body along these pathways, and may cause a loss of hearing, sometimes permanent.

Sleep

Insufficiency of Blood in the Heart, or disturbances of the Spirit may result in restless sleep, much dreaming and palpitations of the Heart. If the Heart Yin is Deficient, the person is irritable and finds it very hard to fall asleep. Excessive sleepiness may be caused by Heat in the Pericardium, Phlegm obstructing the opening of the Heart, or general Deficient Yang.

Medical History

Only by inquiring into the patient's medical past can a doctor place the results of the examination in proper perspective. The doctor should pay attention to minor symptoms from the past that could give a clue as to the root cause of the present condition. A detailed description of the progress of the disease and all medication taken prior to the time of the examination should be obtained. Previous treatment should be noted. (Surgery may hinder the effects of acupuncture.)

Bearing and Living Habits
These factors should be ascertained to the extent possible, since they can prove invaluable in diagnosing an illness. Some elements have been discussed previously under the topics Organs and causes of diseases. The point, again, is that the whole person must be taken into account.

Palpation

Palpation in Chinese medicine has three principal forms. One is the palpation of local areas on the body that are painful, swollen, hot, etc., to determine the nature of a local problem. Swelling which is hot and painful belongs to the Yang type and is caused by Heat. That which is cool to the touch is usually a product of Dampness and therefore is classified as Yin. Hard swellings or nodules are congealed Blood, while those with the elasticity of a balloon, or whose borders are ill-defined, are related to stagnant Qi. In fevers, when the palm is hotter than the back of the hand there is Deficient Yin; if the back of the hand is hotter, there is overactive Yang or Excessive Heat.

Another form of palpation used in diagnosis is at specific acupuncture points on the front and back of the trunk. Usually, a point at which the physician senses a "collapsed" feeling, or which is sore to the touch is most likely to indicate disease in the Organ with which the point is associated.

The last category of diagnosis by palpation in Chinese medicine is palpation of the pulse. There are many places on the body to take the pulse (each channel has at least one) but traditionally it is the pulse of the Lung channel—the radial pulse on the wrist—which is the principal site for pulse diagnosis. The pulse, although specifically related to the Lungs and controlled by the Heart (as are all pulses), nonetheless reflects the condition of all the Organs. Diagnosis by pulse is a subtle art and, even more than other diagnostic procedures, requires a tremendous amount of attentiveness and experience in order to acquire the sensitivity necessary to do it well. While most Chinese doctors would agree that the pulse is best used in conjunction with the other diagnostic methods, doctors well-skilled in pulse diagnosis can discover an enormous amount of information about their patients by this method alone. A student should take as many pulses as possible, because actually feeling the pulse is the only way to learn them; the written word gives only the barest hint.

The *Inner Classic* suggests that the best time to take the pulse is in the early morning, physiologically the calmest time of the day. Although often not possible, it is very important that both the patient and the doctor be relaxed while the pulse is being taken. This means that the patient should wait at least five minutes after arrival at the office before beginning. The doctor must refrain from "quicky" pulse-taking in a hurried frame of mind. If this precaution is not observed, the resulting pulse readings will be misleading.

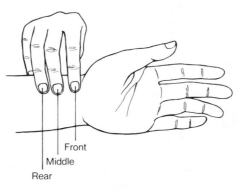

Front
Middle
Rear

Pulse Positions

If possible a patient should face the doctor during pulse diagnosis. The hands should never be above heart level. When taking the pulse three fingers should be used, the middle, index, and ring, with the index finger placed closest to the wrist. This allows for duplication of the pulse sensation and is conducive to acquiring the requisite sensitivity.

In Chinese medicine three pulses are taken on each wrist. The three positions are front, middle, and rear. The middle position is parallel with the lower knob on the posterior side of the ulna (ulnar styloid process), the front position is closer to the hand, and the rear position further from the hand. The middle position is palpated by the middle finger, while the index finger palpates the front, and the ring finger the rear position. The doctor's fingers should be placed where the patient's would; that is, if the patient's hands are smaller than the doctor's, the doctor will have to move her fingers closer together. At first, the three positions are palpated simultaneously, initially lightly, then with medium pressure, then more strongly. After this, each position is checked separately. Different systems are used whereby the pulse at each position is identified with certain Organs. The system most commonly used in China is:

- left hand rear position corresponds to Kidney Yin
- left hand middle position corresponds to Liver
- left hand front position corresponds to Heart
- right hand rear position corresponds to Kidney Yang
- right hand middle position corresponds to Spleen
- right hand front position corresponds to Lungs.

Note that all of the Organs listed here are Yin Organs. According to some systems, the pulse that appears on light pressure is taken to represent the Yang Organs with which the Yin Organs above are paired in the so-called Yin/Yang relationship. (The Triple Burner is linked, for pulse taking purposes, with the Kidney Yang.) Because pulse taking is an art, it should not be surprising that there is no single orthodox set of correspondences. Rather, there are many ways to put together the same pattern.

When the pulse is taken, attention is given to the pace, shape, and quality of the pulse. A normal pulse is distinct, discernible with the fingertip upon medium pressure, and can still be discerned with the application of heavy pressure. It has what is traditionally known as Stomach Qi, Spirit, and Root. The more these qualities are present in the pulse of a sick patient, the less serious is the condition.

'Stomach Qi' is the quality of moderation. The pulse is neither superficial nor submerged, neither too fast nor too slow. It is leisurely and moderately strong. Because the Stomach is the entrepot for nutrition in the body, a patient with Stomach Qi can recover from a disease, whereas a patient without it cannot. 'Spirit' is similarly a quality of moderation, but it is moderation in the shape or strength of the pulse. A weak pulse with Spirit has a core of strength. A strong pulse with Spirit has a feeling of elasticity. 'Root' refers to the rear of the Kidney position. Because the Kidneys are associated with the basal energy of the body, if their pulse has some strength the body has Root.

In a healthy person the front position tends to be floating, while the rear position is usually submerged. Speed averages approximately four beats to each breath, 60-72 heart bearts per minute. Some variations are normal. Athletes often have a slow pulse, 40-54 beats per minute. Young children have quick pulses. Fat people have deep pulses, while thin people have pulses with a tendency to be bigger than normal. Women's pulses are usually softer and slightly quicker than men's. Also, women's right pulses are usually stronger than their left, while the opposite is true of men. Some use these sexual differences in the pulse to predict the sex of a baby. If the mother's pulse is stronger on the right the child will be a girl. If it is stronger on the left, it will be a boy.

There are many pathological pulses. Different schools name seventeen, twenty-eight, even as many as thirty-two different pulse types. Some of these types are very rare and appear only in the late stages of terminal disease. Others vary only slightly from each other, and require considerable experience to differentiate. Generally, the pulses can be grouped together in categories which correspond to the steps in the procedure of taking the pulse. It must be remembered that almost always a person's pulse will be a mixture of the pulse types described below.

Depth

The first quality which the physician searches for is depth. There are two principal abnormal pulses in this category.

Floating. The pulse is distinct when the skin is barely touched with the fingertips, but fades under greater pressure. This pulse is usually associated with Exterior conditions (chills, fever, runny nose, etc.). Since these conditions primarily affect the Lungs, it is ordinarily most pronounced in the Lung position (right front). In a very weak person with a cold this pulse may not appear. In chronic diseases where the Qi and Blood have been seriously depleted (so that the body's Yang Qi is weak and floating, and lacks Yin as a foundation), this pulse will be found, even in the absence of the Exterior symptoms.

Submerged. The pulse is only distinct upon application of considerable pressure. The presence of this pulse signifies that the disorder has advanced to the Interior stage. Specific symptoms accompanying this pulse depend on the nature of the disease.

Pace

The next characteristic of the pulse is pace. The normal pulse should evidence about four beats to each breath of the patient. As mentioned earlier, athletes may have a slower pulse and children a faster one. Usually, however, there are two principal types of pulses which are distinguished by their characteristic pace.

Slow. The pulse rate is three or less heart beats per breath. This signifies Cold or Deficient Yang. Symptoms include pronounced sensitivity to cold, poor circulation, loose bowels, white fur on the tongue and general lassitude.

Quick. The pulse rate is six or more beats per breath. This signifies Heat caused either by the Heat Excess or Deficient Yin. Symptoms include fever, rash, and pronounced thirst.

Length

The length of the pulse is another important characteristic.

Long. This pulse can be felt from above the rear position to below the front position. When a person is sick, this pulse indicates that the disease (usually related to Heat and/or Blood) is well advanced. Symptoms include high fever and irritability. In a healthy person, however, it represents a robust constitution.

Short. The short pulse can only be discerned in the middle position. It signifies insufficiency of Blood and Qi. Symptoms include pale complexion, lack of energy, and the need to sleep more than normal.

Strength

There are two main pulse types in this category.

Weak. This pulse feels weak and hardly presses back at the doctor's fingers. Its presence signifies Deficiency, either generally (Qi and/or Blood) or in the Organ corresponding to the specific pulse location.

Strong. This pulse responds strongly to the touch. It signifies the presence of an Excess in a sick person, but a good condition among the healthy.

Quality

The last and most difficult aspect to ascertain in pulse is its quality. This characteristic includes the texture, smoothness, and regularity of the pulse wave. Such differentiation is often crucial to the accuracy of the diagnosis.

Slippery. This pulse can definitely be discerned, but the boundaries are indistinct, as if feeling a ball through a layer of highly viscous liquid. A slippery pulse usually signifies the presence of Dampness or Phlegm in the body. Symptoms include mucus, sluggish digestion, difficulty in moving the joints, and heavy fur on the tongue. If a healthy woman exhibits this pulse at all positions it usually indicates that she is pregnant.

Rough. The pulse feels choppy as if the waves of the pulse are irregular (in form, not in rhythm). This pulse signifies Congealed Blood (hard, painful nodules in the abdomen, menstrual irregularities), stagnant Qi (upset stomach, headaches, abdominal pains) or Deficient Blood.

Wiry. The feeling of this long and taut pulse is like that of a violin or guitar string. It is a strong pulse that pushes back. A wiry pulse appears in Liver diseases and accompanies pain.

Tight. This pulse feels like a tight clothesline (fuller than wiry), and as if it were fast, but in fact is not. The waves are short and follow each other closely. A tight pulse, when accompanied by a floating pulse, is characteristic of Excessive Cold conditions in particular. Symptoms include severe chills, fever, pain in joints, clear vomit, and a white fur on the tongue.

Huge. This pulse can be felt at all levels and is slightly stronger on top, and at the beginning of the waves. It almost always signifies Excessive Heat conditions and is accompanied by high fever, great thirst, and pronounced sweating. However, if it appears suddenly in a long, debilitating disease, it reflects the exhaustion of Qi and is a very bad sign.

Fine. This pulse is small and thin like a fine thread. It signifies insufficiency of the Blood and Yin. Symptoms include thirst, irritability, low grade fever, and a tongue with a red tip.

Irregular. There are three types of irregular pulses, all of which signify disorders of the Heart Qi. Hasty is fast with irregular pauses, and shows Excessive Heart Yang or congested Qi in the Upper Burner. Knotted is slow with irregular pauses, and signifies obstruction to Blood in the Heart, with Yin in Excess or Phlegm in the Pericardium. Intermittent is systematic but pauses abnormally. It signifies an exhausted condition in the Organs. All three pulses are very dangerous signs when they appear among the sick, but can also occur in relatively healthy people during periods of mental or emotional strain.

CONCLUSION

This introduction has attempted to present the theory and practices of traditional Chinese diagnosis and treatment within its own context. We hope the reader will now be able to begin the main text, where many subjects only briefly noted here are explained, with a clearer idea of its theoretical foundations. Practicing Chinese medicine requires a certain amount of knowledge, but is in many respects an art. This introduction was intended only to provide a bare, theoretical framework within which this art can be practiced and mastered.

REFERENCES

English

Agren, Hans. "Patterns of Tradition and Modernization in Contemporary Chinese Medicine" in Arthur Kleinman, et. al. (Ed.), *Medicine in Chinese Cultures,* pp 37-60. Washington, D.C.: N.I.H., 1975.

Kaptchuk, Ted. *The Web That Has No Weaver: Understanding Chinese Medicine,* New York: Congdon & Weed, 1983.

Porkert, Manfred. *The Theoretical Foundations of Chinese Medicine,* Cambridge, Massachusetts: The MIT Press, 1974.

Chinese

Chinese Academy of Traditional Medicine, Guangdong College of Traditional Medicine, et. al. *Concise Dictionary of Traditional Chinese Medicine, (Jianming Zhongyi Cidian)* Hong Kong, United Press, 1979.

Chinese Academy of Traditional Medicine, Guangdong College of Traditional Medicine, *A Dictionary of Chinese Medical Terms and Nomenclature (Zhongyi Mingzi Shuyu Cidian)* Hong Kong: Commercial Press, 1975.

Shanghai College of Traditional Medicine, *Basics of Chinese Medicine (Zhongyi Jichuxue)* Hong Kong: Commercial Press, 1975.

Shanghai College of Traditional Medicine, *Discerning Patterns and Instituting Treatment (Bianzheng Shizhi),* Shanghai, Shanghai People's Publishing House, 1972.

Section I

Channels

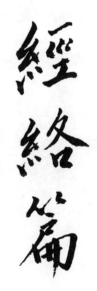

Chapter 1

A Summary of Channel Theory

A study of the channels provides an essential basis for understanding the reciprocal relationships and influences among the various physiological, pathological, diagnostic and therapeutic aspects of traditional Chinese medicine. The theory of the channels summarizes the experience of the Chinese over thousands of years in combatting disease. From ancient times, physicians observed numerous symptoms of disease and the results obtained from various methods of treatment. It was discovered, for example, that by stimulating distinct sites on the body's surface, disease in both the superficial tissues and internal Organs could be treated; that pathology in an internal Organ will often manifest itself in certain external or systemic symptoms; and that disease in one Organ will sometimes affect another. Similarly, it was noted that many diseases follow a predictable course of development. In time, these observations became systematized, forming the basis of Chinese medicine.

According to traditional theory, there exists in the body a system of channels or vessels which integrate all the body's separate parts and functions into a unified organism. Among the channels are major trunks and lesser branches which join internally with the vital Organs, and externally with the limbs, sensory organs and orifices. The Qi and Blood circulate throughout the body via this network of channels. Thus, the intimate relationship between the internal Viscera and the periphery of the body is primarily maintained by means of the channels. Channel theory reflects the holistic attitude of Chinese medicine, with great emphasis placed upon the interrelationships among all parts of the organism.

The theory of the channels is interrelated with the theory of the Organs. Traditionally, the internal Organs have never been regarded as independent anatomical entities. Rather, attention has centered upon the functional and pathological interrelationships between the channel network and the Organs. So close is this identification that each of the twelve traditional Primary channels bears the name of one or another of the vital Organs.

In the clinic, the entire framework of diagnostics, therapeutics and point selection is based upon the theoretical framework of the channels. "It is because of the twelve Primary channels that people live, that disease is formed, that people are treated and disease arises."[1] From the beginning, however, we should recognize that, like other aspects of traditional medicine, channel theory reflects the limitations in the level of scientific development at the time of its formation, and is therefore tainted with the philosophical idealism and metaphysics of its day. That which has continuing clinical value needs to be reexamined through practice and research to determine its true nature.

CLASSIFICATION OF THE CHANNELS

The channels form a web which crisscrosses the body vertically and horizontally. They join the internal Organs with the skin, flesh, ligaments, bones and all other tissues, and integrate each part with

35

the whole. There are two principal types of channels. The main trunks *(jing)* are generally distributed vertically over the body through relatively deep tissues. The connecting branches *(luo)* are distributed horizontally and superficially over the body. The main trunks traverse the limbs peripherally and penetrate the body cavities to connect with the Organs. The connecting branches, distributed largely along the body surface, join the main trunks, connective tissues and cutaneous regions. All the channels but two (along the median line of the body) are bilateral, i.e., duplicated on both sides of the body.

A summary of channel characteristics follows. Detailed descriptions of the pathways of each channel, together with related pathological symptoms will be provided in later chapters.

The Primary, Divergent and Miscellaneous Channels

The main trunks *(jing)* include the twelve Primary, twelve Divergent and eight Miscellaneous channels. Among these, the twelve Primary channels are by far the most important for clinical purposes. Each has been named by combining traditional Yin and Yang polarity with one of the twelve Organs with which it is associated (e.g., the Absolute Yin Liver channel, the Greater Yang Small Intenstine channel, etc.). Peripherally, six of the Primary channels are associated with the leg and the remaining six with the arm. The three leg and three arm channels that traverse the lateral and posterior aspects of the limbs, and join internally with Yang Organs, are referred to as Yang channels. These are commonly translated as the Lesser Yang, Yang Brightness and Greater Yang channels of the arms and legs. The remaining six channels follow the medial and anterior aspects of the limbs, join internally with the Yin Organs, and are called Yin channels. These include the Lesser Yin,Greater Yin and Absolute Yin channels of the arms and legs. Each Yin channel and its related Yin Organ is paired with one of the Yang channels and its related Yang Organ. In addition to providing balance and symmetry to the channel system, each of these complementary Yin/Yang channels and Organs shares a special functional relationship with the other in its pair.*

The twelve Divergent channels are vertical branches of the Primary channels. Each is named after the Primary channel from which it diverges. The principal function of the Divergent channels is to link with the channel and Organ associated with the parent Primary channel in the Yin/Yang relationship. For example, the Divergent branch of the Arm Greater Yin Lung channel joins internally with the Arm Yang Brightness Large Intestine channel, with which the Lung channel is paired in its Yin/Yang relationship. It is the Divergent channel that acts as a go-between in effecting the special functional relationship between pairs of Yin and Yang Primary channels.

Most of the eight Miscellaneous channels are large branch vessels of the Primary channels. They are termed Miscellaneous because their pathways, some of which encircle the body horizontally while others follow the midline vertically, are less uniform than the other main *(jing)* channels.

The Connecting Channels

These include the fifteen (or Great) Connecting channels and their lesser branches: the Minute Connecting channels, the Superficial Connecting channels and the Blood Connecting channels. Twelve of the fifteen Connecting channels separate from the twelve Primary channels at specific points, forming major horizontal or transverse branches. The name of each is derived from the Primary channel from which it separates. The 13th and 14th Connecting channels separate from two of the Miscellaneous channels (the Governing and Conception channels) and the 15th is called the Great Connecting channel of the Spleen. (Sometimes a 16th channel, the Great Connecting channel of the Stomach, is included in this group. However, because the Stomach and Spleen channels are coupled in a Yin/Yang relationship, it is customary to speak only of the fifteen Connecting channels). Like the Divergent channels, the fifteen Connecting channels serve to connect the paired Yin and Yang Primary channels. However, unlike the Divergent channels, this connection is made between

*This is known as the Yin/Yang or Inner/Outer relationship.—*Editors*

Primary channels as they traverse the limbs rather than between their associated Organs internally.

The Minute Connecting channels are smaller branch vessels of the fifteen Connecting channels. The Superficial Connecting channels are smaller branches confined to the surface of the body. Those Connecting channels, particularly the Superficial Connecting channels, which can be seen beneath the skin as blood vessels are called the Blood Connecting channels. There are an unspecified number of these smaller types of Connecting vessels.

The significance of the Connecting channels lies in distributing vital nutrients (Qi and Blood) to those areas not directly traversed by other channels, and in connecting the Yang Primary channels with the Yin Primary channels on the limbs. Such Connecting points, as they are called, are useful in acupuncture therapy.

The External Connections of the Channels:
The Twelve Muscle Channels and Cutaneous Regions

As was said earlier, the channels not only reach into the body cavities to join with associated Viscera, but also circulate through superficial tissues on the surface of the body. Each of the twelve Primary channels is associated with the connective tissues (muscles, tendons, ligaments) and cutaneous areas along its path. Thus, there are twelve Cutaneous Regions and twelve Muscle channels associated with the twelve Primary channels.

CIRCULATION OF QI IN THE CHANNELS

The circulation of Qi and Blood essentially follows the paths of the channels described above. Although Qi and Blood circulate together, it is the Qi that takes the 'leading' role. Qi is said to be the 'commander of the Blood', i.e., the motivating force.

The concept of Qi in the channels is rather complicated. Is it, after all, something material? At the present time it is not certain. Also causing uncertainty are the different interpretations given passages from ancient writings concerning the direction in which Qi moves in the channels. Previously, physicians relied only upon certain sections of the *Spiritual Axis,* such as the following reference which appears in chapter 38:

> [The Qi] in the three Arm Yin [channels] travels from the internal Organs to the hands; [the Qi] in the three Arm Yang [channels] travels from the hands to the head; [the Qi] in the three Leg Yang channels travels from the head to the feet; [the Qi] in the three Leg Yin channels travels from the feet to the abdomen.*

This and other passages concerning the origins, end points and interconnections of the channels would seem to support the theory that the Blood and Qi flow only in one direction. This view, however, is incomplete. In this chapter we will attempt to provide a more comprehensive description of Qi based primarily upon a thorough reading of the *Inner Classic.*

The Qi is variously named according to its functional manifestations. Here we will explain the significance of Nourishing, Protective, Ancestral, and Source Qi. Overall, Nourishing and Protective Qi both flow through the channels to all parts of the body. Ancestral Qi is the force which pushes the Qi and Blood through the channels, and Source Qi provides the basis for the functional activities of the channels.

Nourishing Qi and Blood

The circulation of Blood through the channels bears a close relationship with the Nourishing Qi, frequently called the Blood Qi. According to traditional theory, the Nourishing Qi is created from the

---

*This description of the circulation is the basis for the point numbering system used in the West.—*Editors*

food nutrients in the Stomach and Spleen (the so-called 'middle burner'). The transformation of the Nourishing Qi in turn contributes to the formation of Blood. The Nourishing Qi and Blood then flow inseparably through the channels, nourishing the tissues of the body.

In chapter 16 of the *Spiritual Axis,* the Nourishing Qi is described as circulating sequentially through the Primary channels. It begins with the Arm Greater Yin Lung channel then passes to the Arm Yang Brightness Large Intestine channel, the Leg Yang Brightness Stomach channel, the Leg Greater Yin Spleen channel, the Arm Lesser Yin Heart channel, the Arm Greater Yang Small Intestine channel, the Leg Greater Yang Bladder channel, the Leg Lesser Yin Kidney channel, the Arm Absolute Yin Pericardium channel, the Arm Lesser Yang Triple Burner channel, the Leg Lesser Yang Gall Bladder channel and ends with the Leg Absolute Yin Liver channel, where the cycle begins anew. A second route of circulation joins the Conception and Governing (Miscellaneous) channels along the median line in the front and back of the body. This is regarded as an offshoot of the Lung channel. In this manner, the Nourishing Qi and Blood are continuously circulated, providing nourishment to all parts of the body.

This popular description of the circulation of Qi and Blood, however, is only one of several found in ancient medical writings and must therefore be considered incomplete. For example, the Qi flowing through the channels is comprised of other types in addition to Nourishing Qi. Furthermore, the Qi does not only flow through the Primary channels, but the Miscellaneous, Divergent and Connecting channels as well. Moreover, because of the complex branchings and junctures among the various channels, the order of circulation can neither be as simple nor as symmetrical as the original model suggests. In fact, our discussion in later chapters will show inconsistencies in the description of circulation within individual channels.

Protective Qi

Like Nourishing Qi, the Protective Qi is formed from nutrients in food. However, it is characteristically more 'aggressive' and 'slippery' than the Nourishing Qi which enables it to spread out and penetrate surrounding tissues at will. Whereas the Nourishing Qi is retained within the walls of the channels, the Protective Qi is able to move both inside and outside the channels. Circulating between the skin and flesh, it protects the body from harmful external influences, regulates body warmth and the opening and closing of the pores, and moistens the skin, muscles and hair. It is thus involved in the functions of sweating and urination. Like Nourishing Qi, the Protective Qi may be regulated through acupuncture.

Generally speaking, the Protective Qi is distributed superficially through the tissues of the head, trunk, and limbs during the day, while at night it is stored and circulated deep within the internal Organs.

As in the case of Nourishing Qi, the ancient medical classics contain more than one description of the sequential passage of Protective Qi through the channels of the body. According to one explanation in chapters 62 and 71 of the *Spiritual Axis,* during the day the Protective Qi travels from its inception in the Stomach to the head. From the head it is distributed through the Yang Primary channels, contiguous muscles and other tissues. Reaching the extremities, it enters the Yin Primary channels and moves through the entire network of interconnecting channels and associated Organs. Finally, the Protective Qi returns to the head in the region of the eyes, where the daytime cycle begins anew. At night, the Protective Qi travels first from the eyes to the Kidneys and then to other Yin Organs, circulating via the channels which subsequently join with the Yang Organs. Finally, the Qi returns to the region of the eyes.

An alternative description of the circulation of Protective Qi is that, after first being distributed from the head to the Greater Yang Primary channels of the Arm and Leg, the Protective Qi then passes through the Lesser Yang and Yang Brightness channels of the Arm and Leg. From the Yang Brightness channel of the Leg, it enters the Leg Lesser Yin channel, and returns through the channel system to the region of the eyes, to begin a new cycle. The circulation of the Protective Qi at night is similar to that described in the preceding paragraph.

Although these theories of circulation are said to be based on ancient clinical observation, they lack a material basis and must therefore be further researched.

Source Qi and Ancestral Qi

In order to circulate through the body, the Nourishing and Protective Qi need a motivating force. This is Ancestral Qi, formed from the union of the essence in food, and air inhaled from the atmosphere. The Ancestral Qi collects in the chest and is observable in the rising and falling motions of breathing, and the pulsation of the heart. For example: "The Great Connecting channel of the Stomach...emerging below the left breast, is dependent upon the Ancestral Qi for its movement."[2] Its force is strong enough to pass through the channels, reaching upward toward the throat and downward along the 'path of Qi', through the chest and abdomen to the lower limbs. In this manner, the Protective and Nourishing Qi are spread throughout the body.

The Source Qi* is congenital and is stored in the Kidneys. Traditional medicine maintains that the Kidney Essence is the material basis of the life activities in the human body, and the Kidney Qi the functional basis. All those functions associated with the channels are dependent upon it. Indeed, the Source Qi has been called the "root of the twelve Primary channels."[3]

Taken together, the Source, Ancestral, Protective and Nourishing Qi are called the True Qi, a collective name for the functional bases of life activities.

By way of summary, the Qi of the channels includes the Nourishing, Protective, Source and Ancestral Qi. The Nourishing and Protective Qi circulate through the body motivated by the Ancestral Qi. The Source Qi is the basal energy, the basis for all the functional activities of the channels. The Qi in the channels is the combined functional manifestation of the essence from food and water, the air inhaled from the atmosphere and the vital Essence stored in the Kidneys.

THE FUNCTIONS OF THE CHANNELS

Because of their close relationship with the tissues and organs of the body, the channels have important physiological and pathological functions. These are summarized below.

Transporting the Qi and Blood,
Moistening and Nourishing the Body

According to traditional medicine, the proper functioning of the Organs, muscles, bones, etc., is dependent upon the Qi (a Yang characteristic) and the fluids (a Yin characteristic). Yang Qi thus refers to all varieties of Qi in the body, and Yin fluids to the various nourishing and moistening liquids (Blood, heavy and light fluids). Collectively, these are simply termed Qi and Blood. The Qi is best understood as the energy or force necessary for functional activity, whereas the Blood is the source of moistening, lubrication and nourishment. It is by means of the channels that Qi and Blood spread throughout the body. Only in this manner can each of the body tissues perform its normal activity.

Responding to Dysfunction in the Body

When, for a variety of reasons both internal and external, the normal functioning of the body is disrupted, illness ensues. The channels respond to the presence of disease in a predictable fashion. Certain points along the affected channel may become spontaneously tender or sensitive to the touch. These points are useful not only in diagnosis, but also in acupuncture therapy where they are referred to as "that's it!" points (i.e., the points of pain). Some points more commonly react in this manner to the presence of disease than others. For example: "When there is a disease in the Yin Organs there will be a response in [one of the] twelve Source [points]. Each of the twelve Source [points] has its place of appearance. To know the place and observe its response is to know if its [related] Organ is injured."[4]

---

*As described in the Introduction, Source Qi is the most fundamental variety of Qi and may be regarded as the basal energy of the body.—*Editors*

Recent studies have also demonstrated that the electrical resistance or heat tolerance of the skin at some of the points diminishes. Palpation or electrical measurement of these points are therefore other means of diagnosing disease. For instance, the area just below point GB-34 *(Yanglingquan)* on the lower leg is often tender on patients with cholecystitis; the vicinity of S-37 *(Shangjuxu),* also on the lower leg, becomes particularly tender on patients with appendicitis. Stimulating these points can, through the mediation of the channels, affect the diseased organs. This is one of the theoretical bases of acupuncture therapeutics.

Often, the response to disease is not restricted to specific acupuncture points but will affect a wider area along the path of the channel or its associated domain. This may be evidenced, for example, by changes in the appearance of the skin (discoloration, rash), or abnormal sensations (pain, pressure, distension, etc.). Even though a disease arises in an internal Organ, symptoms may manifest in distant areas traversed by that Organ's associated channel:

> When the Lungs or Heart are diseased, their Qi is detained in the crooks of the elbows. When the Liver is diseased, its Qi is detained in the armpits. When the Spleen is diseased, its Qi is detained in the hips. When the Kidneys are diseased, the Qi is detained behind the knees.[5]

Diseases of the internal Organs may also appear, by means of the channels, as symptoms in the sensory organs of the head. For example, when the Lung Qi is blocked, the nose is congested; when the Heart Fire ascends, the tongue can become dark red and painful; when the Liver Fire rises, the eyes may become inflamed; when the Kidney Qi is exhausted, hearing will diminish. This notion of the connection between Organs by means of the channels was very important in the development of ear acupuncture. (See Section III, chapter 7) Systemic diseases may be accompanied by the appearance of diverse symptoms along the path of an individual channel or, because of the interconnections among the channels, the simultaneous appearance of symptoms associated with more than one channel. For example, in the *Discussion of Cold Induced Disorders* certain disease patterns were described as combinations of the symptoms of two related Primary channels. Thus, one pattern combined deafness, a symptom associated with the Arm Lesser Yang (Triple Burner) channel, with sweating, shivering, tidal fever, dryness in the mouth and pain in the chest and ribs which are all symptoms associated with the Leg Lesser Yang (Gall Bladder) channel. Similarly, symptoms associated with the Arm Greater Yin (Lung) channel and the Leg Greater Yin (Spleen) channel, such as abdominal swelling, vomiting, indigestion, diarrhea, abdominal pain, jaundice, etc., were regarded as the progression of disease along the course of the two channels.

Indeed, the association of an Organ with a wide range of symptoms can only be understood when one is familiar with the course of its related channel. Take the Liver, for example. The Leg Absolute Yin Liver channel begins in the foot and ascends to the genitals, lower abdomen and Stomach before connecting with the Gall Bladder. It then crosses the ribs and continues upward to the eyes and vertex. For this reason, Chinese medicine traces a variety of symptoms to the Liver. Colic is often said to result from the Cold Excess attacking the Liver channel, whose Qi is unable to expel it. If Liver Qi encroaches upon the Stomach, diseases of that Organ may ensue. Illness in the Liver may have a reciprocal effect upon the Gall Bladder, producing Heat and causing a draining of fluids from that Organ, which also appears in symptoms of jaundice and pain in the ribs. Fire in the Liver or insufficient Liver Yin may lead to eye diseases. The ascension of Liver Yang or Wind may cause distant channel symptoms such as vertigo, headache or blurred vision. All of these examples illustrate the numerous interrelationships between the Liver and other parts of the body facilitated through the Liver channel.

Transmitting Disease and Acupuncture Stimulation

When disease besets the body, it may pass to the internal Organs, or from one Organ to another, by means of the channels. An exogenous disease is said to reside first in the pores of the skin from which it enters the Minute Connecting channels, then the larger Connecting channels, the Primary channels and finally, unless it has been successfully treated, the internal Viscera.[6] Each of these stages manifests characteristic symptoms of increasing seriousness, a traditional view which is today still compatible with what we know of the progressive development of some diseases.

Since the compilation of the *Inner Classic* in the 2nd century B.C., other theories have been formulated to account for the complexity in the development of numerous diseases. Yet, fundamental to all traditional theories of disease is the belief that once a disease agent is present in a certain channel, evidenced by characteristic symptoms, it may be transmitted through the channel to other channels, or to the Organ with which the channel is associated. Therefore the channels, in addition to being conduits for the supply of nutrients and energy to the body, are also the passageways of disease. For example, according to the Six Channel Diagnostics, when a disease of exogenous origin affects the Greater Yang channels, it will appear first as symptoms associated with the exterior course of these channels (i.e., an Exterior condition). If the disease is not arrested at this stage it may undergo a transformation as it is transmitted through other channels. Although the Greater Yang symptoms may disappear, symptoms associated with the Lesser Yang or Yang Brightness channels will become evident. Alternatively, the initial symptoms may remain while those associated with other channels appear simultaneously. This phenomenon is explained on the basis of the interconnections among the Yang channels. Furthermore, because of the Yin/Yang reciprocal relationship between the Greater Yang and Lesser Yin channels, when the Normal Qi (that is, the functional health of the body) is weak, lowering the body's resistance to disease, a pathological Excess may be transmitted from the Greater Yang to the reciprocal Lesser Yin channel. The appearance of symptoms along the Lesser Yin channel represents a more serious development of the disease. Also, if a disease which is lodged along the exterior course of a channel is not properly treated it may move inward to attack the Organ associated with the channel. Thus, a disease affecting the Greater Yang channels may, if untreated, affect the Small Intestine (the Organ associated with the Arm Greater Yang channel) and Bladder (associated with the Leg Greater Yang channel).

The stimulation of acupuncture points on the body as a means of treating disease is likewise transmitted through the channels by regulating the Qi. That is, the proper circulation of Qi and Blood can be restored by stimulating points along the channels. When an activity of an Organ or channel is disrupted, points along that or related channels are stimulated with needles, heat, pressure, etc. The therapeutic stimulus is transmitted to the troubled area through the channel. This brings the regulatory effect of the Qi into full play by permitting the Qi and Blood to flow smoothly, and by allowing the Nourishing and Protective Qi to cure the disease. For example, point LI-4 *(Hegu)* is stimulated to relieve toothache, P-6 *(Neiguan)* is needled to treat Stomach pains, SI-3 *(Houxi)* and TB-3 *(Zhongzhu)* are selected for stiff neck, S-36 *(Zusanli)* and S-37 *(Shangjuxu)* for gastrointestinal diseases, etc. The efficacy of stimulating these points on the limbs to treat diseases of the head and trunk is explained by means of transmission through the channel system.

The theory of transmission was undoubtedly strengthened by the occurrence of certain phenomena which frequently accompany acupuncture treatment. For example, a numb, distended sensation extending from the site of needle insertion along the course of the channel, or alteration in the color or moisture of the skin along a channel are commonly experienced after acupuncture therapy. Although reactions of this sort vary from patient to patient, depending both upon constitutional differences and the quality of acupuncture therapy, they have provided an empirical basis for the theory of channel transmission.

THE CLINICAL SIGNIFICANCE OF CHANNEL THEORY

The clinical value of channel theory is closely related to those functions discussed above. In addition to setting forth an holistic view of the interrelationships which exist among all parts of the body, channel theory defines specific laws governing those relationships.

There are three aspects to channel theory. The first focuses upon the relationships between the external parts of the body: between the upper and the lower, the left and the right, the front and the back, the middle and the sides. The second dwells on the laws governing the relationships among the Organs. The third defines the relationships among specific areas on external portions of the body with the internal Organs.

Diagnostically, the application of these laws helps a physician, by a process of induction, to identify disease in an Organ by observing abnormal reactions along external regions of the body with which the Organ is associated. This is done by means of observation or palpation of the body surfaces, and by probing for irregularities on the skin along channels, acupuncture points or Cutaneous Regions.

Therapeutically, the clinical application of channel theory is even greater. In acupuncture therapy, a physician with a knowledge of the distribution of the channels need not only choose acupuncture points in the vicinity of a disease, but may also select distant points on a channel associated with the disease. Such methods as puncturing points on the limbs for diseases of the trunk, points on the sides for diseases in the middle, points on the right side for diseases on the left, and points on the back for disease in the front of the body illustrate this therapeutic principle. The Yin/Yang correspondences among the Primary channels and Organs, points of intersection among the channels, special characteristics of individual points, Cutaneous Regions and the broad domains of the Connecting channels offer further opportunity for therapeutic application of the principles of channel theory.

A few examples should help demonstrate what we have said. In the treatment of febrile diseases, it is common to select Gv-14 *(Dazhui)* to reduce fever. This is because fevers of an exogenous origin are said to arise from an Excess attacking the Yang channels, and Gv-14 *(Dazhui)* is the point of intersection of the Yang channels. When the Yang Qi is insufficient, giving rise to such symptoms as enuresis, chronic diarrhea, etc., Co-4 *(Guanyuan)* is often needled or warmed with moxibustion because it is the point of intersection of the three Leg Yin channels and is associated closely with the Source Qi of the Kidneys. B-67 *(Zhiyin),* on the little toe, can be needled for headache at the vertex because, according to the theory of Root and Branch, Origin and End (see chapter 4), this is the point of Origin on the Leg Greater Yang Bladder channnel whose upper course traverses the top of the head. For respiratory diseases, points along the Lung channel may of course be chosen. Perhaps less obviously, because of the Yin/Yang correspondence between the Lung and Large Intestine channels, points on the latter channel such as LI-4 *(Hegu)* and LI-11 *(Quchi)* are also indicated. Finally, Sp-6 *(Sanyinjiao)* on the lower leg is an example of a point at which the three Leg Yin Primary channels intersect. The location of this point at the junction of these channels makes it particularly efficacious in the treatment of obstetrical and gynecological disorders.

Chinese herbal prescriptions are also based, in large measure, on the principles of channel theory. For example, in the treatment of nephritis*, an herbal prescription would not only call for medication whose effect is to directly treat the Kidneys, but might also include herbs which affect the Spleen and Lungs. On the basis of channel theory, the Spleen, Lungs and Kidneys are interrelated, and the treatment of one will indirectly influence the health of the others. Similarly, in the treatment of eye diseases it is not uncommon to prescribe herbs which strengthen the Liver, since the Liver channel communicates with the eyes.

These illustrations are by no means exhaustive. The theory of the channels has provided a basis for many other important diagnostic and therapeutic precepts and practices in Chinese medicine over the long course of its historical development. Among the more important of these (discussed in the Introduction) are the Five Phases diagnostics and the Eight Parameter diagnostics.

Since the Liberation (1949), there has been further development in diagnostic and therapeutic practices based upon channel theory. This is evidenced by such innovations as the successful treatment of deafmutism and previously thought 'incurable' cases of paralysis, with acupuncture, and by the discovery of new response points on the auricle which are useful in the diagnosis and treatment of disease through ear acupuncture. Of particular note are the discoveries in the area of acupuncture anesthesia, the recent development of which is attributed to modern Chinese science, but whose basis is to be found in the analgesic effects long known to practitioners of acupuncture.

As we have seen, traditional Chinese medicine believes that Qi and Blood circulate through the channels of the body. If the circulation is obstructed, pain and other pathological symptoms are produced. By stimulating the channels at appropriate acupuncture points, the obstruction, and hence the pain and other symptoms, are thereby removed. Similarly, when anesthesia is desired, acupuncture points are selected on channels which traverse, or on channels associated with those which traverse, the site of surgical incision.

There is also a fundamental correspondence between channel theory and the areas of the body

*The Western-defined disease nephritis overlaps with many Kidney disorders in Chinese medicine.—*Editors*

affected by acupuncture anesthesia. Many of the areas which are anesthetized by stimulating points on the Yang channels are on the back. Conversely, many areas anesthetized via points on the Yin channels are on the abdomen. Traditionally, the back is associated with Yang, the abdomen with Yin. More of the Yang than Yin channels are distributed on the shoulders, back, head and back of neck; more of the Yin than Yang channels traverse the abdomen. And just as certain channel phenomena accompany acupuncture therapy in the treatment of disease, these same phenomena occur in acupuncture anesthesia. For example, the sore, numb and swollen sensation that often extends outward from the point of needle insertion along the course of a channel, appears as frequently in the use of acupunture anesthesia as it does in the utilization of acupuncture for the treatment of disease. The pain threshold of the body along the course of a channel which has been stimulated is raised.

We believe that further investigation, both in the laboratory and clinic, into the relationship between acupuncture therapy and anesthesia will ultimately lead to a better understanding of the basis of channel theory.

FOOTNOTES

1. *Spiritual Axis,* chapter 11.

2. *Simple Questions,* chapter 18.

3. *Classic of Difficulties,* chapter 8.

4. *Spiritual Axis,* chapter 1.

5. *Spiritual Axis,* chapter 71.

6. *Simple Questions,* chapter 63.

Chapter 2

The Formation and Development of Channel Theory

The earliest references to the formulation of channel theory are found in the *Inner Classic,* by best estimates written in the 2nd or 3rd century B.C. Naturally, many of the concepts upon which this classic is based must have predated the book by a considerable length of time. Thereafter, through a process of trial and error, and more recently utilizing scientific methodology, the theory of the channels has gradually been reshaped and expanded to better conform with clinical experience. In this chapter we shall discuss the broad contours of this historical development, leaving to later chapters a more detailed elaboration.

ORIGINS

The theory of the channels originated with the observation of the therapeutic effect obtained from stimulating certain points on the body. It has been suggested that some of these points were discovered accidentally when, for example, a person was inadvertently struck or burned and pain or disease elsewhere in the body was spontaneously relieved. Similarly, while probing the exterior of the body for symptoms of disease, it was found that certain discrete locations reacted to the presence of disease, either by becoming tender to the touch, or by manifesting alterations in the color, moisture, consistency or other characteristic of the skin. Massaging these points of reaction would sometimes ameliorate the disease or eliminate it all together. Gradually, it is conjectured, a cause and effect relationship was recognized, such that the stimulation of these sites on the body became associated with treating specific symptoms. The development of finer needles and superior cauterization techniques (see Section III) contributed to the discovery of points in deeper tissue and the localization of heretofore non-specific loci in the superficial skin.

As the locations and therapeutic characteristics of the points become more particularized they were given names. In time, by gathering the characteristics of numerous points, it was discovered that many therapeutic properties were not the exclusive domain of any single point but were common to many points. It was also observed that individual points were often capable of affecting a variety of symptoms, some near and some far from the point's location, including pathologies of the internal Organs. It was therefore quite natural to infer that points with common symptomatology were somehow joined internally, even though they were spatially separated from one another. That is to say, the therapeutic potential of a point was in some way extended over a considerable distance within the body. The idea of separate or isolated points gradually gave way to the concept of lines or channels. This was confirmed by the phenomenon, mentioned earlier, of the transmission of the needle sensation along pathways away from the site of needling, and a similar phenomenon experienced by practitioners of ancient meditation and gymnastic techniques.

From this evidence, the existence of the channels as the connecting vessels, and the Qi as the

44

medium of transmission, was inferred. The acupuncture points were assigned, on the basis of common therapeutic properties, to what are now called the Primary channels. Each of these channels reflects the symptomatological characteristics of both its constituent points, and the internal Organ with which it is said to be connected.

These observations were based upon a relatively broad understanding of human anatomy and physiology. Two thousand years ago dissections were performed on the bodies of executed criminals, as was recorded in the *Book of Han*. The *Inner Classic* and a slightly later work, the *Classic of Difficulties*, contain descriptions of the distribution of blood vessels and blood circulation, the connections between the muscles, tendons, and ligaments with the bones and joints, and the internal Organs.

> The flesh and skin of a man who stands eight [Chinese] feet tall may be observed externally and measured. When the man is dead he can be cut open and [his insides] examined. The strength of the Inner [Yin] Organs, the size of the Outer [Yang] Organs, the amount of Nourishment, the length of the blood vessels, the clarity of the Blood, and the amount of Qi all have their measure.[1]

This anatomical knowledge is one of the sources of channel theory.

The channels are analogous to various modern anatomical systems. The fact that each of the Primary channels has a peripheral pulse suggests a relationship between the vascular system and the channels. Other similarities point to at least a limited degree of correlation between the channels and the nervous system. Foremost among these is that, on the limbs, the channels often follow the paths of nerves. Obstruction to the flow of Qi in the channels is regarded as the cause of pain. There is also a connection between the channels and the brain. The Governing channel is said to travel up the midline of the back to the base of the skull where it enters the brain.[2] The Qi also exits from the brain.[3]

LATER DEVELOPMENTS

The *Inner Classic* is a summary of the theoretical foundations of Chinese medicine at the time of the Former Han Dynasty (founded 202 B.C.), although there are portions which were added as late as the 8th century. This work is comprised of two books, *Simple Questions* and *Spiritual Axis*, the latter of which deals almost exclusively with acupuncture.

The *Inner Classic* contains a description of the pathways of the twelve Primary channels and the internal Organs with which each is associated, the symptomatology of the Primary channels and Organs, and a discussion of the therapeutic properties of the acupuncture points along the channels. It sets out a system of measurement for locating the points based on body proportions, and describes the distribution and function of the Divergent, Connecting and Muscle channels. Reference is made to the Miscellaneous channels. The Roots and Branches, Origins and Ends of the twelve Primary channels are discussed, as are the circulation and functions of the Qi and Blood.

The *Classic of Difficulties,* probably completed in the 3rd century A.D., is essentially a discussion of certain ambiguities found in the *Inner Classic.* The Meeting points are first mentioned in this work. Palpation of the radial artery at the wrist is described as a means of measuring the health of the twelve Primary channels. Several pulse types are delineated.

In the most famous work of the Later Han Dynasty (founded 25 A.D.), *Discussion of Cold Induced Disorders,* the distribution of symptoms among the twelve Primary channels was retained, but a parallel system called the Six Channel Diagnosis combined the symptoms into six symptomatological groupings. Another innovation was the Eight Parameters or Principles of Diagnosis. The Eight Parameters has long been the foundation for diagnosing exogenous, febrile diseases by distinguishing Yang or Yin, Exterior or Interior, Cold or Hot, and Deficient or Excessive characteristics. (See Introduction.)

Charts illustrating the location of acupuncture points first appeared in the Jin (founded 317 A.D.) and Sui (founded 581 A.D.) periods. The first systematic assignment of points along what were later called the Fourteen channels also appeared during the Jin, in a book entitled *Yellow Emperor's Inner Classic: Categorization of the Bright Hall.*

The name, location, depth and associated symptoms of many old and new points were recorded in a Jin book, the *Systematic Classic of Acupuncture and Moxibustion,* which systematized information found in the *Spiritual Axis,* the *Yellow Emperor's Inner Classic: Categorization of the Bright Hall,* and other works. This became an important clinical sourcebook.

From early times, Chinese physicians recognized that abnormality in the tempo and other characteristics of the pulse reflected illness in the Organs or elsewhere along the channels. Physicians of the Jin period made an important contribution to this aspect of traditional medicine. The *Classic of the Pulse* was the earliest treatise exclusively concerned with pulse diagnosis. In this book, all previous knowledge concerning the correlation between pulse and disease was summarized. Pulse diagnosis, one of the Four Diagnostic Methods, is based on this text. (See Introduction.)

Selection of points according to the location of pain (in Chinese, literally, "That's the point!") was first mentioned in the Tang Dynasty (founded 618 A.D.) classic, *Thousand Ducat Prescriptions.* In this system, because any point of tenderness on the body is a legitimate site for acupuncture therapy, the number of acupuncture points is theoretically unlimited. Discrete points of tenderness which responded with a high degree of regularity to the presence of certain diseases in the body were gradually added to the traditional stock of 365 acupuncture points associated with the Primary channels. These were called Miscellaneous points, some of which are among the most commonly selected points in modern practice.

Also in the Tang, the clinical application of the Connecting channels, Muscle channels and Cutaneous Regions was included in discussions of channel theory. Acupuncture charts were, for the first time, printed in five colors.

In the Song Dynasty (founded in 960 A.D.), bronze models of the human body were cast as teaching devices, showing the locations of the Primary channel points. New points were added in two works of that era, the *Illustrated Classic of Acupuncture Points on the Bronze Model* and the *Classic of Nourishing Life with Acupuncture and Moxibustion.* The former book, in particular, had a marked influence on later generations of acupuncture writings.

During the same period, the Governing and Conception channels, which are included among the eight Miscellaneous channels, were added to the twelve traditional Primary channels, which henceforth became known as the Fourteen channels.

In a book of the Yuan Dynasty (founded 1279 A.D.), *Pouch of Precious Pearls,* medicinal herbs were categorized according to their therapeutic effect upon the pathology of one or another of the Primary channels, to which each herb was said to 'belong'. This work provided a guide to herbal prescriptions for later generations. A contemporary discussion of the Primary channels was presented in the *Elucidation of the Fourteen Channels.*

A thorough description of the eight Miscellaneous channels appeared in a Ming Dynasty (founded 1368 A.D.) book entitled *Studies of the Eight Miscellaneous Channels.* Other books of the Ming, especially the *Classic of Categories* and its appendix, provided further elaboration of channel theory. New interpretations of the circulation of Qi through the channels were described in the *Outline of Medicine.* Although all of the aforementioned books are of considerable reference value, perhaps the most important acupuncture textbook is the *Great Compendium of Acupuncture and Moxibustion.* It has remained a popular work down to the present time, and contains an abundance of material concerning the history and clinical application of acupuncture.

There was little development of channel theory in the last of the traditional dynasties, the Qing (founded 1644 A.D.). An exception was the *Illustrated Studies of the Channels* which showed the relation of points to underlying bones, making the points easier to find in the clinic.

The evolution of acupuncture methodology is discussed in Section III.

FOOTNOTES

1. *Spiritual Axis*, chapter 12.

2. *Classic of Difficulties*, chapter 28.

3. *Simple Questions*, chapter 72.

Chapter 3

The Twelve Primary Channels

The twelve Primary channels are the most important constituents of the channel system. The Divergent, Miscellaneous and Connecting channels are but supplementary branches of the Primary trunks.

The names of each of the Primary channels have three parts. The first reflects whether, in its external course on the limbs, the channel traverses the arm or leg. The second part describes the channel's affiliation with either Yin or Yang, depending on whether its course is predominantly along the medial or lateral aspect of the limb. The third part of the name is the Organ with which the channel connects internally. There are three Yang channels (Lesser Yang, Greater Yang and Yang Brightness) and three Yin channels (Lesser Yin, Greater Yin and Absolute Yin) of the Arm, and likewise three Yang and three Yin channels of the Leg, bilaterally.*

When the body is healthy, the Qi and Blood flow through the channels nourishing and protecting body tissues, and helping maintain their functions. If, however, the body is beset with disease or injury, and normal physiology is disrupted, pathological symptoms will appear along the affected channel. Traditional pathology distinguishes symptoms appearing along the external course of a channel from those affecting an internal Organ associated with the channel.

In this chapter, the distribution and symptomatology of each of the Primary channels will be discussed. A useful summary of channel pathology appears at the end of this chapter.

1. Arm Greater Yin Lung Channel   (Dia. 1-1)

This channel begins in the region of the Stomach (1) (the so-called 'middle burner') and passes downward to connect with the Large Intestine. Returning, it follows the cardiac orifice, crosses the diaphragm (2), and enters its associated Organ, the Lung. Emerging transversely from the area between the Lung and the throat (3), the channel descends along the anterior aspect of the upper arm (4), lateral to the Heart and Pericardium channels. Reaching the elbow (5), it continues along the anterior aspect of the forearm to the anterior margin of the styloid process at the wrist (6). From here, it crosses the radial artery at the pulse, and extends over the thenar eminence to the radial side of the tip of the thumb.

A branch splits from the main channel above the styloid process at the wrist (7), and travels directly to the radial side of the tip of the index finger.

---

*For simplicity's sake, we refer only to the Organ when identifying a Primary channel in later parts of this book. For example, the Arm Greater Yin Lung channel is only called the Lung channel. It is important to remember, as noted in the Introduction, that the Chinese do not regard the peripheral pathways of the channels as physiologically separate from the Organ with which each is connected. Rather, they should be seen as the internal and external parts of a single,integrated system.— *Editors*

Legend of Symbols	
———————	Primary channels on which there are points
- - - - - - -	Primary channels and branches without points
•	Points belonging to channel
▲	Points of intersection
—·—·—·—	Connecting lines
✕	Pertaining Organ
𝕊ℕ	Organ belonging to associated channel
⣿⣿⣿	Area of dispersement

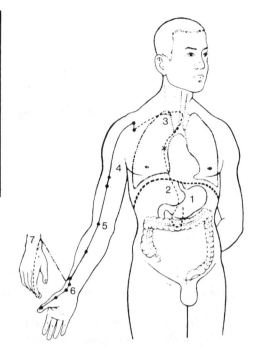

**Dia. 1-1 Arm Greater Yin
Lung Channel**

This channel is associated with the Lung and connects with the Large Intestine. It crosses the diaphragm and is joined with the Stomach, Kidneys and other Organs.

Symptoms associated with the external course of the channel include: fever and sensitivity to cold, nasal congestion, headache, pain in the chest, clavicle, shoulder and back, chills and pain along the channel on the arm.

Symptoms associated with the internal Organ (Lung) include: coughing, asthma, shortness of breath, fullness in the chest, parched throat, changes in the color of urine, irritability, blood in the sputum, palms hot; sometimes accompanied by distended abdomen and loose stool.

2. Arm Yang Brightness Large Intestine Channel (Dia. 1-2)

This channel begins at the radial side of the tip of the index finger (1) and proceeds upward between the first and second metacarpal bones of the hand. It then passes between the tendons of the extensor pollicis longus and brevis at the wrist (2) and continues along the radial margin of the forearm to the lateral side of the elbow (3). From here it rises along the lateral aspect of the upper arm to the shoulder joint (4), then crosses behind the shoulder following the anterior margin of the acromion before turning upward. Just beneath the spinous process of the 7th cervical vertebra, the channel enters directly into the supraclavicular fossa (5), and connects with the Lung before descending across the diaphragm to the Large Intestine (6).

A branch separates from the main channel at the supraclavicular fossa (7) and moves upward through the neck, crosses the cheek and enters the lower gum. From here, it curves around the lip (8) and intersects the same channel coming from the opposite side of the body at the philtrum. The branch finally terminates at the side of the nose.

According to chapter 4 of the *Spiritual Axis*, another branch descends to S-37 *(Shangjuxu)*, the Lower Uniting point of the Large Intestine (9).

48

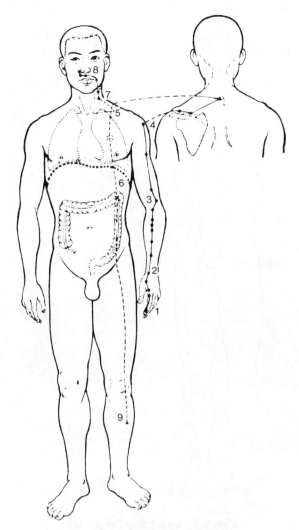

**Dia. 1-2 Arm Yang Brightness
Large Intestine Channel**

This channel is associated with the Large Intestine and connects with the Lung. It also joins directly with the Stomach.

Symptoms associated with the external course of the channel include: fever, parched mouth and thirst, sore throat, nosebleed, toothache, red and painful eyes, swelling of the neck, pain along the course of the channel on the upper arm, shoulder and shoulder blade, motor impairment of the fingers.

Symptoms associated with the internal Organ (Large Intestine) include: abdominal pain, intestinal noises, loose stool; sometimes accompanied by shortness of breath and belching.

3. Leg Yang Brightness Stomach Channel   (Dia. 1-3)

This channel begins beside the nose (1) then ascends to the root of the nose where it intersects with the Bladder channel. Descending along the lateral side of the nose, it enters the upper gum and joins the Governing channel at the philtrum, then (2) circles back around the corner of the mouth, meeting the Conception channel at the mental labial groove on the chin. From here, it follows the angle of the

49

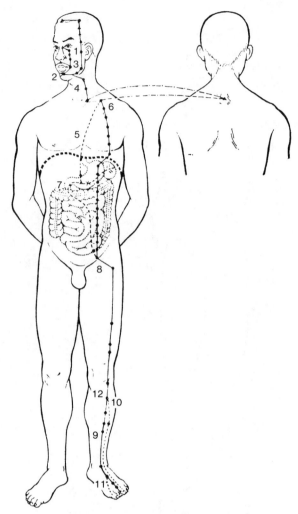

**Dia. 1-3 Leg Yang Brightness
Stomach Channel**

jaw (3) and runs upward in front of the ear. It proceeds along the hairline until it intersects the Gall Bladder channel at GB-6 *(Xuanli)*. Finally, it crosses to the middle of the forehead, parallel with the hairline, where it joins the Governing channel.

One branch separates from the main channel on the lower jaw and descends along the throat (4), entering the supraclavicular fossa. Here, it travels posteriorly to the upper back, where it meets the Governing channel at Gv-14 *(Dazhui)*. It proceeds downward across the diaphragm (5), intersecting the Conception channel internally at points Co-13 *(Shangwan)* and Co-12 *(Zhongwan)* before entering its associated Organ, the Stomach, and communicating with the Spleen.

Another vertical branch descends directly from the supraclavicular fossa (6) along the mammillary line, then passes beside the umbilicus and through the lower abdomen to the inguinal region.

Yet another branch begins at the pylorus (7) and descends internally to the inguinal region where it joins with the vertical branch just described. From here, the channel crosses to point S-31 *(Biguan)* on the anterior aspect of the thigh (8), and descends directly to the patella. It then proceeds along the lateral side of the tibia (9) to the dorsum of the foot, terminating at the lateral side of the tip of the second toe.

A parallel branch separates from the main channel at S-36 *(Zusanli)*, three units below the knee

(10), and terminates at the lateral side of the middle toe. Another branch separates on the dorsum of the foot (11) at point S-42 *(Chongyang)* and terminates at the medial side of the big toe, where it connects with the Spleen channel at point Sp-1 *(Yinbai)*.

This channel is associated with the Stomach and connects with the Spleen. It is also directly joined with the Heart, Large Intestine and Small Intestine.

Symptoms associated with the external course of the channel include: high fever, tidal fevers, flushed face, sweating and delirium, sometimes sensitivity to cold, or pain in the eyes, dry nostrils and nosebleed, fever blisters, sore throat, swelling on the neck, facial paralysis (mouth awry), chest pain, pain or distension along the course of the channel in the leg and foot, coldness in the lower limb.

Symptoms associated with the internal Organ (Stomach) include: abdominal distension, fullness or edema, discomfort when reclining, seizures, persistent hunger, yellow urine.

4. Leg Greater Yin Spleen Channel   (Dia. 1-4)

This channel begins on the medial tip of the big toe (1). From here, it follows the border between the dark and light skin of the medial aspect of the foot. It then passes in front of the medial malleolus and up the leg (2), along the posterior side of the tibia, crossing, and then travelling anterior to, the Liver channel. From here, it crosses over the medial aspect of the knee and continues upward along the anterior, medial aspect of the thigh (3) and into the abdomen. There, after crossing the Conception channel at points Co-3 *(Zhongji)* and Co-4 *(Guanyuan)*, the channel enters its associated Organ, the Spleen (4), and communicates with the Stomach. It then ascends across the diaphragm (5) and intersects the Gall Bladder channel at point GB-24 *(Riyue)*, and the Liver channel at point Li-14 *(Qimen)*. Continuing upward beside the esophagus, it crosses the Lung channel at point L-1 *(Zhongfu)* and finally reaches the root of the tongue, dispersing over its lower surface.

A branch of this channel separates in the Stomach region (6) and advances upward across the diaphragm, transporting Qi into the Heart.

This channel is associated with the Spleen and connects with the Stomach. It is also directly joined with the Heart, Lungs and Intestines.

Symptoms associated with the external course of the channel include: heaviness in the body or head, general feverishness, fatigued limbs and emaciated muscles, stiffness of the tongue, coldness along the medial side of the leg and knee, edema in the foot or leg.

Symptoms associated with the internal Organ (Spleen) include: abdominal pain, fullness or distension, diarrhea, incomplete digestion of food, intestinal noises, vomiting, hard lumps in the abdomen, reduced appetite, jaundice, constipation.

5. Arm Lesser Yin Heart Channel   (Dia. 1-5)

This channel begins in its associated Organ, the Heart (1), then emerges through the blood vessel system surrounding the Heart, and travels downward (2) across the diaphragm where it connects with the Small Intestine.

A branch of the main channel separates in the Heart and ascends alongside the esophagus (3) to the face where it joins the tissues surrounding the eye.

Another branch goes directly from the Heart to the Lung (4), then slants downward to emerge below the axilla (5). From here, the channel descends along the medial border of the anterior aspect of the upper arm, behind the Lung and Pericardium channels, to the antecubital fossa (6), where it continues downward to the capitate bone proximal to the palm. It then enters the palm (7) and follows the medial side of the little finger to the finger tip.

This channel is associated with the Heart and connects with the Small Intestine. It is also directly joined to the Lung and Kidneys.

Symptoms associated with the external course of this channel include: general feverishness, headache, pain in the eyes, pain along the back of the upper arm, dry throat, thirst, hot or painful palms, coldness in the palms and soles of the feet, pain along the scapula and/or medial aspect of the forearm.

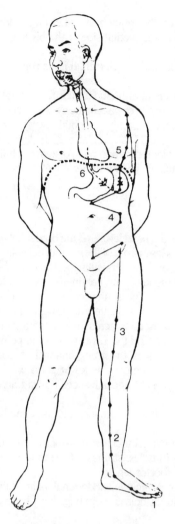

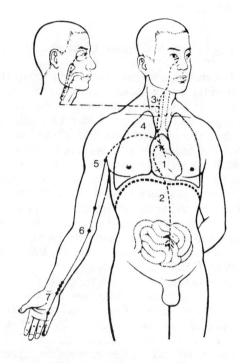

Dia. 1-4 Leg Greater Yin
Spleen Channel

Dia. 1-5 Arm Lesser Yin
Heart Channel

Symptoms associated with the internal Organ (Heart) include: pain or fullness in chest and ribs or below ribs, irritability, shortness of breath, discomfort when reclining, vertigo, mental disorders.

6. Arm Greater Yang Small Intestine Channel   (Dia. 1-6)

This channel originates at the ulnar side of the tip of the little finger and ascends along the ulnar side of the hand (1) to the wrist, emerging at the styloid process of the ulna. From here, it travels directly upward along the posterior aspect of the ulna (2), passing between the olecranon of the ulna and the medial epicondyle of the humerus at the medial side of the elbow. It then proceeds along the posterior border of the lateral aspect of the upper arm (3), emerging behind the shoulder joint and circling around the superior and inferior fossa of the scapula (4). At the top of the shoulder, it crosses the Bladder channel at points B-36 *(Fufen)* and B-11 *(Dazhu),* and the Governing channel at Gv-14 *(Dazhui),* where the channel turns downward into the supraclavicular fossa (5), and connects with the Heart. From here, it descends along the esophagus and crosses the diaphragm to the Stomach (6).

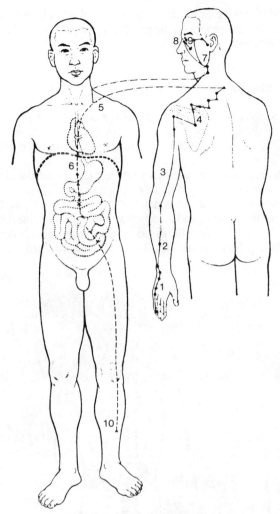

**Dia. 1-6 Arm Greater Yang
Small Intestine Channel**

Before reaching its associated Organ, the Small Intestine, the channel intersects the Conception channel internally, and very deep, at points Co-13 *(Shangwan)* and Co-12 *(Zhongwan)*.

A branch of this channel travels upward from the supraclavicular fossa and crosses the neck and cheek (7) to the outer canthus of the eye, where it meets the Gall Bladder channel at GB-1 *(Tongziliao)*. Then it turns back across the temple and enters the ear at point SI-19 *(Tinggong)*.

Another branch separates from the former branch on the cheek, ascends to the infraorbital region of the eye and then to the inner canthus (8), where it meets the Bladder channel at B-1 *(Jingming)*. It then crosses horizontally to the zygomatic region (9).

According to chapter 4 of the *Spiritual Axis*, another branch descends to S-39 *(Xiajuxu)*, the Lower Uniting point of the Small Intestine (10).

This channel is associated with the Small Intestine and connects with the Heart. It is also joined directly with the Stomach.

Symptoms associated with the external course of this channel include: numbness of the mouth and tongue, pain in the neck or cheek, sore throat, stiff neck, pain along the lateral aspect of the shoulder and upper arm.

Symptoms associated with the internal Organ (Small Intestine) include: pain and distension in the lower abdomen, possibly extending around the waist or to the genitals; diarrhea, or abdominal pain with 'dry' stool or constipation.

7. Leg Greater Yang Bladder Channel   (Dia. 1-7)

This channel begins at point B-1 *(Jingming)* at the inner canthus of the eye (1) and ascends across the forehead, intersecting the Governing channel at point Gv-24 *(Shenting),* and the Gall Bladder channel at point GB-15 *(Toulinqi).* It then crosses to the vertex and again intersects the Governing channel at point Gv-20 *(Baihui).*

From here, a branch descends to the area above the ear (2), joining the Gall Bladder channel at points GB-7 *(Qubin),* GB-8 *(Shuaigu),* GB-12 *(Wangu),* etc.

A vertical branch enters the brain at the vertex (3) and intersects with the Governing channel at point Gv-17 *(Naohu),* before emerging and descending along the nape of the neck (4) and the muscles of the medial aspect of the scapula. Here, the Bladder channel meets the Governing channel at points Gv-14 *(Dazhui)* and Gv-13 *(Taodao),* after which it continues downward, parallel to the spine, to the

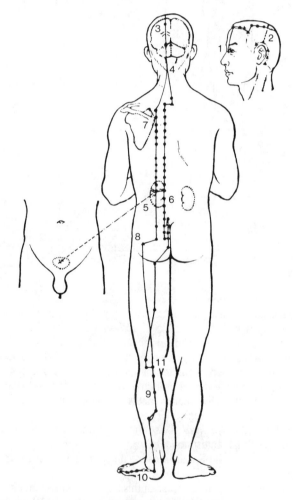

**Dia. 1-7   Leg Greater Yang
Bladder Channel**

lumbar region. The channel then enters the internal cavity (5) via the paravertebral muscles, communicates with the Kidneys, and finally joins its associated Organ, the Bladder.

Another branch (6) separates in the lumbar region, crosses the buttock, and descends to the popliteal fossa of the knee.

Yet another branch separates from the main channel at the back of the neck and descends, parallel to the spine, from the medial side of the scapula to the gluteal region. Here it crosses the buttock (8) to intersect the Gall Bladder channel at point GB-30 *(Huantiao),* and then descends across the lateral, posterior aspect of the thigh to join with the other branch of this channel in the popliteal fossa. Continuing downward through the gastrocnemius muscle (9), the channel emerges behind the external malleolus, then follows the 5th metatarsal bone (10), crossing its tuberosity to the lateral tip of the little toe at point B-67 *(Zhiyin).*

According to chapter 4 of the *Spiritual Axis,* the Bladder channel connects behind the knee with its Lower Uniting point, B-54 *(Weizhong)* (11).

This channel is associated with the Bladder and connects with the Kidneys. It is also joined directly with the Brain and Heart.

Symptoms associated with the external course of this channel include: alternating chills and fever, headache, stiff neck, pain in the lumbar region, nasal congestion, diseases of the eye, pain along the back of the leg and foot.

Symptoms associated with the internal Organ (Bladder) include: pain in the lower abdomen, enuresis, retention of urine, painful urination, mental disorders.

8. Leg Lesser Yin Kidney Channel   (Dia. 1-8)

This channel begins beneath the little toe, crosses the sole of the foot (1) and emerges at point K-2 *(Rangu)* on the inferior aspect of the navicular tuberosity at the instep. From here it travels posterior to the medial malleolus, enters the heel, and proceeds upward along the medial aspect of the lower leg (2) where it intersects the Spleen channel at point Sp-6 *(Sanyinjiao).* Continuing up the leg within the gastrocnemius muscle, the channel traverses the medial aspect of the popliteal fossa (3) and the medial, posterior aspect of the thigh to the base of the spine (4), where it intersects the Governing channel at Gv-1 *(Changqiang).* Here, it threads its way beneath the spine to enter its associated Organ, the Kidney, and to communicate with the Bladder. It intersects the Conception channel at points Co-4 *(Guanyuan)* and Co-3 *(Zhongji).*

A branch ascends directly from the Kidney, crosses the Liver (5) and diaphragm, enters the Lung, and follows the throat to the root of the tongue.

Another branch separates in the Lung (6), connects with the Heart, and disperses in the chest.

This channel is associated with the Kidneys and connects with the Bladder. It is also joined directly with the Liver, Lungs, Heart and other Organs.

Symptoms associated with the external course of the channel include: pain along the lower vertebrae, low back pain, coldness in the feet, motor impairment or muscular atrophy of the foot, dryness in the mouth, sore throat, pain in the sole of the foot or along the posterior aspect of the lower leg or thigh.

Symptoms associated with the internal Organ (Kidney) include: vertigo, facial edema, ashen complexion, blurred vision, shortness of breath, drowsiness and irritability, loose stool, chronic diarrhea or constipation, abdominal distension, vomiting, impotence.

9. Arm Absolute Yin Pericardium Channel   (Dia. 1-9)

This channel begins in the chest (1) where it joins with its associated Organ, the Pericardium. It then descends across the diaphragm and into the abdomen, where it connects successively with the upper, middle and lower burners of the Triple Burner. (See Introduction)

A branch of the main channel runs along the chest (2), emerging superficially in the costal region at point P-1 *(Tianchi)* three units below the anterior axillary fold before ascending to the inferior aspect of the axilla. From here, it descends along the medial aspect of the upper arm (3) between the paths of

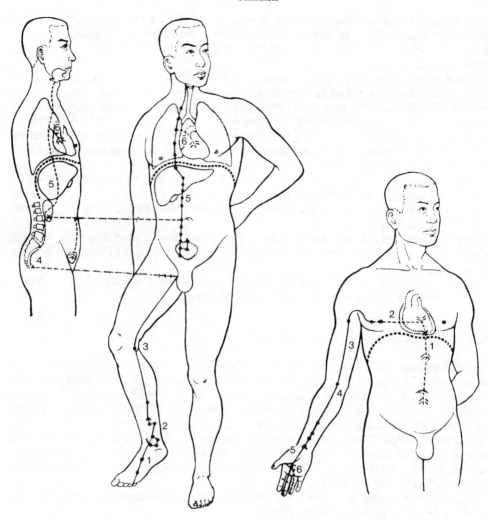

**Dia. 1-8 Leg Lesser Yin
Kidney Channel**

**Dia. 1-9 Arm Absolute Yin
Pericardium Channel**

the Lung and Heart channels to the antecubital fossa (4), and then proceeds down the forearm between the tendons of the palmaris longus and flexor carpi radialis muscles. Entering the palm (5), it follows the ulnar aspect of the middle finger until it reaches the finger tip.

Another branch separates in the palm (6) and proceeds along the lateral aspect of the 4th finger to the finger tip.

This channel is associated with the Pericardium and is connected with the Triple Burner.

Symptoms associated with the external course of this channel include: stiff neck, spasms in the arm or leg, flushed face, pain in the eyes, subaxillary swelling, spasms and contracture of the elbow and arm, restricting movement, hot palms.

Symptoms associated with the internal Organ (Pericardium) include: impaired speech, fainting, irritability, fullness in the chest, motor impairment of the tongue, palpitations, chest pain, mental disorders.

56

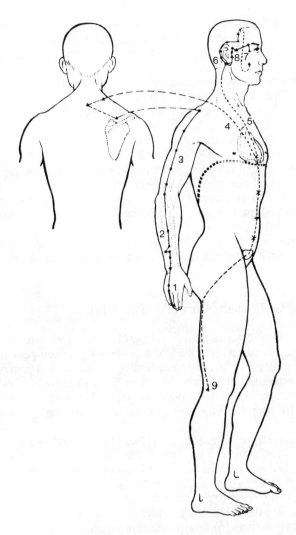

**Dia. 1-10 Arm Lesser Yang
Triple Burner Channel**

10. Arm Lesser Yang Triple Burner Channel   (Dia. 1-10)

This channel originates on the ulnar aspect of the 4th finger tip, ascends between the 4th and 5th metacarpal bones on the dorsum of the wrist (1), traverses the forearm between the ulna and radius (2), and continues upward across the olecranon and the lateral aspect of the upper arm (3) to the shoulder. Here it intersects the Small Intestine channel at point SI-12 *(Bingfeng)* and meets the Governing channel at point Gv-14 *(Dazhui)* before crossing back over the shoulder. It then intersects the Gall Bladder channel at point GB-21 *(Jianjing),* from which it enters the supraclavicular fossa (4) and travels to the mid-chest region at point Co-17 *(Shanzhong).* From here, the channel joins with the Pericardium and descends across the diaphragm to the abdomen linking successively with the upper, middle and lower burners of the Triple Burner, to which this channel belongs. (See Introduction)

A branch of the main channel separates in the chest at point Co-17 *(Shanzhong)* and ascends to

57

emerge superficially from the supraclavicular fossa at the neck (5). Here, it proceeds upward behind the ear (6), intersecting the Gall Bladder channel at points GB-6 *(Xuanli)* and GB-4 *(Hanyan)* on the forehead before winding downward across the cheek to below the eye (7). It intersects the Small Intestine channel at point SI-18 *(Quanliao)*.

Another branch separates behind the auricle and enters the ear. It then emerges in front of the ear (8) where it intersects the Small Intestine channel at point SI-19 *(Tinggong)*, crosses in front of the Gall Bladder channel at point GB-3 *(Shangguan)* and traverses the cheek to terminate at the outer canthus at point TB-23 *(Sizhukong)*.

Chapter 4 of the *Spiritual Axis* states that the Triple Burner channel connects with its Lower Uniting point, B-53 *(Weiyang)* (9). Chapter 2 adds that this branch of the Triple Burner channel emerges from B-53 *(Weiyang)* and follows the course of the Bladder channel to join with the Bladder.

This channel is associated with the Triple Burner and is connected with the Pericardium.

Symptoms associated with the external course of this channel include: swelling and pain in the throat, pain in the cheek and jaw, redness in the eyes, deafness, pain behind the ear or along the lateral aspect of the shoulder and upper arm.

Symptoms associated with the internal Organ (Triple Burner) include: abdominal distension, hardness and fullness in the lower abdomen, enuresis, frequent urination, edema, dysuresis.

11. Leg Lesser Yang Gall Bladder Channel   (Dia. 1-11)

This channel begins at the outer canthus of the eye (1) and traverses the temple to point TB-22 *(Heliao)*. It then ascends to the corner of the forehead where it intersects point S-8 *(Touwei)* before descending behind the ear. From here, it proceeds along the neck (2) in front of the Triple Burner channel, crosses the Small Intestine channel at point SI-17 *(Tianrong)*, then, at the top of the shoulder, turns back and runs behind the Triple Burner channel to intersect the Governing channel at point Gv-14 *(Dazhui)* on the spine. Finally, the channel turns downward (3) into the supraclavicular fossa.

One branch of the main channel emerges behind the auricle (4) and enters the ear at point TB-17 *(Yifeng)*. Emerging in front of the ear, this branch intersects the Small Intestine channel at SI-19 *(Tinggong)*, and the Stomach channel at S-7 *(Xianguan)*, before terminating behind the outer canthus.

Another branch separates at the outer canthus and proceeds downward to point S-5 *(Daying)* on the jaw (5). Then, crossing the Triple Burner channel, it returns upward to the infraorbital region before descending again to the neck (6), where it joins the original channel in the supraclavicular fossa. From here it descends further into the chest, crossing the diaphragm and connecting with the Liver (7) before joining its associated Organ, the Gall Bladder. Continuing along the inside of the ribs, it emerges in the inguinal region of the lower abdomen and winds around the genitals, submerging again in the hip (8) at point GB-30 *(Huantiao)*.

Yet another vertical branch runs downward from the supraclavicular fossa to the axilla (9) and the lateral aspect of the chest. It crosses the ribs and intersects the Liver channel at point Li-13 *(Zhangmen)* before turning back to the sacral region, where it crosses the Bladder channel points B-31 *(Shangliao)* to B-34 *(Xialiao)*. This branch then descends to the hip joint (10) and continues down the lateral side of the thigh and knee, passing along the anterior aspect of the fibula (11) to its lower end. Here, it crosses in front of the lateral malleolus (12) and traverses the dorsum of the foot, entering the seam between the 4th and 5th metatarsal bones before terminating at the lateral side of the tip of the 4th toe, or point GB-44 *(Zuqiaoyin)*.

Finally, a branch separates on the dorsum of the foot (13) at point GB-41 *(Linqi)* and runs between the 1st and 2nd metatarsal bones to the medial tip of the big toe, then crosses under the toenail to join with the Liver channel at point Li-1 *(Dadun)*.

Chapter 4 of *Spiritual Axis* states that this channel connects with its Lower Uniting point, GB-34 *(Yanglingquan)* (14).

This channel is associated with the Gall Bladder and connects with the Liver. It is also joined directly with the Heart.

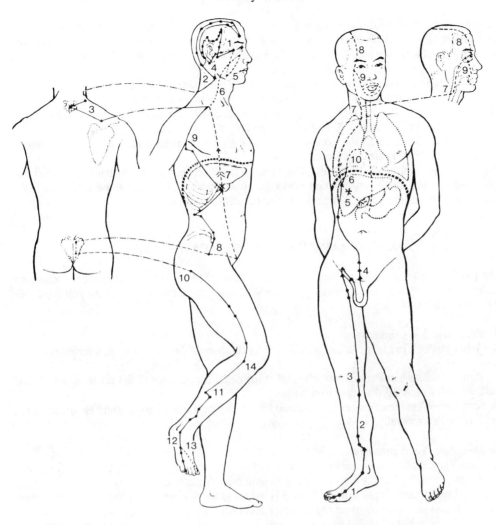

**Dia. 1-11 Leg Lesser Yang
Gall Bladder Channel**

**Dia. 1-12 Leg Absolute Yin
Liver Channel**

Symptoms associated with the external course of this channel include: alternating fever and chills, headache, ashen complexion; pain in the eye or jaw, swelling in the sub-axillary region, scrofula, deafness, pain along the channel in the hip region, leg or foot.

Symptoms associated with the internal Organ (Gall Bladder) include: pain in the ribs, vomiting, bitter taste in the mouth, chest pain.

12. Leg Absolute Yin Liver Channel (Dia. 1-12)

This channel begins on the dorsum of the big toe, continues across the foot (1) to a point one unit in front of the medial malleolus, and proceeds upward to point Sp-6 *(Sanyinjiao)* where it intersects the Spleen channel. From here, it continues up the medial aspect of the lower leg (2), re-crossing the Spleen channel eight units above the medial malleolus, and thereafter running posterior to that channel over the knee (3) and thigh. Winding around the genitals, the channel enters the lower abdomen (4) where it meets the Conception channel at points Co-2 *(Qugu)*, Co-3 *(Zhongji)* and Co-4 *(Guanyuan)* before skirting the Stomach and joining with its associated Organ, the Liver (6), and

59

connecting with the Gall Bladder. Then the channel continues upward across the diaphragm and costal region (6), traverses the neck posterior to the pharynx (7), and enters the nasopharynx, connecting with the tissues surrounding the eye. Finally, the channel ascends across the forehead (8) and meets the Governing channel at the vertex.

A branch separates below the eye (9) and encircles the inside of the lips.

Another branch separates in the Liver, crosses the diaphragm and reaches the Lung (10).

This channel is associated with the Liver and connects with the Gall Bladder. It is also joined directly with the Lungs, Stomach, Kidneys, brain and other Organs.

Symptoms associated with the external course of the channel include: headache, vertigo, blurred vision, tinnitus, fever, spasms in the extremities.

Symptoms associated with the internal Organ (Liver) include: fullness or pain in the costal region or chest, hard lumps in the upper abdomen, abdominal pain, vomiting, jaundice, loose stool, pain in the lower abdomen, hernia, enuresis, retention of urine, dark urine.

A SUMMARY OF CHANNEL PATHOLOGY

Although each of the points along the Primary channels has certain pathological indications peculiar to itself, we may summarize those indications which are common to all of the points on each of the channels as follows:

The three Arm Yin channels

1. Arm Greater Yin Lung channel is indicated for diseases of the chest, throat, trachea, nose and Lung.

2. Arm Absolute Yin Pericardium channel is indicated for diseases of the chest, Stomach and Heart, as well as mental disorders generally.

3. Arm Lesser Yin Heart channel is indicated for diseases of the chest, tongue and Heart, as well as mental disorders generally.

The three Arm Yang channels

1. Arm Yang Brightness Large Intestine channel is indicated for diseases of the face, eyes, ears, nose, gums, throat and Large Intestine, as well as febrile diseases generally.

2. Arm Lesser Yang Triple Burner channel is indicated for diseases of the temporal region, eyes, ears, throat and ribs, as well as febrile diseases generally.

3. Arm Greater Yang Small Intestine channel is indicated for diseases of the vertex, eyes, ears, throat, as well as mental disorders generally.

The three Leg Yang channels

1. Leg Yang Brightness Stomach channel is indicated for diseases of the face, nose, gums, throat, Stomach and Intestines as well as mental and febrile diseases generally.

2. Leg Lesser Yang Gall Bladder channel is indicated for diseases of the temporal region, nose, eyes, throat and ribs, as well as febrile diseases generally.

3. Leg Greater Yang Bladder channel is indicated for diseases affecting the vertex, nose, eyes and lumbar region, as well as febrile and mental diseases generally.

The three Leg Yin channels

1. Leg Greater Yin Spleen channel is indicated for diseases of the upper abdomen, Stomach, Intestines and uro-genital system.

2. Leg Absolute Yin Liver channel is indicated for diseases affecting the hypochondriac region, lower abdomen, uro-genital system and head.

3. Leg Lesser Yin Kidney channel is indicated for diseases affecting the waist, uro-genital system, throat and mental disorders generally.

Chapter 4

Root and Branch, Origin and End, and Path of Qi

THE MEANING OF ROOT AND BRANCH, ORIGIN AND END, AND PATH OF QI

Root and Branch

The theory of the twelve Primary channels encompasses important concepts in addition to those discussed in chapter 3. Among these are Root and Branch, Origin and End and Path of Qi. Based upon the distribution of the Primary channels and the circulation of Qi and Blood, these concepts define the reciprocal relationships existing between channels and points situated on the upper reaches of the body with those on the lower, and between those on the head and trunk with others on the limbs. An understanding of the effects produced on one part of the body by stimulating points on another will be helpful to the physician selecting points in the clinic.

The terms Root and Branch have many different applications in Chinese medicine. They can be used to describe the progress and severity of a disease, the direction and manner of treatment, or to indicate the disease causing agent (Excess) and the body's power of resistance (Normal Qi). According to the theory of the twelve Primary channels, Root and Branch signify the difference between the upper and lower, medial and lateral orientation of the channels and points on the body. At the same time, Root and Branch symbolize the complementary and interdependent nature of the diverse parts of the channel system.

Branch has the meaning of higher, Root of lower. In the context of the channels, the areas of the head, shoulder, back and chest are regarded as Branches, while the extremities of the limbs are the Roots. The specific location of Root and Branch on each of the Primary channels is set forth in the chart below.

There are many allusions to Root and Branch in the *Inner Classic*. For example, in the following passages the lower parts of the limbs (the Roots) are referred to as 'below', and the head (Branch) as 'above.' Thus: "When there is Deficiency below, (the limbs) are cold." And again: "When there is Deficiency above, there is dizziness."

Origin and End

The Origin and End are similar to the Root and Branch. Both signify the physiological relationship between the limbs and trunk, and the therapeutic effect that the stimulation of points in one part of the body has on other parts. The limbs are called the Origins and Roots; the head and trunk are the Ends and Branches. The Origins are the Well points (see Section II, chapter 1) on the four limbs; the Ends are comprised of certain areas on the trunk and head. The Origin and End of each of the Primary

ROOTS AND BRANCHES OF THE PRIMARY CHANNELS

Channel	Root Area	Branch Area
3 Leg Yang channels		
Bladder channel	5 units above heel B-59 *(Fuyang)*	Eye B-1 *(Jingming)*
Gall Bladder channel	In the cleft between the 4th and 5th metatarsal bones GB-43 *(Xiaxi)*, GB-44 *(Qiaoyin)*	In front of the ear GB-2 *(Tinghui)*, SI-19 *(Tinggong)*
Stomach channel	Lateral side of 2nd toe S-45 *(Lidui)*	Frontal area of face S-9 *(Renying)*, S-4 *(Dicang)*
3 Leg Yin channels		
Spleen channel	4 units above internal malleolus Sp-6 *(Sanyinjiao)*	Associated point on back; root of tongue B-20 *(Pishu)*, Co-23 *(Lianquan)*
Kidney channel	2 units below internal malleolus K-6 *(Zhaohai)*, K-2 *(Rangu)*	Associated point on back B-23 *(Shenshu)*
Liver channel	5 units above webbing between 1st and 2nd toes Li-4 *(Zhongfeng)*	Associated point on back B-18 *(Ganshu)*
3 Arm Yang channels		
Small Intestine channel	Above the outer wrist SI-6 *(Yanglao)*	1 unit above the eye M-HN-6 *(Yuyao)*, B-2 *(Zanzhu)*
Triple Burner channel	2 units above webbing between 4th and 5th fingers TB-3 *(Zhongzhu)*	Behind superior angle of the ear; outer canthus of eye TB-19 *(Luxi)*, TB-23 *(Sizhukong)*
Large Intestine channel	Middle of elbow LI-11 *(Quchi)*, LI-14 *(Binao)*	Cheek and mandible LI-20 *(Yingxiang)*, Co-24 *(Chengjiang)*
3 Arm Yin channels		
Lung channel	At the radial 'pulse' L-9 *(Taiyuan)*	Area of axillary artery L-1 *(Zhongfu)*
Heart channel	Ulnar side of wrist H-7 *(Shenmen)*	Associated point on back B-15 *(Xinshu)*
Pericardium channel	2 units proximal to the wrist between the 2 tendons P-6 *(Neiguan)*	3 units below the axilla P-1 *(Tianchi)*

channels of the Leg are listed below.

1. Bladder channel: The Origin is B-67 *(Zhiyin)*, the End is at the eyes. Note that the End is the same as the Branch of this channel, but the Origin and Root are different.
2. Gall Bladder channel: The Origin is GB-44 *(Qiaoyin)*, the End is the area in front of the ear. Each coincides with the channel's Root and Branch, respectively.
3. Stomach channel: The Origin is S-45 *(Lidui)*, the End is in the frontal area of the face. These are identical to the channel's Root and Branch.
4. Spleen channel: The Origin is Sp-1 *(Yinbai)*, the End is in the upper abdomen. Both are different from the channel's Root and Branch.
5. Kidney channel: The Origin is K-1 *(Yongquan)*, the End is Co-23 *(Lianquan)*. The Origin is close to the Root, but the End is different from the Branch.
6. Liver channel: The Origin is Li-1 *(Dadun)*, the End is in the chest. Both are different from the channel's Root and Branch.

Comparison of the Origin and End of each of the six Leg Primary channels with its Root and Branch shows that they are essentially the same. This is because both reflect the close relationship between the upper and lower parts of the channels. Similarly, the Origins and Ends of the six Arm Primary channels are comprised of the Well points (the Origins) of each of the Arm channels on the extremities of the upper limb, and areas on the head, chest and abdomen (the Ends). In the ancient work, *Ode to the Standard of Mystery*, the Origins and Ends are described as the 'four Origins, three Ends'. The four Origins are the lower parts of the four limbs, the three Ends are the head, chest and abdomen.

Roots and Branches, Origins and Ends are ways of signifying the distribution and circulation of Qi through the channels. Origin and End designate the connection existing between one end of a channel and its other end, whereas the concept of Root and Branch describes the dissemination of the Qi in the channels throughout the body. The Root, Branch, Origin, and End of each channel has certain properties distinct from other parts of the channel. Likewise, each acupuncture point found in these different areas along the course of the channel possesses, to some extent, its own, unique properties. Yet, its uniqueness is only relative. Within the framework of the Root/Branch and Origin/End, distinct points at opposite ends of each of the channels complement and mutually reinforce one another, demonstrating the integrative function of the channel system.

Path of Qi

As the Qi circulates through the channels, it passes from the limbs to the head and trunk, and then back again. The course traveled by the Qi in the head, chest, abdomen and back is referred to as the Path of Qi, and is the common causeway through which the Qi travels. This is where the Branches and Ends are situated. The Path of Qi can be divided into four parts: head, chest, abdomen (and back), calf. In the 4th chapter of the *Spiritual Axis* it is said that "[the Qi and Blood of] the twelve Primary channels and 365 Connecting channels rise to the face and through the orifices." This explains why the Branches and Ends of the Yang Primary channels are to be found in the head, face, eyes and ears. It is also written in chapter 52 that "[w]hen the Qi is in the chest it rests in the breast and at the Associated points on the back; when in the abdomen, it rests at the Associated points of the back and at the 'pulse' of the Penetrating channel to the left and right of the umbilicus." This accounts for the placement of the Branches and Ends of the other Primary channels.

The concepts of Root and Branch, Origin and End and the Path of Qi are very important to the clinical application of acupuncture because they can be used to determine which local and/or distant points to select when treating a particular disorder. For example, *Simple Questions*, chapter 70: "When the Qi is rebellious, if the disease is above, select points below; if the disease is below, select points above; if the disease is in the middle, select points on the sides." This expresses the basic principle of treatment utilizing the concept of Root and Branch. It appears often in ancient medical literature.

USING THE ROOT AND ORIGIN POINTS

Transport Points

In the *Inner Classic* the limbs are regarded as the Root, and the trunk as the Branch. The significance of this lies in the selection of points below the elbow and knee, specifically the five Transport points, for treating diseases affecting the trunk.

The names, locations and uses of the particular Transport points are described in detail in Section II, chapter 1.

In the past it was said of the five categories of Transport points that the Well points were used to treat fullness below the heart, the Gushing points to treat fever, the Transporting points for heaviness in the body and pain in the joints and bones, the Penetrating points for asthmatic panting, chills and fever, and the Uniting points for Rebellious Qi and diarrhea. Actually, as we have shown in earlier chapters, each of the Primary channels has its own pathological indications apart from the other channels. Similarly, each of the channel's Transport points has its own symptomatological characteristics, distinct from the rest. Some acupuncture texts also say that the Gushing and Transporting points primarily treat symptoms associated with the external course of the channels, while Uniting points treat disorders of the internal Organs. Practitioners need not, however, be constrained by this advice since the Gushing and Transporting points can also be used for diseases of the Organs.

The Well points are the Origins within the concept of Origin and End. The reason why these points, located at the tips of the fingers and toes, are so important is stated in chapter 62 of the *Spiritual Axis:* "The ends of the four limbs are the meeting places of Yin and Yang. They are the grand connections of Qi." Through the ages, acupuncturists have used the Well points in treating diseases of the trunk. This is based upon the principle of selecting points below for diseases above. Because the End of the Bladder channel is in the head and eyes, and its Origin is the Well point B-67 *(Zhiyin)* on the tip of the little toe, it is observed in *Gatherings from Outstanding Acupuncturists* that: "For diseases of the head, needle B-67 *(Zhiyin)*." Because the Bladder and Kidney channels share a Yin/Yang relationship, this work also advises needling the Well point on the Kidney channel, K-1 *(Yongquan)*, to treat headache at the vertex (traversed by the Bladder channel) and inability to open the eyes. In the *Great Compendium of Acupuncture and Moxibustion* a method using the Well points to treat a variety of disorders is spelled out. For example, the Well point of the Lung channel, L-11 *(Shaoshang)*, is used to treat fullness of the chest, pain in the upper part of the clavicle, coughing, wheezing, sore and swollen throat, irritability, etc. The Well point of the Heart channel, H-9 *(Shaochong)*, is used to treat pain in the Heart, irritability and thirst, extremely cold arms, pain in the sides, depression, mental dullness, mania,etc. In recent clinical practice, the use of Well points—Li-1 *(Dadun)* to treat colic, SI-1 *(Shaoze)* to treat insufficient lactation, P-9 *(Zhongchong)* to treat fainting, etc.—has been both widespread and effective.

Other Points Below the Elbow and Knee

Apart from the Transport points, there are many other points below the elbow and knee in the area of the Root or Origin. Among these are the Source, Connecting, Accumulating and Lower Uniting points, all of which are discussed in greater detail in Section II, chapter 1. A few examples drawn from medical literature (chiefly of the Ming period) will illustrate the importance of these points at the Root or Origin in acupuncture therapy: "For fullness in the chest and pain in the abdomen, needle P-6 *(Neiguan)*." *(Ode to the Standard of Mystery)*. "For severe pain in the Spleen and Heart, use Sp-4 *(Gongsun)*." *(Song of the Glorious Jade)*. "H-5 *(Tongli)* treats palpitations of the Heart." *(Song of the Jade Dragon)*. "B-62 *(Shenmai)* is used for rigidity of the waist and inability to bend backward or forward." *(Illustrated Appendices to the Classic of Categories)*

USING THE BRANCH AND END REGIONS

The Branches and Ends include the regions of the head, chest, abdomen and back through which the Qi is circulated in the channels. These regions, as we have said, are also known collectively as the Path of Qi. The clinical significance of this concept lies in the method by which points are selected according to their location in the Branch or End regions.

The Path of Qi is also understood as a system of lateral association wherein the Path of Qi in the head indicates the relationship between the brain and face, the Path of Qi in the chest suggests the connection among the upper back, neck, chest and upper limbs, the Path of Qi in the abdomen relates the lower back with the abdomen, and the Path of Qi in the lower leg designates the relationship of the lumbar-sacral region, lower abdomen and lower limbs. Disease in one part of the Path can be treated by manipulating points elsewhere in the same segment of the Path.

However, it should be remembered that the circulation of Qi through the channels is both vertical and horizontal. The lateral associations facilitated by the Path of Qi are not separate from the channel system but complement it. The vertical associations between the upper and lower ends of each of the channels, discussed earlier, is yet another aspect of the circulation of Qi in the channel system.

Thus, the Path of Qi, or the Branches and Ends, is essentially a description of the concentration of the Qi from the channels in the trunk and head. As we shall see below, points located in the Branch or End regions may be used for treating local disorders, or they may be selected for diseases in distant parts of the body.

Local Uses of Branch and End Points

There are many examples in acupuncture literature of points on the head and trunk selected for treating local disorders: GB-5 *(Xuanlu)* and GB-4 *(Hanyan)* for migraine headache; Gv-26 *(Renzhong)* and Gv-21 *(Qianding)* for puffiness of the face; SI-19 *(Tinggong)* and TB-17 *(Yifeng)* for deafness, etc.

Points on the trunk, particularly the Alarm points of the chest and abdomen and the Associated points of the back, are commonly selected for diseases of the Organs. Examples include B-13 *(Feishu)*, B-12 *(Fengmen)* and Co-17 *(Shanzhong)* for diseases of the Lungs; B-15 *(Xinshu)*, Co-14 *(Juque)*, Sp-17 *(Shidou)*, B-20 *(Pishu)* and Li-13 *(Zhangmen)* to treat diseases of the chest, ribs, Heart and Spleen; Co-12 *(Zhongwan)*, S-21 *(Liangmen)*, S-25 *(Tianshu)*, B-21 *(Weishu)*, and B-25 *(Dachangshu)* for diseases of the upper abdomen, Stomach and Intestines.

Distant Uses of Branch and End Points

As noted earlier, points at the Root or Origin may be used to treat diseases above at the Branch or End. Points on the sides of the body may be used to treat diseases at the center. The converse is also true and the practice of acupunture can be made more flexible and effective by the use of points in the Branch and End regions to treat diseases of the limbs. For example, atrophy of the muscles of the legs may be treated at point GB-10 *(Fubai)*; rigidity and pain in the joints may be treated at B-42 *(Hunmen)*; moxibustion may be applied at the Associated points on the back for paralysis of the limbs, or at Co-4 *(Guanyuan)* on the abdomen for hemiplegia, etc.

This method of treating disorders below via points above, and diseases at the sides by points at the center demonstrates the theory of reciprocity between Origin and End, Root and Branch. While this method was recorded in many ancient medical works, it was not emphasized by later, post-Sung (after c.1250) physicians. In modern times, however, it has undergone a revival.

65

RECENT DEVELOPMENTS IN THE MATCHING OF
ROOT AND BRANCH, ORIGIN AND END POINTS

In addition to those techniques described above, there is another method that is even more commonly practiced, that of combining Root and Branch or Origin and End points. Illustrations of this method found in the literature can be divided into two categories: those which combine points along the same channel, and those which combine points from different channels.

In the first category, for example, B-65 *(Shugu)* and B-10 *(Tianzhu)*, a Root and a Branch point on the Bladder channel, can be used for treating stiff neck accompanied by high fever *(Ode of a Hundred Syndromes)*. A variation on this method combines Root and Branch points from different channels with the same Yin or Yang prefix. For example, GB-42 *(Diwuhui)*, a point at the Root of the Leg Lesser Yang Gall Bladder channel, could be combined with TB-21 *(Ermen)*, at the Branch of the Arm Lesser Yang Triple Burner channel, for treating tinnitus. Here the points are both from Lesser Yang channels *(Ode of the Essentials of Understanding)*.

In the second category, B-1 *(Jingming)*, at the Branch of the Bladder channel, may be combined with GB-37 *(Guangming)*, at the Root of the Gall Bladder channel, for treating eye diseases *(Ode of Xi Hong)*. Similarly, B-13 *(Feishu)* may be combined with S-40 *(Fenglong)* for coughing with phlegm *(Song of the Jade Dragon)*; or Co-6 *(Qihai)* matched with Sp-6 *(Sanyinjiao)* for treating spermatorrhea *(Ode of a Hundred Syndromes)*.

Since 1949, under the sponsorship of the Party and the Government, acupuncture, like other aspects of traditional medicine, has undergone unprecedented development. The growth in the clinical utilization of Root/Branch and Origin/End is one example. Similarly, the recent development of ear, nose and face acupuncture to treat disorders of the internal Organs and limbs, as well as to induce analgesia, may be regarded as elaborations of the traditional theory of the Path of Qi. For example, using LI-20 *(Yingxiang)* at the sides of the nose to treat roundworm in the bile duct demonstrates the interconnection between the Path of Qi in the head and abdomen. An achievement in the field of head acupuncture has been the successful utilization of Gv-15 *(Yamen)* to cure deaf-mutism. New points have also been discovered on the back: the Barefoot Doctor's points for treating epilepsy and heart problems, N-BW-22 *(Zhongjiaoshu)*, beside the 12th thoracic vertebra, for treating chronic schistosomiasis, and many others. All of these developments illustrate the concept of the Path of Qi and the clinical application of the Branch and End.

The concept of Root and Origin can also be used to understand the recent discovery of important new acupuncture points on the limbs. For example, M-LE-13 *(Lanweixue)* on the lower leg has been used to treat appendicitis and M-LE-23 *(Dannangxue)* to treat cholecystitis. Further, the traditional Primary channel points below the knee and elbow have been used for new purposes. For example, S-37 *(Shangjuxu)* is now used for treating bacillary dysentery, and B-67 *(Zhiyin)* to correct improper position of the fetus. Selection of points for acupuncture anesthesia is likewise based upon the theories of Root/Branch and Origin/End.

Clearly, the traditional concepts of the Path of Qi, Root and Branch, and Origin and End have an important bearing on the selection of acupuncture points in the modern clinic.

Chapter 5

The Eight Miscellaneous and Twelve Divergent Channels

The eight Miscellaneous and twelve Divergent channels comprise an important part of the channel system. The great majority of these vessels branch out from the twelve Primary channels and, sharing the function of circulating Qi throughout the body, form a web of complex interconnections with the Primary channels. Each of these channels has a distinct course which facilitates the functional relationships among the Primary channels. At the same time, each has its own functional characteristics and clinical utility independent of the Primary channels.

THE DISTRIBUTION AND PATHOLOGY OF THE EIGHT MISCELLANEOUS CHANNELS

A single, comprehensive description of the pathways and symptomatology of the eight Miscellaneous channels cannot be found in any one of the traditional medical classics. Here we will summarize the fragmentary accounts found in *Spiritual Axis, Simple Questions, Classic of Difficulties* and later medical commentaries to provide a more complete picture.*

1. Governing Channel   (Dia. 1-13)

This channel is the confluence of all the Yang channels, over which it is said to 'govern'.

There are four paths followed by the channel. The first originates in the perineum and ascends along the middle of the spine until it reaches point Gv-16 *(Fengfu)* at the nape of the neck. Here, it enters the brain, ascends to the vertex, and follows the midline of the forehead across the bridge of the nose, terminating at the upper lip.

The second path begins in the pelvic region, descends to the genitals and perineum, then passes through the tip of the coccyx. Here it diverts into the gluteal region where it intersects the Kidney and Bladder channels before returning to the spinal column and then joining with the Kidneys.

The origin of the third path is in common with that of the Bladder channel at the inner canthus of the

---

*Two of the eight Miscellaneous channels, the Governing and Conception channels, are frequently included with the twelve Primary channels because of their importance and because, like the Primary channels, they have acupuncture points of their own. Together with the twelve Primary channels, they are referred to as the Fourteen channels. The points which are attributed to these two channels are listed in the point index at the end of this book. All the acupuncture points associated with the remaining Miscellaneous channels, as well as a few associated with the Governing and Conception channels, do not strictly 'belong' to these channels. Rather, they are Primary channel points that are intersected by Miscellaneous channels. They are called 'points of intersection' and are listed after the description of the path of each Miscellaneous channel.— *Editors*

67

① Co-1 *(Huiyin)*
② B-12 *(Fengmen)*

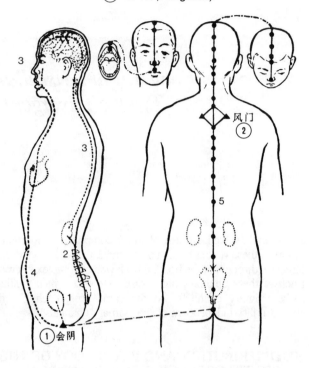

Dia. 1-13 Governing Channel

eye. The two (bilateral) branches, from each of the inner canthi, ascend across the forehead and converge at the vertex where the channel enters the brain. Emerging at the lower end of the nape of the neck, the channel again divides into two branches which descend along opposite sides of the spine to the waist. Here they join with the Kidneys.

Finally, the fourth path of the Governing channel begins in the lower abdomen and rises directly across the navel, passes through the Heart and enters the trachea. Continuing its upward course, the channel crosses the cheek and encircles the mouth, before terminating at a point below the middle of the eye.

This channel intersects the Bladder channel at point B-12 *(Fengmen),* and the Conception channel at point Co-1 *(Huiyin).*

Pathological symptoms: Because this channel supplies the brain and spinal region and intersects the Liver channel at the vertex, obstruction of its Qi may result in symptoms such as stiffness and pain along the spinal column. Deficient Qi in the channel may produce a heavy sensation in the head, vertigo and shaking. Mental disorders may be attributed to Wind entering the brain through this channel. Febrile diseases are commonly associated with the Governing channel. And, because one branch of the channel ascends through the abdomen, when the channel is unbalanced, its Qi rushes upward toward the Heart. Symptoms such as colic, constipation, enuresis, hemorrhoids and functional infertility may result.

2. Conception Channel   (Dia. 1-14)

This channel has two routes. The first arises in the lower abdomen below point Co-3 *(Zhongji),* ascends along the midline of the abdomen and chest, crosses the throat and jaw, and finally winds

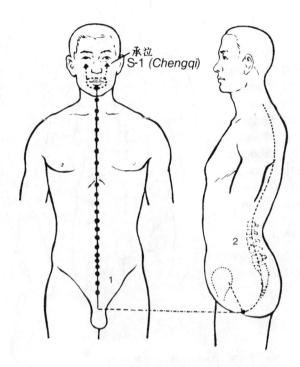

承泣
S-1 *(Chengqi)*

Dia. 1-14 Conception Channel

around the mouth, terminating in the region of the eye.

The second course arises in the pelvic cavity, enters the spine and ascends along the back.

This channel intersects the Stomach channel at point S-1 *(Chengqi)* and the Governing channel at point Gv-28 *(Yinjiao).*

Pathological symptoms: The Conception channel is the confluence of the Yin channels. Therefore, abnormality along the Conception channel will appear principally in pathological symptoms of the Yin channels, especially symptoms associated with the Liver and Kidneys. Its function is closely related with pregnancy and therefore has intimate links with the Kidneys and uterus. If its Qi is Deficient, infertility or other disorders of the urogenital system may result. Leukorrhea, irregular menstruation, colic, etc. are all symptoms associated with the Conception channel.

3. Penetrating Channel   (Dia. 1-15)

This channel has five routes. The first originates in the lower abdomen and emerges along the Path of Qi. From here it tracks the course of the Kidney channel, ascending through the abdomen, skirting the navel and finally dispersing in the chest.

The second route begins where the channel has dispersed in the chest. It ascends across the throat and face and terminates in the nasal cavity.

A third path travels from the lower abdomen to below the Kidney, then emerges along the Path of Qi and descends along the medial aspect of the thigh into the popliteal fossa. From here, it traverses the medial margin of the tibia and the posterior aspect of the medial malleolus before terminating at the bottom of the foot.

The fourth branch separates from the third along the tibia and moves toward the lateral margin of

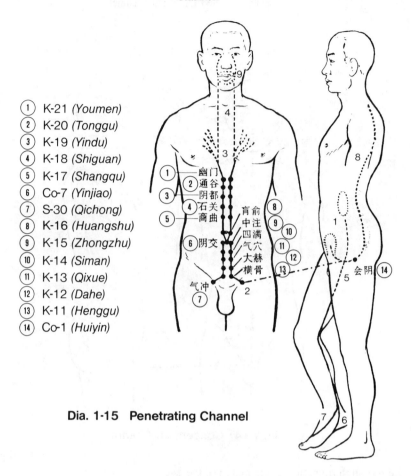

①	K-21 *(Youmen)*
②	K-20 *(Tonggu)*
③	K-19 *(Yindu)*
④	K-18 *(Shiguan)*
⑤	K-17 *(Shangqu)*
⑥	Co-7 *(Yinjiao)*
⑦	S-30 *(Qichong)*
⑧	K-16 *(Huangshu)*
⑨	K-15 *(Zhongzhu)*
⑩	K-14 *(Siman)*
⑪	K-13 *(Qixue)*
⑫	K-12 *(Dahe)*
⑬	K-11 *(Henggu)*
⑭	Co-1 *(Huiyin)*

Dia. 1-15 Penetrating Channel

that bone. It then enters the heel, crosses the tarsal bones of the foot, and finally reaches the big toe.

The fifth branch separates from the main course of the channel in the pelvic cavity. It then inclines backward to enter the spine, and circulates through the back.

This channel intersects the Conception channel at points Co-1 *(Huiyin)* and Co-7 *(Yinjiao),* the Stomach channel at point S-30 *(Qichong),* and the Kidney channel at points K-11 *(Henggu),* K-12 *(Dahe),* K-13 *(Qixue),* K-14 *(Siman),* K-15 *(Zhongzhu),* K-16 *(Huangshu),* K-17 *(Shangqu),* K-18 *(Shiguan),* K-19 *(Yindu),* K-20 *(Tonggu)* and K-21 *(Youmen).*

Pathological symptoms: Because this channel arises in the pelvic cavity, it is intimately associated with gynecological disorders and may also be implicated in male sexual irregularities, including impotence. Abdominal pain or colic may involve this channel as well.

4. Girdle Channel (Dia.1-16)

This channel originates below the hypochondrium at the level of the 2nd lumbar vertebra. From here it turns downward and encircles the body at the waist, like a girdle.

The Girdle channel intersects the Gall Bladder channel at points GB-26 *(Daimai),* GB-27 *(Wushu)* and GB-28 *(Weidao).*

Pathological symptoms: Fullness in the abdomen, irregular menstruation, leukorrhea, pain in the lumbar region, weakness or motor impairment of the lower limb.

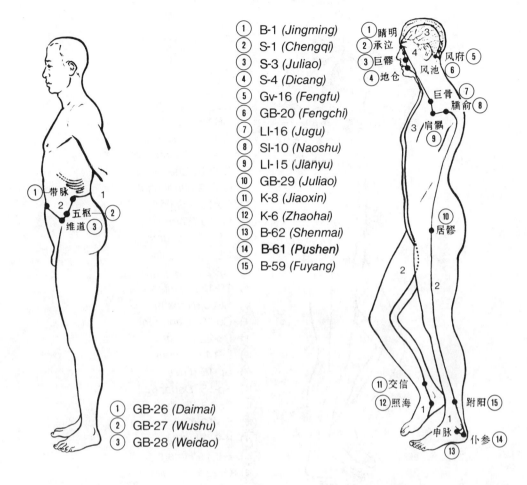

① B-1 *(Jingming)*
② S-1 *(Chengqi)*
③ S-3 *(Juliao)*
④ S-4 *(Dicang)*
⑤ Gv-16 *(Fengfu)*
⑥ GB-20 *(Fengchi)*
⑦ LI-16 *(Jugu)*
⑧ SI-10 *(Naoshu)*
⑨ LI-15 *(Jianyu)*
⑩ GB-29 *(Juliao)*
⑪ K-8 *(Jiaoxin)*
⑫ K-6 *(Zhaohai)*
⑬ B-62 *(Shenmai)*
⑭ **B-61 *(Pushen)***
⑮ B-59 *(Fuyang)*

① GB-26 *(Daimai)*
② GB-27 *(Wushu)*
③ GB-28 *(Weidao)*

Dia. 1-16 Girdle Channel

Dia. 1-17 Yang and Yin Heel Channels

5. Yang Heel Channel   (Dia.1-17)

This channel begins below the lateral malleolus at point B-62 *(Shenmai)* and ascends along the lateral aspect of the leg to the posterior aspect of the hypochondrium. It then continues along the lateral side of the shoulder, traverses the neck and passes beside the mouth before reaching the inner canthus, where it joins the Yin Heel channel and the Bladder channel. From here it ascends across the forehead and winds behind the ear to point GB-20 *(Fengchi)*. It enters the brain at point Gv-16 *(Fengfu)*.

The Yang Heel channel intersects the Bladder channel at points B-62 *(Shenmai)*, B-61 *(Pushen)*, B-59 *(Fuyang)*, and B-1 *(Jingming)*; the Gall Bladder channel at points GB-29 *(Juliao)*, GB-20 *(Fengchi)*; the Small Intestine channel at point SI-10 *(Naoshu)*; the Large Intestine channel at points LI-16 *(Jugu)* and LI-15 *(Jianyu)*; the Stomach channel at points S-4 *(Dicang)*, S-3 *(Juliao)* and S-1 *(Chengqi)*; and the Governing channel at point Gv-16 *(Fengfu)*.

Pathological symptoms: Diseases of the eyes, tightness and spasms of the muscles along the lateral aspect of the lower leg while those along the medial aspect are flaccid or atrophied (found in cases of seizures or paralysis), pain in the lumbar region, stiffness in the lumbar region.

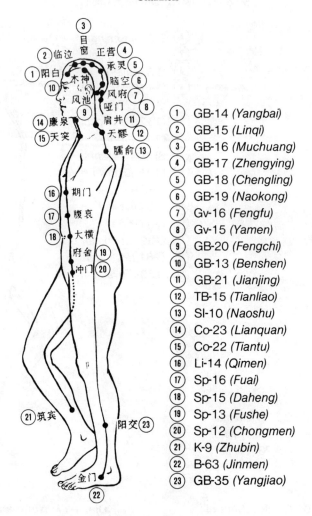

①	GB-14 *(Yangbai)*
②	GB-15 *(Linqi)*
③	GB-16 *(Muchuang)*
④	GB-17 *(Zhengying)*
⑤	GB-18 *(Chengling)*
⑥	GB-19 *(Naokong)*
⑦	Gv-16 *(Fengfu)*
⑧	Gv-15 *(Yamen)*
⑨	GB-20 *(Fengchi)*
⑩	GB-13 *(Benshen)*
⑪	GB-21 *(Jianjing)*
⑫	TB-15 *(Tianliao)*
⑬	SI-10 *(Naoshu)*
⑭	Co-23 *(Lianquan)*
⑮	Co-22 *(Tiantu)*
⑯	Li-14 *(Qimen)*
⑰	Sp-16 *(Fuai)*
⑱	Sp-15 *(Daheng)*
⑲	Sp-13 *(Fushe)*
⑳	Sp-12 *(Chongmen)*
㉑	K-9 *(Zhubin)*
㉒	B-63 *(Jinmen)*
㉓	GB-35 *(Yangjiao)*

**Dia. 1-18 Yang and Yin
Linking Channels**

6. Yin Heel Channel (Dia. 1-17)

This channel originates at point K-6 *(Zhaohai)* below the medial malleolus and extends upward along the medial aspect of the leg, crossing the perineum and chest before entering the supraclavicular fossa. From here, it ascends through the throat and emerges in front of point S-9 *(Renying)*. It then traverses the medial aspect of the cheek before reaching the inner canthus, where it joins the Bladder and Yang Heel channels which together ascend over the head and into the brain.

The Yin Heel channel intersects the Kidney channel at points K-6 *(Zhaohai)* and K-8 *(Jiaoxin)*, and the Bladder channel at point B-1 *(Jingming)*.

Pathological symptoms: Diseases of the eye, tightness and spasms of the muscles along the medial aspect of the lower leg while those along the lateral aspect are flaccid or atrophied (found in cases of seizures or paralysis), lower abdominal pain, pain along the waist to the genitals, hernia, leukorrhagia.

7. Yang Linking Channel   (Dia. 1-18)

This channel begins at point B-63 *(Jinmen)* on the heel, in an area contiguous to all the Leg Yang Primary channels, and ascends along the lateral aspect of the leg. Reaching the lower abdomen, it slants upward across the posterior aspect of the hypochondrium and across the posterior axillary fold to the shoulder. Here, it ascends the neck and crosses behind the ear, proceeding to the forehead. Doubling back over the head, this channel ends at point Gv-16 *(Fengfu)* at the nape of the neck.

The Yang Linking channel intersects the Bladder channel at point B-63 *(Jinmen);* the Gall Bladder channel at points GB-35 *(Yangjiao),* GB-21 *(Jianjing),* GB-20 *(Fengchi),* GB-19 *(Naokong),* GB-18 *(Chengling),* GB-17 *(Zhengying),* GB-16 *(Muchuang),* GB-15 *(Linqi),* GB-14 *(Yangbai)* and GB-13 *(Benshen);* the Triple Burner channel at point TB-15 *(Tianliao);* the Small Intestine channel at point SI-10 *(Naoshu),* the Governing channel at points Gv-15 *(Yamen)* and Gv-16 *(Fengfu);* and the Stomach channel at point S-8 *(Touwei).*

Pathological symptoms: Chills and fever, vertigo; muscular fatigue, stiffness and pain; pain and distension in the waist.

8. Yin Linking Channel   (Dia. 1-18)

This channel begins on the lower leg at point K-9 *(Zhubin)* in an area contiguous to all the Leg Yin Primary channels. Ascending along the medial aspect of the leg, this channel enters the lower abdomen then continues upward across the chest to the throat where it meets the Conception channel at points Co-22 *(Tiantu)* and Co-23 *(Lianquan).*

The Yin Linking channel intersects the Kidney channel at point K-9 *(Zhubin);* the Spleen channel at points Sp-12 *(Chongmen),* Sp-13 *(Fushe),* Sp-15 *(Daheng),* and Sp-16 *(Fuai);* the Liver channel at point Li-14 *(Qimen);* and the Conception channel at points Co-22 *(Tiantu)* and Co-23 *(Lianquan).*

THE FUNCTIONS OF THE EIGHT MISCELLANEOUS CHANNELS

Integrating the Primary Channels

Because many of the Miscellaneous channels branch out from and intersect with the Primary channels, they are regarded as important links which facilitate the interaction among the Primary channels. For example, the Governing channel connects the three Leg Yang Primary channels with the three Arm Yang Primary channels, thereby 'governing' the Qi in all the Yang channels of the body. The principal point of intersection is Gv-14 *(Dazhui),* at the confluence of the three Leg Yang Primary channels on the upper back. Similarly, the Conception channel presides over all the Primary Yin channels. The key points of intersection on this channel are Co-3 *(Zhongji)* and Co-4 *(Guanyuan),* at the confluence of the three Leg Yin Primary channels on the lower abdomen. Of the remaining Miscellaneous channels, the Penetrating channel, arising in the lower abdomen near the path of the Kidney channel and ascending to the navel in the domain of the Stomach channel, is regarded as an important link between these two Primary channels. Furthermore because, like the Conception channel, it originates in the pelvic cavity and, like the Governing channel, sends a branch up through the spine, the Penetrating channel is considered a vital link between these two Miscellaneous channels and, through them, to all the Primary channels. The Girdle channel encircles the body at the waist, joining the vertical paths of all the Primary channels. The Yin and Yang Linking and Heel channels provide many connections between paired Yin and Yang Primary channels and their associated Viscera.

Linking and Supervising the Primary Channels

Although each of the Primary channels has its own peculiar functions, each one also shares certain functional characteristics with other Primary channels. The Miscellaneous channels serve to link those Primary channels which share common characteristics. For example, the Primary Yang channels are linked internally one to another, as are the Yin channels, by the Miscellaneous Yang and Yin Linking channels, respectively.

Furthermore, by linking Primary channels which share similar functions, the Miscellaneous channels play a commanding or supervisory role over them. For example, the Governing channel, in addition to being the confluence of all the Primary Yang channels, is also closely associated with the Kidneys and brain, and has a strong influence on the Liver channel. Its principal functions, therefore, encompass both the overall supervision of Qi in the Primary Yang channels and consolidation of the Source Qi in the Kidneys. Similarly, the Conception channel nourishes and regulates the Qi in the Primary Yin channels. Because Blood is associated with Yin, the Conception channel 'commands' diseases related to conception and gynecology as well as diseases of the Blood.

The Penetrating channel originates in the pelvic cavity, the so-called 'sea of Blood', and influences the activities of the Viscera connected with all the Primary channels. It is therefore referred to as the 'sea of the twelve Primary channels'. Its importance with respect to the internal Viscera is attributed to its connection with the Kidney and Stomach channels, and to its common origin with the Governing and Conception channels in the pelvic cavity. There are three principal reasons for this. First, the Kidneys are the congenital root from which the Source Qi is issued. Second, the Stomach is the source of nutrients from which Nourishing and Protective Qi are produced, and which are then distributed through the channels to all the Viscera. Third, the Stomach has an intimate association with the Conception and Governing channels, the 'commanders' of the Qi in the Yin and Yang channels.

The Girdle channel encircles the body at the waist and intersects all the channels which traverse the trunk. It thereby assists in regulating the circulation of Qi in those channels, especially from the waist down. The distribution of the Yin and Yang Heel channels on the legs and trunk lends them a supervisory function over the Primary channels which traverse these domains. Because the Heel channels intersect the Bladder channel at the inner canthus, and continue over the head and into the brain, they serve an integrative function in these areas. Finally, the Yin Linking channel is said to supervise the functions of the Yin Primary channels, while the Yang Linking channel supervises the functions of the Yang Primary channels.

To summarize, the Primary channels may be regarded as the main trunks of the channel system, and the Miscellaneous channels as branches which diverge from these trunks. Each of the Miscellaneous channels, after separating from a Primary channel, intersects and forms linkages with other channels. Therefore, the functions of each Miscellaneous channel are often a composite of the functions of those channels with which it communicates and over which the Miscellaneous channel exercises an integrative and supervisory role.

Regulating the Supply of Qi and Blood in the Primary Channels

As a network of conduits criss-crossing the Primary channels, the Miscellaneous channels drain and store Qi and Blood from the Primary channels when it is excessive, and supply Qi and Blood when it is deficient. In this way, the Miscellaneous channels monitor and regulate the activity in the Primary channels. For example, menstruation is governed in part by the Kidney Qi. Since the Conception and Penetrating channels can store excess Kidney Qi, they can regulate menstrual flow each month by supplying this additional, stored Qi at the proper time.

THE CLINICAL SIGNIFICANCE OF THE MISCELLANEOUS CHANNELS

Because each of the Miscellaneous channels diverges from or intersects with one or more of the Primary channels, its symptomatology is not distinct from, but is rather a composite of the pathological symptoms associated with those Primary channels which it joins.

For example, the Yin Linking channel has connections with the Kidney, Spleen and Liver channels, and is also associated with the Conception and Stomach channels. Therefore, diseases affecting the Yin Linking channel usually involve symptoms in one or more of these other channels and their related Viscera. Similarly, gynecological and obstetric disorders in Chinese medicine are often associated with the Penetrating, Conception and Girdle channels, all of which are Miscellaneous channels. At the same time, however, such disorders are reflected in symptoms of the Liver, Spleen, Heart, Kidney and other Primary channels and their related Organs, with which the Miscellaneous channels are intimately connected. The pathology of a Miscellaneous channel, therefore, is characterized by patterns of symptoms encompassing several channels.

Based on these principles, it follows that the method of treating diseases affecting a Miscellaneous channel is to stimulate points on related Primary channels. In fact, among the Miscellaneous channels only the Governing and Conception channels possess their own acupuncture points. The remaining Miscellaneous channels are treated by stimulating points of intersection with Primary channels. In ancient times, each of the Miscellaneous channels was assigned a special point of intersection at one of its principal junctures with a Primary channel on the limbs. These Meeting points of the eight channels, as they are called (see Section II, chapter 1), were found to be particularly efficacious in the treatment of diseases associated with the Miscellaneous channels. However, we should not limit our attention, as did many physicians in the past, to only these special points. Any point of intersection between a Miscellaneous channel and another channel may be utilized for therapy, depending only on the symptoms. For example, the point Gv-15 *(Yamen)* on the Governing channel is now frequently used for treating mutism. Yet nowhere in the ancient literature is mutism listed as a pathological symptom associated with the Governing channel. It was, however, mentioned as a symptom of the Yang Linking channel which intersects the Governing channel at this point.

THE DISTRIBUTION AND PATHOLOGY OF THE
TWELVE DIVERGENT CHANNELS

In addition to its own internal linkage with one of the Organs and its external pathway on the limbs, each of the twelve Primary channels has one or more branches which penetrate into the body cavities. These are called Divergent channels.

The distribution of the Divergent channels may be summarized as follows. Most of those belonging to the Primary Yang channels, after entering the Organs in the abdominal or thoracic cavities from their points of origin on the limbs, resurface at the neck where they rejoin the Primary Yang channel from which they diverged. Those belonging to the Primary Yin channels, after separating from their parent channel, converge with the Divergent Yang channel with which each is associated in the Yin/Yang relationship, and then join with the Primary Yang channel itself. Note that the Divergent Yin channels, unlike the Divergent Yang channels, do not return to their parent Primary channel. Instead, they connect to the Primary Yang channel with which the Primary Yin channel is associated in the Yin/Yang relationship. That is to say, in the end all the Divergent channels join with the six Primary Yang channels, thereby providing an important link between the Yin and Yang Primary channels and Organs. This is called the 'six confluences'. Furthermore, each of the Divergent Yang channels, after entering the abdominal or thoracic cavity, joins the Organ of its parent Primary Yang channel with the Organ of the Primary Yin channel with which the first is associated in the Yin/Yang relationship. The Primary Yin and Yang Organs are thus connected.

Each of the Divergent channels from the three Leg Yang Primary channels traverses the cardiac region and ascends to the head. Likewise, each of the Divergent channels from the three Arm Yin Primary channels, after crossing the axilla and entering its pertaining Organ, traverses the throat to the head and face.

These common characteristics will be clearer when we examine the paths of each of the Divergent channels set forth below.

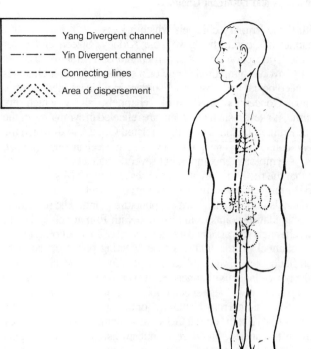

Yang Divergent channel
Yin Divergent channel
Connecting lines
Area of dispersement

**Dia. 1-19 Divergent Channels of the
Bladder and Kidney Primary Channels**

1. Divergent Channel of the Leg Greater Yang (Bladder) Primary Channel   (Dia. 1-19)

After diverging from the Primary channel in the popliteal fossa, this Divergent channel travels to a point 5 units below the sacrum. It then detours to the anal region, connects with the Bladder and disperses in the Kidneys. From here it follows the spine and disperses in the cardiac region before emerging at the neck where it rejoins the Bladder Primary channel.

2. Divergent Channel of the Leg Lesser Yin (Kidney) Primary Channel   (Dia. 1-19)

After separating from the Primary channel in the popliteal fossa, this Divergent channel intersects the Divergent channel of the Bladder on the thigh. It then proceeds upward, connecting first with the Kidney before crossing the Girdle channel at about the 7th thoracic vertebra. Here, the channel ascends to the base of the tongue and continues upward, emerging at the nape of the neck to converge with the Bladder Primary channel.

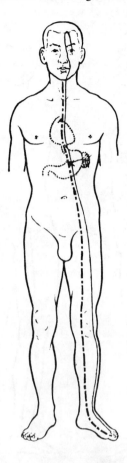

**Dia. 1-20 Divergent Channels of the
Stomach and Spleen Primary Channels**

3. Divergent Channel of the Leg Yang Brightness (Stomach) Primary Channel   (Dia. 1-20)

After diverging from the Primary channel on the thigh, this Divergent channel enters the abdomen, connects with the Stomach, and then disperses through the Spleen. From there, it ascends across the Heart and follows the esophagus until it reaches the mouth. It then continues upward beside the nose and connects with the eye before rejoining the Stomach Primary channel.

4. Divergent Channel of the Leg Greater Yin (Spleen) Primary Channel   (Dia. 1-20)

After separating from the Primary channel on the thigh, this Divergent channel converges with the Divergent channel of the Stomach and proceeds upward to the throat, after which it enters the tongue.

5. Divergent Channnel of the Leg Lesser Yang (Gall Bladder) Primary Channel   (Dia. 1-21)

After diverging from the Primary channel on the thigh, this Divergent channel crosses over and enters the lower abdomen in the pelvic region where it converges with the Divergent channel of the

77

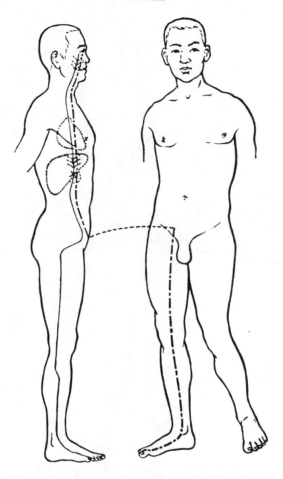

**Dia. 1-21 Divergent Channels of the
Gall Bladder and Liver Primary Channels**

Liver. From here, it crosses between the lower ribs, connects with the Gall Bladder and spreads through the Liver before proceeding upward across the Heart and esophagus, dispersing in the face. Here it connects with the eye and rejoins the Gall Bladder Primary channel at the outer canthus.

6. Divergent Channel of the Leg Absolute Yin (Liver) Primary Channel (Dia. 1-21)

This Divergent channel separates from the Primary channel on the foot and continues upward to the pubic region, where it converges with the Gall Bladder Primary channel.

7. Divergent Channel of the Arm Greater Yang (Small Intestine) Primary Channel (Dia. 1-21)

After separating from the Primary channel at the shoulder, this channel enters the axilla, crosses the Heart, and descends to the abdomen where it connects with the Small Intestine.

78

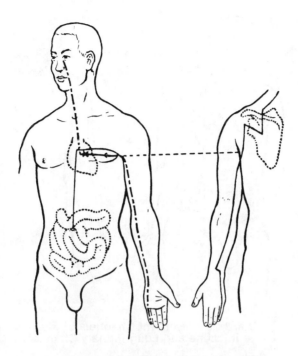

**Dia. 1-22   Divergent Channels of the
Small Intestine and Heart Primary Channels**

8. Divergent Channel of the Arm Lesser Yin (Heart) Primary Channel   (Dia. 1-22)

After diverging from the Primary channel in the axillary fossa, this Divergent channel enters the chest and connects with the Heart. It then ascends across the throat and emerges on the face, joining with the Small Intestine channel at the inner canthus.

9. Divergent Channel of the Arm Yang Brightness (Large Intestine) Primary Channel (Dia. 1-23)

After separating from the Primary channel on the hand, this Divergent channel continues upward across the arm and shoulder to the breast. A branch diverges at the top of the shoulder, enters the spine at the nape of the neck, and proceeds downward to join with the Large Intestine and Lung. Another branch ascends from the shoulder along the throat, emerging at the supraclavicular fossa where it rejoins the Primary channel.

10. Divergent Channel of the Arm Greater Yin (Lung) Primary Channel   (Dia. 1-23)

After diverging from the Primary channel at the axilla, this Divergent channel travels anterior to the path of the Pericardium channel into the chest, where it connects with the Lung before dispersing in the Large Intestine. A branch proceeds upward from the Lung, emerging at the collar bone. From here, it ascends across the throat where it converges with the Large Intestine channel.

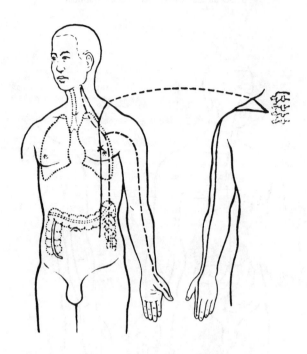

**Dia. 1-23 Divergent Channels of the
Large Intestine and Lung Primary Channels**

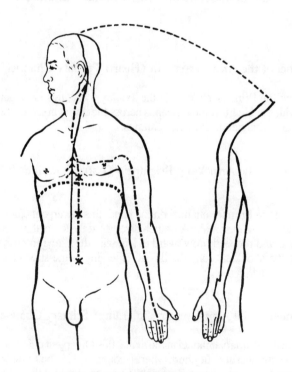

**Dia. 1-24 Divergent Channels of the
Triple Burner and Pericardium Primary Channels**

11. Divergent Channel of the Arm Lesser Yang (Triple Burner) Primary Channel   (Dia. 1-24)

After separating from the Primary channel at the vertex, this Divergent channel descends into the supraclavicular fossa and across the Triple Burner, dispersing in the chest.

12. Divergent Channel of the Arm Absolute Yin (Pericardium) Primary Channel   (Dia. 1-24)

After separating from the Primary channel at a point three units below the axilla, this Divergent channel enters the chest and communicates with the Triple Burner. A branch ascends across the throat, emerging behind the ear where it converges with the Triple Burner channel.

THE FUNCTIONS AND CLINICAL SIGNIFICANCE OF THE TWELVE DIVERGENT CHANNELS

The Divergent channels are branches of the twelve Primary channels. However, because they possess characteristics distinct from the Primary channels, and because the area over which their Qi is distributed is rather extensive, they are considered a separate component of the channel system. Some important aspects are discussed below.

Strengthening the Yin/Yang Relationship Among the Primary Channels

As discussed earlier, six of the twelve Primary channels are Yang and are associated with the Yang Organs internally. Each of these six channels is paired with one of the six Primary Yin channels, which are associated internally with the Yin Organs. One of the principal functions of the Divergent channels is to facilitate the connection between pairs of Yang and Yin Primary channels and Organs. As we have shown, each of the Yin Divergent channels, after separating from its Primary channel on the limbs, ultimately converges with the Yang channel (either Divergent or Primary) with which it is associated in the Yin/Yang relationship. Similarly, within the body cavities most of the Divergent channels first join with their pertaining Organ, and then connect with the Organ belonging to the other channel in the Yin/Yang pair. In this manner, the bonds between paired Yin and Yang Organs and channels are strengthened.

When selecting acupuncture points for therapy, this relationship between paired Yin and Yang channels is very important. Often, a disease affecting a Yang channel will be treated by selecting points on the Yin channel with which it is linked, and vice versa. For example, a headache within the domain of the Large Intestine channel (Yang) may be treated at point L-7 *(Lieque)* on the Lung channel (Yin); conversely, a fever affecting the Lung channel may be treated at point LI-4 *(Hegu)* on the Large Intestine channel. The same holds true for diseases of the internal Organs. A disease of the Stomach (a Yang Organ) may, on occasion, be treated through a point on the channel associated with the Spleen (the Yin Organ paired with the Stomach).

Of course, the linkages among the Primary channels themselves should not be ignored. And the role that the Miscellaneous and Connecting channels play in effecting the Yin/Yang relationship between paired channels and Organs must also be taken into account. Nevertheless, the Divergent channels play an important part in strengthening these bonds.

Distributing Qi to the Face and Head

Among the twelve Primary channels, it is principally the Yang channels that circulate to the head and face. Among the Yin channels, only the Liver and Heart channels directly traverse the head. Among the Divergent channels, however, not only do the Yang channels circulate to the head, but the three Yin Divergent channels of the Leg travel there after converging with their respective Yang

Divergent channels, and the three Yin Divergent channels of the Arm join with the head after entering their pertaining Organs and traversing the throat. In this manner, together with other channels, the Divergent channels serve to distribute the body's Qi to the head.

The importance of the Qi circulating in the head is described in the following passage from chapter 4 of the *Spiritual Axis:*

> The Blood and Qi of the twelve Primary channels and 365 Connecting channels circulates upward where it reaches the orifices [of the sensory organs]. The Essence and Yang Qi travel to the eyes so that they may see. The Divergent [channel] Qi travels to the ears so that they may hear. The Ancestral Qi opens the nose so that it may smell. The coarse Qi from the Stomach travels to the lips and tongue so that they may taste, and the Qi of the Fluids ascends to imbue the face.

The convergence of Qi in the head underscores the importance of the points on the head in acupuncture therapy. Recent developments in acupuncture methodology, such as ear, nose and facial acupuncture, which treat diseases of the limbs and internal Organs by stimulating points on the head, further illustrate the importance of this part of the body. As an integral part of the channel system that distributes Qi to the head, the Divergent channels play an important role.

Integrating Otherwise Neglected Areas of the Body Into the Channel System

The Divergent channels serve to integrate all parts of the body with the Primary channels. Areas which are not traversed by the paths of the Primary channels, and Organs which are otherwise unconnected or only remotely connected by the Primary channels, are more securely linked by the Divergent channels. For example, in traditional medicine the physiological and pathological relationship between the Heart and Kidneys is considered very important. According to Primary channel theory, although the Kidneys are said to be connected with the Heart, there is no corresponding link from the Heart to the Kidneys. The Divergent channel of the Bladder, however, after joining with the Bladder itself, travels from the Kidneys to the Heart, strengthening the link between these two Organs. To use another example, traditional medical doctrine maintains that the Stomach and Heart mutually influence each other, such that medicine which calms the Stomach may be prescribed for its effect in pacifying the Spirit in the Heart as well. Yet Primary channel theory shows no connection between the Stomach and Heart whatsoever. It is the Divergent channel of the Stomach which joins the Stomach to the Heart via the Spleen, and which explains the physiological effect that the one Organ may have upon the other.

The Divergent channels are also instrumental in strengthening the bonds between Primary channels and areas contiguous to their paths. For example, the Divergent channel of the Bladder circulates through the rectal area, strengthening the connection between that region of the body and the Bladder Primary channel. This accounts for the ability of certain points on the Bladder channel to treat hemorrhoids.

In this chapter we have not attempted to provide an exhaustive study of the Miscellaneous and Divergent channels, but to outline their significance within the channel system as a whole. In the next chapter we will consider the remaining constituents of the channel system, the Connecting channels, Muscle channels and Cutaneous Regions.

Chapter 6

The Connecting Channels, Muscle Channels, and Cutaneous Regions

The Connecting channels, Muscle channels and Cutaneous Regions are superficial branches of the channel system. The Connecting channels branch out from the Primary channels, the Muscle channels connect with muscle tissues, and the Cutaneous Regions are superficially distributed over broad surfaces of the skin. All are interconnected, yet each has its own distinctive functional properties and domain.

THE DISTRIBUTION AND PATHOLOGY OF THE FIFTEEN CONNECTING CHANNELS

The Connecting channels are vessels which branch out from the Primary channels. The great majority are distributed superficially over the body. Each of the twelve Primary channels, as well as the Governing and Conception channels, is joined with one of the major Connecting channels. In addition, there is a Great Connecting channel of the Spleen. Sometimes a sixteenth channel, the Great Connecting channel of the Stomach, is included in the list.

The distribution of the Connecting channels may be summarized as follows. On the limbs, the Connecting branches of the Primary Yin channels travel toward the Primary Yang channels with which each is associated in the Yin/Yang relationship. The Connecting branches of the Primary Yang channels likewise travel toward the Primary Yin channels. On the trunk, the Connecting branch of the Conception channel disperses in the abdominal region, while that of the Governing channel disperses in the head, as well as joining with the Bladder channel. The Great Connecting channels of the Spleen and Stomach disperse in the chest.

The larger Connecting branches are termed, simply, Connecting channels. Smaller, sub-branches are called Minute Connecting channels. The superficial blood vessels which can be observed with the naked eye are regarded as part of the Superficial Connecting channels and are called Blood channels. The larger Connecting channels branch out from the Primary channels. The smaller vessels, down to the Minute Connecting channels, branch out in turn from the larger Connecting channels, spreading over wide surfaces and linking all the body tissues to the channel system.

The pathways and symptomatology[1] of the fifteen larger Connecting channels are described in detail below.

1. The Connecting Channel of the Lung   (Dia. 1-25)

After separating from the Primary channel at point L-7 *(Lieque)* on the wrist, this Connecting channel travels to the Large Intestine channel. Another branch follows the Lung channel into the palm of the hand, where it spreads through the thenar eminence.

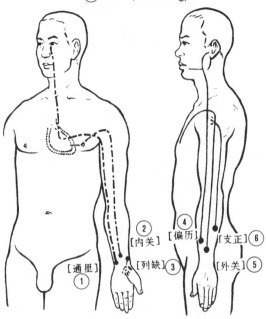

① H-5 *(Tongli)*
② P-6 *(Neiguan)*
③ L-7 *(Lieque)*
④ LI-6 *(Pianli)*
⑤ TB-5 *(Waiguan)*
⑥ SI-7 *(Zhizheng)*

**Dia. 1-25 Yin and Yang Connecting
Channels of the Arm**

Symptoms of Excess: hot palms or wrist.
Symptoms of Deficiency: shortness of breath, frequent micturation, enuresis.

2. The Connecting Channel of the Heart   (Dia. 1-25)

After separating from the Primary channel at point H-5 *(Tongli)* on the wrist, this channel joins the Small Intestine channel. At about 1½ units above the transverse crease of the wrist, the channel again separates from the Small Intestine channel and follows the Heart channel to the Heart itself. It then proceeds to the base of the tongue and connects with the eye.
Symptoms of Excess: fullness and pressure in the chest.
Symptom of Deficiency: aphasia.

3. The Connecting Channel of the Pericardium   (Dia. 1-25)

After separating from the Primary channel at point P-6 *(Neiguan)* on the wrist, this channel spreads out between the two tendons and follows the Pericardium channel upward to the Pericardium, after which it connects with the Heart.
Symptom of Excess: chest pains.
Symptom of Deficiency: irritability.

4. The Connecting Channel of the Large Intestine   (Dia. 1-25)

After separating from the Primary channel at point LI-6 *(Pianli)* on the wrist, this channel joins with the Lung channel. Another branch follows the arm to the shoulder, crosses the jaw and extends to the teeth. Still another branch separates at the jaw and enters the ear region.

Symptoms of Excess: toothache, deafness.

Symptoms of Deficiency: sensation of coldness in the teeth, fullness and congestion in the chest.

5. The Connecting Channel of the Small Intestine   (Dia. 1-25)

After separating from the Primary channel at point SI-7 *(Zhizheng)* on the forearm, this channel connects with the Heart channel. Another branch continues up the arm, crosses the elbow and joins with the shoulder.

Symptoms of Excess: looseness in the joints, atrophy of the muscles in the elbow and arm.

Symptoms of Deficiency: long, finger-shaped warts, scabies.

6. The Connecting Channel of the Triple Burner   (Dia. 1-25)

After separating from the Primary channel at point TB-5 *(Waiguan)* on the wrist, this channel proceeds up the posterior aspect of the arm and over the shoulder, converging with the Pericardium channel in the chest.

Symptom of Excess: spasms of the elbow.

Symptom of Deficiency: flaccid muscles in the arm and elbow.

7. The Connecting Channel of the Stomach   (Dia. 1-26)

After separating from the Primary channel at point S-40 *(Fenglong)* on the lower leg, this channel connects with the Spleen channel. A branch follows the lateral margin of the tibia upward across the thigh and trunk to the top of the head, where it converges with the other Yang channels. Another branch separates in the neck and connects with the throat.

Symptoms of Excess: epilepsy, insanity.

Symptoms of Deficiency: flaccid or atrophied muscles in the legs or feet, pharyngitis, sudden aphasia.

8. The Connecting Channel of the Bladder   (Dia. 1-26)

This channel separates from the Primary channel at point B-58 *(Feiyang)* on the lateral aspect of the lower leg, then connects with the Kidney channel.

Symptoms of Excess: nasal congestion, headache, back pain.

Symptoms of Deficiency: clear nasal discharge, nosebleed.

9. The Connecting Channel of the Gall Bladder   (Dia. 1-26)

After separating from the Primary channel at point GB-37 *(Guangming)* on the lateral aspect of the lower leg, this channel connects with the Liver channel, proceeds downward and disperses over the dorsum of the foot.

Symptom of Excess: fainting.

Symptom of Deficiency: weak and flaccid muscles of the foot, making it difficult to stand.

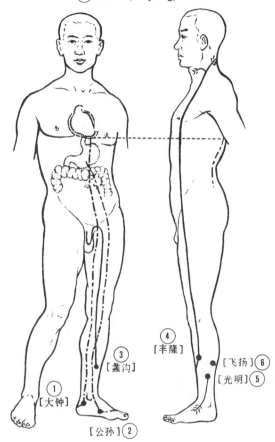

1 K-4 *(Dazhong)*
2 Sp-4 *(Gongsun)*
3 Li-5 *(Ligou)*
4 S-40 *(Fenglong)*
5 GB-37 *(Guangming)*
6 B-58 *(Feiyang)*

**Dia. 1-26 Yin and Yang Connecting
Channels of the Leg**

10. The Connecting Channel of the Spleen   (Dia. 1-26)

After separating from the Primary channel at point Sp-4 *(Gongsun)* on the instep of the foot, this channel connects with the Stomach channel. A branch ascends to the abdomen and connects with the Stomach and Intestines.

Symptoms of Excess: vomiting and diarrhea, sharp intestinal pains.

Symptom of Deficiency: abdominal swelling.

11. The Connecting Channel of the Kidney   (Dia. 1-26)

After separating from the Primary channel at point K-4 *(Dazhong)* on the medial aspect of the ankle, this channel connects with the Bladder channel. A branch follows the Kidney channel upward

① Gv-1 *(Changqiang)*
② Co-15 *(Jiuwei)*

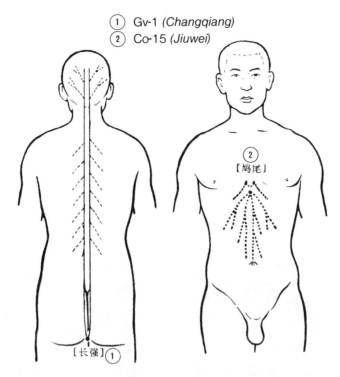

**Dia. 1-27 Connecting Channels of the
Conception and Governing Channels**

to a point below the perineum, then threads its way through the lumbar vertebrae.
   Symptoms of Excess: irritability, depression, enuresis.
   Symptom of Deficiency: low back pain.

12. The Connecting Channel of the Liver   (Dia. 1-26)

After separating from the Primary channel at point Li-5 *(Ligou)* on the medial aspect of the lower leg, this channel connects with the Gall Bladder channel. A branch proceeds up the leg to the genitals.
   Symptoms of Excess: colic, swelling of the testicles.
   Symptom of Deficiency: itching in the pubic region.

13. The Connecting Channel of the Conception Channel   (Dia. 1-27)

This channel separates from the Conception channel at the lower part of the sternum. From point Co-15 *(Jiuwei)*, the channel spreads over the abdomen.
   Symptom of Excess: pain in the skin of the abdomen.
   Symptom of Deficiency: itching on the skin of the abdomen.

14. The Connecting Channel of the Governing Channel   (Dia. 1-27)

After separating from the Governing channel at point Gv-1 *(Changqiang)* in the perineum, this channel travels upward along both sides of the spine to the nape of the neck, where it spreads over the

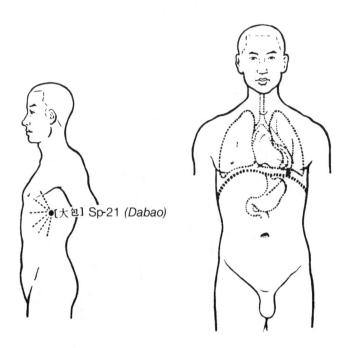

[大包] Sp-21 *(Dabao)*

**Dia. 1-28 Great Connecting Channels
of the Spleen and Stomach**

top of the head. When the channel reaches the level of the shoulder blades, it joins with the Bladder channel and threads through the spine.

Symptom of Excess: stiffness along the spine.

Symptom of Deficiency: heaviness or dizziness in the head.

15. The Great Connecting Channel of the Spleen   (Dia. 1-28)

After separating from the Primary channel at point Sp-21 *(Dabao)* on the lateral aspect of the chest, this Connecting channel spreads through the hypochondria, gathering the Blood around the circumference of the body.

Symptom of Excess: general aches and pains throughout the body.

Symptom of Deficiency: weakness in the muscles of the limbs and joints.

16. The Great Connecting Channel of the Stomach   (Dia. 1-28)

Below the left breast, the Qi of this channel is said to throb ceaselessly, a phenomenon which can be felt with the hand. The channel originates in the stomach cavity and crosses the diaphragm, connecting with the Lung.

Pathological symptoms: rapid breathing, irregular breathing, the sensation of a knot-like obstruction to breathing in the chest.

88

THE FUNCTIONS OF THE CONNECTING CHANNELS

One of the functions of the Connecting channels is to strengthen the Yin/Yang relationship between associated pairs of Primary channels. In this respect, the Connecting channels are similar to the Divergent channels. However, although the Divergent channels connect the Primary channels during the course of their peripheral circulation of the limbs, the principal effect is to strengthen the Yin/Yang relationship between associated pairs of internal Organs (e.g., the Stomach with the Spleen, the Heart with the Small Intestine, etc.). On the other hand, although the Connecting channels join with the Organs internally, they do not necessarily join the Organs one to another. Instead, they serve mainly to connect associated Yang and Yin channels, peripherally (e.g., the Stomach channel with the Spleen channel). The manner of connection is also different. The Yin Divergent channels ultimately converge with the Yang channels and are essentially subordinate to them. The Yang and Yin Connecting channels, however, each connect with a Primary channel of opposite polarity, the Yin to the Yang and vice versa. In this sense, the Yin and Yang Connecting channels are coequal.

Another function of the Connecting channels is that which is performed by the larger fifteen (or sixteen) Connecting channels in supervising the activities of all the lesser Connecting channels (the Superficial, Blood and Minute Connecting channels). The Connecting points of the Connecting channels (see Section II, chapter 1) are significant in that they mark the convergence of all the contributing channels' Qi. Co-15 *(Jiuwei)*, the Connecting point of the Conception channel, for instance, has a supervisory function over all the Yin Connecting channels in the abdomen. Gv-1 *(Changqiang)*, the Connecting point of the Governing channel, supervises all the activities of the Yang Connecting channels on the head and back. Sp-21 *(Dabao)*, the Connecting Point of the Great Connecting channel of the Spleen, has the power of supervising all the Blood in the body (one of the reasons for the designation of the Spleen as the 'ruler of the Blood').

In addition, the Connecting channels assist in the distribution of Qi and Blood to all the tissues of the body, particularly through the extensive network of Minute channels which suffuse the superficial layers of skin and penetrate into the body cavities. Symptoms of bleeding frequently involve the Connecting channels. The Protective Qi, which circulates through the Primary channels to protect, warm and nourish body tissues, first circulates through the superficial layers of skin and muscle via the network of Connecting channels. Although the Primary channels are the principal arteries in this system of distribution, the Connecting channels spread out over broad surfaces, filling in the spaces between the Primary channels.

THE CLINICAL SIGNIFICANCE OF THE CONNECTING CHANNELS

Although there is very little information about the pathology of the Connecting channels in the *Inner Classic*, what few references there are suggest that the diseases reflected along these channels basically fall within the realms of the Primary channels with which each is connected. As we have seen, the *Inner Classic* usually mentions only two or three symptoms or diseases for each of the major Connecting channels.

However, these symptoms are not merely limited to those shared by the parent Primary channel and Organ with which each is connected. Often, symptoms of another Primary channel with which the first is associated in its Yin/Yang relationship can be found as well. This is reflected in the use of Connecting points in treating certain diseases. For example, stimulation of the Connecting point of the Stomach channel, S-40 *(Fenglong)*, is recommended for pharyngitis, insanity, and abdominal pains. These are all symptoms associated with the Stomach channel. However, this same Connecting point is also recommended for treating edema, chest pains, vomiting, and irregular menstruation. These symptoms are associated with the Stomach channel's counterpart in the Yin/Yang relationship, the Spleen channel. Furthermore, because the Qi in the Stomach channel is joined with that of the Lung channel, a Lung symptom, excessive Phlegm, can also be treated through this Connecting point.

The Connecting channels may therefore be thought of as reflecting in a broad manner the symptoms of their parent Primary channels, as well as those of associated Primary channels in the Yin/Yang and other relationships. Based on this principle, later generations of physicians devised a very useful system of point selection, whereby the Source point on the Primary channel principally affected by a disease would be chosen in addition to the Connecting point of its associated Primary channel. For example, a disease affecting the Heart channel could be treated by needling H-7 *(Shenmen)*, the Source point of the Heart channel, together with SI-7 *(Zhizheng)*, the Connecting point of the Small Intestine channel.

There are also brief instructions in the *Inner Classic* concerning the pathology of the smaller Connecting channels: the Superficial channels, Blood channels and Minute channels. For instance, diseases can be diagnosed by observing irregularities over the Superficial connecting channels on the surface of the skin. A greenish discoloration indicates the presence of Cold and pain, while a reddish discoloration evidences Heat. As for therapy, there are several references to pricking the Blood channels so as to bleed the patient. For example, to treat stiffness in the lower back, pricking the Blood channels contiguous to the Bladder channel in the popliteal fossa at the back of the knee is recommended. More recently, based upon guidelines in the *Inner Classic*, other effective methods of letting blood, or drawing blood to the surface of the skin for therapeutic purposes have been developed. These include cupping and application of the cutaneous needle. (See Section III)

THE DISTRIBUTION AND PATHOLOGY OF THE TWELVE MUSCLE CHANNELS

The twelve Muscle channels constitute a part of the channel system on the periphery of the body. Although they enter the body cavities on the trunk, they do not reach the internal Organs. The twelve Muscle channels take their names from the twelve Primary channels whose external courses they generally follow. Accordingly, there are three Yin and three Yang Muscle channels of the Arm, and three Yin and three Yang Muscle channels of the Leg. The Yang Muscle channels are distributed along the back, head and posterior aspect of the limbs, while the Yin Muscle channels are distributed along the anterior aspect of the limbs and enter the thoracic and abdominal cavities.

By way of general description, the Muscle channels originate in the extremities and ascend to the head and trunk. The Greater Yang and Lesser Yin Muscle channels are oriented along the posterior aspect of the body, the Lesser Yang and Absolute Yin channels along the sides, and the Yang Brightness and Greater Yin channels along the anterior aspect. The Muscle channels have points of connection and points of convergence, and each of the Muscle channels connects with at least one other Muscle channel. For example, the Leg Greater Yang (Bladder) Muscle channel connects with points LI-15 *(Jianyu)* on the shoulder and GB-12 *(Wangu)* on the head, and converges with the Yang Brightness and Lesser Yang Muscle channels. The three Leg Yin Muscle channels, as well as the Leg Yang Brightness channel, all converge in the genital region. The Leg Greater Yin channel ascends to the abdomen, and then proceeds to the spine. The Leg Lesser Yin Muscle channel also follows the spine as far as the nape of the neck, where it joins with the Leg Greater Yin Muscle channel. The Arm Yang Muscle channels ascend to the head and converge at the hairline above the temple. The Arm Yin Muscle channels all extend into the thoracic cavity. One of them, the Arm Greater Yin, travels to the ribs. Another, the Arm Lesser Yin, extends into the umbilical region.

The distribution and pathological symptoms of each of the twelve Muscle channels is discussed below.

1. The Leg Greater Yang (Bladder) Muscle Channel   (Dia. 1-29)

This channel originates at the little toe (1), proceeds upward to the external malleolus (2) and then to the knee (3). A lower branch extends below the external malleolus to the heel (4), then ascends to the lateral margin of the popliteal fossa (5). Another branch separates at the convergence of the medial

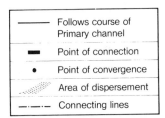

———	Follows course of Primary channel
▬	Point of connection
•	Point of convergence
⣿	Area of dispersement
—·—·—	Connecting lines

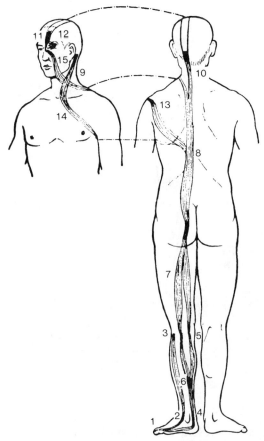

Dia. 1-29 Leg Greater Yang (Bladder) Muscle Channel

and lateral heads of the gastrocnemius muscle (6) and ascends to the medial margin of the popliteal fossa. These two branches join in the gluteal region (7) and continue upward along the side of the spine (8) to the nape of the neck, where a branch reaches inward to the root of the tongue (9). Above the neck, the channel joins with the occipital bone (10) and proceeds over the head to the bridge of the nose (11). A branch crosses the top of the eye and connects at the side of the nose below (12). Another branch extends from the lateral margin of the posterior axillary crease to point LI-15 *(Jianyu)* on the shoulder (13). Another branch crosses below the axilla and over the chest (14), emerging at the supraclavicular fossa and ascending to point GB-12 *(Wangu)* behind the ear. Still another branch, after emerging from the supraclavicular fossa, traverses the face to a site beside the nose (15).

Pathological symptoms: strained muscles of the big toe, swelling and pain in the heel, spasms in the joints, stiffness along the spine, spasms of the back, inability to raise the arm at the shoulder, stiffness or pulled muscle in the axillary region, strained muscles at the clavicle.

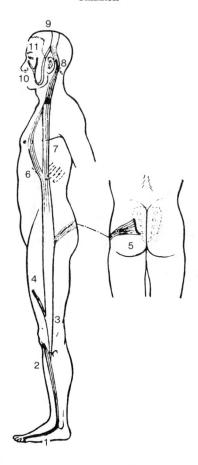

**Dia. 1-30 Leg Lesser Yang (Gall Bladder)
Muscle Channel**

2. The Leg Lesser Yang (Gall Bladder) Muscle Channel (Dia. 1-30)

This channel begins on the fourth toe (1), joins with the external malleolus, then proceeds up the lateral aspect of the leg where it connects with the knee (2). A branch starts at the upper part of the fibula and ascends along the thigh (3). One of its sub-branches travels anteriorly, joining the thigh above point S-32 *(Futu)* (4). Another sub-branch travels posteriorly, and joins with the sacrum (5).

The main channel proceeds upward (6) across the ribs and anterior to the axilla, connecting first in the breast region and then above the collar bone. Another part of the main channel (7) extends from the axilla upward across the clavicle, emerging in front of the Leg Greater Yang channel, then continues upward behind the ear to the temple (8). From here, it continues to the vertex (9), where it joins its bilateral counterpart. A branch descends from the temple across the cheek before joining with the bridge of the nose (10). A sub-branch connects with the outer canthus (11).

Pathological symptoms: strained muscles of the fourth toe, strained muscles of rotation on the lateral aspect of the knee, inability to bend the knee, muscle spasm in the popliteal fossa, strained muscles of the pelvis, strained muscles of the sacrum extending upward to below the ribs, pain in the hypochondria, strained muscles in the breast, clavicle, and neck regions, inability to turn eyes left or right.

92

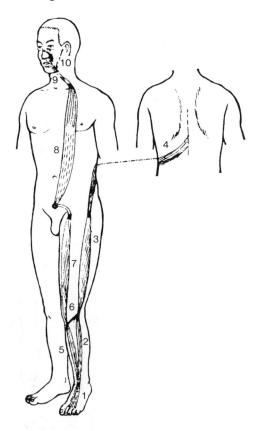

Dia. 1-31   Leg Yang Brightness (Stomach)
Muscle Channel

3. The Leg Yang Brightness (Stomach) Channel   (Dia. 1-31)

This channel originates at the second, fourth and middle toes, crosses the dorsum of the foot (1), and slants upward along the lateral aspect of the leg (2), joining at the knee. From here, this branch of the channel crosses the hip (3) and lower ribs before circling behind the body to connect with the spine (4). Another branch separates from the first branch above the ankle and follows the tibia (5) to the knee. A sub-branch crosses to the head of the fibula, where it joins with the Leg Lesser Yang channel (6). From the knee, the channel ascends across the thigh (7) and connects again in the pelvic region where it joins with the reproductive organs. Continuing upward across the abdomen and chest (8), the channel connects with the clavicle then extends up the neck (9) and around the mouth, connecting at the side of the nose. Above, it joins with the Leg Greater Yang Muscle channel to form a muscular 'net' around the eye. A sub-branch separates at the jaw and traverses the face, connecting in front of the ear (10).

Pathological symptoms: strained muscles of the middle toe, twisted muscles in the lower leg, spasms or hardening of the muscles in the foot, twisted muscles in the thigh, swelling in the anterior pelvic region, hernia, spasms of the abdominal muscles, strained muscles of the neck and cheek, sudden appearance of mouth awry with inability to close the eye because of muscle spasm, muscles of eyelid flaccid, preventing their opening (a Hot symptom), muscles of the cheek tightly contracted, pulling on the sides of the mouth (a Cold symptom), muscles of cheek flaccid and unable to contract, causing mouth to appear awry (a Hot symptom).

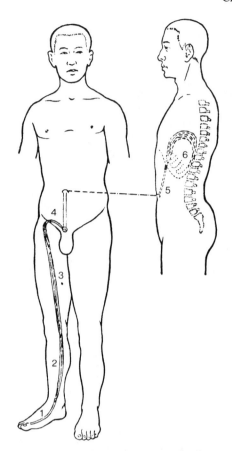
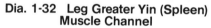

**Dia. 1-32 Leg Greater Yin (Spleen)
Muscle Channel**

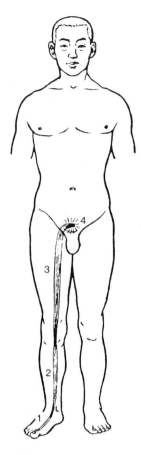

**Dia. 1-33 Leg Absolute Yin (Liver)
Muscle Channel**

4. Leg Greater Yin (Spleen) Muscle Channel (Dia. 1-32)

This channel originates on the medial side of the big toe and ascends across the foot (1), connecting with the internal malleolus. From here, the channel proceeds upward (2) and connects with the medial side of the knee, then traverses the medial aspect of the thigh (3), and connects with the hip before joining with the reproductive organs (4). After crossing the abdomen and connecting with the umbilicus, the channel enters the abdominal cavity (5), connects with the ribs and then disperses through the chest. An internal branch adheres to the spine (6).

Pathological symptoms: strained muscles of the big toe, pain in the internal malleolus, pain in the muscles of rotation in the ankle, pain along the medial aspect of the knee, pain in the adductor muscles of the thigh, pain due to muscle strain of the groin, pain due to strained upper abdominal muscles, pain due to pulled muscles of the mid-thoracic vertebrae.

5. Leg Absolute Yin (Liver) Muscle Channel (Dia. 1-33)

This channel begins on the dorsum of the big toe (1), crosses in front of the internal malleolus and ascends along the medial aspect of the tibia (2), connecting at the inside of the knee. From here, it

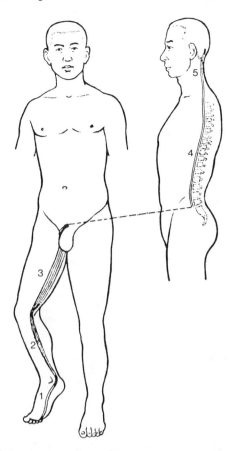

**Dia. 1-34 Leg Lesser Yin (Kidney)
Muscle Channel**

proceeds up the medial aspect of the thigh (3) to the genitals, where it joins with other Muscle channels (4).

Pathological symptoms: strained muscles of the big toe, pain in the area anterior to the internal malleolus, pain at the medial aspect of the knee, pain due to twisted muscles along the medial aspect of the thigh, dysfunction of the genitals (impotence from excessive sexual indulgence, contraction of the genitals if injured by Cold, flaccidness if injured by Heat).

6. Leg Lesser Yin (Kidney) Muscle Channel (Dia. 1-34)

This channel originates beneath the little toe and, together with the Leg Greater Yin (Spleen) Muscle channel, crosses below the internal malleolus (1) and connects at the heel, where it converges with the Leg Greater Yang (Bladder) Muscle channel. From here, it proceeds up the leg (2) and connects at the lower, medial aspect of the knee. It then joins with the Leg Greater Yin channel and proceeds upward along the medial aspect of the thigh (3) to the genital region. A branch ascends along the side of the spine (4) to the nape of the neck, where it connects with the occipital bone and converges with the Leg Greater Yang (Bladder) Muscle channel (5).

Pathological symptoms: twisted muscles on the bottom of the foot, pain or twisted muscles along

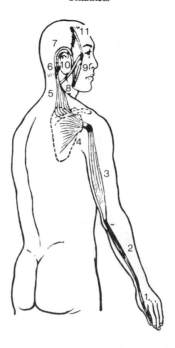

**Dia. 1-35 Arm Greater Yang (Small Intestine)
Muscle Channel**

the course of the channel, as well as other symptoms of disease which appear along the channel (most importantly, those symptoms associated with epilepsy or infantile convulsion).

If the disease is an Exterior condition, it is difficult to flex the head. If the disease in an Interior condition, the head cannot be extended. Similarly, a Yang disorder is one in which the back will not bend forward. In a Yin disorder the back cannot bend backward.

7. The Arm Greater Yang (Small Intestine) Muscle Channel   (Dia. 1-35)

This channel begins on the dorsum of the little finger, connects at the wrist (1), and ascends along the forearm (2) to the elbow, where it connects with the medial condyle of the humerus. From here, the channel proceeds up the arm (3) and connects below the axilla.

A branch travels behind the axilla, surrounds the scapula (4) and follows in front of the Leg Greater Yang (Bladder) Muscle channel on the neck (5), connecting behind the ear. A branch separates behind the auricle and enters the ear itself (6). After emerging above the auricle (7), this branch descends across the face and connects beneath the mandible (8), then ascends to connect at the outer canthus and temple (9). Another branch separates at the mandible, ascends around the teeth and in front of the ear (10), connecting at the outer canthus and the angle of the natural hairline (11).

Pathological symptoms: Stiffness or pain in the muscles of the little finger, pain along the medial and posterior aspects of the elbow, pain below and on the posterior aspect of the axilla caused by pulled muscles along the medial aspect of the arm, pain in the neck caused by pulled muscles surrounding the scapula, tinnitus related to ear ache, pain reaching from the ear to the mandible, poor vision.

If there are spasms in the muscles of the neck it is due to weakness or atrophy of this Muscle channel. Swelling on the neck along the course of this channel may be related to the presence of Cold or Heat.

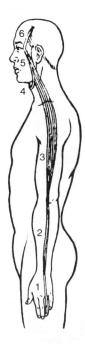

**Dia. 1-36 Arm Lesser Yang (Triple Burner)
Muscle Channel**

8. The Arm Lesser Yang (Triple Burner) Muscle Channel   (Dia. 1-36)

This channel arises at the tip of the fourth finger and connects at the dorsum of the wrist (1). From here, the channel proceeds upward along the forearm (2) and connects with the olecranon of the elbow before continuing upward along the lateral aspect of the upper arm (3). It then passes over the shoulder to the neck, where it joins with the Arm Greater Yang (Small Intestine) Muscle channel.

A branch separates at the angle of the mandible and connects with the base of the tongue (4). Another branch travels upward in front of the ear to the outer canthus (5), then across the temple where it connects at the side of the forehead (6).

Pathological symptoms: stiff, strained or twisted muscles and pain along the course of the channel, curled tongue.

9. The Arm Yang Brightness (Large Intestine) Muscle Channel   (Dia. 1-37)

This channel originates at the tip of the index finger and connects at the dorsum of the wrist (1). From here, it ascends across the forearm (2), and connects at the lateral aspect of the elbow before continuing up the arm (3), where it connects at the shoulder.

A branch encircles the scapula and attaches to the spine (4). The main channel proceeds from the top of the shoulder to the neck (5), where a branch separates and connects at the side of the nose (6). The main channel continues upward, anterior to the Arm Greater Yang (Small Intestine) Muscle channel, and crosses over the head (7), connecting at the mandible on the opposite side of the face (8).

Pathological symptoms: stiff, strained or twisted muscles and pain along the course of the channel, inability to raise the arm at the shoulder, inability to rotate the neck from side to side.

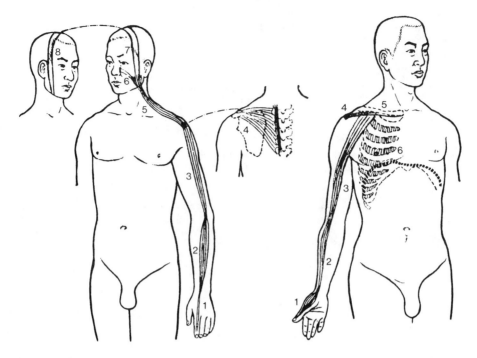

**Dia. 1-37 Arm Yang Brightness (Large
Intestine) Muscle Channel**

**Dia. 1-38 Arm Greater Yin (Lung)
Muscle Channel**

10. The Arm Greater Yin (Lung) Muscle Channel   (Dia. 1-38)

This channel begins on the thumb and, after connecting at the thenar eminence (1), crosses the wrist at the 'pulse'. It then proceeds upward along the forearm (2), connecting at the elbow. From here, the channel continues up the medial aspect of the arm (3) and enters the chest cavity below the axilla. Emerging again in front of the clavicle, the channel connects at the front of the shoulder (4). Above, it connects with the clavicle (5), and below it connects in the Lungs, spreading over the diaphragm (6) and converging again at the lowest rib.

Pathological symptoms: stiff, strained or twisted muscles and pain along the course of the channel, in serious cases, muscle spasms over the area of the ribs, spitting blood.

11. The Arm Absolute Yin (Pericardium) Muscle Channel   (Dia. 1-39)

This channel begins on the palmar aspect of the middle finger and accompanies the Arm Greater Yin (Lung) Muscle channel upward (1), connecting first at the medial aspect of the elbow, and again below the axilla (2). From here, the channel descends, spreading over the ribs both front and back (3). A branch enters the body below the axilla and spreads over the chest, connecting at the diaphragm (4).

Pathological symptoms: stiff, strained or twisted muscles and pain along the course of the channel. When such muscular strain extends into the chest area, chest pain and spasms may be associated symptoms.

12. Arm Lesser Yin (Heart) Muscle Channel   (Dia. 1-40)

This channel originates on the medial aspect of the little finger, connects first with the pisiform bone

98

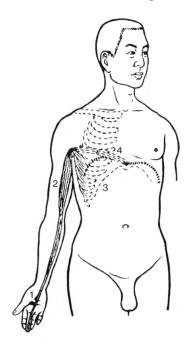

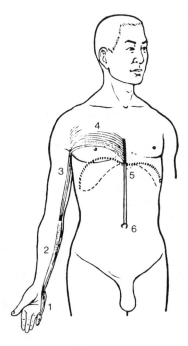

Dia. 1-39 Arm Absolute Yin (Pericardium) Muscle Channel

Dia. 1-40 Arm Lesser Yin (Heart) Muscle Channel

of the hand (1), and again at the medial aspect of the elbow (2). From here, the channel proceeds upward and enters the chest cavity below the axilla (3). It crosses the Arm Greater Yin (Lung) Muscle channel in the breast region, and connects in the chest (4). Descending across the diaphragm (5), the channel connects at the umbilicus (6).

Pathological symptoms: internal cramping sensation, stiff, strained or twisted muscles and pain along the course of the channel.

THE FUNCTION AND CLINICAL SIGNIFICANCE OF THE TWELVE MUSCLE CHANNELS

To understand the function of the Muscle channels, it is first necessary to understand their nature. The Muscle channels are a constituent of the channel system, and depend upon the nourishment of Blood and Qi circulating through the other channels for their functional activity. Thus, the orientation of the Muscle channels by and large coincides with the pathways of the twelve Primary channels. At the same time, the Muscle channels illustrate the correspondence between anatomical features of the body, in this case the muscles, tendons, ligaments and other connective tissues, and traditional features of the channel system. The Muscle channels are not viewed as distinct anatomical entities, but rather represent an early description of the structure and function of the body's musculature within the larger framework of the traditional channel system. The pathology of the Muscle channels likewise reflects those symptoms which affect corresponding groups of muscles and other connective tissues as they are presently understood.

The functions of the Muscle channels parallel the functions of muscles and other sinews generally. "The muscles restrain the bones and are useful in moving the joints."[2] The connective tissues are divided into three groups: the large, the small, and the membranous connective tissues. Although the origins and insertions of individual muscles and their particular functions are not too clearly defined in

99

the early texts, the gross description of muscle distribution and function is quite accurate.

The clinical significance of the Muscle channels is to be found in their function and pathology. It is the Muscle channels that extend and flex the muscles and joints, and move the limbs. Their pathology is therefore reflected in symptoms of impaired movement: pulled, twisted, strained or atrophied muscles, muscle spasms, cramps, etc.

Viewing the distribution of muscles on the body, it can be seen that every joint has basically two groups of counter-functioning, yet complementary muscles (i.e., muscles of extension and flexion, abduction and adduction, internal and external rotation) whose balanced interaction maintains normal movement. In traditional medicine, these contrasting, yet mutually interdependent muscle groups and actions are ascribed the characteristics of Yin and Yang. When the Yin and Yang fail to balance and regulate one another, Muscle channel dysfunction results. It has been described: "When the Yang is distressed, [the muscles] over-extend; when the Yin is distressed, [the muscles] over-contract."[3] And again: "When there is Cold, the muscles become tense; when there is Heat, the muscles become lax."[4]

Therapeutically, a local Muscle channel symptom can generally be treated by stimulating an area contiguous to the pain. In addition, because of the intimate relationship between the Primary channels and Muscle channels, an acupuncture point on the related Primary channel may be selected. (E.g., see the treatment for sequelae of infantile paralysis in Section IV.) The principle that when the Yang is overactive, the Yin will be underactive, and vice versa,[5] refers to imbalance between muscle groups on the medial (Yin) and lateral (Yang) aspects of the limbs. Treatment of such conditions is directed toward restoring the prior balance between the counteracting groups of Yin and Yang muscles.

THE TWELVE CUTANEOUS REGIONS

The Cutaneous Regions refer to that part of the channel system located in the superficial layers of the skin. The significance of the Cutaneous Regions is two-fold, systemic and local. Systemically, as the most superficial of the body tissues, the skin maintains continuous and direct contact with the external environment. It is therefore the area of the body most sensitive to climatic change, to which it must adapt in order to protect the organism from the harmful effects of exogenous influences. To this end, the skin relies principally upon the strength of the body's Normal Qi, and more specifically, the Protective Qi which permeates the skin and resists invasion of harmful influences which must first penetrate the skin before they can affect internal tissues and organs. At the same time, the skin has a particularly close relationship with the Lungs whose Qi, like the Protective Qi, circulates through and warms the skin. If the Lung Qi is weak, harmful influences may penetrate the skin and affect the Lungs (influenza, coughing, etc.). Traditional medicine regards the early stages of any exogenous disease as an Exterior condition. This means that the disease agent is lodged in the superficial layers of the skin where it spawns symptoms characteristic of the onset of certain diseases. If successfully treated at this stage, the disease will be unable to advance further inward along the channel system. If the treatment is unsuccessful, the disease will penetrate to the internal Organs. This Interior condition, as it is called, represents a more serious stage of the disease.

Locally, the Cutaneous Regions are twelve distinct areas on the skin within the domains of the twelve Primary and Connecting channels, and particularly the Superficial Connecting channels. Each of the broad surfaces of the Cutaneous Regions (see Dia. 1-41 and 42) is superficially juxtaposed over the more sparse network of its related Connecting channels, which in turn overlay and interconnect with the trunk-like arteries of the Primary channels. Pathological symptoms associated with the Primary and Connecting channels will often appear as local manifestations along the surface of their related Cutaneous Regions.

Because of the connections between a local Cutaneous Region and the organism generally, a disease of external origin may penetrate the superficial Cutaneous Regions of the channel system and spread inward through the body. Conversely, a disease which has penetrated a Cutaneous Region and has begun to manifest more serious, Interior symptoms may, if properly treated, be expelled to the Exterior regions of the channel system. In acupuncture therapy, an Interior disease may sometimes be treated through its associated Exterior position in the Cutaneous Regions. Likewise, an Exterior disease may be remedied by means of its Interior correlate in the channel system. This demonstrates the close interrelationships among all parts of the channel system.

Clinically, the use of the Cutaneous Regions is quite extensive. In diagnosis, the surface of the skin is examined for evidence of discoloration. Bluish-purple indicates local pain, a darkish hue reflects obstruction, yellow to red evidences Heat, and a pallid complexion usually signifies Cold or Deficiency, etc. Pimples (particularly on the back), hardened lumps or nodules beneath the surface of the skin, abnormal skin sensations and, more recently, local fluctuations in the electroconductivity of the skin are all useful signs in diagnosing disease associated with the channels traversing the affected Cutaneous Region.

Therapeutically, methods were devised in ancient times which utilized specially designed needles for superficial stimulation of the skin. The cutaneous needle (see Section III) is a more recent development of these earlier instruments. As the Protective Qi circulates through the superficial layers of skin, it is theorized that a disease of external origin which first lodges in the skin can be expelled by stimulating the Protective Qi in the affected Cutaneous Region with the cutaneous needle. Application of medicinal ointments and the lancing of boils are based on the same principle. The effect of moxibustion in curing disease also depends upon the mediation of the appropriate Cutaneous Region. It should be evident from even this brief discussion that the Cutaneous Regions play an important part in acupuncture and moxibustion therapy.

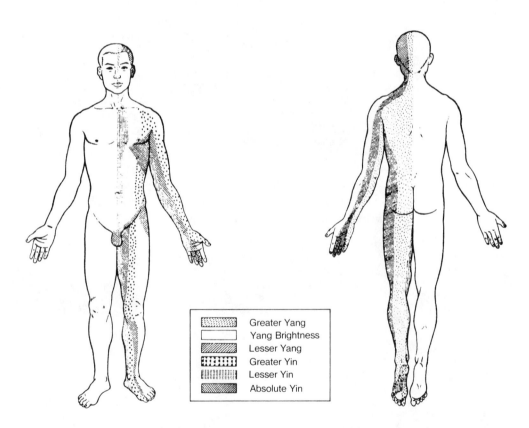

Greater Yang
Yang Brightness
Lesser Yang
Greater Yin
Lesser Yin
Absolute Yin

**Dia. 1-41 Cutaneous Regions
(Front View)**

**Dia. 1-42 Cutaneous Regions
(Back View)**

FOOTNOTES

1. The pathological symptoms are drawn from *Spiritual Axis*, chapter 10.

2. *Simple Questions*, chapter 44.

3. *Spiritual Axis*, chapter 13.

4. Ibid.

5. *Classic of Difficulties*, chapter 29.

Chapter 7

A Summary of Research Concerning the Channels and Points

The gradual formation of the traditional theory of the channels and points has been discussed in previous chapters. Since the Chinese Revolution in 1949, a considerable amount of research has been done in the medical and scientific communities to determine the empirical basis of these phenomena. Significant results have been obtained and are introduced in summary form in this chapter. A companion summary of research concerning the effects of acupuncture on each of the major physiological systems of the body is presented in Section III.

VIEWING THE CHANNELS AND POINTS AS PRESSURE SENSITIVE SITES ON THE BODY SURFACE

Since ancient times, a patient's disease could be diagnosed by observing and probing with the fingers along the course of the channels for areas of tenderness or pain. It is believed that the warmth and strength of the internal Organs can be discerned thereby. Frequently, when disease is present in the body, certain sites along the channels become spontaneously tender and painful to the touch. It was therefore theorized that these channels are connections between the surface of the body and the internal Organs, and between one area of the body and another. By carefully examining these points of 'pressure pain', as they are called, a diagnosis of the disease can be made. Acupuncture can then be performed to treat the illness, often at these same points of 'pressure pain'. This phenomenon has provided an important basis for research.

Such areas on the body surface which react to the presence of disease may be small points or larger areas. Sometimes the underlying tissues become hardened, such that a physician may feel small nodules or lumps, particularly on the back. This method of diagnosis, and the treatment based upon it, has been of particular value in cutaneous acupuncture, and the more recently developed ear acupuncture. (See Section III)

In addition to the ear, these reactive points are also found on the trunk and limbs. Some conspicuous examples on the abdomen include vicinity of Co-13 *(Shangwan)* or Co-12 *(Zhongwan)* for Stomach diseases; Li-14 *(Qimen)* and GB-24 *(Riyue)* (both on the right side) for diseases of the Liver and Gall Bladder; the right side of the abdomen generally for appendicitis. On the back: B-11 *(Dazhu)* and B-12 *(Fengmen)* or B-13 *(Feishu)* for diseases of the respiratory organs; B-17 *(Geshu)*, B-18 *(Ganshu)* and B-19 *(Danshu)* for diseases of the Liver and Gall Bladder; B-20 *(Pishu)* and B-21 *(Weishu)* for Stomach diseases; B-22 *(Sanjiaoshu)* and B-23 *(Shenshu)* for Kidney diseases. On the limbs: P-4 *(Ximen)* for Heart disease; S-34 *(Liangqiu)* and S-36 *(Zusanli)* for Stomach diseases; S-36 *(Zusanli)*, S-37 *(Shangjuxu)*, Sp-9 *(Yinlingquan)* and Sp-8 *(Diji)* for diseases of the Intestines.

Most acupuncture points share this reactive characteristic. When pressed with the finger, there is a feeling of soreness in the underlying tissues. ("When they are pressed, there should be pain and a

103

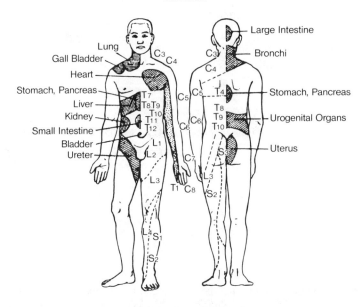

Dia. 1-43   Head's Zones

sunken sensation."[1]) This phenomenon is particularly evident in the special point groupings, such as the Associated, Alarm, Accumulating and Connecting points, etc., as well as those points mentioned in the preceding paragraph (see Section II, chap. 1). Diagnosis based upon palpation of these sensitive points along the channels is called 'channel diagnosis'. From the perspective of pathology, the channels may be seen as a cutaneous and subcutaneous network which reacts to the presence of disease. The points may be regarded as specific sites of reaction along this network. These points have also been observed to alter their position slightly along the channels, depending upon the functional condition of the body. The points which react most distinctly to disease are those which should be chosen for purposes of diagnosis.

This is, however, only one method of traditional diagnosis. It has its shortcomings: the same diseases may often cause different points to react; stages in the development of a disease may not necessarily be reflected in a corresponding increase or decrease in sensitivity at the points; different diseases may affect the same points. Therefore, other means of diagnosis must be used in conjunction with this one, both to confirm its accuracy and to more carefully determine the source of the problem. It should be remembered that the symptoms associated with the channels, as discussed in previous chapters, are quite broad in scope and that the specific points along the pathways of the channels reflect the functional relationships within the body as a whole. Channel diagnosis might therefore best be considered as a point of departure for further examination.

Since 1959, various medical units in Shanghai have studied the alterations in certain points on the ear and in the vicinity of point S-37 *(Shangjuxu)* on the lower leg of patients with acute appendicitis. These studies have shown that when this disease is present, certain specific points react with pain. And, as the inflammation subsides, the reaction diminishes with it. In a report describing the investigation of one hundred cases of infectious hepatitis, the Accumulating point on the Liver channel, Li-6 *(Zhongdu)*, consistently showed the highest rate of positive response (73%), whereas other related points such as B-18 *(Ganshu)*, B-19 *(Danshu)*, GB-36 *(Waiqiu)* and GB-34 *(Yanglingquan)* exhibited very little tenderness, and Li-14 *(Qimen)* and GB-24 *(Riyue)* were tender only on the same side as the liver. Similarly, among fifty patients with infectious hepatitis whose ears were probed for points of reaction, 94% showed a positive response at the Liver point in the cymba conchae on the auricle.

The Shanghai Institute of Physiology performed experiments on the ears of monkeys to determine the cause of the reactive points. Using a variety of pain stimuli, reactive pain was elicited at specific sites on the ear. After removing the cerebral cortex from both sides, the pain stimuli still produced the characteristic reaction, proving that the existence of the cortex is not essential for this response. Injecting procaine into the fourth ventricle of the brain accelerated the subsidence of the reactive pain, whereas injecting a preparation made from *Strychnos nux-vomica (maqianzi)* strengthened the reaction. In both cases, as the effects of the medicine wore off, the reactive pain returned as before. This suggests that the area within the central nervous system responsible for reactive pain points on the ear is in the center of the brain stem near the fourth ventricle.

Modern medicine has also identified certain regions on the surface of the body, such as Head's zones, which react to diseases of the internal organs. (Dia. 1-43) These areas are segmental in nature, appearing within the dermatome associated with a disease in a particular organ. Within these areas themselves are certain sites which become particularly sensitive. These may be found by probing with the head of a needle or other instrument along the surface of the skin, or by raising and gently pinching the skin and underlying tissue, or gently pulling on body hair.

A look at Dia. 1-43 shows that the Head's zones and the area traversed by the channels frequently overlap. For example, B-13 *(Feishu)* and B-21 *(Weishu)*, the Associated points of the Lung and Stomach on the Bladder channel, as well as other back points are located at the most sensitive sites within areas corresponding to the same organs in Head's zones. The Alarm points Co-12 *(Zhongwan)* for the Stomach, Co-4 *(Guanyuan)* for the Small Intestine, Co-3 *(Zhongji)* for the Bladder, Li-14 *(Qimen)* for the Liver, and GB-25 *(Jingmen)* for the Kidneys also fall within the areas of sensitivity which modern medicine has identified with these organs. The consensus is that these reactive points can be explained by referred pain from the affected organ. Despite significant positional changes in the development of the embryo, those regions which were related in the earliest stages of embryological development maintain their relationships, via neurological connections, in the fully developed organism. It is for this reason that specific areas on the surface of the body react to diseases of the internal organs—through the mechanism of referred pain. Points of 'pressure pain' in acupuncture are those sites at which areas of referred pain conjoin with acupuncture loci. In acupuncture therapy, these points are frequently stimulated to treat diseases in the affected organs.

VIEWING THE CHANNELS AND POINTS AS ELECTRICAL PHENOMENA OF THE SKIN

According to traditional theory, the Qi and Blood circulate through the channels, communicating with acupuncture points in the skin. The channels and points thus serve a conducting function which has led modern researchers to investigate their electrical properties.

Studies of the electrical phenomena of the skin are of two kinds. In the first, an electric current is applied externally, and the electroconductivity and resistance of the skin are measured. In the second, no external source of current is used. The electric current of the skin itself is measured and fluctuations in current or electrical potential are recorded. Both of these methods have been employed in investigations of the relationship between the channels and points.

As experiments with the first method have shown, there are places on the skin with higher electroconductivity than surrounding areas, much like the Ryoduraku points ('points of excellent capacity', developed in the 1950's by Japanese physician, Yoshio Nakatani). However, there are differences between these and acupuncture points. Some of the Ryoduraku points coincided with traditional acupuncture loci, while others did not. For example, according to materials gathered in Shanghai, when the area along the Stomach channel from the lateral, inferior margin of the knee to S-37 *(Shangjuxu)* was measured on both healthy subjects and others with appendicitis, the position of the Ryoduraku point varied. On some, it corresponded to the location of point S-36 *(Zusanli)*, but on others it did not. Most researchers have found that the electroconductivity of the skin over the acupuncture points is not always greater than in other areas. The Physiology Instruction and Research Group at our own institute (Shanghai College of Traditional Medicine) selected 28 acupuncture points on various parts of the body for study. The electroconductivity of the skin over some of these points was higher than surrounding areas; at other points it was similar or lower. It is also said that the Ryoduraku points are aligned along 'vessels of excellent capacity', some of which correspond to the channels of acupuncture. The Fujian Institute of Chinese Medicine found in their own investigations that the distribution of these vessels coincided, for the most part, with traditional acupuncture channels. However, a careful study of the medial aspect of the limbs below the elbow and knee was conducted by the Shanghai Institute of Physiology among patients with nephritis, hepatitis, pulmonary tuberculosis and lobar pneumonia. Results failed to turn up such 'vessels of excellent capacity' within the regions which, according to traditional theory, are traversed by the Kidney, Liver and Lung channels.

Furthermore, as many studies within China have proved, the amount of electroconductivity at certain areas of the skin does not increase or decrease according to the paths of the channels *per se*, but is instead related to anatomical location. For example, measurements by the Physiology Instruction and Research Group of our own college demonstrated that the electroconductivity on the surface of the head is highest of any place on the body, with the trunk being second and the extremities last. On the trunk, electroconductivity in the sacral region is greater than other areas of the back, and the chest is greater than the abdomen on the front of the body. As for the limbs, there is a gradual increase in electroconductivity as one approaches the head. Points along the flexor surfaces of the elbow and knee showed a higher degree of electroconductivity relative to other points on the limbs. There was also a uniform relationship between electroconductivity and differences in the temperature of the skin. Most importantly, this reflected the relation between sweating and electrical resistance in the skin. But it also suggested that dilation of the blood vessels in the skin may account for an increase in electroconductivity.

Some observers believe that, because the conductivity over some of the Source points does not approximate the average value of other points on the same channels, the Source points should not be considered representative 'points of excellent capacity'. However, in studies at the Shanghai No. 1 Medical School, the Zhongshan Medical School, and elsewhere, the electroconductivity over the Source points was shown to be similar to the average values recorded over the Five Transport points along each channel, if not to other ordinary points along the channels. Investigations within China have measured the fluctuations in conductivity not only at the Source points, but also at other point groupings considered to be particularly important in traditional acupuncture theory, e.g., the Transport, Alarm, Meeting, Connecting and other points on the body, as well as some points on the ear. Additionally, investigations have been made on cadavers and experimental animals. The findings, however, vary widely.

Using the second method to measure the amount of electric current in the skin, it was found that there were points, similar to the so-called 'cutaneous motor points', which registered particularly large amounts of current. The distribution of these points is the same as those with heightened electroconductivity. Again, the amount of current appears to be related to the anatomical location of the measurement, such that the current increases the closer one probes to the head. The Physiology Instruction and Research Group of Shanghai No. 1 Medical School made a general examination (excluding the top of the head) of a group of healthy students, and observed the relationship between these motor points and acupuncture loci. Their preliminary findings are that the number of such motor points exceeds the number of acupuncture points. On the back, there were eleven rather distinct lines of motor points, on the chest nine lines, and on the abdomen seven, with approximate bilateral orientation. The distribution of such lines on the limbs was neither as distinct nor as numerous as those on the trunk. The motor points on the hands, feet and face were more scattered than they were arranged along vertical lines. They were also, for the most part, bilaterally oriented. Along the median line of the chest and back was a band about two centimeters in width, and net-like in appearance, wherein the electric current was uniformly rather large. Within this area, points of greatest current could be distinguished. Along the transverse creases of the elbow and knee (flexor surfaces), the current was likewise uniformly rather large, with the motor points forming a line roughly corresponding to the crease itself. With each measurement, the absolute number of motor points varied. However, the great majority of them reappeared. Some of the locations of motor points were identical to those of important acupuncture loci. These included Gv-14 *(Dazhui)*, Co-15 *(Jiuwei)*, LI-20 *(Yingxiang)*, S-4 *(Dicang)*, Gv-26 *(Renzhong)*, S-3 *(Juliao)*, S-2 *(Sibai)*, L-5 *(Chize)*, L-6 *(Kongzui)*, L-9 *(Taiyuan)*, Li-1 *(Dadun)* and S-44 *(Neiting)*.

Studies at the Hebei Medical School and elsewhere showed that fluctuations in cutaneous electric current over acupuncture points on certain channels coincided with variations in the functional activity of those internal Organs associated with the channel. For example, the strength of the urinating function of the Bladder was reflected in the cutaneous electric current at points B-60 *(Kunlun)* and B-28 *(Pangguangshu)* on the Bladder channel; the strength of the digestive function of the Stomach, at S-44 *(Neiting),* S-43 *(Xiangu),* S-42 *(Chongyang),* S-41 *(Jiexi)* and S-36 *(Zusanli)* as well as other points along the Stomach channel, in addition to B-21 *(Weishu)* and Co-12 *(Zhongwan),* the Associated and Alarm points of the Stomach, respectively; and the strength of the defecating function of the rectum at B-25 *(Dachangshu)* on the left, the Large Intestine Associated point.

Acupuncture stimulation rather strongly affects both the electroconductivity and electric current of the skin. Needling acupuncture points can cause certain changes in the electric current of the skin at both acupuncture and non-acupuncture sites. However, the changes over the acupuncture loci themselves are somewhat more distinct than those over neighboring non-acupuncture sites. Similarly, although needling non-acupuncture sites may cause changes in the electric current of the skin at distant locations, these changes are not as distinct as when acupuncture points are needled. The electric potential at acupuncture points is greater than that of non-acupuncture sites, or areas contiguous to the points. Electric potential varies regularly according to whether the measurement is made at night or during the day, and also fluctuates according to the functional condition of the body.

Some researchers discovered the existence of special electric currents along the pathways of the channels. When the Qi sensation characteristic of acupuncture stimulation was obtained (see Section III), distinctive electrical waves were recorded along the respective channels at both acupuncture and non-acupuncture sites. Along some of the channels, this wave could be discerned over a relatively long segment. However, this phenomenon was either considerably weaker or altogether absent on either side of the channel. Some researchers, using an electrocardiograph to measure the shape of the waves conducted along a particular channel, obtained similar results. However, it has already been demonstrated that the waves in the first case were those of the electric current in the muscles, and in the second case, of the heart.

Because the results of observing the electric phenomena of the skin along the channels do not point to a unanimous conclusion, many opinions have been voiced among researchers in China. One view holds that the amount of electroconductivity and current in the skin reflects the normal or abnormal functioning of the body. And, because there is a certain degree of similarity in electric current among points along any particular channel, the existence of distinctive 'channel phenomena' must be admitted. Although the results of measurement are extremely complex, if one were to consider all the possible fluctuations in each channel, and their interrelationships, it may be possible to discern laws which accurately describe the manner of activity of each channel. It is suggested further that the channels are a kind of axis for the biological electricity of the body, or an electric circuit, a special kind of electron or electron 'bundle' which passes electromagnetic waves along a fixed course; that the electric phenomena of the skin reflect the electromagnetic field within the body, and just as the magnetic field within the body corresponds to that of the cosmos, changes in the cosmos may then be reflected in fluctuations in the electrical activity along the chanels; and that the Qi in traditional Chinese medicine is the equivalent of modern electromagnetic phenomena, etc.

Another body of opinion maintains that the wide differences in measurements of electroconductivity and current in the skin primarily reflects the numerous physical variables whenever the methods are applied. This is to say, what is being measured is only the electrical phenomena of the external cutaneous tissues. From the variations in these measurements, one may only assume that there have been changes in the external skin, rather than inferring some connection with the hypothetical channels located in deeper tissues. It is because of these conceptual and methodological shortcomings that many results appear irregular. This has caused some to be skeptical about whether or not such measurements reflect the nature of the channels, and even whether such data is a useful tool in studying the channels.

However, regardless of whether the electrical phenomena of the skin can reflect the activities of the channels, it is the majority opinion that electrical phenomena at the acupuncture points is due to neural involvement and regulation. The electrical activity of the skin was early used as an indicator of autonomic nervous function. For example, the appearance of the 'points of excellent capacity' is related to the opening and closing of skin pores, which in turn is controlled by autonomic nerves.

Similarly, the relationship between the 'cutaneous motor points' and the internal organs may be explained through the mediation of the sympathetic nerves.

VIEWING THE CHANNELS FROM THE PERSPECTIVE OF THE PATHWAYS OF RESPONSE TO NEEDLING AND MEDITATION

A patient's perception of a sore, distended, heavy sensation associated with 'obtaining Qi' at the site of acupuncture stimulation, may be accompanied by the feeling that this sensation is being conducted outward along the path of the needled channel. Generally, such conduction is perceived only along a portion of the channel, and it is the exceptionally sensitive patient who feels this sensation conducted over a great distance. This phenomenon has naturally stirred much investigative interest.

According to recent reports based upon examinations of several thousand subjects, there have been only 13 cases in which this conduction phenomenon was experienced along all twelve Primary channels, one case along the twelve Primary channels as well as the Governing and Conception channels, and one case along the twelve Primary channels and all eight Miscellaneous channels. These exceptional cases have been called 'channel sensitive people'. The measurements were taken after using various modes of stimulation, including both regular and electro-acupuncture, and moxibustion. Both healthy and ill subjects were studied, and among the latter were paraplegics. Generally, measurements were made after stimulating the Well and Source points on the extremities. Among those who responded to stimulation at these points, many also experienced the conduction phenomenon to some extent along the pathway of the stimulated channel.

Some reports distinguish between the 'electric flash' sensation of needling one of the sensory nerves directly, which is common, and the perception of the needle sensation along the channels themselves, the occurrence of which is limited to those who are more sensitive. The reaction time to the latter is slower and the subjects can trace the path of conduction. In a book entitled *Studies of the Channels,* published in 1949 by two Japanese researchers, this channel phenomenon was described with respect to a patient suffering optic nerve atrophy who was particularly sensitive to needle stimulation. It was found that the perception of the conduction of the needle sensation was rather slow, progressing from 15-48 millimeters per second to as much as 27-120 millimeters per second along the paths of the stimulated channels. Needling the Source point of each channel, it was found that the sensation extended along the entire length of almost every Primary channel. Needling other points also demonstrated, by the conduction phenomenon, the pathways of certain Miscellaneous channels. The existence of paths of conduction other than the traditional channels was also discovered. Needling a point approximately three finger-widths beside the 8th thoracic vertebra, the needle sensation was found to extend along a course similar, but not identical to, that of the Bladder channel, terminating at the third toe. This uncharted channel was called the 'Eighth Associated *(Shu)* channel', and the point on the back from which it originated the 'Eighth Associated *(Shu)* point'. When a point three finger-widths beside the 7th thoracic vertebra (corresponding to B-17 *(Geshu)*) was needled, the needle sensation extended into the region of the heart, and terminated beside the lateral corner of the cuticle of the middle finger. This so-called channel was given the name 'Diaphragm Associated *(Geshu)* channel'.

Many studies have been undertaken in China concerning the common phenomenon of 'obtaining Qi' at the site of needling. For example, a study was done by the Qingdao Medical School Anatomical Teaching and Research Group in which LI-4 *(Hegu)* was needled and the Qi sensation obtained. It was generally found that by using massage, and increasing local blood pressure to about 120 mm of mercury, the characteristic needle sensation disappeared. Injecting .2-.3 milliliters of normal saline caused the sensation to cease, only to return 1-4 minutes later to previous levels. Experiments performed by the Physiology Teaching and Research Group of the Peking Medical School and elsewhere, in which the deep tissues at the site of an acupuncture point received a procaine bloc, showed that subsequent needling at the point failed to 'obtain Qi'. Needling S-36 *(Zusanli)* on the lower leg when the lumbar region is anesthetized likewise inhibits the Qi sensation at that point.

From these experiments it is concluded that the Qi sensation is conducted via the nervous system, and that the conduction of this sensation, although occurring on the periphery of the body, is mediated through the central nervous system. It has been suggested that the needling causes excitation of the central nervous system, which in turn causes the needling sensation to expand and spread in a particular direction.

The phenomenon reported among practitioners of traditional meditation *(Qigong)* is most certainly related to channel theory. In the *Inner Classic* this is referred to as 'leading the Qi'. Those who practice this technique have reported feeling the conduction of the Qi sensation along the Conception and Governing channels, and sometimes along other channels as well. In materials gathered in 1959 at the Shanghai Municipal Meditation Treatment Bureau, 16 instances of this phenomenon were recorded, affecting the Conception, Governing, Yang and Yin Linking, and Girdle Miscellaneous channels, as well as the Stomach, Spleen, Gall Bladder and Bladder Primary channels. Among these, the highest incidence was reported along the Conception, Governing and Girdle channels.

Finally, there have been clinical reports of spontaneously occurring sensations conducted along the paths of the channels. These have been described as feeling like a 'flow of water' or 'flow of air', occasionally painful. Sometimes, this feeling is accompanied by alterations of the skin such as rashes, nodules or striations along the paths of the channels. Although such reports are rare, it is important that they be investigated to discern their true nature. There are many aspects of channel phenomena whose specific circumstances must be further investigated.

RESEARCH CONCERNING THE SPECIAL CHARACTERISTICS OF ACUPUNCTURE POINTS

In recent years there has been a growing body of research published in China concerning the characteristics of acupuncture points and their relation to non-acupuncture points, the channels, and the functional activities of the internal organs. However, the results still lack uniformity as a result of differences in both the purpose and method of experimentation.

The great majority of research has demonstrated a prominent difference between acupuncture points and other, non-acupuncture sites. The effects of stimulating acupuncture points are pronounced, whereas those at non-acupuncture sites are either ineffectual or relatively weak. For example, researchers at the No. 2 Medical School of Shanghai needled the equivalent of S-36 *(Zusanli)* and M-LE-13 *(Lanwei)* on laboratory rabbits and found that peristaltic movements were accelerated in most cases, whereas needling non-acupuncture sites showed no significant change. In similar studies at the Yangpu Central Hospital in Shanghai, although there was an increase in peristaltic movement after needling non-acupuncture sites, the continuation of these movements was of a shorter duration than when acupuncture points were needled.

The Microbiology Teaching and Research Group of Peking Medical School studied the effect of acupuncture on the phagocytic function of white blood cells. Needling S-36 *(Zusanli)* and LI-4 *(Hegu)* produced significant increases in phagocytosis, whereas needling non-acupuncture sites produced no significant change. If a nerve bloc is injected at the acupuncture point, there is no increase in phagocytosis. The researchers concluded that the resulting increase was a reaction to stimulating the nervous system.

Various reports have also indicated that the specific functional characteristics of different points is relative. The Physiology Teaching and Research Group of Shanghai No. 1 Medical School needled LI-4 *(Hegu)* and L-7 *(Lieque)* to compare the effects of the two points on toothache. In the more than ten cases selected for study, the analgesic effect of needling LI-4 *(Hegu)* was more pronounced than L-7 *(Lieque)*. In another study, acupuncture was performed on patients who had no palpable brachial or radial pulses. In the first group of 19 patients, 15 responded with a distinct pulse when points along the Pericardium channel were needled. In a second group of 19 patients, 12 responded when points along the Lung channel were needled. And in a final group of 12 patients, only 5 responded to needling of Heart channel points. This study shows that the effectiveness of treating disease with different acupuncture points is relative. In a study of the effects of acupuncture on patients with stomach ulcers performed at a hospital affiliated with the Shanghai No. 2 Medical School, it was found that when S-36 *(Zusanli)* was needled, a majority of cases showed an increase in gastric acid secretion, but when Sp-4 *(Gongsun)*, P-6 *(Neiguan)* or S-34 *(Liangqiu)* were needled, the secretion of gastric acid was inhibited. When utilizing injection therapy (see Section III) to treat abdominal pain, it was observed that the results of injecting S-36 *(Zusanli)*, a point on the Stomach channel, were best; injecting S-6

(Jiache), a different point on the same channel, was somewhat less effective; P-6 *(Neiguan)* and B-60 *(Kunlun),* points on different channels, was less effective still; injecting non-acupuncture sites was by and large ineffective. As these studies show, there are significant differences among the points which are most pronounced under pathological circumstances.

With regard to the varying effects that needling the same point will have on different diseases, most research has demonstrated that the general effect of needling an acupuncture point is to regulate or restore stability in the diseased organ with which the point is associated. For instance, in experiments performed by the Shanghai College of Traditional Medicine on laboratory rabbits, it was shown that needling the equivalent of S-36 *(Zusanli)* and S-37 *(Shangjuxu)* generally caused an excitation of rectal motility in those cases which were previously abnormally low, and an inhibition of motility in those cases which were previously high. Similarly, needling B-54 *(Weizhong)* on rabbits with a high degree of bladder tone causes relaxation, and in cases of low bladder tone, contraction of the bladder. Needling points related to organs which are functioning normally has no significant effect on those organs. For example, at the Shanghai No. 1 Medical School it was found that needling S-36 *(Zusanli)* and M-LE-13 *(Lanweixue)* on patients with appendicitis resulted in a slowing of rapid pulses and a normalization of bowel sounds, along with a marked increase in blood cortisol. There was either no change or extremely little change in these parameters when healthy people where needled.

The medical units mentioned here have also found that there are groups of points with similar functions. For example, S-36 *(Zusanli),* S-37 *(Shangjuxu),* S-39 *(Xiajuxu)* and M-LE-13 *(Lanweixue)* all affect the movement of the appendix; they differ only in the extent to which they exert that influence. However, it cannot yet be explained why points along the same channel, but located at radically different parts of the body, share certain functional characteristics in common, albeit there exists a certain relationship to their anatomical locations.

Clinical experience with acupuncture anesthesia has also demonstrated the relative effectiveness among different points which share similar indications. For example, when the First People's Hospital of Shanghai began using acupuncture anesthesia for tonsillectomy in 1959, two pair of points were selected for needling on the upper limbs and two pair on the lower limbs. The result was not considered ideal. After repeated experimentation on their own bodies, the medical personnel at this hospital discovered that both the needle sensation ('obtaining Qi') and analgesic properties were strongest at LI-4 *(Hegu)* and P-6 *(Neiguan)* on the forearm. The points on the lower limbs were therefore discarded and the subsequent degree of effectiveness of the treatment improved significantly. It is believed that the needle sensation at the two points on the upper limb was communicated through nerves in the arm to the same or neighboring segment of the spinal cord as that of the cervical nerves at the site of the operation. The nerves coming from the lower limbs, however, were considered to be separated by too great a distance to match the effectiveness of upper limb points on cervical analgesia. With this understanding, LI-18 *(Futu),* located directly on a cervical spinal nerve, was stimulated with a slight electric current until the patient experienced a sensation 'as if the neck had become thicker'. By this means, the degree of effectiveness of the acupuncture anesthesia was raised to more than 95%. From our experiences with acupuncture anesthesia at the Shanghai College of Traditional Medicine, points on the upper limb are considered primary for surgery on the neck and chest, and points on the lower limb for abdominal surgery. Once again, this evidences the relative differences in the analgesic and regulatory functions among the points. The Shanghai Physiology Research Institute has demonstrated in their experiments with laboratory animals the particular significance of selecting points according to segmental proximity. They believe that since the pain sensation conducted along the splanchnic nerves from organs in the abdominal cavity enters the central nervous system at the lower half of the thoracic section of the spinal cord, the most effective analgesia can therefore be obtained by needling points in the area innervated by spinal nerves in the same or neighboring spinal segment as that shared by the splanchnic nerve of the affected organ.

STUDIES OF THE ANATOMICAL STRUCTURE OF THE CHANNELS AND ACUPUNCTURE POINTS

In recent times, considerable research has been done with respect to the anatomical structure of the channels and acupuncture points. Presently, most research is directed at establishing the relationship between the points and anatomical structures. Certain references in the *Inner Classic* have given impetus to these investigations: "The twelve Primary channels circulate deep within the muscle and cannot be seen. The one that is commonly seen is the Leg Greater Yin (Spleen) channel as it passes above the inner ankle, since there is no place for it to hide. Those vessels that are commonly seen are all Connecting channels." [2] And also: "The circulation [within the channels] can be measured externally by palpation of the pulse. After death, [the channels] can be seen by dissection." [3]

The Relationship Between the Acupuncture Points and Peripheral Nerves

According to numerous reports, the closest relationship exists between the peripheral nerves in the tissues and the acupuncture points. In anatomical dissections performed at 309 traditional acupuncture points by the Anatomical Teaching and Research Group of the Shanghai College of Traditional Medicine in 1959, it was found that 152 points could be stimulated directly over nerves, while 73 additional points could be stimulated within .5 cm. of a nerve. In another study of 324 acupuncture points by the Anatomical Teaching and Research Group of Shanghai No. 1 Medical School in 1960, it was found that 323 were supplied by nerves. Among these, 304 were associated with superficial cutaneous nerves, 155 with deep nerves and 137 points were found to have both superficial and deep neural involvement. Observation under the microscope showed that all layers of the skin and muscle tissues at acupuncture sites contained numerous and varied nerve branches, plexi and endings.

As for the distribution of the channels, there is a particularly close relationship between the paths of the channels on the limbs and the pathways of peripheral nerves. For instance, in anatomical investigations by the Shanghai College of Traditional Medicine, the course of the Lung channel on the upper limb was found to be similar to the path of the musculocutaneous nerve, the Pericardium channel similar to the median nerve, and the Heart channel similar to the paths of the ulnar and medial cutaneous nerves of the arm.

The Relationship Between the Acupuncture Channels and Points, and the Blood Vessels and Lymph Vessels

Anatomical investigation by the Shanghai College of Traditional Medicine of 309 acupuncture points after needling, showed that 24 points were directly over arterial branches and an additional 262 points were with .5 cm. of either arterial or veinous branches. This would suggest that the relationship between acupuncture points and blood vessels is secondary to that between the points and the peripheral nerves. Investigation by the Harbin Medical Science University of points B-60 *(Kunlun)*, B-54 *(Weizhong)* and B-57 *(Chengshan)* on the Bladder channel on the lower leg showed that in most cases the same lymph vessel crossed all three points mentioned. Of the points Sp-6 *(Sanyinjiao)*, Sp-9 *(Yinlingquan)* and Sp-10 *(Xuehai)* on the Spleen channel, two to three are commonly joined by the same lymph vessel. However, in only a few cases were lymph vessels found at or near S-36 *(Zusanli)* or S-31 *(Biguan)*, and at GB-34 *(Yanglingquan)*, GB-31 *(Fengshi)*, B-50 *(Chengfu)* and other points, no lymph vessels were found at all. The relationship between acupuncture points and the distribution of lymph vessels apparently has less importance than either nerves or blood vessels.

SOME VIEWS ON THE NATURE OF THE CHANNELS

Traditional medicine offered its own theories, discussed in earlier chapters, concerning the phenomenon of the channels. However, there is no definitive explanation of the material nature of the channels, despite continuing research. Below, several prominent opinions are offered in the spirit of 'letting a hundred flowers blossom, a hundred schools contend'.

The Relationship Between the Channels and the Peripheral Nervous System

The peripheral nervous system includes nerves which connect with the brain and spinal cord. The upper spinal nerves include the cervical plexus and the brachial plexus, which are distributed over the upper limbs and connect with sympathetic ganglia in the cervical and thoracic regions. The lower spinal nerves are comprised of the lumbar plexus and sacral plexus, distributed over the lower limbs and connecting with sympathetic ganglia in the lumbosacral region. It is believed that the functions of the points along the channels are related to these nerves. The three Primary Yin channels of the Arm (Heart, Pericardium and Lung) traverse the medial aspect of the upper limb and reach the Heart and Lungs. They are therefore stimulated to treat disease in the thoracic region. The three Primary Yang channels of the Arm (Large Intestine, Small Intestine and Triple Burner) traverse the dorsal aspect of the upper limb, the cervical spinal nerves and the cervical sympathetic nerve ganglia, and the internal carotid artery, linking with the cranial nerves and sensory organs of the head. These channels are therefore stimulated for diseases of the head. The three Primary Yin channels of the Leg (Spleen, Liver and Kidney) traverse the medial aspect of the lower limb, linking with the sympathetic ganglia and the lumbosacral nerves. These channels are stimulated for diseases of the abdominal region. The three Primary Yang channels of the Leg (Bladder, Gall Bladder and Stomach) traverse the lateral aspect of the lower limb, linking with the spinal and sympathetic nerves in the lumbosacral region, and reach up the back, joining with nerves in the head. These channels might therefore be stimulated for diseases of the head and sensory organs.

Modern anatomical studies have shown that the distribution of nerve fibers around the blood vessels and other tissues is very dense. For this reason it has been suggested that the neural involvement in such tissues, and in particular the peripheral nerves, is the actual material basis for the channels. Research at the Fujian Medical School and elsewhere has demonstrated that the principle underlying the effect of acupuncture is nerve reflex action. During acupuncture, the nerve trunk beneath the point, or receptors in the skin, connective tissue or blood vessels are stimulated. A reflexive action is initiated through these receptors. The afferent nerves include somatic (motor and sensory) and autonomic nerves. The involvement of the central nervous system includes the excitory and inhibitory processes of the cortex, as well as sub-cortical visceral reflex actions. The reflexive relationship between the acupuncture points and the internal organs is realized through the participation of the autonomic nerves.

The Relationship Between the Channels and the Neural Segments

Looking at the distribution of channels and nerves, it can be seen that the former have a vertical, and the latter a horizontal orientation. This anomaly is particularly conspicuous on the trunk. However, numerous studies have shown that the functional characteristics of the acupuncture points along the channels correspond with the neural segment within which each is located. This suggests a correspondence between the channels and neural segments. References in the medical classics to separate 'paths of Qi' for the head, chest, abdomen and legs, or the functional division of the trunk into three 'burners', have also been taken as proof that even in ancient times the horizontal relationships pertaining to the points on the channels were recognized. For example, the functional connections between the Associated or Alarm points on the back and chest, and the internal Organ with which each is associated (see Section II), could not be determined solely from the vertical orientation of the channels. On the contrary, the location and function of these points vis a vis the internal Organs may only be satisfactorily explained by the respective neural segment, or 'dermatome', in which each is located. For example, Co-17 *(Shanzhong)* is within the dermatome of the 4th thoracic nerve and is stimulated to treat diseases of the respiratory system. Co-12 *(Zhongwan)* is in the dermatome of the 8th thoracic nerve and is selected for diseases of the Stomach. Co-4 *(Guanyuan)* is in the 12th thoracic dermatome and may be used for diseases of the urogenital system.

The Relationship Between the Channels and the
Function of the Central Nervous System

The appearance of intersegmental reactions, whereby stimulating points at one place causes a response across entirely different neural segments, has been examined in the light of modern anatomical analysis. This phenomenon is believed not to result from the existence of functional pathways along the surface of the skin which conduct local stimulation; rather, it is due to the excitation of specific areas in the central nervous system, possibly the cerebral cortex, which are arranged together by function. According to this view, the channels are projections of this specific functional arrangement within the central nervous system distributed over the body. It has been hypothesized that stimulating any point on the body will cause excitation of a corresponding point within the central nervous system which corresponds to specific body functions, and the excitation of which may be transmitted along the pathways of nerve cells to other parts of the body. Therefore, the stimulation of an acupuncture point distant from a diseased organ, which produces a therapeutic effect, is possibly a result of the needle stimulation causing excitation of a site within the central nervous system which has a regulatory relationship with that organ. Among 15 amputees examined at the Peking Medical School, 12 had phantom pain or feeling in that part of the limb which had been amputated. After needling acupuncture points on the affected limb, it was found that the conduction of the needle sensation was still evident. Moreover, it was perceived to reach to the already amputated extremity of the limb. One explanation is that the sensation of conductivity is related to the existence of a site of residual excitation in the cerebral cortex.

The Relationship Among the Channels, the Internal Organs and the Cerebral Cortex

In studies at colleges of traditional medicine in China, connections between the channels and the internal organs have been established. Similar connections between the cerebral cortex and the internal organs have also been proven. From this, it has been inferred that there exists a relationship among the channels, cerebral cortex and internal organs. During experiments performed on laboratory dogs, S-36 *(Zusanli)* was needled until a conditioned reflex was established in the dogs' behaviour, associating the needling of this point with the presence of food. When other points on the same channel (Stomach) were needled, although never before combined with the presence of food, there was still, in most cases, a conditioned reflexive secretion of saliva. Yet, when points on the Bladder channel were needled, the secretions were either reduced or altogether absent. And when GB-34 *(Yanglingquan),* located only a few centimeters from S-36 *(Zusanli),* was needled, there was likewise no salivation. It has been suggested that the conditioned reflex was conducted only along the path of the channel. From the perspective of gross anatomy, the course along which this reflexive phenomenon travelled has no uniform relationship to the distribution of nerve trunks. Therefore, it is believed that although the channels and nerves are related, the channels themselves have an independent system of conduction through which specific response can be elicited from various stimuli (mechanical, electric, chemical, etc.). However, a description of the basic structures of this system of conduction must await further investigation.

The Relationship Between the Channels and the Neurohumoral Regulatory Functions

It is said in the *Inner Classic:* "The Qi and Blood which flow through the channels nourishes the Yin and Yang [i.e., the internal Organs] and moistens the muscles, bones and joints."[4] In the view of modern physiology, the proper regulation of the functions of each part of the body is effected through the combined neurohumoral system.

The stimulation provided by acupuncture of the nervous system causes a reflex effect which is conducted either along the nerves, or along a combination of nerves and body fluids, to the effector organ. There has, accordingly, been considerable experimentation concerning the relationship between the channels and the neurohumoral system. The effect of stimulating an acupuncture point in a certain area will disappear if the related nerve reflex arc is broken, e.g., after severing or anesthetizing the afferant or efferant nerves in that area. If there are changes in the state of the nervous system the effect of acupuncture also varies: hyperactive function may be inhibited and hypoactive function stimulated. Acupuncture thus encourages a tendency toward normalization of function. The specific mechanism may occur along an axon reflex, through sympathetic neural involvement, or through spinal segment linkage. Sometimes there may be nearby segmental or intersegmental linkages due to physiologic or pathologic reflexes. It also may be relayed through specific and non-specific projection systems, affecting high level areas of the central nervous system, or possibly influencing the cerebral cortex and causing more distant or systemic effects. If there is humoral involvement, the effects are even broader and more protracted.

As an explanation of the theoretical basis of the effects of acupuncture, the neurohumoral system is rather inclusive. However, certain problems concerning channel phenomena are still not satisfactorily explained on the basis of present knowledge.

The Channels and Conductivity

Investigations by the Physiology and Pathology Teaching and Research Groups of Shenyang Medical School concluded that needling any acupuncture point will cause various levels of nervous and humoral activity. However, different points have their own specific 'sphere of influence' and, judging from experiments performed on laboratory animals, although the acupuncture channels are closely related to the nervous sytem it is hypothesized that the channels constitute a similar, though independent system of conduction.

Observations were made of the rate at which certain substances were absorbed into the lymphatic system from inflammation in the ears of the laboratory rabbits. It was discovered that when S-36 *(Zusanli)* on the Stomach channel was needled, there was in improvement in blood circulation at the site of inflammation, manifested as an acceleration in the rate of absorption of certain substances. The researchers believe that this shows an effect which is peculiar to the channels, and which they call the 'absorption phenomenon' of the channels. When Sp-9 *(Yinlingquan)* on the Spleen channel (associated with the Stomach channel in the Yin/Yang relationship) was needled, a similar response occurred. However, when GB-40 *(Qiuxu)* on the Gall Bladder channel was needled, either subsequent to or simultaneous with needling S-36 *(Zusanli),* there was a clear reduction in the rate of absorption. This the researchers call the 'absorption inhibition phenomenon' of the channels. Yet, if the degree of needle stimulation is altered, e.g., mild stimulation at S-36 *(Zusanli)* and strong stimulation at GB-40 *(Qiuxu),* the inhibition is eliminated. This is referred to as 'eliminating the absorption inhibition phenomenon'. In later experiments, the possibility that this kind of absorption phenomenon of the channels can be blocked by a certain non-anesthetic bloc was discovered.

To resolve the problem of different 'spheres of influence' possessed by each of the points, as well as the existence of mutual control relationships between different points or channels, experiments were performed in which the nerve supply in the vicinity of a certain point was severed. It was found that the so-called 'absorption phenomenon' of the channels almost completely disappeared. If only a part of the nerve supply was retained, then the absorption phenomenon was likewise retained in part. This shows the close relationship between the 'absorption phenomenon' of the channels and the nervous system.

On the basis of the phenomena described above, researchers believe that the channels comprise a kind of conduction system, possibly distributed superficially over the body, which is relatively independent and obeys strict laws. It is regulated by the nervous system, but does not embody those functional activities of the central nervous system described in the classical anatomy. It seems to possess certain physiological as well as material and chemical properties, and can be obstructed by certain substances. It is believed quite possible that the channels are a system of conduction which evolved very early and was differentiated at a relatively early stage.

The Channels and Bio-electricity

The electrical properties of the skin along the paths of the channels and at the acupuncture points was spoken of earlier. Studies in Fujian Province show that as Organ function is strengthened, the electric potential at the Source point on the related channel increases. But, if the organ is removed, or if the tissues traversed by the channel are destroyed, the electric potential decreases, even to zero. Studies of the effects of surgery, wounds and broken bones likewise showed diminished electric potential at the Source point of those channels which traversed the injured tissues. Based on these observations, the researchers believe that fluctuation in the electric potential at the Source points is determined by the existence and functional health of its related Organ, as well as the continued communication with the Organ along the parent channel. Further, it is believed that the channels are, in actuality, electrical pathways within the body, and that the electric current emitted from the tissues and Organs, depending on its strength, amplitude, etc., criss-crosses the entire body along specific pathways of electric conduction. As for the material basis of conduction within the tissues, they believe that since any tissue within the body has the capacity to conduct electricity, there is a wide variety of tissues that do serve this function. The system of channels, thus formed, exists independently, and although closely connected with the nervous system, is not identical with it.

In addition to the theories described above, there are others which maintain that the channels are related to the vascular and lymphatic systems; that the channels are a system that controls the combined activities of the body and that, drawing from cybernetics, the body should be considered as an automatic control system wherein the channels are likened to 'pathways of conduction', the acupuncture points to 'effector organs', and acupuncture and other forms of stimulation as 'sources of information'. Signals are transmitted and returned between the channels in this control system and the object of control. These researchers feel that channel theory was a "black box" method by which the ancients conceptualized the integrative functions of the body. Channel theory provided the general rules of structure and function.

The importance of the channels in traditional physiology, pathology, diagnosis, and treatment cannot be overstated. The functional relationship among the channels, physiology and pathology contains much that modern medicine cannot explain or perhaps has not yet discovered. This understanding awaits our further efforts.

FOOTNOTES

1. *Spiritual Axis*, chapter 51.

2. *Spiritual Axis*, chapter 10.

3. *Spiritual Axis*, chapter12.

4. *Spiritual Axis*, chapter 47.

Section II

Points

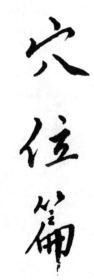

Note: The World Health Organization (WHO) adopted identification numbers for several points on the Bladder channel that differ from those used in this book. The WHO numbers are now more widely used. A comparative list of the points is set forth below.

Acupuncture: A Comprehensive Text	World Health Organization
B-36 *(Fufen)*	BL-41 *(Fufen)*
B-37 *(Pohu)*	BL-42 *(Pohu)*
B-38 *(Gaohuangshu)*	BL-43 *(Gaohuangshu)*
B-39 *(Shentang)*	BL-44 *(Shentang)*
B-40 *(Yixi)*	BL-45 *(Yixi)*
B-41 *(Geguan)*	BL-46 *(Geguan)*
B-42 *(Hunmen)*	BL-47 *(Hunmen)*
B-43 *(Yanggang)*	BL-48 *(Yanggang)*
B-44 *(Yishe)*	BL-49 *(Yishe)*
B-45 *(Weicang)*	BL-50 *(Weicang)*
B-46 *(Huangmen)*	BL-51 *(Huangmen)*
B-47 *(Zhishi)*	BL-52 *(Zhishi)*
B-48 *(Baohuang)*	BL-53 *(Baohuang)*
B-49 *(Zhibian)*	BL-54 *(Zhibian)*
B-50 *(Chengfu)*	BL-36 *(Chengfu)*
B-51 *(Yinmen)*	BL-37 *(Yinmen)*
B-52 *(Fuxi)*	BL-38 *(Fuxi)*
B-53 *(Weiyang)*	BL-39 *(Weiyang)*
B-54 *(Weizhong)*	BL-40 *(Weizhong)*

Chapter 1

An Overview of the Points

The channels and points are the foundation of acupuncture and moxibustion. In this Section the location, pathological indications and other characteristics of each of the acupuncture points will be discussed.

In the historical development of acupuncture, the actual utilization of points in the treatment of disease has contributed to the formation of channel theory. This theory has, in turn, provided a framework for the selection of points in the clinic.

THE DEVELOPMENT AND CLASSIFICATION OF THE POINTS

The words 'acupuncture point' are derived from the Chinese characters meaning hole or orifice, and position—the 'position of the hole'. Traditionally, the word hole was combined with other terms such as hollow, passageway, transport, and Qi. This suggests that the holes on the surface of the body were regarded as routes of access to the body's internal cavities.

It is conjectured that from very early times, man, suffering from one ailment or another, was fortuitously cured by a sharp blow, burn or other accident; or that, feeling pain in some part of his body, he massaged the tender area with his hands and felt better. Over a period of time, this experience was recognized as more than coincidental, and such heretofore random observations were recorded in a more systematic fashion. Gradually, there emerged a methodical system of needling and moxibustion to treat disease. In the beginning, the unnamed acupuncture points were generally referred to as "stone and burning places," a sharp stone being the original needle, and "burning" a reference to the earliest form of moxibustion.

Three phases have been discerned in the historical development of the concept of the acupuncture point.

The first was that of unspecified location. In this earliest phase, people would needle or cauterize whatever area on their body was uncomfortable, i.e., "whatever hurts is the point." Such points of pain included those which were spontaneously tender, as well as those which were painful only when pressed with the hand. Because there were no specific locations for the points, they had no names.

In the second phase, after a long period of practice and experience, certain points became identified with specific diseases. The capacity of distinct points to affect and be affected by local or distant pain and disease, was perceived as a predictable, physiological feature of the body. As the correlation between point and disease became established, names were assigned to certain points to distinguish them from other, random points of pain.

In the final phase, what were previously isolated, localized points, each with a singular function, became integrated in a larger system which related and grouped diverse points systematically according to similar functions. The vehicle of integration was the channel system. It is difficult to grasp

119

TABLE 2-1
AGGREGATION OF CHANNEL POINTS

Book and Dynasty	Midline points	Bilateral points	Total
Yellow Emperor's Inner Classic (Han)	25	135	160
Therapeutic Importance of Acupuncture Points from the Bright Hall; and *Systematic Classic of Acupuncture and Moxibustion* (Jin)*	49	300	349
Illustrated Classic of Acupuncture Points as found on the Bronze Model (Song); and *Elucidation of the Fourteen Channels* (Yuan)[1]	51	303	354
Classic of Nourishing Life with Acupuncture and Moxibustion (Song); and *Great Compendium of Acupuncture and Moxibustion* (Ming)[2]	51	308	359
Illustrated Appendices to the Classic of Categories (Ming); and *Golden Mirror of Medicine* (Qing)[3]	52	309	361

* After the *Inner Classic,* there was a book devoted to description of the points entitled *Therapeutic Importance of Acupuncture Points from the Bright Hall.* Although this work was lost before the 10th century, its contents had been entirely incorporated into the *Systematic Classic of Acupuncture and Moxibustion,* written by Huangfu Mi in 282. —*Editors*

the concept of the channels without referring to the points. On the other hand, to look at the points independently of the channel system would be to return acupuncture to the first stage of its development, when each of the points was regarded as a random, isolated phenomenon. The two concepts must be considered together, the points being an important basis upon which channel theory was formulated.

We move now to the classification of the points, of which there are four types.

The channel points

The earliest exposition of the channels, points and methodology of acupuncture is found in the *Yellow Emperor's Inner Classic* (2nd century, B.C.). In this book, many points were assigned to one or another of the channels according to similar curative properties. The names of the twelve Primary channels, six of which traverse the arms, and an equal number the legs, are derived in part from the twelve traditional Organs with which they are joined. Thus, the name of each channel reflects those parts of the body with which the channel, and its constituent points, is therapeutically linked. In the *Inner Classic,* usually only the name of the channel is mentioned in connection with treating a certain disease, since it was known that the points along the channel shared the same therapeutic properties. This illustrates how systematized acupuncture had become by this time.

The channel points include all those on the twelve Primary channels, bilaterally, as well as the points on the Conception and Governing channels which follow the median line of the body in front and back. As Table 2-1 indicates, although an occasional point was added during later dynasties, more than 95% of the channel points had been identified by the 3rd century.

Among these points there are differences between those which are important or less important, and between those which are commonly or rarely used. In order to emphasize the importance of certain channel points, ancient physicians further differentiated among them. Some of the more important categories of channel points are discussed later in this chapter.

Miscellaneous or 'off-channel' points

The channel points are so named because they are located along the paths of the twelve Primary channels plus the Conception and Governing channels (the so-called Fourteen channels). As time passed, new points were discovered or confusion arose when one name was used to designate two or more distinct points, only one of which was situated along a channel. In this manner, a new category of points emerged called miscellaneous or off-channel points. The evolution of these points was similar to that of the channel points. In the beginning, a site on the body was needled or cauterized according to the traditional principle of "whatever hurts is the point." Then, as the effectiveness of a particular point became established, it was given a name. Later generations of practitioners, familiar with the location and curative properties of a miscellaneous point, might then add it to the list of channel points. For example, B-38 *(Gaohuangshu)* was originally a miscellaneous point on the back used for moxibustion. Its properties were fully described in the T'ang Dynasty work, *Thousand Ducat Prescriptions.* By the Song Dynasty, it was listed as one of the channel points in the *Illustrated Classic of Acupuncture Points as found on the Bronze Model,* and has remained so ever since.

Some miscellaneous points like M-HN-9 *(Taiyang),* because of their proximity to convenient physical landmarks, are more easily located than neighboring channel points. For this reason, they are preferred in the clinic. Other miscellaneous points, however, are more difficult to locate. Some even require special measuring techniques, such as the use of string. As for these, channel points with similar characteristics are preferred. Finally, there are some miscellaneous points which are not individual points at all, but are groupings or clusters of channel and off-channel points.

Points of pain

This general name is given to those sites on the body that become spontaneously tender when disease or injury occurs, but which are not among the channel or miscellaneous points. Their locations are not fixed. A physician may find a point of tenderness when, palpating for other conventional points, the patient winces or suddenly starts. (The Chinese call these "Aah! is the point.") They were first recognized as a separate category of points in the previously mentioned, *Thousand Ducat Prescriptions.*

New points

Traditionally, all acupuncture points were distributed among the three categories discussed above. Since the establishment of the People's Republic of China in 1949, however, and particularly during the period from the Cultural Revolution to the present, many new and effective points were discovered, both by professional medical personnel as well as paramedics ("barefoot doctors") and others who have been encouraged to experiment on themselves in order to further the knowledge of acupuncture.

The discovery of new points has closely paralleled the development of medical practice. For example, the use of acupuncture in recent years to treat deaf-mutism, eye diseases, sequelae of infantile paralysis, etc. has focused attention upon the discovery of new points around the ears, eyes and lower limbs. Some of these new points, discovered by people in one part of the country, differ only in name from those discovered elsewhere; others differ only slightly in location on the body, but basically share the same therapeutic indications. In the course of practice, these differences should be reconciled. In this book a number of new points are presented whose locations and effectiveness have been clearly established. It is our hope that by listing them here, we may contribute to the standardization of nomenclature and encourage further research.

Many of the new points were discovered by combining Western and Chinese medicine, for example, by comparing the anatomical description of the nervous system with traditional channel theory. Because acupuncture points are presently understood to be surface projections of distinct internal structures, including nerves and other tissues, it was suspected, and later confirmed, that new points might be found along major nerve trunks or at those places where nerve branches converged with the main trunk.

Another method of exploration utilizes an electric probe that measures the electrical conductivity of the skin to identify certain 'reactive points'. This method has been particularly useful in charting the points on the ear. Similarly, the probe can be used to measure electrically excitable 'motor points' in the nerves and muscles. For example, when using the 'embedding thread' method to treat sequelae of infantile paralysis, the most important point for stimulation may be selected from among those in the paralyzed muscle which best responds to the probe.

Using a combined Chinese and Western approach to discover new points has opened new vistas for traditional acupuncture.

LOCATING THE POINTS

When locating the precise position of an acupuncture point, the most important single guide is sensitivity. Generally speaking, as mentioned in the *Thousand Ducat Prescriptions,* acupuncture points are found in depressions in the muscles or joints, and are often sensitive to finger pressure, particularly where an illness or symptom with which a certain point is associated is present in the body.

For gross measurements, the muscle and bone structures provide useful landmarks. The ancients devised a system called 'bone measurement', whereby the length of certain bones provided a standard of measurement relative to the body proportions of the individual patient. The standard of measurement is defined in terms of units and tenths of a unit. When a finger is used to measure these distances it is called a finger unit.

In this book, the location of points will be described in the terms set out below.

External features

These may be divided into fixed and movable features. Fixed features include the orifices of the five senses, the hairline, finger nails, nipples of breasts, the navel and certain muscle and bone features.

Movable features include the creases on the skin above the joints, depressions in the muscles and tendons which become visible when moved, and the utilization of certain actions in measuring (e.g., see the methods for finding Gv-20 *(Baihui)*, L-7 *(Lieque)*, and Sp-10 *(Xuehai)* in later chapters).

Proportional measurement

When locating points from physical landmarks, a system of unit measurements is applied. The length of a unit is relative to the physical proportions of the individual.

The proportional measurements of each part of the body were originally set out in *Spiritual Axis*. But because later generations of physicians altered these somewhat, it is not uncommon today to find differences in reckoning. For instance, the distance from the elbow to the wrist is generally counted as twelve units, but some measure it as ten. To take another example, *Spiritual Axis* originally fixed the distance from the navel to the pubic bone as six and one-half units, yet counting from point to point on the lower abdomen one reaches the sum of only five units. However, the distance between each of these points is actually longer than the length of each of the eight units on the upper abdomen. So, as a compromise, one could say there are six units on the lower abdomen. That is to say, distances are more conveniently expressed as whole numbers, and often as even numbers since these are easier to divide. Similarly, the distance on the forehead between the two corners of the hairline is said to be nine

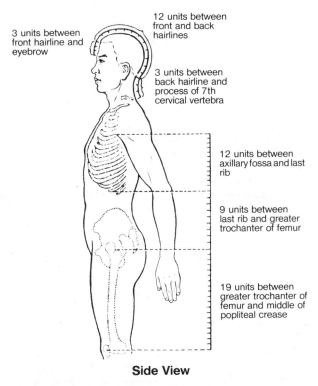

Side View

**Dia. 2-1 Unit Measurements Between
Gross Anatomical Features**

Points

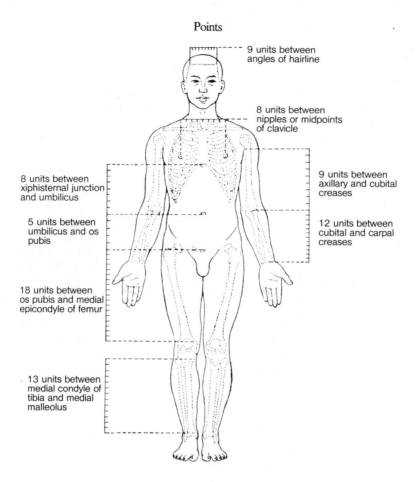

9 units between
angles of hairline

8 units between
nipples or midpoints
of clavicle

8 units between
xiphisternal junction
and umbilicus

5 units between
umbilicus and os
pubis

18 units between
os pubis and medial
epicondyle of femur

13 units between
medial condyle of
tibia and medial
malleolus

9 units between
axillary and cubital
creases

12 units between
cubital and carpal
creases

Front View

units. Compare this with the twelve units from the anterior hairline to the posterior hairline, and it is immediately apparent that the units on the forehead are of a much smaller scale, in fact only about two-thirds the length of the units which measure the vertical distance over the head.

Despite these differences in the scale of unit measurements among various parts of the body, it should be remembered that the purpose of proportional measurement is to facilitate the finding of the approximate locations of points over gross distances on the body, rather than to establish a single, absolute standard for making fine measurements.

For purposes of this book, proportional measurements between major physical landmarks are shown in Diagram 2-1.

Finger measurement

Beginning with the physical landmarks and the gross unit proportions described above, practitioners will often then use their fingers to make more precise measurements in the clinic. Because the length of a unit is relative to the size of one's fingers, a practitioner must compensate for the differences between the size of her own fingers and those of her patients.

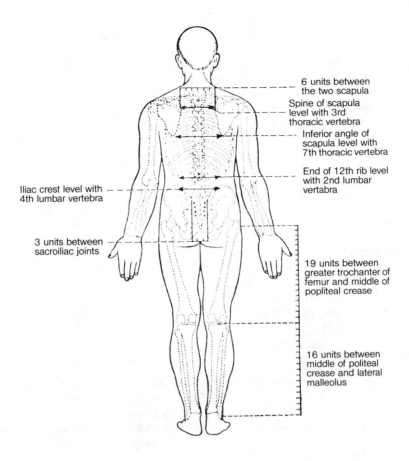

6 units between
the two scapula

Spine of scapula
level with 3rd
thoracic vertebra

Inferior angle of
scapula level with
7th thoracic vertebra

End of 12th rib level
with 2nd lumbar
vertabra

Iliac crest level with
4th lumbar vertebra

3 units between
sacroiliac joints

19 units between
greater trochanter of
femur and middle of
popliteal crease

16 units between
middle of politeal
crease and lateral
malleolus

Back View

Units can be measured with the length or breadth of the fingers (see Diagram 2-2). The length of the index finger from the second joint to the tip is considered to be two units, and from the distal joint to the tip is one unit. The length of the middle phalangeal bone of the middle finger is also one unit.

The breadth of four fingers (excluding the thumb) placed side by side, and measured at the distal joint, is three units; the index and middle fingers are one and one-half units; and the breadth of the thumb at the middle joint is one unit.

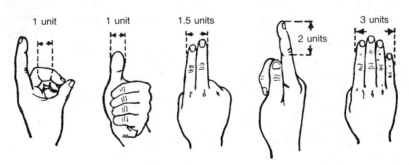

1 unit   1 unit   1.5 units   2 units   3 units

Dia. 2-2 Finger Units

125

CHARACTERISTICS OF THE POINTS AND
SPECIAL POINT GROUPINGS

Generally speaking, the points along the Primary channels on the limbs reflect the symptoms characteristic of their respective channels (see Section I, chapters 3-6). The points along the Primary channels on the trunk and head, however, reflect the symptoms of neighboring Organs.

The Conception channel bisects the head and trunk anteriorly, the Governing channel posteriorly. These channels may be divided into upper, middle, and lower sections on the trunk. The points in each section control diseases in that region of the body along its horizontal plane. The same is true for points along the other channels traversing the trunk. For example, points on the chest and back in the plane between the 1st and the 4th thoracic vertebra affect diseases of the Lungs, Heart and Pericardium; points on the upper abdomen and back in the plane between the 8th and the 12th thoracic vertebra affect diseases of the Liver, Gall Bladder, Spleen and Stomach; and points on the lower abdomen and back in the plane of the lumbar and sacral vertebrae affect diseases of the Kidneys, Intestines and Bladder.*

Of particular importance to the functioning of the body as a whole are the regions of the upper back, where many of the Yang channels join with the Governing channel, and the lower abdomen, where many Yin channels join with the Conception channel. The head, which is the meeting place for all the Primary Yang channels, is also of considerable systemic importance.

Below are several groups of points which have traditionally been regarded as special because of their locations or functional characteristics.

The Five Transport points

Five points on each of the twelve Primary channels below the knee or elbow are designated as the Well, Gushing, Transporting, Traversing and Uniting points. The points are named sequentially such that the Well points are the most distal, and the Uniting points the most proximal. Together, they represent the 'growth' of Qi in the channels from its small, shallow and distant beginnings on the extremities (the Well points) to its large, deep and swelling presence further up the limbs (the Uniting points) using the image of flowing water.

'Well' refers to the source or spring and suggests that in its beginnings, the Qi in the channels is rather small and shallow. Most of the Well points are located next to a finger or toenail. 'Gushing' suggests that the Qi has begun to flow and is slightly larger than at its source. These points are found on the foot or hand. 'Transporting' indicates that the flow of Qi is rapid enough to carry other things with it. Most Transporting points are near the wrist or ankle. 'Traversing' suggests that the Qi has flowed over a long distance. Most of these points are located on the lower leg or forearm. 'Uniting' means to collect or come together, as a stream finally unites with a lake or ocean. The Qi here is vast and deep. Most of the Uniting points are near the elbow or knee. (See Table 2-2.)

The functions of these points were first discussed in *Spiritual Axis* and elaborated upon in the *Classic of Difficulties*. The Well points are used to treat diseases of the Viscera generally, and fullness in the region below the Heart specifically. If a disease causes changes in the patient's complexion, or if the body is feverish, the Gushing points are needled. If the disease is prolonged, or if there is heaviness in the body and pain in the joints, the Transporting points are stimulated. When a disease affects the sound of the voice, or if there is wheezing or panting with chills and fever, the Traversing points are selected. Bleeding, diseases of the Stomach, or disorders accompanied by irregular appetite or diarrhea may be treated via the Uniting points. The particular properties of these points provide a useful reference for application in the clinic.

The Lower Uniting points

Related to the Uniting points (above), and of special significance in treating diseases of the six Yang

*This scheme follows that of the placement of Organs in the Triple Burner. See Introduction. —*Editors.*

TABLE 2-2 THE FIVE TRANSPORTING POINTS

Channel	Well	Gushing	Transporting	Traversing	Uniting
Lung	L-11 (Shaoshang)	L-10 (Yuji)	L-9 (Taiyuan)	L-8 (Jingqu)	L-5 (Chize)
Pericardium	P-9 (Zhongchong)	P-8 (Laogong)	P-7 (Daling)	P-5 (Jianshi)	P-3 (Quze)
Heart	H-9 (Shaochong)	H-8 (Shaofu)	H-7 (Shenmen)	H-4 (Lingdao)	H-3 (Shaohai)
Spleen	Sp-1 (Yinbai)	Sp-2 (Dadu)	Sp-3 (Taibai)	Sp-5 (Shangqiu)	Sp-9 (Yinlingquan)
Liver	Li-1 (Dadun)	Li-2 (Xingjian)	Li-3 (Taichong)	Li-4 (Zhongfeng)	Li-8 (Ququan)
Kidney	K-1 (Yongquan)	K-2 (Rangu)	K-3 (Taixi)	K-7 (Fuliu)	K-10 (Yingu)
Large Intestine	LI-1 (Shangyang)	LI-2 (Erjian)	LI-3 (Sanjian)	LI-5 (Yangxi)	LI-11 (Quchi)
Triple Burner	TB-1 (Guanchong)	TB-2 (Yemen)	TB-3 (Zhongzhu)	TB-6 (Zhigou)	TB-10 (Tianjing)
Small Intestine	SI-1 (Shaoze)	SI-2 (Qiangu)	SI-3 (Houxi)	SI-5 (Yanggu)	SI-8 (Xiaohai)
Stomach	S-45 (Lidui)	S-44 (Neiting)	S-43 (Xiangu)	S-41 (Jiexi)	S-36 (Zusanli)
Gall Bladder	GB-44 (Qiaoyin)	GB-43 (Xiaxi)	GB-41 (Linqi)	GB-38 (Yangfu)	GB-34 (Yanglingquan)
Bladder	B-67 (Zhiyin)	B-66 (Tonggu)	B-65 (Shugu)	B-60 (Kunlun)	B-54 (Weizhong)

Organs (Stomach, Bladder, Gall Bladder, Large Intestine, Small Intestine, Triple Burner), are the six Lower Uniting points. Among these, the Lower Uniting points of the three Leg Yang channels are considered most important. Because all the Organs associated with the Yang channels are located in the abdominal cavity, and since the three Leg Yang channels are connected with the three Arm Yang channels (in the head), stimulation of the Lower Uniting points on the Leg Yang channels will therefore affect all the Yang Organs in the abdomen. This category was first mentioned in the *Spiritual Axis.*

In addition to the Lower Uniting points of the three Leg Yang channels, each of the Organs associated with the three Arm Yang channels is assigned a Lower Uniting point on one of the Yang channels of the Leg. This makes a total of six Lower Uniting points for treating the six Yang Organs in the abdomen. The Lower Uniting points for the Large Intestine, Small Intestine and Stomach are all located on the Stomach channel, while those of the Triple Burner and Bladder are on the Bladder channel. This is because the functions of these Organs are most closely related. (See Table 2-3.)

Table 2-3 Lower Uniting Points of the Six Yang Organs

Stomach	S-36 *(Zusanli)*
Large Intestine	S-37 *(Shangjuxu)*
Small Intestine	S-39 *(Xiajuxu)*
Bladder	B-54 *(Weizhong)*
Triple Burner	B-53 *(Weiyang)*
Gall Bladder	GB-34 *(Yanglingquan)*

The twelve Source points

The Source points are said to be those points where the Source Qi of the various Organs flows and is detained. The Source point of each of the Yin channels is identical with the Transporting point of that channel, whereas on the Yang channels the Source point is immediately proximal to the Transporting point.

In the *Spiritual Axis,* it is said that the Source points generally reflect an Excess or Deficiency of Qi in their respective channels and are useful in diagnosing, by means of palpation, the presence of disease in Organs associated with the channels.

Table 2-4 The Twelve Source Points

Lung channel	L-9 *(Taiyuan)*
Pericardium channel	P-7 *(Daling)*
Heart channel	H-7 *(Shenmen)*
Spleen channel	Sp-3 *(Taibai)*

Liver channel	Li-3 *(Taichong)*
Kidney channel	K-3 *(Taixi)*
Large Intestine channel	LI-4 *(Hegu)*
Triple Burner channel	TB-4 *(Yangchi)*
Small Intestine channel	SI-4 *(Wangu)*
Stomach channel	S-42 *(Chongyang)*
Gall Bladder channel	GB-40 *(Qiuxu)*
Bladder channel	B-64 *(Jinggu)*

The fifteen Connecting points

These are fifteen points, one of which belongs to each of the twelve Primary channels on the limbs, and one each on the front, back and side of the trunk for the Conception, Governing, and Great Spleen Connecting channels, respectively. Since a principal function of the Connecting channels is to join a Yang Primary channel with its paired Yin Primary channel (see Section I, chapter 6), the Connecting points are used to regulate diseases affecting both of the coupled channels. For example, if there are symptoms affecting both the Gall Bladder (Yang) and Liver (Yin) channels, stimulation of the Connecting point on either of these channels will help control the symptoms in both. Generally, if Liver symptoms predominate and Gall Bladder symptoms are secondary, the Liver channel Connecting point is selected; conversely, if symptoms associated with the Gall Bladder channel are more evident than those of the Liver, the Gall Bladder channel Connecting point is preferred.

Table 2-5   The Fifteen Connecting Points

Lung channel	L-7 *(Lieque)*
Pericardium channel	P-6 *(Neiguan)*
Heart channel	H-5 *(Tongli)*
Spleen channel	Sp-4 *(Gongsun)*
Liver channel	Li-5 *(Ligou)*
Kidney channel	K-4 *(Dazhong)*
Conception channel	Co-15 *(Jiuwei)*
Great Connecting channel of the Spleen	Sp-21 *(Dabao)*
Large Intestine	LI-6 *(Pianli)*
Triple Burner channel	TB-5 *(Waiguan)*

Small Intestine channel   SI-7 *(Zhizheng)*

Stomach channel   S-40 *(Fenglong)*

Gall Bladder channel   GB-37 *(Guangming)*

Bladder channel   B-58 *(Feiyang)*

Governing channel   Gv-1 *(Changqiang)*

The sixteen Accumulating points

There are sixteen Accumulating points which are holes or crevices located at the sites where Qi and Blood in the channels converge and accumulate as they circulate through the body. One of these points can be found on each of the Primary channels, in addition to the Yin and Yang Linking and Heel (Miscellaneous) channels. The Accumulating points are used primarily in the treatment of acute diseases, or as diagnostic tools, whereby the points are palpated to determine whether a disease in the related channel is Deficient or Excessive.

Table 2-6   The Sixteen Accumulating Points

Lung channel   L-6 *(Kongzui)*

Pericardium channel   P-4 *(Ximen)*

Heart channel   H-6 *(Yinxi)*

Large Intestine channel   LI-7 *(Wenliu)*

Triple Burner channel   TB-7 *(Huizong)*

Small Intestine channel   SI-6 *(Yanglao)*

Stomach channel   S-34 *(Liangqiu)*

Gall Bladder channel   GB-36 *(Waiqiu)*

Bladder channel   B-63 *(Jinmen)*

Spleen channel   Sp-8 *(Diji)*

Liver channel   Li-6 *(Zhongdu)*

Kidney channel   K-5 *(Shuiquan)*

Yin Linking channel   K-9 *(Zhubin)*

Yang Linking channel   GB-35 *(Yangjiao)*

Yin Heel channel   K-8 *(Jiaoxin)*

Yang Heel channel   B-59 *(Fuyang)*

The Meeting points of the eight Miscellaneous channels

Each of the eight Miscellaneous channels has a Meeting point on the upper or lower limb. Although it is true that not all of the Miscellaneous channels circulate extensively through the limbs, nevertheless each is indirectly linked through its 'meeting' with one of the twelve Primary channels. These points are utilized in accordance with the symptomatology of the Miscellaneous channels (Section 1, chapter 5). Ordinarily, a Meeting point on the upper limb is combined with a related Meeting point on the lower limb, as in Table 2-7. For example, Sp-4 *(Gongsun)* would be used in combination with P-6 *(Neiguan)* for a disease of the Stomach.

Table 2-7 The Meeting Points of the Eight Miscellaneous Channels			
Primary channel	Meeting point	Miscellaneous channel	Indications
Spleen channel	Sp-4 *(Gongsun)*	Penetrating channel	Diseases of Heart, chest and Stomach
Pericardium channel	P-6 *(Neiguan)*	Yin Linking channel	
Small Intestine	SI-3 *(Houxi)*	Governing channel	Diseases of the inner canthus, neck, ear, shoulder, Small Intestine, Bladder
Bladder channel	B-62 *(Shenmai)*	Yang Heel channel	
Gall Bladder channel	GB-41 *(Zulinqi)*	Girdle channel	Diseases of the outer canthus, back of ear, cheek, neck, and shoulder
Triple Burner channel	TB-5 *(Waiguan)*	Yang Linking channel	
Lung channel	L-7 *(Lieque)*	Conception channel	Diseases of the respiratory system, throat, chest and diaphragm
Kidney channel	K-6 *(Zhaohai)*	Yin Heel channel	

The Associated points of the back

The Associated points of the back, one for each of the twelve primary Organs, are situated in a row along the Bladder channel roughly parallel to the spine. They are described as points through which the circulating Qi of the Organs passes. In *Spiritual Axis,* it is said that the presence of a disease in an Organ 'associated' with one of these points may be diagnosed by means of palpation at the Associated point. Tenderness at the point indicates a disorder in the associated Organ. E.g., in chapter 39 of *Simple Questions* it is written: "When Cold Qi lodges in the vessels [connected with] the points of the back, the flow of Blood through the vessels becomes rough. When the flow through the vessels is rough, the Blood is Deficient. When the Blood is Deficient there is pain. When the flow gathers in the point of the Heart then the point responds with pain."

Each of the Associated points is positioned in approximately the same horizontal plane as its related Organ. For example, the Associated point of the Kidneys is at the same level on the back as the

Kidneys themselves.

The use of acupuncture and moxibustion at the Associated points of the back is particularly efficacious in the treatment of the Organs, as well as the distant manifestations of Organ disorders in the sensory organs and elsewhere.

Table 2-8   The Associated Points of the Back

Organ	Associated point
Lung	B-13 *(Feishu)*
Pericardium	B-14 *(Jueyinshu)*
Heart	B-15 *(Xinshu)*
Liver	B-18 *(Ganshu)*
Gall Bladder	B-19 *(Danshu)*
Spleen	B-20 *(Pishu)*
Stomach	B-21 *(Weishu)*
Triple Burner	B-22 *(Sanjiaoshu)*
Kidneys	B-23 *(Shenshu)*
Large Intestine	B-25 *(Dachangshu)*
Small Intestine	B-27 *(Xiaochangshu)*
Bladder	B-28 *(Pangguangshu)*

Alarm points

The Alarm points are situated on the chest and abdomen. Like the Associated points, the points of Alarm are twelve in number, corresponding to the twelve primary Organs. Similarly, tenderness on or near an Alarm point is a useful diagnostic indicator of disease in the Organ associated with that point. Since the Alarm points are located near the Organs, they are sensitive to imbalances therein. For example, *Simple Questions,* chapter 47: "When the Gall Bladder is Deficient, the Qi overflows and there is a bitter taste in the mouth. To treat this condition, use the Alarm point of the Gall Bladder."

Table 2-9   Alarm Points

Organ	Alarm point
Lung	L-1 *(Zhongfu)*
Pericardium	Co-17 *(Shanzhong)*

Liver	Li-14 *(Qimen)*
Heart	Co-14 *(Juque)*
Gall Bladder	GB-24 *(Riyue)*
Stomach	Co-12 *(Zhongwan)*
Spleen	Li-13 *(Zhangmen)*
Triple Burner	Co-5 *(Shimen)*
Kidneys	GB-25 *(Jingmen)*
Small Intestine	Co-4 *(Guanyuan)*
Large Intestine	S-25 *(Tianshu)*
Bladder	Co-3 *(Zhongji)*

The eight Meeting points

The points in this group have proven particularly effective in the treatment of diseaes of certain Organs, tissues, Blood and Qi. For example, chapter 45 of the *Classic of Difficulties* provides: "For Interior Heat, select the Meeting point of Qi." (In practice, this point may be used for other internal diseases as well.) Depending on the nature of the disease, select the related point.

Table 2-10   The Eight Meeting Points

Yin Organs	Li-13 *(Zhangmen)*
Yang Organs	Co-12 *(Zhongwan)*
Qi	Co-17 *(Shanzhong)*
Blood	B-17 *(Geshu)*
Muscles and Tendons	GB-34 *(Yanglingquan)*
Blood Vessels	L-9 *(Taiyuan)*
Bones	B-11 *(Dazhu)*
Marrow	GB-39 *(Xuanzhong)*

The points of intersection

Acupuncture points located at the intersection of two or more channels are called points of intersection. The channel to which the point belongs is called the channel of origin, and the other channels which intersect at this point are called intersecting channels.

Channels are linked to each other at points of intersection. These points are indicated both for diseases associated with their channels of origin, as well as for diseases affecting intersecting channels. Selection of a point of intersection may be particularly beneficial when the symptom or disease is one for which all the intersecting channels are indicated. For example, on the lower abdomen are two important points of intersection, Co-3 *(Zhongji)* and Co-4 *(Guanyuan).* The channel of origin is the Conception channel; the intersecting channels include the three Leg Yin channels (Spleen, Kidney and Liver). Because all of these channels are indicated for uro-genital disorders, Co-3 *(Zhongji)* and Co-4 *(Guanyuan)* figure prominently in most acupuncture prescriptions for such diseases.

Tables 2-11 and 2-12 provide a master reference list of the numerous points of intersection, indicating the channel of origin and the channels which intersect each point.

TABLE 2-11 POINTS OF INTERSECTION ON THE YANG CHANNELS										
Key: "O" indicates channel of origin "X" indicates intersecting channels	Governing	Bladder	Small Intestine	Gall Bladder	Triple Burner	Stomach	Large Intestine	Yang Linking	Yang Heel	Girdle
Gv-24 *(Shenting)*	O	X				X				
Gv-26 *(Renzhong)*	O					X	X			
Gv-20 *(Baihui)*	O	X								
Gv-17 *(Naohu)*	O	X								
Gv-16 *(Fengfu)*	O							X		
Gv-15 *(Yamen)*	O							X		
Gv-14 *(Dazhui)*	O	X		X		X				
Gv-13 *(Taodao)*	O	X								
Gv-1 *(Changqiang)*	O									
B-1 *(Jingming)*		O	X			X				
B-11 *(Dazhu)*		O	X							
B-12 *(Fengmen)*		O								
B-36 *(Fufen)*		O	X							
B-59 *(Fuyang)*		O							X	

	Governing	Bladder	Small Intestine	Gall Bladder	Triple Burner	Stomach	Large Intestine	Yang Linking	Yang Heel	Girdle
B-62 *(Shenmai)*		O							X	
B-61 *(Pushen)*		O							X	
B-63 *(Jinmen)*		O						X		
SI-10 *(Naoshu)*			O					X	X	
SI-12 *(Bingfeng)*			O	X	X		X			
SI-18 *(Quanliao)*			O		X					
SI-19 *(Tinggong)*			O	X	X					
GB-1 *(Tongziliao)*			X	O	X					
GB-3 *(Shangguan)*				O	X	X				
GB-4 *(Hanyan)*				O	X	X				
GB-6 *(Xuanli)*				O	X	X				
GB-7 *(Qubin)*		X		O						
GB-8 *(Shuaigu)*		X		O						
GB-10 *(Fubai)*		X		O						
GB-11 *(Qiaoyin)*		X		O						
GB-12 *(Wangu)*		X		O						
GB-13 *(Benshen)*				O				X		
GB-14 *(Yangbai)*				O				X		
GB-15 *(Linqi)*		X		O				X		
GB-16 *(Muchuang)*				O				X		
GB-17 *(Zhengying)*				O				X		

	Governing	Bladder	Small Intestine	Gall Bladder	Triple Burner	Stomach	Large Intestine	Yang Linking	Yang Heel	Girdle
GB-18 *(Chengling)*				O				X		
GB-19 *(Naokong)*				O				X		
GB-20 *(Fengchi)*				O				X		
GB-21 *(Jianjing)*				O	X			X		
GB-24 *(Riyue)*				O						
GB-30 *(Huantiao)*		X		O						
GB-26 *(Daimai)*				O						X
GB-27 *(Wushu)*				O						X
GB-28 *(Weidao)*				O						X
GB-29 *(Juliao)*				O					X	
GB-35 *(Yangjiao)*				O				X		
TB-15 *(Tianliao)*					O				X	
TB-17 *(Yifeng)*				X	O					
TB-20 *(Jiaosun)*				X	O		X			
TB-22 *(Heliao)*			X	X	O					
S-1 *(Chengqi)*						O			X	
S-3 *(Juliao)*						O			X	
S-4 *(Dicang)*						O	X		X	
S-7 *(Xiaguan)*				X		O				
S-8 *(Touwei)*				X		O		X		
S-30 *(Qichong)*						O				

	Governing	Bladder	Small Intestine	Gall Bladder	Triple Burner	Stomach	Large Intestine	Yang Linking	Yang Heel	Girdle
LI-14 (Binao)							O			
LI-15 (Jianyu)							O		X	
LI-16 (Jugu)							O		X	
LI-20 (Yingxiang)						X	O			

TABLE 2-12
POINTS OF INTERSECTION ON THE YIN CHANNELS

Key: "O" indicates channel of origin "X" indicates intersecting channels	Conception	Spleen	Lung	Liver	Pericardium	Kidney	Heart	Yin Linking	Yin Heel	Penetrating
Co-24 (Chengjiang)	O									
Co-23 (Lianquan)	O							X		
Co-22 (Tiantu)	O							X		
Co-13 (Shangwan)	O									
Co-12 (Zhongwan)	O									
Co-10 (Xiawan)	O	X								
Co-7 (Yinjiao)	O									X
Co-4 (Guanyuan)	O	X		X		X				
Co-3 (Zhongji)	O	X		X		X				
Co-2 (Qugu)	O			X						
Co-1 (Huiyin)	O									X
Sp-6 (Sanyinjiao)		O		X		X				

	Conception	Spleen	Lung	Liver	Pericardium	Kidney	Heart	Yin Linking	Yin Heel	Penetrating
Sp-12 *(Chongmen)*		O		X						
Sp-13 *(Fushe)*		O		X				X		
Sp-15 *(Daheng)*		O						X		
Sp-16 *(Fuai)*		O						X		
L-1 *(Zhongfu)*		X	O							
Li-13 *(Zhangmen)*				O						
Li-14 *(Qimen)*		X		O				X		
P-1 *(Tianchi)*					O					
K-11 *(Henggu)*						O				X
K-12 *(Dahe)*						O				X
K-13 *(Qixue)*						O				X
K-14 *(Siman)*						O				X
K-15 *(Zhongzhu)*						O				X
K-16 *(Huangshu)*						O				X
K-17 *(Shangqu)*						O				X
K-18 *(Shiguan)*						O				X
K-19 *(Yindu)*						O				X
K-20 *(Tonggu)*						O				X
K-21 *(Youmen)*						O				X
K-6 *(Zhaohai)*						O			X	
K-8 *(Jiaoxin)*						O			X	
K-9 *(Zhubin)*						O		X		

Editors' Preface to the Points: There follow seven chapters devoted to description of the points. Chapters 2 through 6 introduce 215 of the most commonly used points. The format of presentation is designed to provide the student with a wealth of useful information.

First, each of the points has been assigned an alphabetical abbreviation and code number in accordance with widely accepted form. The alphabetical abbreviations for points located on the channels are as follows:

L- (Lung channel points)   K- (Kidney channel points)
LI- (Large Intestine channel points)   P- (Pericardium channel points)
S- (Stomach channel points)   TB- (Triple Burner channel points)
Sp- (Spleen channel points)   GB- (Gall Bladder channel points)
H- (Heart channel points)   Li- (Liver channel points)
SI- (Small Intestine channel points)   Gv- (Governing channel points)
B- (Bladder channel points)   Co- (Conception channel points)

Each of these letters indicating a channel is followed by a number which identifies a point's sequence on the channel. For example, S-36 signifies the 36th point on the Stomach channel.

The remaining, non-channel points are either miscellaneous (M-) or new (N-). Such points have been assigned two additional letters which designate their general location on the body:

HN- (Head and Neck)
CA- (Chest and Abdomen)
BW- (Back and Waist)
UE- (Upper Extremity)
LE- (Lower Extremity)

Like the channel points, each of the new or miscellaneous points has been given a number. For example, M-HN-9 signifies the 9th miscellaneous point which is situated in the region of the head and neck.

In addition to these abbreviations, we have chosen to add the transliteration of the original Chinese name in parentheses after each point. The purpose for this is two-fold: first, for the benefit of those students (or teachers) who learned their acupuncture from Chinese sources, or who intend to pursue further studies with Chinese textbooks or with a Chinese instructor; and second, to remove any doubt about the identity of a point should it be given another abbreviation under a different numbering system. (Alternate names for the same point are cross-referenced in Appendix IV, Cross Index of Acupuncture Points. A guide to pronunciation of the *Pinyin* system of transliteration is provided in Appendix II.)

When first introduced, the Chinese characters for each point are also given, together with an English translation. Although not always the case, knowing the meaning of the point's original name provides the student with a clue to its location or therapeutic properties, and is another way to remember the point.

After the name, the location and anatomical structures in the vicinity of the point are described. This is followed by a statement of the traditional function of the point expressed in terms of Chinese patterns (e.g., 'Disperses Wind in the Liver and clears the channels').

Two sets of indications are given, the first couched in terms of Western-defined symptoms and diseases, the second according to traditional patterns of disease. (Many of the traditional terms are explained elsewhere in the text. Consult the general index.) The lists of indications are not intended to be exhaustive.

Recommended combinations or prescriptions incorporating the subject point are set out under the heading 'Illustrative combinations.' (Abbreviations of textual sources are amplified in Appendix I, Table of Abbreviated Titles.) Many other prescriptions appear in Section IV, Therapy.

Under the heading 'Needling method,' the suggested angle and depth of needle insertion is specified, followed by a brief description of the sensation generally experienced by the patient. We have chosen to delete instructions regarding the use of moxibustion at each point, as we believe the information provided in Sections III and IV is sufficient in this respect.

Chapters 7 and 8 list the remaining 540+ channel and non-channel points on the body. The description of these less frequently used points is limited to location, indications, and needling method.

The special ear, face, nose, head, hand and foot acupuncture points are described separately in Section III, chapters 7 and 8.

FOOTNOTES

1. The new points included Gv-3 *(Yaoyangguan)*, Gv-10 *(Lingtai)*, B-38 *(Gaohuangshu)*, B-14 *(Jueyinshu)*, and H-2 *(Qingling)*.

2. The new points included B-16 *(Dushu)*, B-24 *(Qihaishu)*, B-26 *(Guanyuanshu)*, GB-31 *(Fengshi)*, and B-3 *(Meichong)*.

3. The new points included Gv-7 *(Zhongshu)* and Li-12 *(Jimai)*.

4. *Simple Questions,* chapter 47.

Chapter 2

Common Points of the Head and Neck

Gv-20 *(Baihui)* 百会 "Hundred Meetings"

Location

At the intersection of the median line at the vertex of the head with a line drawn from the tip of one ear to the other. (Dia. 2-3)

Anatomy

In the galea aponeurotica, to the left and right of which are commonly found parietal foramen. Supplied by the plexus at the anastomosis of the left and right superficial temporal artery and vein; in its deep position commonly supplied by the emissary vein. Supplied by branches of the greater occipital and frontal nerves.

Traditional functions

Clears the senses and calms the Spirit, extinguishes the Liver Wind, stabilizes the ascending Yang.

Indications

Headache, dizziness, shock, hypertension, insomnia, seizures, prolapsed anus.

Traditional indications

Headache, pain at the vertex, dizziness, tinnitus, deafness, nasal congestion, stroke, locked jaw, hemiplegia, madness, prolapsed anus, prolapsed uterus, hemorrhoids.

Illustrative combinations

With Gv-16 *(Fengfu)*, Gv-14 *(Dazhui)* and LI-11 *(Quchi)* for type B infectious encephilitis; with Gv-26 *(Renzhong)*, P-6 *(Neiguan)* for shock; with M-HN-3 *(Yintang)*, M-HN-9 *(Taiyang)*, LI-4 *(Hegu)* for headache; with Gv-1 *(Changqiang)*, B-57 *(Chengshan)* for prolapsed anus; with Co-6 *(Qihai)*, M-CA-16 *(Weibao)*, S-36 *(Zusanli)* for prolapsed uterus.

Classical combinations

With Co-15 *(Jiuwei)* and Gv-1 *(Changqiang)* for prolapsed anus. (Source: OHS)

Needling method

Transverse insertion, either front to back or left to right, 0.5-1.5 units. Sensation: local distension and pain. CAUTION: Extreme care should be taken when using this point on infants whose skulls have not fully grown together, or patients with hydrocephalus.

**Dia. 2-3 Points on
Top of Head**

① Gv-20 *(Baihui)*
② B-7 *(Tongtian)*
③ Gv-23 *(Shangxing)*
④ S-8 *(Touwei)*

Remarks

Point of intersection of the Bladder channel with the Governing channel.

Gv-23 *(Shangxing)* 上星 "Upper Star"

Location

On the median line of the head, 1 unit behind the natural hairline at the forehead. (Dia. 2-3)

Anatomy

At the border between the left and right frontalis muscles. Supplied by branches of the superficial temporal and frontal arteries and veins, and by a branch of the frontal nerve.

Traditional functions

Disperses Wind Heat conditions, clears the nasal cavity.

Indications

Headache, rhinitis, nosebleed, rhinopolypus, keratitis, sore eyes.

Traditional indications

Severe headache, facial edema, extra tissue in nose, nosebleed, sinus problems, dizziness, sore eyes, myopia, febrile diseases in which there is no sweating, seizures.

Illustrative combinations

With Gv-25 *(Suliao)*, LI-20 *(Yingxiang)* for nosebleed; with LI-4 *(Hegu)*, Li-3 *(Taichong)* for rhinitis; with Gv-20 *(Baihui)*, LI-4 *(Hegu)* for headache.

Classical combinations

With GB-40 *(Qiuxu)* and S-43 *(Xiangu)* for tidal fevers. (Source: GCAM)

Needling method

Slanted insertion, 0.5-1 unit. Sensation: local distension and pain.

Remarks

Older books caution against using moxibustion at this point.

142

B-7 *(Tongtian)* 通天 "Reaching Heaven"

Location
1 unit anterior and 1.5 units lateral to Gv-20 *(Baihui)*. (Dia. 2-3)

Anatomy
In the galea aponeurotica. Supplied by the plexus at the anastomosis of the superficial temporal and occipital arteries and veins, and by a branch of the frontal nerve.

Indications
Rhinitis, headache.

Traditional indications
Congested 'runny nose', loss of sense of smell; pain and heaviness at the vertex, dizziness; mouth awry, hemiplegia.

Illustrative combinations
With Gv-23 *(Shangxing)*, M-HN-3 *(Yintang)*, LI-4 *(Hegu)* for rhinitis; with M-HN-9 *(Taiyang)*, GB-20 *(Fengchi)*, LI-4 *(Hegu)* for headache.

Classical combinations
With B-6 *(Chengguang)* for mouth awry and watery, nasal discharge. (Source: CNLAM)

Needling method
Transverse insertion, toward the front or back of the head, 0.5-1 unit. Sensation: local distension.

S-8 *(Touwei)* 头维 "Head Support"

Location
At the angle of the forehead, 4.5 units lateral to the median line of the head at the hairline. (Dia. 2-3)

Anatomy
In the galea aponeurotica on the superior margin of the temporalis muscle. Supplied by frontal branches of the superficial temporal artery and vein, and by a branch of the zygomaticotemporalis nerve and ramus of the facial nerve.

Indications
Headache, migraine headache, psychosis, facial paralysis.

Traditional indications
Sore eyes with excessive tearing, blurred vision, spasms of the eyelid; headache, wheezing accompanied by irritability and fullness in the chest.

Illustrative combinations
With LI-4 *(Hegu)* joined to SI-3 *(Houxi)*, and Li-3 *(Taichong)* joined to K-1 *(Yongquan)* for psychosis; with L-7 *(Lieque)* for migraine headaches; with GB-14 *(Yangbai)*, TB-17 *(Yifeng)*, S-4 *(Dicang)* and LI-20 *(Yingxiang)* for facial paralysis.

Classical combinations
With B-2 *(Zanzhu)* for eye tics. (Source: GCAM)

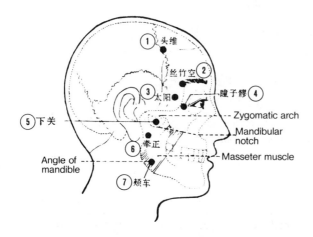

① S-8 (Touwei)
② TB-23 (Sizhukong)
③ M-HN-9 (Taiyang)
④ GB-1 (Tongziliao)
⑤ S-7 (Xiaguan)
⑥ N-HN-20 (Qianzheng)
⑦ S-6 (Jiache)

**Dia. 2-4 Points on
Side of Head**

Needling method
Transverse insertion, front to back, 0.8-1.5 units. Sensation: pain and distension extending outward from point of insertion.

Remarks
Ancient texts prohibit the use of moxibustion at this point. Point of intersection of the Gall Bladder channel with the Stomach channel.

M-HN-3 *(Yintang)*   印堂   "Seal Hall"

Location
At the midpoint between the two eyebrows. (Dia. 2-5)

Anatomy
In the procerus muscle. Supplied on either side by branches of the medial frontal artery and vein, and by a superior palpebral branch of the supratrochlearis nerve.

Traditional functions
Eliminates Wind Heat, calms the Spirit.

Indications
Headache, vertigo, rhinitis, common cold, hypertension, insomnia, infantile convulsions.

Traditional indications
Headache, dizziness, diseases of the nose, sore eyes; acute or chronic infantile convulsions; unconsciousness due to loss of blood in childbirth.

Illustrative combinations
With LI-20 *(Yingxiang)*, LI-4 *(Hegu)* for rhinitis; with M-HN-9 *(Taiyang)*, GB-20 *(Fengchi)* for headache; with LI-11 *(Quchi)*, S-40 *(Fenglong)* for hypertension; with H-7 *(Shenmen)*, Sp-6 *(Sanyinjiao)* for insomnia.

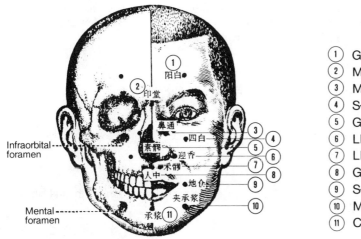

①	GB-14 *(Yangbai)*
②	M-HN-3 *(Yintang)*
③	M-HN-14 *(Bitong)*
④	S-2 *(Sibai)*
⑤	Gv-25 *(Suliao)*
⑥	LI-20 *(Yingxiang)*
⑦	LI-19 *(Heliao)*
⑧	Gv-26 *(Renzhong)*
⑨	S-4 *(Dicang)*
⑩	M-HN-18 *(Jiachengjiang)*
⑪	Co-24 *(Chengjiang)*

Dia. 2-5 Points on Face

Needling method

Transverse insertion, pointed downward (pinch the skin while inserting the needle); or point toward the left or right joined to B-2 *(Zanzhu)* or B-1 *(Jingming),* etc., 0.5-1 unit. Sensation: local distension and soreness, sometimes extending to the tip of the nose.

M-HN-9 *(Taiyang)* 太陽 "Sun"

Location

At the temple, approximately 1 unit posterior to the midpoint between the outer canthus of the eye and the tip of the eyebrow. (Dia. 2-4)

Anatomy

In the fascia temporalis and temporalis muscle. Supplied by the venous plexus within the temporalis fascia, the zygomaticoorbital and deep temporal arteries and veins. Supplied in its superficial position by the auriculotemporal and facial nerves, and in its deep position by the zygomaticotemporalis nerve.

Traditional functions

Disperses Wind in the head, cools and clears the eyes.

Indications

Headache, migraine headache, common cold, facial paralysis, trigeminal neuralgia, eye diseases.

Traditional indications

Lateral and midline headaches, sore, red and swollen eyes, sty, membrane over eye.

Illustrative combinations

With M-HN-3 *(Yintang),* LI-4 *(Hegu)* for headache or colds; with pricking the tip of ear for acute conjunctivitis; with pricking B-2 *(Zanzhu)* for inflammation of eyelid; with TB-17 *(Yifeng)* for toothache.

Needling method

(1) Straight insertion, 0.5-1 unit. Sensation: local distension and soreness. (2) Transverse insertion to treat migraine headache, point needle backward to join GB-8 *(Shuaigu),* 1-2 units. Sensation: distension and soreness extending throughout the temple. (3) Transverse insertion, to treat facial

145

paralysis, point needle downward to join with S-6 *(Jiache),* 3 units. Sensation: distension and soreness, possibly extending as far as the tongue. (4) The point can be pricked for a few drops of blood when treating either acute conjunctivitis or headache.

GB-14 *(Yangbai)*　陽白　"Yang White"

Location
1 unit above the middle of the eyebrow on a line directly above the pupil of the eye, in the depression on the superciliary arch. (Dia. 2-5)

Anatomy
In the frontalis muscle. Supplied by lateral branches of the frontal artery and vein, and situated directly on a lateral branch of the frontal nerve.

Traditional functions
Eliminates Wind, clears the vision.

Indications
Supraorbital neuralgia, facial paralysis, ptosis, eye diseases.

Traditional indications
Headache, sore eyes, eyelid tic, night blindness, itching eyelids; vomiting, chills, stiff neck.

Illustrative combinations
With B-2 *(Zanzhu),* LI-4 *(Hegu)* and K-7 *(Fuliu)* for diplopia; with M-HN-9 *(Taiyang),* S-8 *(Touwei),* GB-20 *(Fengchi)* for ptosis; with S-2 *(Sibai),* N-HN-20 *(Qianzheng),* and S-4 *(Dicang)* for facial paralysis.

Needling method
Transverse insertion, pointed downward, may join to M-HN-6 *(Yuyao).* For facial paralysis the needle may be pointed left or right, joining with B-2 *(Zanzhu)* or TB-23 *(Sizhukong),* 1-1.5 units. Sensation: distension in the forehead, sometimes extending to the vertex.

Remarks
Point of intersection of the Stomach and Yang Linking channels with the Gall Bladder channel.

M-HN-6 *(Yuyao)*　鱼腰　"Fish Waist"

Location
In the hollow at the middle of the eyebrow, directly above the pupil of the eye. (Dia. 2-6)

Anatomy
In the orbicularis oculi muscle. Supplied by lateral branches of the frontal artery and vein, and situated directly on a lateral branch of the frontal nerve.

Indications
Myopia, acute conjunctivitis, ophthalmoplegia, facial paralysis, supraorbital neuralgia.

Illustrative combinations
With LI-4 *(Hegu)* for myopia; with B-2 *(Zanzhu),* TB-9 *(Sidu),* P-6 *(Neiguan)* for supraorbital neuralgia; with GB-1 *(Tongziliao),* B-2 *(Zanzhu)* and B-1 *(Jingming)* for cataracts.

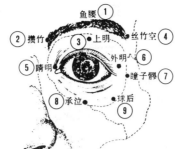

① M-HN-6 *(Yuyao)*
② B-2 *(Zanzhu)*
③ N-HN-4 *(Shangming)*
④ TB-23 *(Sizhukong)*

⑤ B-1 *(Jingming)*
⑥ N-HN-6 *(Waiming)*
⑦ GB-1 *(Tongziliao)*
⑧ S-1 *(Chengqi)*
⑨ M-HN-8 *(Qiuhou)*

Dia. 2-6 Points in Vicinity of Eye

Needling method

Transverse insertion for supraorbital neuralgia, direct needle toward either side; may also be joined to B-2 *(Zanzhu)* or TB-23 *(Sizhukong)*, 0.5-1 unit. Sensation: local distension and soreness, sometimes extending to the eyeball.

B-2 *(Zanzhu)*   攒竹   "Gathered Bamboo"

Location

In the hollow at the medial end of the eyebrow, in the supraorbital notch. (Dia. 2-6)

Anatomy

In the frontalis and corrugator supercillii muscles. Supplied by the frontal artery and vein, and by a medial branch of the frontal nerve.

Indications

Headache, myopia, acute conjunctivitis, keratoleukoma, excessive lacrimation, spasms of the eyelid, facial paralysis.

Traditional indications

Cold and Hot headaches, headache in the area around the eyebrows, eyes red, swollen and sore, dizziness, excessive tearing; insanity; infantile convulsions.

Illustrative combinations

With GB-20 *(Fengchi)*, LI-4 *(Hegu)* and joined to M-HN-6 *(Yuyao)* for frontal headache; with M-HN-9 *(Taiyang)*, GB-20 *(Fengchi)*, LI-4 *(Hegu)* for acute conjunctivitis; with S-2 *(Sibai)*, Co-24 *(Chengjiang)* for facial muscle spasm; with M-HN-7 *(Yuwei)*, LI-14 *(Binao)* for sore eyes; with M-HN-13 *(Yiming)*, B-1 *(Jingming)* and S-36 *(Zusanli)* for opacity of the vitreous body.

Classical combinations

With S-8 *(Touwei)* for painful eyes. (Source: OSM)

Needling method

(1) Straight insertion, 0.3-0.5 unit. Sensation: local distension. (2) For eye diseases, the needle may be inserted at a slant and joined to B-1 *(Jingming)*, 0.5-1 unit. Sensation: distension and pain locally and around the eye. (3) For headache or facial paralysis, the needle should be transversally inserted and joined to M-HN-6 *(Yuyao)*, 1-1.5 units. Sensation: distension and pain locally and around the eye. (4) For supraorbital neuralgia insert needle transversely toward the inner canthus, 0.5 unit. Sensation: possibly an electric, numb sensation extending toward the neck.

Remarks

Ancient books prohibit the use of moxibustion at this point.

TB-23 *(Sizhukong)* 丝竹空 "Silken Bamboo Hollow"

Location

In the depression at the lateral end of the eyebrow. (Dia. 2-6)

Anatomy

On the lateral border of the zygomatic process of the frontal bone, in the orbicularis oculi muscle. Supplied by frontal branches of the superficial temporal artery and vein, and by a zygomaticotemporalis nerve.

Indictions

Headache, eye diseases, facial paralysis.

Traditional indications

Lateral and midline headaches, reddened eyes, vertigo, ingrown eyelash, blurred vision, seizures, insanity.

Illustrative combinations

With TB-3 *(Zhongzhu)*, GB-20 *(Fengchi)* for migraine headache; with B-2 *(Zanzhu)*, S-2 *(Sibai)*, S-4 *(Dicang)* for facial paralysis.

Classical combinations

With B-2 *(Zanzhu)* for red, swollen eyes. (Source: SGJ)

Needling method

Transverse insertion, directed either posteriorly or toward M-HN-6 *(Yuyao)*, 0.5-1 unit. Sensation: local distension.

Remarks

Ancient books prohibit the use of moxibustion at this point.

B-1 *(Jingming)* 睛明 "Eyes Bright"

Location

0.1 unit above the inner canthus of the eye. (Dia. 2-6)

Anatomy

In the medial palpebral ligament; at its deep position in the rectus medialis bulbi. Supplied by the medial angular artery and vein and the supratrochlear and infratrochlear arteries and veins; at its deep position, and above the point, by the ophthalmic artery and vein. Supplied by the supratrochlearis and infratrochlearis nerves, in its deep position by a branch of the ophthalmic nerve, and above the point by the nasociliary nerve.

Traditional functions

Disperses Wind, cools Heat, opens the channels and clears the vision.

Indications

Acute and chronic conjunctivitis, myopia, hypermetropia, astigmatism, color blindness, night blindness, atrophy of the optic nerve, optic neuritis, inflammation of the ora serrata, glaucoma, early stages of cataract, keratoleukoma, pterygium.

Traditional Indications

Red and sore eyes, polypus extending into the eye, excessive tearing on exposure to wind, glaucoma, opacity of cornea, obstructive membranes inside or outside the eye.

Illustrative combinations

With M-HN-8 *(Qiuhou)*, M-HN-9 *(Taiyang)*, M-HN-13 *(Yiming)*, SI-1 *(Shaoze)*, LI-4 *(Hegu)* for cataracts or keratoleukoma; with SI-1 *(Shaoze)*, M-HN-9 *(Taiyang)*, LI-4 *(Hegu)* for pterygium; with M-HN-8 *(Qiuhou)*, GB-20 *(Fengchi)*, Li-3 *(Taichong)* for glaucoma; with LI-4 *(Hegu)*, S-36 *(Zusanli)*, and GB-37 *(Guangming)* for atrophy of optic nerve.

Classical combinations

With M-HN-9 *(Taiyang)* and M-HN-7 *(Yuwei)* for eye disorders. (Source: SJD)

Needling method

Straight insertion. After instructing the patient to close the eyes, gently push the eyeball laterally and away from the point, where it is held with one finger. The needle is then slowly inserted, with a minimum of agitation or twirling, between the orbit and the nose to a depth of 1-1.5 units. Sensation: local distension and soreness, extending both behind and around the eyeball. CAUTION: It is very common for this point to bleed a bit after needling. This can be stopped by applying pressure for a few moments after the needle is withdrawn. When there is bleeding, there may appear a 'purpling' of the skin around the eye. For this reason a cold compress can be used first, to stop the bleeding, followed by a hot compress. After a week, the purple should disappear; in any event, it will not affect the vision. Care should be taken not to insert the needle too deeply, to avoid entering the cranial cavity.

Remarks

Older books prohibit moxibustion at this point. B-1 *(Jingming)* is the point of intersection of the Stomach, Triple Burner, Yang and Yin Heel channels at the Bladder channel.

S-1 *(Chengqi)*   承泣   "Contain Tears"

Location

Directly below the pupil of the eye, between the inferior border of the orbit and the eyeball. (Dia. 2-6)

Anatomy

Above the inferior border of the orbit, in the orbicularis oculi muscle; in its deep position within the orbit are the rectus inferior bulbi and obliquus inferior bulbi muscles. Supplied by branches of the infraorbital and ophthalmic arteries and veins. Supplied by a branch of the infraorbital nerve, and an inferior, muscle branch of the oculomotor nerve.

Indications

Acute and chronic conjunctivitis, myopia, hypermetropia, astigmatism, convergent squint (esotropia), color blindness, night blindness, glaucoma, inflammation or atrophy of the optic nerve, cataract, keratitis, retinitis pigmentosa.

Traditional indications

Eyes red and sore, excessive tearing, opacity of cornea, myopia, eyelid tic, mouth and eyes awry.

Illustrative combinations

With B-1 *(Jingming)*, GB-20 *(Fengchi)*, LI-4 *(Hegu)*, S-36 *(Zusanli)*, B-18 *(Ganshu)*, B-23 *(Shenshu)* for optic nerve atrophy; join with B-1 *(Jingming)* by transverse insertion for myopia; with N-HN-3 *(Jianming)*, N-BW-12 *(Jianming #5)*, GB-20 *(Fengchi)*, B-20 *(Pishu)*, B-23 *(Shenshu)*, B-18 *(Ganshu)* for retinitis pigmentosa.

Needling method

Straight insertion. Ask the patient to look upward, then hold the eyeball secure from below with a finger, and slowly insert the needle along the lower wall of the orbit to a depth of 1-1.5 units. (Dia. 2-7) For myopia, the needle should be inserted transverely toward the inner canthus. Sensation: local distension and soreness, occasionally some lacrimation. CAUTION: See note under B-1 *(Jingming)*.

Remarks
Older books prohibit moxibustion at this point. S-1 *(Chengqi)* is the point of intersection of the Yang Heel and Conception channels at the Stomach channel.

M-HN-8 (Qiuhou)　球后　"Behind the Ball"

Location
At the inferior border of the orbit, approximately one-fourth the distance from the lateral to the medial side of the orbit. (Dia. 2-6)

Anatomy
At the lateral, inferior side of the inferior tarsus, in the orbicularis oculi muscle. In its deep position supplied by the infraorbital artery and vein, and by the infraorbital nerve. In its superficial position supplied by a branch of the facial nerve and by the ramus zygomaticofacialis.

Indications
Myopia, inflammation or atrophy of the optic nerve, glaucoma, retinitis pigmentosa, opacity of the vitreous body, convergent squint (esotropia).

Illustrative combinations
With B-1 *(Jingming)*, GB-20 *(Fengchi)*, SI-6 *(Yanglao)*, GB-37 *(Guangming)* for inflammation of the optic nerve.

Needling method
Straight insertion. Ask the patient to look upward, then secure eyeball in place from below with a finger, and slowly insert the needle in a slightly medial and upward direction toward the optic nerve, 1.5-2 units. Sensation: distension and soreness throughout the eye, and a protruding sensation. CAUTION: See note under B-1 *(Jingming)*.

N-HN-4 (Shangming)　上明　"Upper Brightness"

Location
Directly below the midpoint of the arch of the eyebrow, just under the superior border of the orbit. (Dia. 2-6)

Anatomy
At the superior aspect of the superior tarsus, in the orbicularis oculi muscle; in its deep position in the levator palpebrae superioris and rectus superior bulbi muscles. Supplied by branches of the supraorbital artery and vein, and by the frontal and oculomotor nerves.

Indications
Ametropia, keratoleukoma, atrophy of the optic nerve.

Illustrative combinations
With M-HN-8 *(Qiuhou)*, N-HN-1 *(Shangjingming)* and LI-4 *(Hegu)* for keratoleukoma; with N-HN-3(a) *(Jianming #1)*, N-HN-3(b) *(Jianming #2)*, GB-20 *(Fengchi)*, GB-37 *(Guangming)* and S-36 *(Zusanli)* for atrophy of optic nerve.

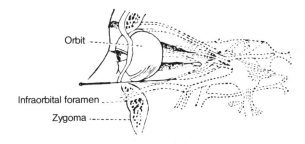

**Dia. 2-7 Direction of Needle
Insertion at S-1 *(Chengqi)***

Needling method

Straight insertion, along the superior border of the orbit, 1-1.5 units. Sensation: distension around the eyeball.

N-HN-6 *(Waiming)*　外明　"Outer Brightness"

Location

Approximately 0.3 unit above the outer canthus of the eye. (Dia. 2-6)

Anatomy

At the superior aspect of the superior tarsus, in the orbicularis oculi muscle; in its deep position are the lacrimal gland and the rectus lateralis bulbi. Supplied by the lacrimal artery and vein, and by the lacrimal nerve.

Indications

Same as N-HN-4 *(Shangming)* above.

Illustrative combinations

Same as N-HN-4 *(Shangming)* above.

Needling method

Same as N-HN-4 *(Shangming)* above. Sensation: local distension and soreness.

GB-1 *(Tongziliao)*　瞳子髎　"Pupil Seam"

Location

Approximately 0.5 unit lateral to the outer canthus of the eye. (Dia. 2-6)

Anatomy

In the orbicularis oculi muscle, and in its deep position, in the temporalis muscle. Supplied by the zygomaticoorbital artery and vein. Supplied by the zygomaticofacialis nerve, the zygomaticotemporalis nerve, and temporal and frontal branches of the facial nerve.

Indications

Headache, keratitis, ametropia, night blindness, atrophy of the optic nerve.

151

Traditional indications
Glaucoma, membranes over the eye, excessive tearing, headache, sore throat.

Illustrative combinations
With N-HN-4 *(Shangming)*, LI-4 *(Hegu)* for ametropia; with B-1 *(Jingming)*, SI-6 *(Yanglao)*, S-36 *(Zusanli)* for night blindness; with B-2 *(Zanzhu)*, GB-20 *(Fengchi)*, GB-38 *(Yangfu)* for headache.

Classical combinations
With GB-40 *(Qiuxu)* for membrane on the eye. (Source: CNLAM)

Needling method
Transverse insertion directed toward M-HN-9 *(Taiyang)*, 0.5-1 unit. Sensation: local distension, sometimes extending to the ear canal.

Remarks
Point of intersection of the Small Intestine and Triple Burner channels at the Gall Bladder channel.

S-2 *(Sibai)*   四白   "Four Whites"

Location
Approximately 1 unit directly below the pupil of the eye, at the infraorbital foramen. (Dia. 2-5)

Anatomy
At the infraorbital foramen, between the orbicularis oculi and quadratus labii superioris muscles. Supplied by branches of the facial and infraorbital arteries and veins. Supplied by a branch of the facial nerve, and situated directly on the infraorbital nerve.

Traditional functions
Eliminates Wind, clears the vision, spreads the Liver Qi, and benefits the Gall Bladder.

Indications
Facial paralysis or spasms, trigeminal neuralgia, keratitis, myopia, sinusitis, round worms in the bile duct, allergic facial swelling.

Traditional indications
Eyes red and sore, membrane over the eye; headache, dizziness; mouth and eyes awry.

Illustrative combinations
With M-LE-23 *(Dannangxue)*, S-25 *(Tianshu)*, Co-4 *(Guanyuan)* for round worm in the bile duct; with S-4 *(Dicang)*, GB-20 *(Fengchi)*, LI-4 *(Hegu)* for facial paralysis.

Needling method
(1) Straight insertion, 0.3-0.8 unit, or transverse insertion, 0.8-1 unit. Sensation: local distension and soreness. (2) For trigeminal neuralgia, the needle may be inserted from below in a lateral, upward direction, 0.3-0.5 unit, entering the infraorbital foramen. Sensation: possibly a numb, electric sensation extending to the upper lip. CAUTION: When needling upward, care must be taken not to penetrate too deeply, to avoid puncturing the eyeball.

Remarks
Older books prohibit moxibustion at this point.

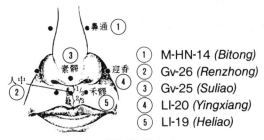

① M-HN-14 *(Bitong)*
② Gv-26 *(Renzhong)*
③ Gv-25 *(Suliao)*
④ LI-20 *(Yingxiang)*
⑤ LI-19 *(Heliao)*

**Dia. 2-8 Points in
Vicinity of Nose**

Gv-25 *(Suliao)*　素髎　"Plain Seam"

Location

At the center of the tip of the nose. (Dia. 2-8)

Anatomy

In the nasal cartilage at the tip of the nose. Supplied by branches of the facial artery and vein on the dorsal side of the nose, and by a lateral nasal branch of the anterior ethmoidal nerve.

Traditional functions

Raises the Yang and restores the Qi, clears the senses and drains Heat.

Indications

Shock, low blood pressure, bradycardia, brandy nose, nosebleed, rhinitis.

Traditional indications

Extra tissue in nose, runny nose, infantile convulsions.

Illustrative combinations

With P-6 *(Neiguan)*, S-36 *(Zusanli)* for septic shock; with N-HN-23 *(Xingfen)*, P-6 *(Neiguan)* for bradycardia or low blood pressure; with LI-20 *(Yingxiang)*, LI-4 *(Hegu)* for brandy nose; with Gv-23 *(Shangxing)*, LI-20 *(Yingxiang)* for nosebleed; with P-6 *(Neiguan)* and K-1 *(Yongquan)* for electrical shock.

Needling method

Slanted insertion, from the tip of the nose upward, 0.5-1 unit. Sensation: soreness and numbness extending throughout the nose.

LI-20 *(Yingxiang)*　迎香　"Welcome Fragrance"

Location

0.5 unit lateral to the nostril, in the nasolabial sulcus. (Dia. 2-8)

Anatomy

At the center of the nasolabial sulcus on the lateral margin of the ala nasi, in the quadratus labii superioris muscle; in its deep position at the border of the apertura piriformis. Supplied by branches of the facial and infraorbital arteries and veins, and by the nerve plexus at the anastomosis of the facial and infraorbital nerves.

153

Traditional functions
Opens the nasal passages, disperses Wind Heat conditions.

Indications
Rhinitis, nasosinusitis, facial paralysis, round worm in the bile duct.

Traditional indications
Nosebleed, tissue in nose, runny nose, inability to distinguish odors, facial swelling and itching, mouth and eyes awry.

Illustrative combinations
Join to S-2 *(Sibai)* with Gv-26 *(Renzhong)*, M-LE-23 *(Dannangxue)*, S-36 *(Zusanli)*, Co-12 *(Zhongwan)* for round worm in bile duct; with Gv-23 *(Shangxing)*, LI-20 *(Yingxiang)* joined to M-HN-14 *(Bitong)*, with LI-11 *(Quchi)*, LI-4 *(Hegu)* for nasosinusitis.

Classical combinations
With LI-4 *(Hegu)* for itchy, swollen face. (Source: GCAM)

Needling method
For round worm of the bile duct, transverse insertion joined to S-2 *(Sibai)*, 0.5-1 unit; for diseases of the nose, join to M-HN-14 *(Bitong)*, 0.5-0.8 unit. Sensation: local distension and soreness, lacrimation; sometimes sensation extends throughout the nose.

Remarks
Older books prohibit moxibustion. Point of intersection of the Stomach channel at the Large Intestine channel.

LI-19 *(Heliao)* 禾髎 "Grain Seam"

Location
Directly below the lateral margin of the nostril, level with Gv-26 *(Renzhong)*. (Dia. 2-8)

Anatomy
In the fossa canina of the superior maxilla, at the insertion of the quadratus labii superioris muscle. Supplied by superior labium branches of the facial artery and vein, and by the nerve plexus at the anastomosis of the facial and infraorbital nerves.

Indications
Rhinitis, nose bleed, facial paralysis.

Traditional indications
Ulceration of the nose, extra tissue in the nose, nosebleed, "locked" jaw.

Illustrative combinations
With N-HN-20 *(Qianzheng)*, S-4 *(Dicang)*, S-2 *(Sibai)*, GB-14 *(Yangbai)* for facial paralysis; with M-HN-3 *(Yintang)*, L-7 *(Lieque)* for nosebleed.

Needling method
Transverse insertion, directed medially, 0.3-0.5 unit. Sensation: local pain.

Remarks
Older books prohibit moxibustion.

M-HN-14 *(Bitong)*　鼻通　"Nose Passage"

Location

In the depression below the nasal bone, at the superior end of the nasolabial sulcus. (Dia. 2-5, 2-8)

Anatomy

At the lateral, inferior side of the nasal bone and dorsal nasal cartilage, in the quadratus labii superioris muscle. Supplied by branches of the facial artery and vein, and by the anterior ethmoidal nerve, the infratrochlearis nerve, and a branch of the infraorbital nerve.

Indications

Allergic rhinitis, hypertrophic rhinitis, atrophic rhinitis, rhinopolypus, nasosinusitis.

Illustrative combinations

With Gv-23 *(Shangxing)*, M-HN-3 *(Yintang)*, LI-4 *(Hegu)* for chronic rhinitis; with B-2 *(Zanzhu)*, L-7 *(Lieque)* for nasosinusitis.

Needling method

Transverse insertion, directed upward toward the nose, 0.5-0.8 unit. Sensation: local distension and soreness, sometimes extending to the nasofrontal region.

S-7 *(Xiaguan)*　下关　"Lower Hinge"

Location

With the mouth closed, in the hollow formed between the zygomatic arch and the mandibular notch. (Dia. 2-4)

Anatomy

At the inferior margin of the zygomatic arch, below which is the parotid gland, and in the origin of the masseter muscle. Supplied by the facial artery and vein, and in its deepest position by the maxillary artery and vein. Situated directly on a zygomaticoorbital branch of the facial nerve and a branch of the auriculotemporal nerve; in its deepest position supplied by the mandibular nerve.

Indications

Toothache, temporomandibular arthritis, spasms of the masseter muscle, facial paralysis, trigeminal neuralgia, otitis media, deaf-mutism.

Traditional indications

Toothache, tinnitus, earache, pus in the ear, deafness, dislocated jaw, mouth and eyes awry.

Illustrative combinations

With LI-4 *(Hegu)* for temporomandibular arthritis; with S-6 *(Jiache)*, TB-17 *(Yifeng)* for spasms of masseter muscle; with TB-21 *(Ermen)*, TB-17 *(Yifeng)*, TB-3 *(Zhongzhu)* for deaf-mutism.

Needling method

(1) Straight insertion, for trigeminal neuralgia, needle pointed slightly downward, 1.5 units. Sensation: distension and soreness in the vicinity of the point, or an electric, numb sensation extending to the lower gums. (2) Slanted insertion, for temporomandibular arthritis, needle directed either backward or forward, 0.8-1 unit. Sensation: distension and soreness extending throughout the jaw. (3) Transverse insertion, for toothache, needle directed toward either the upper or lower teeth (in the direction of S-6 *(Jiache)*, 1.5-2 units. Sensation: distension and soreness extending to the upper and lower teeth. (4) Slanted insertion, for ear diseases, directed toward the ear, 1.5 units. Sensation: distension and soreness possibly extending into the ear. (5) Slanted insertion, for spasms of the masseter muscle, needle directed downward, 1.5-2 units. Sensation: local distension and soreness.

N-HN-20 *(Qianzheng)*　牵正　"Pull Aright"

Location

0.5-1 unit anterior to the earlobe. (Dia. 2-4)

Anatomy

In the masseter muscle, under which is the parotid gland. Situated directly on the buccal branch of the facial nerve. Above and anterior to the point is a parotid duct. In its deep position supplied by branches of the masseteric artery and vein, and by the masseteric nerve.

Indications

Facial paralysis, parotitis, ulcers in the mouth.

Illustrative combinations

With S-4 *(Dicang)*, GB-20 *(Fengchi)*, GB-14 *(Yangbai)* for facial paralysis; with TB-17 *(Yifeng)*, LI-4 *(Hegu)* for parotitis; with Co-24 *(Chengjiang)*, Gv-28 *(Yinjiao)*, S-4 *(Dicang)*, LI-4 *(Hegu)* for ulcers in the mouth.

Needling method

Slanted insertion, needle directed forward, 0.5-1 unit. Sensation: local distension and soreness, sometimes extending throughout the cheek.

S-6 *(Jiache)*　頰车　"Jaw Vehicle"

Location

Approximately 1 finger width above and anterior to the angle of the mandible, at the prominence of the masseter muscle when teeth are clenched. (Dia. 2-4)

Anatomy

In the masseter muscle. Supplied by the masseteric artery and vein, and by the great auricular, facial and masseteric nerves.

Traditional functions

Disperses Wind and opens the channels, benefits the teeth and jaws.

Indications

Toothache, parotitis, temperomandibular arthritis, spasm of the masseter muscle, facial paralysis.

Traditional indications

Toothache, "locked" jaw, mouth and eyes awry, stiff neck.

Illustrative combinations

With N-UE-1 *(Yatong)*, S-7 *(Xiaguan)*, LI-4 *(Hegu)*, S-44 *(Neiting)* for toothache; with TB-17 *(Yifeng)*, LI-4 *(Hegu)* for acute parotitis.

Classical combinations

With Co-24 *(Chengjiang)* and LI-4 *(Hegu)* for locked jaw. (Source: GCAM)

Needling method

(1) Straight insertion, 0.5 unit. Sensation: local distension and soreness. (2) Transverse insertion, for facial paralysis, join to S-4 *(Dicang)*, 2-3 units. Sensation: local distension and soreness extending around the point. (3) For spasm of the masseter muscle, direct the needle upward. (4) For toothache in the upper or lower jaw, direct the needle toward the upper or lower teeth, respectively.

S-4 *(Dicang)* 地仓 "Earth Granary"

Location
0.4 unit lateral to the corner of the mouth. (Dia. 2-5)

Anatomy
In the orbicularis oris muscle, and in its deep position in the buccinator muscle. Supplied by the facial artery and vein, and by branches of the facial and infraorbital nerves; in its deep position, supplied by a terminal branch of the buccal nerve.

Indications
Facial paralysis, trigeminal neuralgia, excessive salivation, spasm of the eyelid.

Traditional indications
Mouth and eyes awry, muteness, drooling, eye tic.

Illustrative combinations
With M-HN-6 *(Yuyao)*, S-2 *(Sibai)* for trigeminal neuralgia; with S-6 *(Jiache)*, LI-20 *(Yingxiang)*, LI-4 *(Hegu)* for facial paralysis; with Co-24 *(Chengjiang)*, LI-4 *(Hegu)* for excessive salivation.

Needling method
Transverse insertion. For facial paralysis, this point may be joined to S-6 *(Jiache)*, 1.5-2.5 units. For trigeminal neuralgia, join to LI-20 *(Yingxiang)*, 1-2 units. Sensation: distension and soreness or pain, either locally or throughout the side of the face.

Remarks
Point of intersection of the Yang Heel and Large Intestine channels on the Stomach channel.

Gv-26 *(Renzhong)* 人中 "Philtrum"

Location
In the philtrum, approximately 1/3 the distance from the bottom of the nose to the top of the lip. (Dia. 2-8)

Anatomy
In the philtrum, in the orbicularis oris muscle. Supplied by a buccal branch of the facial nerve and a branch of the infraorbital nerve.

Traditional functions
Clears the senses and cools Heat, calms the Spirit, benefits the lumbar spine.

Indications
Shock, coma, heat exhaustion, seizures, hysteria, psychosis, motion sickness, acute lower back sprain, facial edema, nose diseases, halitosis, spasm of the muscles in the region of the mouth or eyes.

Traditional indications
Apoplectic locked jaw, unconsciousness, convulsions, seizures and insanity; mouth and eyes awry, facial edema, lip tremor, emaciation and thirst, even after drinking, jaundice, edema, twisting pain in the vicinity of the heart and abdomen.

Illustrative combinations
With P-6 *(Neiguan)*, K-1 *(Yongquan)*, S-36 *(Zusanli)* for septic shock; with Co-1 *(Huiyin)*, P-9

157

(Zhongchong) for revival from drowning; with LI-4 *(Hegu)* joined to P-8 *(Laogong)* for hysteria; with B-54 *(Weizhong)* for lower back sprain; with M-UE-1 *(Shixuan)*, K-1 *(Yongquan)*, B-54 *(Weizhong)* for heat exhaustion.

Classical combinations

With P-9 *(Zhongchong)*, LI-4 *(Hegu)* for apoplexy with unconsciousness (Source: GCAM); with Gv-21 *(Qianding)* for Deficient floating facial edema (Source: OHS); with B-54 *(Weizhong)* for pain in the lumbar spine. (Source: SJD)

Needling method

(1) Transverse insertion, directed upward, 0.5-1 unit. Sensation: local pain, possibly distension. (2) For excessive salivation, first insert the needle upward toward the septum of the nose, then withdraw slightly (keeping the needle under the skin) and direct first toward one of the nostrils, then the other. Sensation: local distension and pain.

Remarks

Point of intersection of the Stomach and Large Intestine channels on the Governing channel.

Co-24 *(Chengjiang)* 承浆 "Contain Fluid"

Location

On the chin in the depression below the middle of the lower lip. (Dia. 2-5)

Anatomy

Between the orbicularis oris and mentalis muscles. Supplied by branches of the inferior labial artery and vein, and by branches of the facial and mental nerves.

Indications

Facial paralysis, hemiplegia, toothache, ulcers in the mouth, excessive salivation.

Traditional indications

Mouth and eyes awry, facial edema, emaciation and thirst, hemiplegia.

Illustrative combinations

With LI-19 *(Heliao)*, N-HN-20 *(Qianzheng)*, GB-20 *(Fengchi)* for facial paralysis; with S-4 *(Dicang)*, S-45 *(Lidui)* for fever blisters on lip and mouth; with Gv-16 *(Fengfu)* for stiff neck.

Classical combinations

With Gv-16 *(Fengfu)* for headache and stiff neck. (Source: GCAM)

Needling method

Slanted insertion, directed upward, 0.3-0.5 unit. Sensation: local distension and pain.

Remarks

Point of intersection of the Large Intestine, Stomach and Governing channels on the Conception channel.

M-HN-18 *(Jiachengjiang)* 夹承浆 "Grasping 'Contain Fluid'"

Location

1 unit lateral to Co-24 *(Chengjiang)*, directly below S-4 *(Dicang)*, under which can be felt the mental foramen of the mandible. (Dia. 2-5)

Anatomy

In the orbicularis oris and quadratus labii inferioris muscles. Supplied by branches of the facial and mental arteries, veins and nerves.

Indications

Trigeminal neuralgia, facial paralysis or spasm.

Illustrative combinations

With B-2 *(Zanzhu),* S-2 *(Sibai)* for facial spasm; with S-7 *(Xiaguan),* LI-4 *(Hegu)* for trigeminal neuralgia.

Needling method

(1) Straight insertion, 0.2-0.5 unit. Sensation: local distension and soreness. (2) For trigeminal neuralgia, after finding the mental foramen in the mandible, slanted insertion in a medial, downward direction, 0.5 unit. Sensation: electric, numb sensation extending to the lower lip.

TB-21 *(Ermen)*   耳门   "Ear's Door"

Location

At the front of the tuberculum supratragicum, in the depression formed when the mouth is opened. (Dia. 2-9)

Anatomy

Supplied by the superficial temporal artery and vein at the inferior margin of the zygomatic arch, and by the auriculotemporal nerve and a branch of the facial nerve.

Traditional functions

Opens the ear, disperses Heat.

Indications

Tinnitus, deafness, deaf-mutism, otitis media, toothache, temperomandibular arthritis.

Traditional indications

Tinnitus, deafness, pus in the ear, toothache in the upper jaw, pain in the jaw and headache.

Illustrative combinations

Join to SI-19 *(Tinggong)* and GB-2 *(Tinghui),* also with TB-17 *(Yifeng)* and TB-3 *(Zhongzhu)* for deafness; with N-HN-15 *(Yilong),* N-LE-16 *(Zuyicong)* and other points for deaf-mutism; with TB-17 *(Yifeng),* LI-4 *(Hegu)* for otitis media.

Classical combinations

With TB-23 *(Sizhukong)* for headache (Source: OHS); with TB-17 *(Yifeng)* and LI-4 *(Hegu)* for pressure ear. (Source: GCAM)

Needling method

With the mouth open, join below to SI-19 *(Tinggong)* and GB-2 *(Tinghui),* 1.5-2.5 units. Sensation: local distension and soreness, sometimes extending throughout the side of the face.

Remarks

Ancient books prohibit the use of moxibustion when treating patients with pus in the ear.

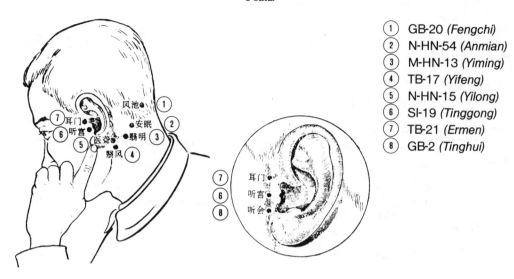

① GB-20 *(Fengchi)*
② N-HN-54 *(Anmian)*
③ M-HN-13 *(Yiming)*
④ TB-17 *(Yifeng)*
⑤ N-HN-15 *(Yilong)*
⑥ SI-19 *(Tinggong)*
⑦ TB-21 *(Ermen)*
⑧ GB-2 *(Tinghui)*

Dia. 2-9 Points in Vicinity of Ear

SI-19 *(Tinggong)*   听宫   "Palace of Hearing"

Location
In the depression anterior to the middle of the tragus of the ear when the mouth is open. (Dia. 2-9)

Anatomy
At the anterior margin of the tragus, and the posterior margin of the condyle of the mandible. Supplied by anterior aural branches of the superficial temporal artery and vein, and by branches of the facial and auriculotemporal nerves.

Indications
Tinnitus, deafness, deaf-mutism, otitis media, inflammation of the external ear canal.

Traditional indications
Seizures and insanity; tinnitus, deafness, pus in the ear, toothache, pain in the chest and abdomen.

Illustrative combinations
With TB-17 *(Yifeng)*, LI-4 *(Hegu)* for otitis media; with GB-2 *(Tinghui)*, TB-17 *(Yifeng)*, TB-7 *(Huizong)* for deafness.

Needling method
Straight insertion with mouth open, direct needle slightly downward, 1.5-2 units. Sensation: local distension and soreness, possibly extending throughout the side of the face; sometimes a distended sensation in the eardrum, expanding outward.

Remarks
Point of intersection of the Triple Burner and Gall Bladder channels on the Small Intestine channel.

160

GB-2 *(Tinghui)* 听会 "Confluence of Hearing"

Location
In the depression anterior to the intertragic notch of the ear, below SI-19 *(Tinggong).* (Dia. 2-9)

Anatomy
Supplied by an anterior aural branch of the superficial temporal artery, and in its deep position by the external carotid artery and posterior facial vein. Supplied by the great auricular nerve and a branch of the facial nerve.

Indications
Tinnitus, deafness, otitis media, deaf-mutism, toothache, facial paralysis.

Traditional indications
Mouth and eyes awry, hemiplegia, madly running away, seizure in which the body is alternately tense and limp, dislocation of the jaw, swelling of the parotid glands, tinnitus, deafness, toothache.

Illustrative combinations
With N-HN-11 *(Tingmin),* N-HN-17 *(Chiqian)* for deafness; with S-6 *(Jiache),* S-4 *(Dicang)* for apoplectic facial paralysis.

Classical combinations
With TB-4 *(Yangchi)* for deafness. (Source: OSM)

Needling method
Straight insertion with mouth open, direct needle slightly backward, 1-1.5 units. Sensation: local distension and soreness.

TB-17 *(Yifeng)* 翳风 "Shielding Wind"

Location
In the depression between the mastoid process and the mandible, behind the earlobe. (Dia. 2-9)

Anatomy
Supplied by the posterior auricular artery and the superficial external jugular vein, and by the great auricular nerve; in its deep position supplied by the trunk of the facial nerve where it emerges from the stylomastoid foramen.

Traditional functions
Benefits hearing and vision, disperses Wind and clears the channels.

Indications
Tinnitus, deafness, deaf-mutism, parotitis, temporomandibular arthritis, toothache, sore eyes, facial paralysis.

Traditional indications
Tinnitus, deafness, swelling in the cheeks, convulsions (generally with headache and an arched and rigid back), mouth and eyes awry, locked jaw, blurred vision, membrane over the eye.

Illustrative combinations
With S-6 *(Jiache),* LI-4 *(Hegu)* for parotitis; with S-7 *(Xiaguan)* for temporomandibular arthritis; with N-HN-20 *(Qianzheng),* S-4 *(Dicang),* LI-20 *(Yingxiang)* for facial paralysis; with SI-19 *(Tinggong),* N-HN-10 *(Tingcong),* N-HN-8 *(Tingxue)* for tinnitus.

Classical combinations
With H-5 *(Tongli)* for sudden loss of voice. (Source: CNLAM)

Needling method
(1) Slanted insertion, for deaf-mutism, needle pointed in a medial, downward direction, 1.5-2 units. Sensation: local distension and soreness, sometimes extending toward the pharynx causing a constricted, hot feeling. (2) Straight insertion, for facial paralysis or parotitis, needle pointed toward the eyeball of the opposite side, 0.5-1 unit. Sensation: distension and pain at the bottom of the ear, sometimes distension and soreness extending to the anterior part of the tongue.

Remarks
Point of intersection of the Gall Bladder channel on the Triple Burner channel.

N-HN-15 *(Yilong)*　医聋　"Shielding Deafness"

Location
In the depression 0.5 unit above TB-17 *(Yifeng)* behind the ear. (Dia. 2-9)

Anatomy
In the posterior auricularis muscle. Supplied by branches of the posterior auricular artery and vein, by the great auricular nerve, and situated directly on a posterior auricular branch of the facial nerve.

Indications
Tinnitus, deafness, deaf-mutism.

Illustrative combinations
With N-HN-8 *(Tingxue)*, N-HN-10 *(Tingcong)*, N-HN-18 *(Yimingxia)* for tinnitus or deafness; with TB-21 *(Ermen)* joined to SI-19 *(Tinggong)* and GB-2 *(Tinghui)* for deaf-mutism.

Needling method
Slanted insertion, directed slightly forward and downward, 1.5-2 units. Sensation: distension and soreness in the lower ear, sometimes extending to the root of the tongue.

M-HN-13 *(Yiming)*　翳明　"Shielding Brightness"

Location
1 unit posterior to TB-17 *(Yifeng)* behind the ear. (Dia. 2-9)

Anatomy
In the anterior part of the insertion of the tendon of the sternocleidomastoid muscle. Supplied by the great auricular and lesser occipital nerves, and by branches of the posterior auricular artery and vein; in its deep position between the internal carotid artery and internal jugular vein, and supplied by the vagus nerve and a superior cervical ganglion of the sympathetic trunk.

Indications
Myopia, hypermetropia, night blindness, atrophy of the optic nerve, cataract, tinnitus, vertigo, parotitis, headache, insomnia, mental illness.

Illustrative combinations
With M-HN-3 *(Yintang)*, P-6 *(Neiguan)*, Sp-6 *(Sanyinjiao)* for insomnia; with M-HN-8 *(Qiuhou)*, B-1 *(Jingming)* for early stage of cataract; with TB-9 *(Sidu)*, GB-20 *(Fengchi)*, Gv-15 *(Yamen)*, P-6 *(Neiguan)*, Li-3 *(Taichong)* for aural vertigo.

Needling method

Straight insertion, 1-1.5 units. Sensation: distended, electric sensation on the side of the head needled.

N-HN-54 *(Anmian)*   安眠   "Peaceful Sleep"

Location

Midway between GB-20 *(Fengchi)* and TB 17 *(Yifeng)* behind the ear. (Dia. 2-9)

Anatomy

In the midpoint at the insertion of the tendon of the sternocleidomastoid muscle; in its deep position is the splenius capitis muscle. Supplied by the occipital artery and vein, and by the minor occipital and a branch of the great auricular nerves.

Indications

Insomnia, vertigo, headache, palpitations, mental illness, hysteria.

Illustrative combinations

With P-6 *(Neiguan)*, Sp-6 *(Sanyinjiao)* for insomnia; with Gv-26 *(Renzhong)*, Gv-14 *(Dazhui)*, Gv-13 *(Taodao)* for psychosis; with LI-11 *(Quchi)*, S-40 *(Fenglong)* for vertigo.

Needling method

Straight insertion, 1-1.5 units. Sensation: local distension and soreness, sometimes extending throughout the side of the face needled.

SI-17 *(Tianrong)*   天容   "Heaven's Contents"

Location

Posterior and inferior to the angle of the mandible at the anterior margin of the sternocleidomastoid muscle. (Dia. 2-13)

Anatomy

Posterior to the angle of the mandible, in the anterior margin at the insertion of the sternocleidomastoid muscle, and the inferior margin in the posterior belly of the digastric muscle. Anterior to the point is the superficial, external jugular vein and the internal carotid artery and vein. Supplied by an anterior branch of the great auricular nerve, a cervical branch of the facial nerve, and in its deep position by a superior cervical ganglion of the sympathetic trunk.

Indications

Tonsillitis, pharyngitis, distension and soreness of the neck, asthma.

Traditional indications

Deafness, tinnitus, throat constricted and difficulty in swallowing, swelling and soreness of the neck, severe coughing.

Illustrative combinations

With LI-4 *(Hegu)* for tonsillitis; with B-10 *(Tianzhu)*, LI-4 *(Hegu)* for pharyngitis.

Classical combinations

With LI-5 *(Yangxi)* for fullness in the chest and shortness of breath. (Source: CNLAM)

Needling method

Straight insertion, toward the root of the tongue, 1-1.5 units. Sensation: distension and soreness extending to the root of the tongue or into the throat region.

TB-16 *(Tianyou)* 天牖 "Heaven's Window"

Location

Posterior and inferior to the mastoid process at the posterior border of the sternocleidomastoid muscle, near the hairline. (Dia. 2-13)

Anatomy

Posterior and inferior to the mastoid process, in the posterior margin at the insertion of the sternocleidomastoid muscle. Supplied by the occipital artery, and by the lesser occipital nerve.

Indications

Tinnitus, deafness, stiff neck, sore throat.

Traditional indications

Sudden deafness, sore eyes, constricted throat, excessive dreaming, scrofula.

Illustrative combinations

With SI-19 *(Tinggong)*, TB-2 *(Yemen)* for deafness; with TB-17 *(Yifeng)*, LI-4 *(Hegu)* for sore throat.

Classical combinations

With SI-3 *(Houxi)* for stiff neck with inability to rotate the head. (Source: CNLAM)

Needling method

Straight insertion, 0.5-1 unit. Sensation: local distension and soreness.

S-9 *(Renying)* 人迎 "Man's Welcome"

Location

1.5 units lateral to the laryngeal prominence. (Dia. 2-13)

Anatomy

In the platysma muscle, at the meeting of the anterior margin of the sternocleidomastoid muscle and the thyroid cartilage. Supplied by the superior thyroid artery, at the bifurcation of the external and internal carotid arteries, by the superficial anterior jugular vein, and medial to the internal jugular vein. Supplied by the cutaneous colli nerve and a cervical branch of the facial nerve; in its deep position by the glomus caroticum, and in its deepest position by the sympathetic trunk, and laterally by a descending branch of the sublingual and the vagus nerves.

Traditional functions

Regulates the Blood and Qi, benefits the throat.

Indications

High or low blood pressure, asthma, goiter, distension and soreness in the throat, speech impediment.

Traditional indications

Swollen throat, cough, wheezing, swellings on the neck, scrofula, delirium.

164

Illustrative combinations

Joined to SI-17 *(Tianrong),* and with LI-4 *(Hegu),* S-36 *(Zusanli),* M-UE-32 *(Zeqian),* K-3 *(Taixi),* P-6 *(Neiguan),* Sp-6 *(Sanyinjiao)* for goiter; with LI-11 *(Quchi),* S-36 *(Zusanli)* for hypertension; with Gv-26 *(Renzhong),* Li-3 *(Taichong),* P-6 *(Neiguan),* Gv-25 *(Suliao)* for low blood pressure.

Needling method

Straight or slanted insertion, 0.5-1 unit. Sensation: local distension and soreness, extending toward the shoulder.

Remarks

Point of intersection of the Gall Bladder channel on the Stomach channel. CAUTION: Moxibustion is prohibited. Care must be taken not to insert the needle too deeply, puncturing an artery.

LI-18 *(Futu)* 扶突 "Support the Prominence"

Location

3 units beside the laryngeal prominence, lateral to S-9 *(Renying)* and in the posterior margin of the sternocleidomastoid muscle. (Dia. 2-13)

Anatomy

In the posterior margin of the sternocleidomastoid muscle, in its deep position at the origin of the levator scapulae muscle. In its deep position, medial side, supplied by the ascending cervical artery. Supplied by the great auricular, the cutaneous colli, and the lesser occipital and accessory nerves.

Indications

Wheezing, excessive mucous, hoarse voice, distension and soreness in the throat, difficult swallowing. Used for anesthesia during thyroid operation.

Traditional indications

Coughing and wheezing, excessive mucous, difficulty in swallowing, sounds in throat "like a duck".

Illustrative combinations

With Co-22 *(Tiantu),* K-3 *(Taixi)* for wheezing; with Co-22 *(Tiantu),* LI-4 *(Hegu)* for hoarse voice.

Classical combinations

With Co-22 *(Tiantu)* and K-3 *(Taixi)* for sounds in the throat. (Source: CNLAM)

Needling method

Straight insertion, 0.5-1 unit. Sensation: distended and constricted feeling in the throat.

M-HN-21 *(Shanglianquan)* 上廉泉 "Upper Spring of Integrity"

Location

1 unit above the laryngeal prominence, in the depression between the mandible and the hyoid bone. (Dia. 2-13)

Anatomy

Between the hyoid bone and the margin of the mandible in the mylohyoid muscle, between the geniohyoid muscle and the root of the tongue. Supplied by the lingual artery and vein, and by the lingual nerve and a branch of the sublingual nerve.

Indications
Slurred speech, mutism, salivation, stomatitis, acute or chronic pharyngitis.

Illustrative combinations
With Co-24 *(Chengjiang)*, S-4 *(Dicang)* for excessive salivation; with Gv-15 *(Yamen)*, LI-4 *(Hegu)* for slurred speech; with M-HN-24 *(Panglianquan)*, LI-4 *(Hegu)* for hysterical aphasia.

Needling method
Slanted insertion, toward the root of the tongue, 1-1.5 units; or, partially withdraw the needle and direct toward the left, then repeat toward the right. Sensation: alternately distended and constricted sensation around the root of the tongue and pharynx.

M-HN-26 *(Biantao)*　扁桃　"Tonsil"

Location
Below the inferior border at the angle of the mandible, anterior to the carotid artery. (Dia. 2-13)

Anatomy
In the triangle below the mandible, in the platysma muscle. Supplied by the cutaneous colli nerve and a cervical branch of the facial nerve, above the submandibular gland, and the facial artery and vein. In its deep position in the geniohyoid and hyoglossus muscles; supplied by the lingual and glossopharyngeus nerve, and the rami tonsillares.

Indications
Tonsillitis, pharyngitis.

Illustrative combinations
With LI-4 *(Hegu)* for tonsillitis; with B-10 *(Tianzhu)*, L-11 *(Shaoshang)* for pharyngitis.

Needling method
Straight insertion, 1-1.5 units. Sensation: heavy, distended feeling in the neck, sometimes extending into the throat.

Gv-15 *(Yamen)*　哑门　"Door of Muteness"

Location
About 0.5 unit above the natural hairline on the nape of the neck, between the spinous processes of the 1st and 2nd cervical vertebrae. (Dia. 2-10)

Anatomy
Between the spinous processes of the 1st and 2nd cervical vertebrae. Supplied by a branch of the occipital artery and vein, the internal vertebral venous plexus, and by the 3rd occipital nerve.

Traditional functions
Clears the senses and consciousness.

Indications
Headache, deaf-mutism, seizures, cerebral palsy, incomplete maturation of the brain, hysteria, convulsions.

Traditional indications
Occipital headache, stiff neck, nosebleed, stiff tongue inhibiting speech, apoplexy, insanity, convulsions.

① B-10 *(Tianzhu)*
② Gv-15 *(Yamen)*
③ GB-20 *(Fengchi)*

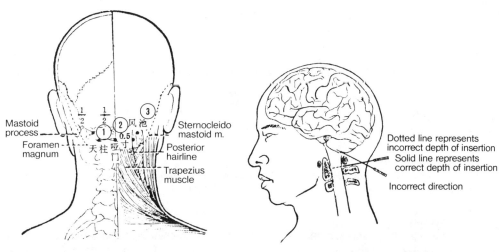

Dia. 2-10 Points on Back of Neck

Dia. 2-11 Direction of Needle Insertion at Gv-15 *(Yamen)*

Illustrative combinations

With Gv-26 *(Renzhong)*, SI-3 *(Houxi)*, S-40 *(Fenglong)* for seizures; with Gv-14 *(Dazhui)*, M-HN-13 *(Yiming)*, P-6 *(Neiguan)*, S-36 *(Zusanli)*, and the Three Vertebral Points for incomplete maturation of the brain.

Classical combinations

With TB-1 *(Guanchong)* for flaccid tongue and inability to speak (Source: OHS); with Gv-16 *(Fengfu)* for excessive extension of the spine. (Source: GCAM)

Needling method

Straight insertion, 1-2 units. Needle should be inserted level with the mouth or earlobe, and should not be rotated or otherwise agitated after insertion. Sensation: local distension. When the needle is inserted too deeply there will be a strong electric sensation indicating that the spinal cord has been touched. In this case the needle should be at least partially withdrawn. CAUTION: In addition to avoiding an excessively deep insertion, extreme care must be exercised so as to avoid inserting the needle upward into the medulla oblongata, where it could cause death. (Dia. 2-11)

Remarks

Point of intersection of the Yang Linking channel on the Governing channel.

B-10 *(Tianzhu)*   天柱   "Heaven's Pillar"

Location

Approximately 1.3 units lateral to Gv-15 *(Yamen)* on the back of the neck. (Dia. 2-10)

Anatomy
In the origin of the trapezius muscle, and in its deep position in the semispinalis capitis muscle. Supplied by the trunk of the occipital artery and vein, and the trunk of the greater occipital nerve.

Indications
Occipital headache, stiffness and soreness in the back of the neck, pharyngitis, hysteria, neurasthenia.

Traditional indications
Heavy, dizzy, and painful head, nasal congestion and swelling of the larynx, eye diseases, seizures, infantile convulsions.

Illustrative combinations
With L-11 *(Shaoshang)* for pharyngitis; with M-UE-24 *(Luozhen)* for stiff neck.

Classical combinations
With Gv-13 *(Taodao)* and B-60 *(Kunlun)* for severe dizziness (as if about to fall) (Source: CNLAM); with L-11 *(Shaoshang)* for chronic cough. (Source: CNLAM)

Needling method
Straight insertion, 0.5-1 unit. Sensation: local distension and soreness, sometimes extending to the top of the head. CAUTION: Do not point needle upward where it might puncture the medulla oblongata.

GB-20 *(Fengchi)*　风池　"Pool of Wind"

Location
Between the hollow below the tuberosity of the occipital bone at the back of the head and the mastoid process, and between the trapezius and sternocleidomastoid muscles. (Dia. 2-10)

Anatomy
In the hollow between the sterocleidomastoid and trapezius muscles, and in its deep position in the splenius capitis muscle. Supplied by branches of the occipital artery and vein, and by a branch of the lesser occipital nerve.

Traditional functions
Disperses Wind Hot conditions, benefits the hearing and vision.

Indications
Common cold, vertigo, headache, stiff neck, eye diseases, rhinitis, tinnitus, deafness, hypertension, seizures, hemiplegia, brain diseases.

Traditional indications
Sinusitis, eyes red and sore, deafness, tinnitus, lateral and midline headaches, insomnia, common cold, tidal fevers, swellings or tumors on the neck.

Illustrative combinations
With Gv-14 *(Dazhui)*, LI-4 *(Hegu)* for common cold; with M-BW-29 *(Yaoqi)*, Gv-26 *(Renzhong)*, P-6 *(Neiguan)* for seizures; with LI-11 *(Quchi)*, S-36 *(Zusanli)*, Li-3 *(Taichong)* for hypertension.

Classical combinations
With B-13 *(Feishu)* for spinal kyphosis (Source: GCAM); with B-5 *(Wuchu)* for problems with vision. (Source: CNLAM)

168

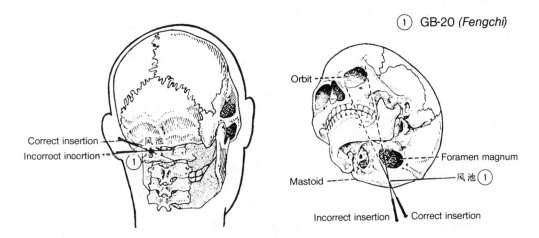

Dia. 2-12 Direction of Needle Insertion at GB-20 *(Fengchi)*

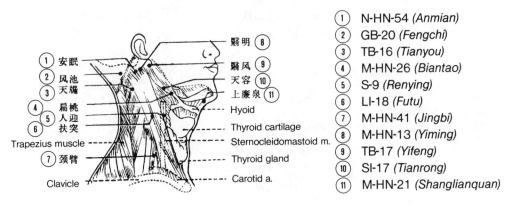

① N-HN-54 *(Anmian)*
② GB-20 *(Fengchi)*
③ TB-16 *(Tianyou)*
④ M-HN-26 *(Biantao)*
⑤ S-9 *(Renying)*
⑥ LI-18 *(Futu)*
⑦ M-HN-41 *(Jingbi)*
⑧ M-HN-13 *(Yiming)*
⑨ TB-17 *(Yifeng)*
⑩ SI-17 *(Tianrong)*
⑪ M-HN-21 *(Shanglianquan)*

Dia. 2-13 Neck Points

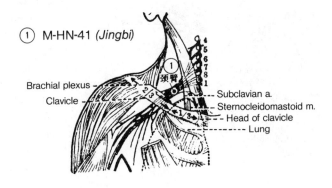

① M-HN-41 *(Jingbi)*

Dia. 2-14 Location of M-HN-41 *(Jingbi)*

169

Needling method

(1) Straight insertion, level with the ear lobe, pointed slighty downward, 1-1.5 units. Sensation: local distension and soreness, possibly extending to the top of the head, the temple, forehead or eyes. (Dia. 2-12) (2) Slanted insertion, joined to opposite GB-20 *(Fengchi),* 2-3 units. Sensation: local distension and soreness, sometimes extending throughout the back of the neck. CAUTION: Caution must be exercised to avoid inserting the needle too deeply, puncturing the medulla oblongata.

Remarks

Point of intersection of the Yang Linking and Triple Burner channels on the Gall Bladder channel.

1. Gv-20 *(Baihui)*
2. B-7 *(Tongtian)*
3. S-8 *(Touwei)*
4. TB-23 *(Sizhukong)*
5. M-HN-9 *(Taiyang)*
6. TB-21 *(Ermen)*
7. SI-19 *(Tinggong)*
8. S-7 *(Xiaguan)*
9. N-HN-20 *(Qianzheng)*
10. S-6 *(Jiache)*
11. SI-17 *(Tianrong)*
12. M-HN-26 *(Biantao)*
13. GB-2 *(Tinghui)*
14. N-HN-15 *(Yilong)*
15. GB-20 *(Fengchi)*
16. N-HN-54 *(Anmian)*
17. Gv-15 *(Yamen)*
18. B-10 *(Tianzhu)*
19. TB-16 *(Tianyou)*
20. M-HN-13 *(Yiming)*
21. TB-17 *(Yifeng)*
22. LI-18 *(Futu)*
23. M-HN-41 *(Jingbi)*
24. S-9 *(Renying)*
25. M-HN-21 *(Shanglianquan)*
26. M-HN-18 *(Jiachengjiang)*
27. Co-24 *(Chengjiang)*
28. S-4 *(Dicang)*
29. LI-19 *(Heliao)*
30. Gv-26 *(Renzhong)*
31. LI-20 *(Yingxiang)*
32. Gv-25 *(Suliao)*
33. S-2 *(Sibai)*
34. M-HN-14 *(Bitong)*
35. S-1 *(Chengqi)*
36. M-HN-8 *(Qiuhou)*
37. GB-1 *(Tongziliao)*
38. N-HN-6 *(Waiming)*
39. B-1 *(Jingming)*
40. N-HN-4 *(Shangming)*
41. M-HN-3 *(Yintang)*
42. B-2 *(Zanzhu)*
43. M-HN-6 *(Yuyao)*
44. GB-14 *(Yangbai)*
45. Gv-23 *(Shangxing)*

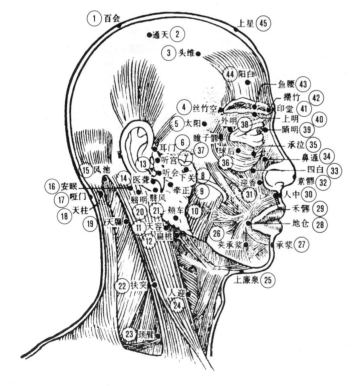

Dia. 2-15 Relationship of Head and Neck Points with Musculature

M-HN-41 *(Jingbi)* 颈臂 "Neck and Arm"

Location
One third the distance from the medial end of the clavicle to its lateral end, up 1 unit, at the posterior margin of the sternocleidomastoid muscle. (Dia. 2-14)

Anatomy
At the posterior margin of the sternocleidomastoid muscle, and in the platysma muscle, situated directly on an anterior branch of the supraclavicular nerve. In its deep position, slightly medial to the lateral margin of the anterior scalenus muscle, directly on the brachial plexus root. Supplied by branches of the superficial carotid and transverse cervical arteries and veins.

Indications
Numbness in the arm, paralysis of the upper limb.

Illustrative combinations
With LI-11 *(Quchi)*, LI-5 *(Yangxi)* for radial nerve paralysis; with M-UE-30 *(Bizhong)*, P-6 *(Neiguan)* for median nerve paralysis; with SI-8 *(Xiaohai)*, SI-7 *(Zhizhong)* for ulnar nerve paralysis.

Needling method
Straight insertion, 0.5-0.8 unit. Sensation: numb, electric sensation extending down the length of the arm. CAUTION: Avoid pointing the needle downward which may puncture the top of the lung.

SUMMARY OF COMMON POINTS OF HEAD AND NECK

Region	Points	Common Characteristics	Particular Characteristics
Head			
Top	Gv-20 (Baihui), B-7 (Tongtian), Gv-23 (Shangxing)	Diseases of head; headache at vertex	Gv-20 (Baihui): shock, brain diseases, prolapsed anus; B-7 (Tongtian) and Gv-23 (Shangxing): nose diseases
Side	S-8 (Touwei), M-HN-9 (Taiyang)	Lateral headache	S-8 (Touwei): facial paralysis; M-HN-9 (Taiyang): eye diseases, trigeminal neuralgia
Front	GB-14 (Yangbai), M-HN-3 (Yintang)	Frontal headache	GB-14 (Yangbai): eye diseases, facial paralysis; M-HN-3 (Yintang): nose diseases, brain diseases
Face	S-2 (Sibai), S-7 (Xiaguan), N-HN-20 (Qianzheng), S-6 (Jiache)	Diseases of the face and jaw, facial and trigeminal nerves	S-2 (Sibai): diseases of nose and eyes; S-7 (Xiaguan): diseases of ear, toothache, temporomandibular arthritis; S-6 (Jiache): parotitis, toothache
Eye	B-1 (Jingming), S-1 (Chengqi), M-HN-8 (Qiuhou), N-HN-4 (Shangming), N-HN-6 (Waiming), GB-1 (Tongziliao), B-2 (Zanzhu), M-HN-6 (Yuyao), TB-23 (Sizhukong)	Eye diseases	GB-1 (Tongziliao) and TB-23 (Sizhukong): lateral headache; B-2 (Zanzhu): facial paralysis, frontal headache; M-HN-6 (Yuyao): facial paralysis, neuralgia of supraorbital nerve
Nose	Gv-25 (Suliao), LI-20 (Yingxiang), M-HN-14 (Bitong)	Nose diseases	Gv-25 (Suliao): shock; LI-20 (Yingxiang): facial paralysis, round worm in bile duct

Region	Points	Common Characteristics	Particular Characteristics
Ear	TB-21 (Ermen), SI-19 (Tinggong), GB-2 (Tinghui), TB-17 (Yifeng), N-HN-15 (Yilong)	Ear diseases	TB-17 (Yifeng): parotitis, facial paralysis, toothache
Mouth	Gv-26 (Renzhong), LI-19 (Heliao), S-4 (Dicang), Co-24 (Chengjiang), M-HN-18 (Jiachengjiang)	Facial paralysis, diseases of mouth and teeth	Gv-26 (Renzhong): shock, coma, acute lower back pain, mental illness; LI-19 (Heliao): nose diseases; S-4 (Dicang): salivation, trigeminal neuralgia; M-HN-18 (Jiachengjiang): facial spasms, trigeminal neuralgia
Neck			
Back	Gv-15 (Yamen), GB-20 (Fengchi), B-10 (Tianzhu)	Diseases of back of head and nape of neck	Gv-15 (Yamen): mutism, brain diseases; GB-20 (Fengchi): brain diseases, hypertension, eye diseases, common cold
Side	M-HN-13 (Yiming), N-HN-54 (Anmian), SI-17 (Tianrong), TB-16 (Tianyou)	Diseases of the side of the neck	M-HN-13 (Yiming): diseases of eyes and ears, parotitis, insomnia; N-HN-54 (Anmian): insomnia, mental illness, hysteria; SI-17 (Tianrong): sore throat; TB-16 (Tianyou): diseases of ears and throat
Front	S-9 (Renying), LI-18 (Futu), M-HN-21 (Shanglianquan), M-HN-26 (Biantao)	Diseases of the front of the neck	S-9 (Renying): hypertension; LI-18 (Futu): diseases of vocal chords; M-HN-21 (Shanglianquan): paralysis of tongue, mutism; M-HN-26 (Biantao): tonsillitis
Other	M-HN-41 (Jingbi)		M-HN-41 (Jingbi): numbness, pain or paralysis of upper limb

Chapter 3

Common Points of the Chest and Abdomen

Co-22 *(Tiantu)*   天突   "Heaven's Prominence"

Location

0.5 unit above the suprasternal notch in the middle of the depression. (Dia. 2-16)

Anatomy

In the middle of the superior margin of the jugular notch of the sternum, between the left and right sternocleidomastoid muscles; in its deep position in the sternohyoid and sternothyroid muscles. Supplied by the arch of the jugular vein and a branch of the inferior thyroid artery. In its deep position is the trachea. The posterior side of the manubrium sterni is supplied by the anonyma artery and the aortic arch, and by an anterior branch of the supraclavicular nerve.

Traditional functions

Facilitates and regulates movement of Lung Qi, cools the throat and clears the voice.

Indications

Bronchial asthma, bronchitis, pharyngitis, goiter, hiccoughs, nervous vomiting, spasms of the esophagus, diseases of the vocal cords.

Traditional indications

Heavy wheezing, coughing blood and pus in the sputum, hoarse voice ('like the sound of a duck'), early stages of tumors or nodular growths on the neck.

Illustrative combinations

With M-BW-1 *(Dingchuan),* Co-17 *(Shanzhong),* S-40 *(Fenglong)* for bronchial asthma; with K-27 *(Shufu),* Co-17 *(Shanzhong),* L-1 *(Zhongfu)* for coughing and wheezing induced by rheumatic heart disease; with P-6 *(Neiguan),* Co-12 *(Zhongwan)* for hiccoughs.

Needling method

(1) Transverse insertion, first insert perpendicularly for 0.2-0.3 unit, then point needle downward along the posterior side of the manubrium sterni, anterior to the trachea, approximately 1-1.5 units. Sensation: local distension and soreness and a constricted sensation around the pharynx. (2) Straight insertion, 0.3-0.5 unit. Sensation: location distension and soreness. CAUTION: When making the transverse insertion caution must be exercised to avoid inserting the needle too deeply, puncturing the

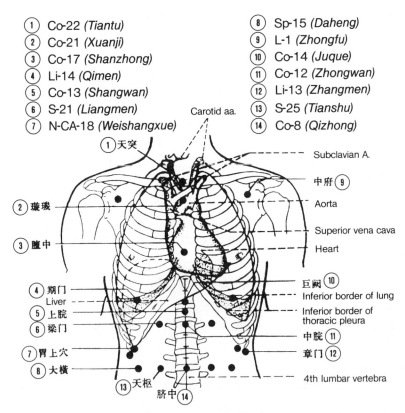

①	Co-22 *(Tiantu)*	⑧	Sp-15 *(Daheng)*
②	Co-21 *(Xuanji)*	⑨	L-1 *(Zhongfu)*
③	Co-17 *(Shanzhong)*	⑩	Co-14 *(Juque)*
④	Li-14 *(Qimen)*	⑪	Co-12 *(Zhongwan)*
⑤	Co-13 *(Shangwan)*	⑫	Li-13 *(Zhangmen)*
⑥	S-21 *(Liangmen)*	⑬	S-25 *(Tianshu)*
⑦	N-CA-18 *(Weishangxue)*	⑭	Co-8 *(Qizhong)*

Carotid aa.

① 天突

② 璇璣

③ 膻中

④ 期门
Liver
⑤ 上脘
⑥ 梁门
⑦ 胃上穴
⑧ 大横

⑬ 天枢
脐中 ⑭

Subclavian A.

中府 ⑨

Aorta

Superior vena cava

Heart

巨阙 ⑩
Inferior border of lung

Inferior border of thoracic pleura

中脘 ⑪

章门 ⑫

4th lumbar vertebra

Dia. 2-16 Points on Chest and Upper Abdomen

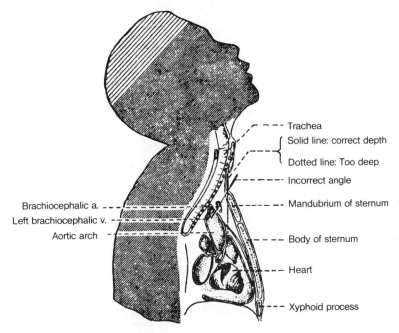

Trachea
Solid line: correct depth
Dotted line: Too deep
Incorrect angle
Mandubrium of sternum
Body of sternum
Heart
Xyphoid process

Brachiocephalic a.
Left brachiocephalic v.
Aortic arch

Dia. 2-17 Direction and Depth of Insertion at Co-22 *(Tiantu)*

175

aorta or anonyma arteries. Similarly, an excessively deep straight insertion will puncture the trachea. Finally, one should avoid straying too far to the left or right, particularly in cases of emphysema, where the needle may puncture the lung or subclavian artery. (See Dia. 2-17).

Remarks
Point of intersection of the Yin Linking channel at the Conception channel.

Co-21 *(Xuanji)* 璇玑 "North Star"

Location
1 unit below Co-22 *(Tiantu)* on the midline of the sternum, midway between the articulations of the left and right first rib with the sternum. (Dia. 2-16)

Anatomy
In the middle of the manubrium sterni, supplied by anterior perforating branches of the internal thoracic artery and vein, and an anterior branch of the supraclavicular nerve.

Indications
Bronchial asthma, chronic bronchitis, spasms of the esophagus, cardiac spasm.

Traditional indications
Swollen pharynx, throat blockage; coughing, fullness and pain in the chest and ribs, laryngeal stridor in children.

Illustrative combinations
With Co-22 *(Tiantu),* P-6 *(Neiguan)* for esophageal spasm.

Classical combinations
With Co-6 *(Qihai)* for emaciation and wheezing. (Source: SJD)

Needling method
Transverse insertion, pointed downward, 0.5-1 unit. Sensation: local distension and soreness.

L-1 *(Zhongfu)* 中府 "Central Residence"

Location
Approximately 1 unit below the lateral end of the clavicle in the lateral part of the first intercostal space. (Dia. 2-16)

Anatomy
In the pectoralis major and minor muscles; in its deep position, in the internal and external intercostal muscles. On its superior, lateral side supplied by the axillary artery and vein, and by the thoracoacromial artery and vein. Supplied by an intermediate branch of the supraclavicular nerve, a branch of the anterior thoracic nerve, and the first intercostal nerve.

Indications
Bronchitis, pneumonia, asthma, pulmonary tuberculosis.

Traditional indications
Coughing and wheezing, coughing blood and pus; throat blockage, congested nose; excessive sweating, tumors and nodular growths on the neck.

Illustrative combinations
With B-13 *(Feishu),* L-6 *(Kongzui)* for chronic bronchitis; with M-BW-1 *(Dingchuan),* P-6

(Neiguan), Co-17 *(Shanzhong)* for bronchial asthma; with N-BW-6 *(Jiehexue),* N-BW-20 *(Feirexue),* B-13 *(Feishu)* for pulmonary tuberculosis.

Classical combinations
With B-44 *(Yishe)* for fullness in the chest and throat (Source: OHS); with H-9 *(Shaochong)* for chest pain (Source: CNLAM).

Needling method
Slanted insertion, pointed upward, 0.5-1 unit. Sensation: distension and soreness extending into the chest and upper arm.

Remarks
Point of intersection of the Spleen channel on the Lung channel. Alarm point of the Lung channel.

Co-17 *(Shanzhong)*　膻中　"Penetrating Odor"

Location
On the sternum, level with the nipples of the breasts; or between and just above the articulations of the right and left fifth rib with the sternum. (Dia. 2-16)

Anatomy
Supplied by anterior, perforating branches of the internal thoracic artery and vein, and by a medial, anterior cutaneous branch of the fourth intercostal nerve.

Traditional functions
Regulates and suppresses rebellious Qi; expands the chest, benefits the diaphragm.

Indications
Bronchial asthma, bronchitis, chest pain, mastitis, insufficient lactation, intercostal neuralgia.

Traditional indications
Wheezing, panting, spitting and coughing blood, difficulty or inability to swallow food (due to constriction or dryness in the esophagus), tumors on the neck, lung abcess, chest pain.

Illustrative combinations
With M-BW-1 *(Dingchuan),* Co-22 *(Tiantu),* P-6 *(Neiguan)* for bronchial asthma; with S-18 *(Rugen),* S-36 *(Zusanli),* SI-1 *(Shaoze)* for insufficient lactation; with LI-4 *(Hegu),* LI-11 *(Quchi)* for mastitis.

Classical combinations
With SI-1 *(Shaoze)* and S-18 *(Rugen)* for insufficient milk (Source: GCAM); with TB-10 *(Tianjing)* to treat blockage of the chest with heart pain. (Source: CNLAM)

Needling method
Transverse insertion, pointed upward or toward the breasts, 0.5-1.5 units. Sensation: local distension and soreness, or a deep, heavy feeling in the front of the chest.

Remarks
Point of intersection of the Spleen, Kidney, Small Intestine and Triple Burner channels on the Conception channel.

Co-14 *(Juque)*　巨闕　"Great Palace"

Location
On the sternum, 1 unit below Co-15 *(Jiuwei),* or approximately 6 units above the navel. (Dia. 2-16)

Anatomy

Supplied by branches of the superior epigastric artery and vein, and by a medial, anterior cutaneous branch of the seventh intercostal nerve.

Traditional functions

Calms the Spirit and regulates the Qi, pacifies the Stomach and benefits the diaphragm.

Indications

Mental diseases, seizures, angina pectoris, stomach-ache, vomiting, hiccough, round worms in the bile duct, chronic hepatitis.

Traditional indications

Coughing due to rebellious ascension of Qi, palpitations due to fright, vomiting long after ingestion of food, seizures, jaundice, chest pain related to round worms.

Illustrative combinations

With B-15 *(Xinshu)*, P-4 *(Ximen)*, H-5 *(Tongli)* for angina pectoris; with Gv-14 *(Dazhui)*, Gv-26 *(Renzhong)*, M-BW-29 *(Yaoqi)*, P-6 *(Neiguan)* for seizures.

Classical combinations

With TB-10 *(Tianjing)* and B-15 *(Xinshu)* to treat mental instability (Source: GCAM); with B-15 *(Xinshu)* to treat irritability of the Heart. (Source: CNLAM)

Needling method

Straight insertion, 1.5-2 units. Sensation: local distension and discomfort, sometimes extending upward. CAUTION: When needling patients in whom the left lobe of the liver, or the heart, is enlarged, caution must be taken not to insert the needle too deeply, or to slant it in an upward direction.

Remarks

Alarm point of the Heart. The functions of this point and Co-15 *(Jiuwei)* are basically the same.

Co-13 *(Shangwan)*   上脘   "Upper Cavity"

Location

5 units directly above the navel. (Dia. 2-16)

Anatomy

Supplied by branches of the superior epigastric artery and vein, and by a branch of the seventh intercostal nerve.

Indications

Acute and chronic gastritis, dilated stomach, stomach spasms, cardiac spasms.

Traditional indications

Feverishness with no sweating, irritable and feverish Heart, chest pain, distension of the abdomen, excessive salivation, jaundice.

Illustrative combinations

With P-6 *(Neiguan)*, Sp-4 *(Gongsun)* for cardiac spasm; with P-6 *(Neiguan)*, S-36 *(Zusanli)*, LI-10 *(Shousanli)* for acute gastritis.

Classical combinations

With Co-12 *(Zhongwan)* for stomach pain. (Source: SJD)

Needling method
Straight insertion, 1.5-2 units. Sensation: distension and heavy feeling in the upper abdomen.

Remarks
Point of intersection of the Stomach and Small Intestine channels on the Conception channel.

Co-12 *(Zhongwan)*　中脘　"Middle Cavity"

Location
4 units directly above the navel. (Dia. 2 16)

Anatomy
Supplied by the superior epigastric artery and vein, and by a medial, anterior cutaneous branch of the seventh intercostal nerve (in the pyloric region of the stomach).

Traditional functions
Regulates the Stomach Qi, transforms and suppresses rebellious Qi.

Indications
Acute or chronic gastritis, gastric ulcers, prolapsed stomach, acute intestinal obstruction, stomachache, vomiting, abdominal distension, diarrhea, constipation, indigestion, hypertension, neurasthenia, mental diseases.

Traditional indications
Pain in the stomach cavity, vomiting food long after ingestion, sour taste upon swallowing, indigestion, lack of appetite, abdominal pain, abdominal distension, dysentery, constipation, spitting blood related to consumptive illnesses, madness, jaundice.

Illustrative combinations
With N-CA-18 *(Weishang)*, S-36 *(Zusanli)* for prolapsed stomach; with S-25 *(Tianshu)*, P-6 *(Neiguan)*, Co-6 *(Qihai)* for acute intestinal obstruction.

Classical combinations
With Co-6 *(Qihai)* and Co-17 *(Shanzhong)* for vomiting (Source: NPA); with Li-14 *(Qimen)* and S-37 *(Shangjuxu)* for asthma. (Source: GCAM)

Needling method
Straight insertion, 1-2 units, or the needle may be inserted at a slant in all directions around the point. Sensation: a heavy, distended feeling in the upper abdomen, or a feeling of contraction in the stomach region. CAUTION: Because of the location of the stomach, pancreas, and abdominal aorta in the deep position beneath this point, caution must be exercised to avoid an excessively deep insertion. This is particularly the case when treating thin patients. Furthermore, when needling patients who have an enlarged liver or spleen, a slanted insertion of the needle in a direction to the left or right of the point is strongly discouraged.

Remarks
Point of intersection of the Small Intestine, Triple Burner and Stomach channels on the Conception channel.

S-21 *(Liangmen)*　梁门　"Door of the Beam"

Location
4 units above the navel and 2 units lateral to Co-12 *(Zhongwan)*. (Dia. 2-16)

Anatomy

In the rectus abdominis muscle and its sheath; in its deep position, in the fascia transversalis. Supplied by branches of the seventh intercostal artery and vein and the superior epigastric artery and vein. Situated on a branch of the eighth intercostal nerve.

Indications

Stomach-ache, stomach ulcers, acute and chronic gastritis, nervous dysfunction of the stomach.

Traditional indications

Pain in the stomach cavity, abdominal pain caused by an accumulation of Qi, diarrhea, colic, prolapsed anus.

Illustrative combinations

With Co-12 *(Zhongwan)*, S-36 *(Zusanli)*, LI-10 *(Shousanli)* for stomach ulcers; with P-6 *(Neiguan)*, S-34 *(Liangqiu)* for nervous dysfunction of the stomach.

Needling method

Straight insertion, 1-2 units. Sensation: a heavy, distended feeling in the upper abdomen.

N-CA-18 *(Weishangxue)* 胃上穴 "Above the Stomach Orifice"

Location

2 units above the navel, 4 units lateral to Co-10 *(Xiawan)*. (Dia. 2-16)

Anatomy

In the internal and external oblique muscles, and the transversus abdominis muscle. Supplied by the ninth intercostal nerve, artery and vein.

Indications

Prolapsed stomach, abdominal distension.

Illustrative combinations

Join to Co-8 *(Qizhong)*, and also needle Co-12 *(Zhongwan)*, Co-6 *(Qihai)*, S-36 *(Zusanli)* for prolapsed stomach; with Co-6 *(Qihai)* joined to Co-3 *(Zhongji)* for abdominal distension.

Needling method

Transverse insertion, pointed toward either the navel or S-25 *(Tianshu)*, 2-3 units. Sensation: abdomen feels distended, the navel pulled taut and the stomach contracted.

Remarks

Another source situates this point 2.5 units lateral to Co-10 *(Xiawan)*.

Li-14 *(Qimen)* 期门 "Expectation's Door"

Location

6 units above the navel and 3.5 units lateral to Co-14 *(Juque)* in the sixth intercostal space. (Dia. 2-16)

Anatomy

Near the medial end of the sixth intercostal space in the internal and external oblique muscles and the aponeurosis of the transversus abdominis muscle. Supplied by the sixth intercostal artery, vein and nerve.

Traditional functions
Facilitates the spreading of Liver Qi, transforms and removes Congealed Blood.

Indications
Intercostal neuralgia, hepatitis, enlarged liver, cholecystitis, pleurisy, nervous dysfunction of the stomach.

Traditional indications
Distension around the ribs, chest pain, vomiting, tidal fevers, enlargement of the spleen as a result of prolonged tidal fevers, failure to discharge the placenta.

Illustrative combinations
With B-17 *(Geshu)*, B-18 *(Ganshu)* and moxibustion at S-36 *(Zusanli)* for intercostal neuralgia; with Li-4 *(Zhongfeng)*, GB-34 *(Yanglingquan)* for hepatitis.

Classical combinations
With Li-1 *(Dadun)* to treat hard nodules and pain in the flanks. (Source: SJD)

Needling method
Slanted insertion, 0.5 unit. Sensation: slight pain, sometimes extending to the back of the abdominal wall.

Remarks
Point of intersection of the Spleen and Yin Linking channels on the Liver channel. Alarm point of the Liver. Another source situates this point in the costal cartilage of the ninth rib, directly below the breast.

Li-13 *(Zhangmen)*　章门　"System's Door"

Location
At the anterior end of the eleventh rib on the mid-axillary line. (When the arm is bent at the elbow and held against the side, the tip of the elbow roughly corresponds to the position of the point.) (Dia. 2-16)

Anatomy
In the internal and external oblique muscles. Supplied by the tenth intercostal nerve.

Indications
Enlargement of the liver and spleen, hepatitis, enteritis, vomiting, abdominal distension, pain in the chest and ribs.

Traditional indications
Diarrhea due to Cold in the Middle Burner, turbid and cloudy urine, fullness in the chest and ribs, lumps and distension in the chest due to accumulation of Qi; prolonged jaundice that becomes black jaundice, yellow skin and dark facial complexion.

Illustrative combinations
With Li-14 *(Qimen)*, M-BW-16 *(Pigen)*, B-21 *(Weishu)* for enlargement of the spleen and liver due to schistosomiasis; with B-20 *(Pishu)*, S-25 *(Tianshu)*, S-36 *(Zusanli)* for chronic enteritis.

Classical combinations
With Sp-3 *(Taibai)* and K-6 *(Zhaohai)* to treat constipation. (Source: GCAM)

Needling method

Straight or slanted insertion, 0.8-1 unit. Sensation: distended feeling at the side of the abdomen, possibly extending to the posterior abdominal wall. CAUTION: The right lobe of the liver is below this point on the right side of the body. Therefore caution must be exercised to avoid needling too deeply. Deep below this point, on the left side, is the lower end of the spleen. Excessively deep insertion on this side must also be avoided, particularly in cases of patients with enlarged liver or spleen.

Remarks

Point of intersection of the Gall Bladder channel on the Liver channel. Alarm point of the Spleen. Meeting point of the Yin Organs.

Co-8 *(Qizhong)*   脐中   "Middle of the Navel"

Location

In the middle of the navel. (Dia. 2-18)

Anatomy

Supplied by branches of the inferior epigastric artery and vein, and by a medial, anterior cutaneous branch of the tenth intercostal nerve.

Traditional functions

Warms and stabilizes the Yang, strengthens the transporting function of the Spleen and Stomach.

Indications

Acute and chronic enteritis, chronic diarrhea, intestinal tuberculosis, shock resulting from intestinal adhesions, edema, prolapsed anus.

Traditional indications

Apoplexy, heat stroke (or exhaustion), loss of consciousness, intestinal noises and pain, continuous diarrhea, prolapsed anus, simultaneous vomiting and diarrhea.

Illustrative combinations

With S-25 *(Tianshu)*, Co-13 *(Shangwan)*, P-6 *(Neiguan)*, S-36 *(Zusanli)* for acute gastritis or enteritis; with S-25 *(Tianshu)* and B-25 *(Dachangshu)* for chronic enteritis (use moxibustion).

Classical combinations

With Co-9 *(Shuifen)* and Co-6 *(Qihai)* for pain around the navel. (Source: GCAM)

Needling method

Moxibustion only, 20-30 minutes. CAUTION: Do not use needles at this point.

S-25 *(Tianshu)*   天枢   "Heaven's Axis"

Location

2 units lateral to the navel. (Dia. 2-18)

Anatomy

In the sheath of the rectus abdominis muscle. Supplied by the ninth intercostal artery and vein, branches of the inferior epigastric artery and vein, and by a branch of the tenth intercostal nerve.

Traditional functions

Regulates and facilitates the functioning of the Intestines, regulates the Qi and eliminates stagnation.

①	S-21 *(Liangmen)*	⑦	M-CA-16 *(Weibao)*	⑬	S-25 *(Tianshu)*
②	N-CA-18 *(Weishangxue)*	⑧	N-CA-4 *(Tituoxue)*	⑭	Co-8 *(Qizhong)*
③	Li-13 *(Zhangmen)*	⑨	M-CA-18 *(Zigong)*	⑮	Co-4 *(Guanyuan)*
④	GB-26 *(Daimai)*	⑩	S-30 *(Qichong)*	⑯	Co-3 *(Zhongji)*
⑤	Co-6 *(Qihai)*	⑪	Co-12 *(Zhongwan)*	⑰	S-28 *(Shuidao)*
⑥	GB-27 *(Wushu)*	⑫	Sp-15 *(Daheng)*	⑱	S-29 *(Guilai)*

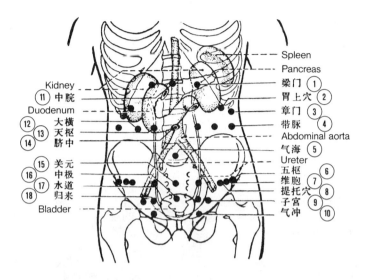

Dia. 2-18 Points on Abdomen

Indications
Acute and chronic gastritis or enteritis, dysentery, intestinal paralysis, peritonitis, round worm in the intestinal tract, endometritis, constipation, low back pain.

Traditional indications
Vomiting, diarrhea, abdominal pain, constipation, vaginal discharge with blood, irregular menstruation, dripping of turbid urine, infertility, abdominal obstruction or lumps due to accumulation of Qi or Blood.

Illustrative combinations
With S-37 *(Shangjuxu)* for acute dysentery; with Co-7 *(Yinjiao)*, Co-4 *(Guanyuan)* for dysmenorrhea.

Classical combinations
With K-5 *(Shuiquan)* for irregular menstruation (Source: OHS); with TB-6 *(Zhigou)* for vomiting with or without diarrhea. (Source: GCAM)

Needling method
Straight insertion, 1.5-2.5 units. Sensation: local distension and soreness, possibly extending throughout the side of the abdomen that is needled.

Remarks
Alarm point of the Large Intestine.

Sp-15 *(Daheng)*   大横   "Big Horizontal"

Location
3.5 units lateral to the navel. (Dia. 2-18)

Anatomy
In the external and internal oblique, and the transversus abdominis muscles. Supplied by the tenth intercostal artery and vein, and by the tenth intercostal nerve.

Indications
Abdominal distension, diarrhea, constipation, intestinal paralysis, parasitic worms in the intestines.

Traditional indications
Diarrhea, constipation, Cold pain in the lower abdomen, severe diarrhea.

Illustrative combinations
With M-UE-9 *(Sifeng)* or S-36 *(Zusanli)* for roundworm in the intestines; with GB-34 *(Yanglingquan)* for habitual constipation.

Needling method
(1) Straight insertion, 1-1.5 units. Sensation: local distension and soreness. (2) Transverse insertion, for parasitic worms in the intestines, the needle is inserted toward the navel, 2-2.5 units. Sensation: local distension and soreness, possibly extending throughout the side of the abdomen on which this point is needled.

Remarks
Point of intersection of the Yin Linking channel on the Spleen channel.

Co-6 *(Qihai)*   气海   "Sea of Qi"

Location
1.5 units directly below the navel. (Dia. 2-18)

Anatomy
Supplied by branches of the superficial and inferior epigastric arteries and veins and by a medial, anterior cutaneous branch of the eleventh intercostal nerve.

Traditional functions
Regulates the Qi functions, strengthens Deficient Kidneys.

Indications
Neurasthenia, abdominal distension, abdominal pain, irregular menstruation, dysmenorrhea, intestinal paralysis, incontinence, polyuria, urinary retention, spermatorrhea, impotence.

Traditional indications
Vaginal discharge with blood, irregular menstruation, excessive bleeding, infertility, colic, incontinence among children, heat stroke (or exhaustion), 'abandoned' stroke.

Illustrative combinations
With Co-3 *(Zhongji)*, Sp-6 *(Sanyinjiao)* for dysmenorrhea; with Gv-4 *(Mingmen)*, Gv-2 *(Yaoshu)* for incontinence.

Classical combinations
With Sp-6 *(Sanyinjiao)* for cloudy urine with loss of sperm (Source: OHS); with B-54 *(Weizhong)* for Deficient Qi. (Source: NPA)

Needling method
Slanted insertion, pointed downward, 2-3 units. Sensation: local distension and soreness possibly extending into the genital region. CAUTION: Do not needle or use moxibustion at this point on pregnant women. When the bladder is full, do not insert the needle downward too deeply.

Co-4 *(Guanyuan)*　关元　"Hinge at the Source"

Location
3 units directly below the navel. (Dia. 2-18)

Anatomy
Supplied by branches of the superficial and inferior epigastric artery and vein, and by a medial, anterior cutaneous branch of the intercostal nerve.

Traditional functions
Nourishes and stabilizes the Kidneys, regulates the Qi and restores the Yang.

Indications
Abdominal pain, diarrhea, dysentery, urinary tract infections, nephritis, irregular menstruation, dysmenorrhea, leukorrhea, pelveoperitonitis, functional uterine bleeding, prolapsed uterus, sperma-torrhea, impotence, enuresis, roundworms in the intestinal tract.

Traditional indications
'Abandoned' stroke, general weakness, vaginal discharge, lack of menstruation, infertility, twisting pain below the navel, loss of sperm, hernia, blood in the urine, enuresis, blood in the stool, tidal fever accompanied by coughing blood, emaciation and constant thirst, dysentery.

Illustrative combinations
With Sp-1 *(Yinbai)*, Sp-10 *(Xuehai)*, S-36 *(Zusanli)* for functional uterine bleeding; join to Co-2 *(Qugu)*, and also needle S-36 *(Zusanli)*, Sp-6 *(Sanyinjiao)* for spermatorrhea or impotence; with Sp-9 *(Yinlingquan)*, Sp-6 *(Sanyinjiao)* for urinary tract infection.

Classical combinations
With Li-1 *(Dadun)* for unilateral distension of testicle (Source: GCAM); with K-1 *(Yongquan)* for acute pain with inability to urinate. (Source: CNLAM)

Needling method
Slanted insertion, pointed downward, 1.5-2 units. Sensation: local distension and soreness, sometimes extending to the genital region.

S-28 *(Shuidao)*　水道　"Waterway"

Location
3 units directly below the navel, and 2 units lateral to Co-4 *(Guanyuan)*. (Dia. 2-18)

Anatomy
In the rectus abdominis muscle and its sheath. Supplied by branches of the twelfth intercostal artery and vein, and on its lateral side by the inferior epigastric artery and vein. Supplied by the twelfth intercostal nerve.

Traditional functions
Cools Damp Heat and benefits the Bladder.

Indications
Nephritis, cystitis, urinary retention, ascites, orchitis.

Traditional indications
Distension and fullness in the lower abdomen, Heat and constriction in the Triple Burner, lack of urine, pain leading to the genitals.

Illustrative combinations
With Co-9 *(Shuifen)*, Sp-9 *(Yinlingquan)*, S-36 *(Zusanli)* for ascites; with B-23 *(Shenshu)*, B-28 *(Pangguangshu)*, Sp-6 *(Sanyinjiao)* for nephritis.

Needling method
Straight insertion, 1-1.5 units. Sensation: distension and soreness, possibly extending to the lower side of the abdomen on which the point is needled.

N-CA-4 *(Tituoxue)* 提托穴 "Lift and Support Orifice"

Location
4 units lateral to Co-4 *(Guanyuan)* on the lower abdomen. (Dia. 2-18)

Anatomy
In the external and internal oblique muscles, and the transversus abdominis muscle. Supplied by the iliohypogastric nerve and accompanying veins and arteries.

Indications
Prolapsed uterus, pain in the lower abdomen, hernia.

Illustrative combinations
With Co-3 *(Zhongji)* joined to Co-2 *(Qugu)*; and S-36 *(Zusanli)*, Sp-6 *(Sanyinjiao)* for prolapsed uterus.

Needling method
Straight insertion, 1-1.5 units. Sensation: distension and soreness in the lower abdomen, sometimes a lifting sensation in the uterus.

GB-26 *(Daimai)* 带脉 "Girdle Vessel"

Location
Directly below Li-13 *(Zhangmen)* and level with the navel. (Dia. 2-18)

Anatomy
In the external and internal oblique muscles, and the transversus abdominis muscle. Supplied by the twelfth intercostal artery and vein, and by the twelfth intercostal nerve.

Traditional functions
Regulates the Girdle channel and alleviates Damp Heat.

Indications
Endometritis, cystitis, irregular menstruation, profuse blood and leukorrhea, paraplegia due to trauma.

Traditional indications
Irregular menstruation, red and white vaginal discharge, intestinal colic, diarrhea, convulsions.

Illustrative combinations
With B-30 *(Baihuanshu)*, Sp-9 *(Yinlingquan)*, Sp-6 *(Sanyinjiao)* for leukorrhea; with Co-3 *(Zhongji)* joined to Co-2 *(Qugu)*, Sp-8 *(Diji)*, and Sp-6 *(Sanyinjiao)* for endometritis; with N-BW-15 *(Shenji)*, GB-30 *(Huantiao)*, N-BW-16 *(Tiaoyue)* and N-LE-19 *(Siqiang)* for paraplegia.

Classical combinations
With GB-43 *(Jiaxi)* for pain and stiffness in the lower abdomen, lack of menstruation (Source: CNLAM); with Sp-10 *(Xuehai)* for irregular menstruation. (Source: CNLAM)

Needling method
Straight insertion, 1-1.5 units. Sensation: distension and soreness on the side of the waist that is needled.

Remarks
Point of intersection of the Girdle channel on the Gall Bladder channel.

GB-27 *(Wushu)* 五枢 "Five Pivots"

Location
On the anterior side of the anterior superior iliac spine, approximately level with Co-4 *(Guanyuan)*. (Dia. 2-18)

Anatomy
In the external and internal oblique muscles, and the transversus abdominis muscle. Supplied by the deep and superficial iliac arteries and veins, and by the iliohypogastric nerve.

Indications
Endometritis, leukorrhea, hernia, orchitis, low back pain.

Traditional indications
Colic, vaginal discharge containing blood, low back pain, abdominal pain, constipation, infantile convulsions.

Illustrative combinations
With GB-26 *(Daimai)*, M-CA-18 *(Zigong)* for endometritis; with Li-8 *(Ququan)*, Li-3 *(Taichong)* for orchitis.

Classical combinations
With S-29 *(Guilai)* for retraction of the testicles. (Source: CNLAM)

Needling method
Straight insertion, 1-2 units. Sensation: local distension and soreness.

Remarks
Point of intersection of the Girdle channel on the Gall Bladder channel.

M-CA-16 *(Weibao)* 维胞 "Support Uterus"

Location
In the depression below and medial to the anterior superior iliac spine, approximately level with Co-4 *(Guanyuan)*. (Dia. 2-18)

187

Anatomy

On the superior side of the inguinal ligament and the medial side of the anterior superior iliac spine, in the external and internal oblique muscles, and the transversus abdominis muscle. Situated directly on the ilioinguinal nerve. In its deep position, supplied by the internal iliac artery and vein, and the lateral cutaneous nerve of the thigh.

Indications

Prolapsed uterus, hernia, dysfunction of the intestines.

Illustrative combinations

With Co-6 *(Qihai)*, Co-3 *(Zhongji)*, S-36 *(Zusanli)*, Sp-6 *(Sanyinjiao)* for prolapsed uterus.

Needling method

Slanted insertion, along the inguinal ligament, 2-3 units. Sensation: distension and soreness in the lower abdomen and a contracting sensation in the uterus.

Co-3 *(Zhongji)*　中极　"Middle Summit"

Location

4 units directly below the navel. (Dia. 2-18)

Anatomy

Supplied by branches of the superficial epigastric and inferior epigastric arteries and veins, and by a branch of the iliohypogastric nerve.

Traditional functions

Assists the transforming functions of Qi, regulates the uterus, and alleviates Damp Heat.

Indications

Spermatorrhea, enuresis, retention of urine, impotence, premature ejaculation, irregular menstruation, leukorrhea, female sterility, nephritis, urethritis, pelveoperitonitis, dysmenorrhea, sciatica.

Traditional indications

Irregular menstruation, lack of menses, excessive bleeding, vaginal discharge containing blood, itching in the vagina, vaginal pain, spontaneous loss of sperm, edema, frequent urination, lack of urine.

Illustrative combinations

With Co-2 *(Qugu)*, K-5 *(Shuiquan)*, Co-9 *(Shuifen)*, Sp-6 *(Sanyinjiao)*, and GB-39 *(Xuanzhong)* joined with K-7 *(Fuliu)* for ascites due to rheumatic heart disease; with K-11 *(Henggu)*, Sp-9 *(Yinlingquan)* for spermatorrhea, impotence and premature ejaculation; with Sp-9 *(Yinlingquan)*, Sp-6 *(Sanyinjiao)* for enuresis; with M-CA-18 *(Zigong)*, Sp-6 *(Sanyinjiao)* for irregular menstruation.

Classical combinations

With B-23 *(Shenshu)*, LI-4 *(Hegu)*, Sp-6 *(Sanyinjiao)* for lack of menses. (Source: GCAM)

Needling method

Straight insertion, 1-2 units. Sensation: local distension and soreness, possibly extending into the genital region.

Remarks

Point of intersection of the three Leg Yin channels (Liver, Spleen, Kidney) on the Conception channel. Alarm point of the Bladder.

S-29 *(Guilai)* 归來 "Return"

Location

4 units below the navel and 2 units lateral to Co-3 *(Zhongji)*. (Dia. 2-18)

Anatomy

In the lateral margin of the rectus abdominis muscle, the internal oblique muscle, and the aponeurosis of the transversus abdominis muscle. Supplied on its lateral side by the inferior epigastric artery and vein, and by the iliohypogastric nerve.

Indications

Irregular menstruation, inflammation of the adnexa, endometritis, orchitis.

Traditional indications

Colic, lack of menses, infertility, vaginal discharge, impotence.

Illustrative combinations

With Co-3 *(Zhongji)*, Co-2 *(Qugu)*, M-CA-18 *(Zigong)*, Sp-6 *(Sanyinjiao)* for irregular menstruation; with K-3 *(Taixi)*, Co-6 *(Qihai)*, K-7 *(Fuliu)* for trichomonas vaginitis.

Needling method

Straight insertion, or transverse insertion toward the pubic symphysis, 1.5-2 units. Sensation: distension and soreness in the lower abdomen, sometimes extending into the genital region.

M-CA-18 *(Zigong)* 子宮 "Uterus"

Location

4 units below the navel and 3 units lateral to Co-3 *(Zhongji)*. (Dia. 2-18)

Anatomy

In the external and internal oblique muscles, and the transversus abdominis muscle. Supplied by the superficial epigastric artery and vein. Situated directly on the iliohypogastric nerve, and supplied by its accompanying arteries and veins.

Indications

Prolapsed uterus, irregular menstruation, dysmenorrhea, pelveoperitonitis, female sterility, pyelonephritis, cystitis, orchitis, appendicitis.

Illustrative combinations

With Co-4 *(Guanyuan)*, Sp-10 *(Xuehai)*, Sp-9 *(Yinlingquan)* for chronic pelveoperitonitis; with Co-3 *(Zhongji)*, Sp-9 *(Yinlingquan)* for leukorrhea.

S-30 *(Qichong)* 气冲 "Pouring Qi"

Location

At the lateral, superior side of the pubic tubercle, 2 units lateral to the median line of the abdomen in the upper inguinal region, medial to the common iliac artery. (Dia. 2-18)

Anatomy

In the aponeurosis of the external and internal oblique muscles, and the lower region of the transversus abdominis muscle. Supplied by branches of the superficial epigastric artery and vein, and laterally by the interior epigastric artery. Supplied by the ilioinguinal nerve.

Indications
Diseases of the reproductive organs, hernia.

Traditional indications
Pain in the penis or testicles, colic, excessive bleeding, infertility, disorders related to childbirth.

Illustrative combinations
With Li-8 *(Ququan)*, Li-3 *(Taichong)* for hernia; with Co-4 *(Guanyuan)* joined to Co-3 *(Zhongji)*, Sp-6 *(Sanyinjiao)* for urinary tract infection.

Needling method
(1) Straight insertion, 0.5-1 unit. Sensation: local heavy, distended feeling. (2) Slanted insertion, toward the genitals, 1-2 units. Sensation: local distension and soreness extending to the genitals. CAUTION: Internally, the presence of the spermatic cord in men, or the round ligament in women makes a deep insertion dangerous.

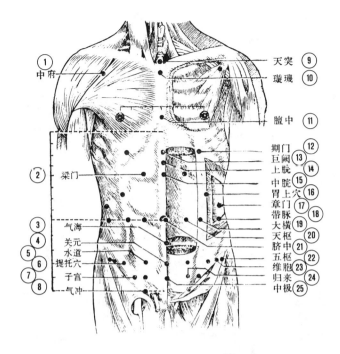

中府 ① 中府
天突 ⑨
璇璣 ⑩
膻中 ⑪
② 梁门
期门 ⑫
巨闕 ⑬
上脘 ⑭
中脘 ⑮
胃上穴 ⑯
章门 ⑰
带脉 ⑱
大横 ⑲
天枢 ⑳
脐中 ㉑
五枢 ㉒
维胞 ㉓
归来 ㉔
中极 ㉕
③ 气海
④ 关元
⑤ 水道
⑥ 提托穴
⑦ 子宫
⑧ 气冲

① L-1 *(Zhongfu)*
② S-21 *(Liangmen)*
③ Co-6 *(Qihai)*
④ Co-4 *(Guanyuan)*
⑤ S-28 *(Shuidao)*
⑥ N-CA-4 *(Tituoxue)*
⑦ M-CA-18 *(Zigong)*
⑧ S-30 *(Qichong)*
⑨ Co-22 *(Tiantu)*
⑩ Co-21 *(Xuanji)*
⑪ Co-17 *(Shanzhong)*
⑫ Li-14 *(Qimen)*
⑬ Co-14 *(Juque)*

⑭ Co-13 *(Shangwan)*
⑮ Co-12 *(Zhongwan)*
⑯ N-CA-18 *(Weishangxue)*
⑰ Li-13 *(Zhangmen)*
⑱ GB-26 *(Daimai)*
⑲ Sp-15 *(Daheng)*
⑳ S-25 *(Tianshu)*
㉑ Co-8 *(Qizhong)*
㉒ GB-27 *(Wushu)*
㉓ M-CA-16 *(Weibao)*
㉔ S-29 *(Guilai)*
㉕ Co-3 *(Zhongji)*

**Dia. 2-19 Relationship Between Points on
Chest and Abdomen with Musculature**

191

SUMMARY OF COMMON POINTS OF THE CHEST AND ABDOMEN

Region	Points	Common Characteristics	Particular Characteristics
Chest	Co-22 (Tiantu), Co-21 (Xuanji), L-1 (Zhongfu), Co-17 (Shanzhong), Li-14 (Qimen)	Disease of the chest (including respiratory system)	Co-22 (Tiantu): throat disease, vomiting, belching; L-1 (Zhongfu): pulmonary T.B., pleurisy, spitting blood; Co-17 (Shanzhong) and Li-14 (Qimen): diseases of Lung and Gall Bladder
Upper Abdomen	Co-14 (Juque), Co-13 (Shangwan), Co-12 (Zhongwan), S-21 (Liangmen), N-CA-18 (Weishang)	Disease of upper abdomen (most importantly, the Stomach)	Co-14 (Juque): mental disease, seizures, angina pectoris; Co-13 (Shangwan): stops vomiting; Co-12 (Zhongwan) and S-21 (Liangmen): gastro-intestinal disease; N-CA-18 (Weishang): prolapsed stomach
Lower Abdomen	Co-8 (Qizhong), S-25 (Tianshu), Sp-15 (Daheng)	Intestinal diseases	Co-8 (Qizhong): shock; S-25 (Tianshu): menstrual disorders; Sp-15 (Daheng): roundworms
	Co-6 (Qihai), Co-4 (Guanyuan), Co-3 (Zhongji)	Disease of urogenital system	Co-6 (Qihai) and Co-4 (Guanyuan): Intestinal diseases
	S-28 (Shuidao), N-CA-4 (Tituoxue), M-CA-16 (Weibao), S-29 (Guilai), M-CA-18 (Zigong), S-30 (Qichong)	Disease of urogenital system	N-CA-4 (Tituoxue) and M-CA-16 (Weibao): prolapsed uterus; M-CA-18 (Zigong): disease of female reproductive system; S-30 (Qichong): hernia
Flanks	Li-13 (Zhangmen), GB-26 (Daimai), GB-27 (Wushu)	Diseases of the flanks	Li-13 (Zhangmen): enlargement of the Liver and Spleen; GB-26 (Daimai): disease of female reproductive system; GB-27 (Wushu): disease of reproductive system

Chapter 4

Common Points of the Back

Gv-14 *(Dazhui)* 大维 "Big Vertebra"

Location
Between the spinous processes of the 7th cervical and 1st thoracic vertebrae. (Dia. 2-20)

Anatomy
In the supraspinal ligaments. Supplied by the vertebral venous plexus, and by the medial branch of the dorsal ramus of the eighth cervical nerve.

Traditional functions
Relieves Exterior conditions and opens the Yang, clears the brain and calms the Spirit.

Indications
Fever, heat stroke, malaria, psychosis, seizures, bronchitis, asthma, pulmonary tuberculosis, emphysema, hepatitis, blood diseases, eczema, hemiplegia, pain in the back of the shoulder.

Traditional indications
Cold-induced diseases, fever and chills, tidal fevers, cough, constricted feeling in chest and soreness in ribs, hot sensation in bones with recurrent fever (associated with Deficient Yin conditions), seizures, congested throat.

Illustrative combinations
With GB-20 *(Fengchi)*, LI-11 *(Quchi)* for influenza; with N-BW-8 *(Ganrexue)*, S-40 *(Fenglong)* for bronchitis; with LI-11 *(Quchi)*, S-36 *(Zusanli)*, B-20 *(Pishu)*, Sp-6 *(Sanyinjiao)* for leukopenia; with Gv-13 *(Taodao)*, M-BW-5 *(Erzhuixia)*, Gv-12 *(Shenzhu)* for psychosis.

Classical combinations
With Gv-2 *(Yaoshu)* for tidal fevers. (Source: CNLAM)

Needling method
Straight insertion, slanted slightly upward, 1-1.5 units. Sensation: local distension and soreness extending downward or to both shoulders. CAUTION: Do not insert the needle too deeply. If an electric, numb sensation is felt in the limbs, the needle should be immediately withdrawn and any further agitation of the needle ceased.

193

Remarks
Point of intersection of the Yang channels on the Governing channel.

M-BW-1 *(Dingchuan)*　定喘　"Stop Wheezing"

Location
0.5-1 unit lateral to the lower end of the spinous process of the 7th cervical vertebra. (Dia. 2-20)

Anatomy
In thick skin, supplied by a cutaneous branch of the dorsal ramus of the seventh cervical nerve. Below are the trapezius, rhomboid, posterior superior serratus, splenius, longissimus and semispinalis muscles. In its deep position, this point is situated directly on the medial branch of the dorsal ramus of the eighth cervical nerve. Also supplied by the transverse and deep cervical arteries and veins.

Indications
Cough, bronchitis, asthma, urticaria, stiff neck.

Illustrative combinations
With Co-22 *(Tiantu)*, Gv-14 *(Dazhui)*, S-40 *(Fenglong)*, for pertussis; with B-12 *(Fengmen)*, B-13 *(Feishu)*, LI-4 *(Hegu)* for bronchitis; with Co-22 *(Tiantu)*, Co-21 *(Xuanji)*, Co-17 *(Shanzhong)*, P-6 *(Neiguan)*, S-40 *(Fenglong)* for bronchial asthma.

Needling method
Straight insertion, pointed slightly toward the spine, 0.5-1 unit. Sensation: local distension and soreness, sometimes extending to the shoulders or chest.

GB-21 *(Jianjing)*　肩井　"Shoulder Well"

Location
Midway between Gv-14 *(Dazhui)* and the acromion of the shoulder. (Dia. 2-20)

Anatomy
In the posterior margin of the deltoid and trapezius muscles. In its deep position between the levator scapulae and supraspinatus muscles. Supplied by the transverse cervical artery and vein, by a posterior branch of the supraclavicular nerve, and in its deep position by the accessory nerve.

Indications
Hemiplegia due to stroke, mastitis, functinal uterine bleeding, scrofula, pain in the back of the shoulder.

Traditional indications
Vertigo, stiff neck, cough caused by rebellious Qi, aphasia due to apoplexy, breast abcess, difficult labor, scrofula.

Illustrative combinations
With SI-11 *(Tianzong)*, SI-1 *(Shaoze)* for mastitis; with GB-20 *(Fengchi)*, LI-15 *(Jianyu)* for pain in shoulder.

Classical combinations
With LI-11 *(Quchi)* for painful shoulder. (Source: OSM)

Needling method

Straight insertion, 0.5-1 unit. Sensation: distension and soreness extending to shoulder region. CAUTION: Care should be taken not to insert needle too deeply, to avoid puncturing the lung.

SI-15 *(Jianzhongshu)*　肩中俞　"Mid-Shoulder Hollow"

Location

2 units lateral to Gv-14 *(Dazhui)* on the upper back. (Dia. 2-20)

Anatomy

At the end of the transverse process of the first thoracic vertebra, superficially in the trapezius muscle, and in its deep position in the levator scapulae muscle. Supplied by a transverse cervical artery and vein, by the medial branch of the dorsal ramus of the first thoracic spinal nerve, the dorsal scapular nerve and the accessory nerve.

Indications

Bronchitis, asthma, bronchiectasis, stiff neck, pain in the back and shoulder.

Traditional indications

Coughing, spitting blood, blurred vision, fever and chills, consumption from milk in infants, pain in the back and shoulder.

Illustrative combinations

With Gv-12 *(Shenzhu),* Gv-9 *(Zhiyang),* L-6 *(Kongzui)* for bronchiectasis; with B-13 *(Feishu),* P-6 *(Neiguan),* S-36 *(Zusanli)* for bronchitis.

Needling method

Straight insertion, 0.5-0.8 unit. Sensation: distension and soreness reaching deeply.

Gv-13 *(Taodao)*　陶道　"Way of Happiness"

Location

Between the spinous processes of the 1st and 2nd thoracic vertebrae. (Dia. 2-20)

Anatomy

In the supraspinal and interspinal ligaments. Supplied by a posterior branch of the first intercostal artery, and the vertebral venous plexus. Supplied by the medial branch of the dorsal ramus of the first thoracic spinal nerve.

Traditional functions

Relieves Exterior conditions, cools Heat and calms the Spirit.

Indications

Fever, malaria, headache, seizures, psychosis, pulmonary tuberculosis, head and neck muscle spasms.

Traditional indications

Fever and chills, absence of sweating, tidal fevers, headache, heaviness in the head and dizziness, infantile convulsions, consumptive conditions, hot sensations in the bones (associated with Deficient Yin conditions), stiffness along the spine.

195

Illustrative combinations
With P-5 *(Jianshi)*, P-6 *(Neiguan)*, LI-11 *(Quchi)* for malaria; with M-BW-29 *(Yaoqi)*, Gv-26 *(Renzhong)*, P-6 *(Neiguan)*, S-40 *(Fenglong)* for seizures.

Classical combinations
With B-13 *(Feishu)* for fever. (Source: OHS)

Needling method
Straight insertion, pointed slightly upward, 1-1.5 units. Sensation: same as Gv-14 *(Dazhui)*.

Remarks
Point of intersection of the Bladder channel on the Governing channel.

B-11 *(Dazhu)*   大杼   "Big Shuttle"

Location
1.5 units lateral to the lower end of the spinous process of the 1st thoracic vertebra. (Dia. 2-20)

Anatomy
Superficially located in the trapezius, rhomboid, posterior superior serratus muscles, and in its deepest position in the longissimus muscle. Supplied by a posterior branch of the first intercostal artery and vein, and by the medial branch of the dorsal ramus of the first thoracic spinal nerve, and in its deepest postion by the lateral branch of that nerve.

Indications
Common cold, bronchitis, pneumonia, pleurisy, neck and back pain, tuberculosis of the bones, arthritis, numbness in the limbs.

Traditional indications
Headache accompanied by chills, low back pain, throat blockage, fullness in the chest and shortness of breath, tidal fevers, infantile convulsions, pain and inability to bend the knee, stiffness along the spine.

Illustrative combinations
With Co-17 *(Shanzhong)*, S-40 *(Fenglong)* for asthma; with B-13 *(Feishu)*, L-1 *(Zhongfu)*, L-6 *(Kongzui)* for pneumonia; with GB-20 *(Fengchi)*, B-12 *(Fengmen)*, B-13 *(Feishu)* for the common cold.

Classical combinations
With B-41 *(Geguan)* and Co-9 *(Shuifen)* for acute stiff back. (Source: CNLAM)

Needling method
Slanted insertion toward the spine, 0.7-1 unit. Sensation: local distension, soreness and numbness sometimes extending between the ribs.

Remarks
Point of intersection of the Small Intestine channel on the Bladder channel. Meeting point for the bones.

B-12 *(Fengmen)*   风门   "Wind's Door"

Location
1.5 units lateral to the lower end of the spinous process of the 2nd thoracic vertebra. (Dia. 2-20)

Anatomy

In the trapezius, rhomboid and posterior superior serratus muscles; in its deep position in the longissimus muscle. Supplied by a medial, posterior branch of the second intercostal artery and vein, by the medial branch of the dorsal ramus of the second thoracic spinal nerve, and in its deep position by a lateral branch of this nerve.

Traditional functions

Opens the Lungs, disperses Wind, regulates the Qi.

Indications

Common cold, bronchitis, pneumonia, pleurisy, asthma, urticaria, shoulder sprain.

Traditional indications

Headache, congested nose, cough due to cold, vomiting, belching, stiff neck, pain in the chest and back.

Illustrative combinations

With Gv-14 *(Dazhui)*, LI-4 *(Hegu)* for influenza (cups may be applied after needling); with LI-11 *(Quchi)*, L-7 *(Lieque)*, Sp-10 *(Xuehai)* for urticaria; with B-13 *(Feishu)*, L-6 *(Kongzui)* for pleurisy.

Needling method

(1) Straight insertion, slanted slightly toward the spine, 1-1.5 units. Sensation: local distension and soreness, sometimes extending between the ribs. (2) Transverse insertion, pointed downward along the muscle, 1-2 units. Sensation: local distension and soreness. CAUTION: Care should be taken not to insert needle too deeply, to avoid puncturing the lung.

Remarks

Point of intersection of the Governing channel on the Bladder channel.

Gv-12 *(Shenzhu)*　身柱　"Body's Pillar"

Location

Between the spinous processes of the 3rd and 4th thoracic vertebrae. (Dia. 2-20)

Anatomy

In the supraspinal and interspinal ligaments. Supplied by posterior branches of the third intercostal artery and vein, the vertebral venous plexus, and by the medial branch of the dorsal ramus of the third thoracic spinal nerve.

Indications

Bronchitis, pneumonia, asthma, pulmonary tuberculosis, chest and back pain, mental diseases, hysteria.

Traditional indications

Wheezing cough associated with a consumptive condition, Heat in the chest, aphasia due to apoplexy, seizures, infantile convulsions, stiffness and pain in the lumbar region.

Illustrative combinations

With Gv-14 *(Dazhui)*, B-12 *(Fengmen)* for pertussis; with Co-4 *(Guanyuan)*, S-36 *(Zusanli)* for rickets (use moxibustion); with Gv-14 *(Dazhui)*, B-13 *(Feishu)* for chronic bronchitis (use moxibustion).

Needling method

Slanted insertion, pointed slightly upward, 0.7-1 unit. Sensation: distension and soreness, or heavy, sinking feeling extending toward the lower back.

B-13 *(Feishu)*   肺俞   "Lung's Hollow"

Location

1.5 units lateral to the lower end of the spinous process of the 3rd thoracic vertebra. (Dia. 2-20)

Anatomy

In the trapezius and rhomboid muscles; in its deep position in the longissimus muscle. Supplied by medial, posterior branches of the third intercostal artery and vein, and by a medial branch of the dorsal ramus of the third thoracic spinal nerve, and in its deep position by the lateral branch of that nerve.

Traditional functions

Regulates the Lung Qi, reduces fever.

Indications

Bronchitis, asthma, pneumonia, pulmonary tuberculosis, pleurisy, spontaneous sweating, night sweats.

Traditional indications

Hot sensation in the bones (associated with Deficient Yin conditions) and night sweats, spitting blood, wheezing cough, fullness in chest and difficult breathing, throat blockage, insanity, convulsions, goiter.

Illustrative combinations

With N-BW-20 *(Feirexue)*, Co-17 *(Shanzhong)*, L-1 *(Zhongfu)*, P-6 *(Neiguan)* for bronchial asthma; join B-10 *(Tianzhu)* to B-13 *(Feishu)*, Gv-14 *(Dazhui)* to N-BW-6 *(Jiehexue)*, Co-17 *(Shanzhong)* to Co-18 *(Yutang)*, or Co-20 *(Huagai)* to Co-21 *(Xuanji)*, and also needle L-5 *(Chize)* and S-36 *(Zusanli)* for pulmonary tuberculosis; with Gv-14 *(Dazhui)* and B-38 *(Gaohuangshu)* for chronic bronchitis (use moxibustion).

Classical combinations

With Co-22 *(Tiantu)* for coughing (Source: OHS); with Co-14 *(Juque)* for fullness in the chest. (Source: CNLAM)

Needling method

Same as B-12 *(Fengmen)* above. CAUTION: Care should be taken not to insert needle too deeply, to avoid puncturing the lung.

Remarks

Associated point of the Lung.

SI-13 *(Quyuan)*   曲垣   "Crooked Wall"

Location

In the depression at the extreme medial end and above the spine of the scapula, in the supraspinous fossa. (Dia. 2-20)

Anatomy

On the superior margin of the spine of the scapula, in the trapezius and supraspinatus muscles. Supplied by descending branches of the transverse cervical artery and vein, and in its deep position by muscle branches of the suprascapular artery and vein. Supplied by a medial branch of the dorsal ramus of the second thoracic spinal nerve, the accessory nerve, and in its deep position by a muscle branch of the suprascapular nerve.

Indications

Inflammation of the tendon of the supraspinatus muscle, diseases of the soft tissues of the shoulder joint.

Traditional indications

Pain in the shoulder and shoulder blade, blockage conditions, muscle spasms.

Illustrative combinations

With LI-14 *(Binao)*, GB-34 *(Yanglingquan)* for inflammation of the tendon of the supraspinatus muscle, on the affected side.

Needling method

Straight insertion, 0.5-0.8 unit. Sensation: local distension and soreness.

SI-11 *(Tianzong)*   天宗   "Heaven's Ancestor"

Location

In the center of the infraspinous fossa of the shoulder blade. (Dia. 2-20)

Anatomy

In the infraspinatus muscle at the center of the infraspinous fossa. Supplied by muscle branches of the circumflex artery and vein of the scapula, and by the suprascapular nerve.

Indication

Pain in the shoulder, upper arm and shoulder blade.

Traditional indications

Pain in the shoulder and shoulder blade, fullness in the chest and ribs, severe painful hiccoughs, swelling in the cheek and jaw.

Illustrative combinations

With LI-15 *(Jianyu)*, TB-14 *(Jianliao)*, GB-34 *(Yanglingquan)* for inflammation of the shoulder joint; with Co-17 *(Shanzhong)*, S-18 *(Rugen)*, SI-1 *(Shaoze)* for insufficient lactation or mastitis.

Needling method

Straight insertion, or slanted in different directions, 0.5-1.5 units. Sensation: local distension and soreness.

B-14 *(Jueyinshu)*   厥阴俞   "Absolute Yin Hollow"

Location

1.5 units lateral to the lower end of the spinous process of the 4th thoracic vertebra. (Dia. 2-20)

Anatomy

In the trapezius and rhomboid muscles; its deep position is in the longissimus muscle. Supplied by medial posterior branches of the fourth intercostal artery and vein. Situated directly on a medial, cutaneous branch of the dorsal ramus of the fourth thoracic spinal nerve, and in its deep position on a lateral branch of that nerve.

Indications

Rheumatic heart disease, neurasthenia, intercostal neuralgia.

① Gv-14 *(Dazhui)*
② SI-15 *(Jianzhongshu)*
③ B-11 *(Dashu)*
④ B-12 *(Fengmen)*
⑤ SI-13 *(Quyuan)*
⑥ B-14 *(Jueyinshu)*
⑦ SI-11 *(Tianzong)*
⑧ B-15 *(Xinshu)*
⑨ B-17 *(Geshu)*
⑩ Gv-9 *(Zhiyang)*
⑪ B-18 *(Ganshu)*

⑫ B-19 *(Danshu)*
⑬ B-20 *(Pishu)*
⑭ B-21 *(Weishu)*
⑮ M-BW-1 *(Dingchuan)*
⑯ GB-21 *(Jianjing)*
⑰ Gv-13 *(Taodao)*
⑱ B-13 *(Feishu)*
⑲ Gv-12 *(Shenzhu)*
⑳ B-38 *(Gaohuangshu)*
㉑ B-16 *(Dushu)*
㉒ Gv-10 *(Lingtai)*

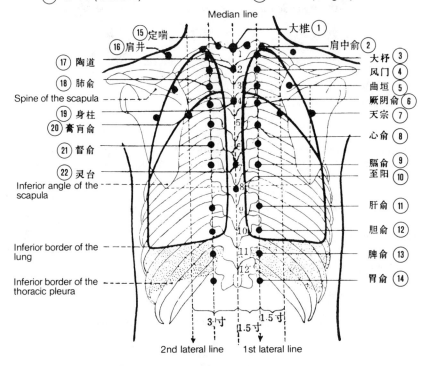

Dia. 2-20 Back Points

Traditional indications

Pain in chest caused by accumulation of Qi in the diaphragm, vomiting caused by rebellious Qi, coughing, toothache.

Illustrative combinations

With B-15 *(Xinshu)*, Sp-6 *(Sanyinjiao)* for rheumatic heart disease; with H-8 *(Shaofu)*, H-5 *(Tongli)* for tachycardia; with B-15 *(Xinshu)*, B-18 *(Ganshu)*, B-23 *(Shenshu)* for neurasthenia.

Classical combinations

With H-7 *(Shenmen)* and GB-15 *(Linqi)* for chest pain. (Source: CNLAM)

Needling method

Same as B-12 *(Fengmen)* above. CAUTION: Care should be taken not to insert needle too deeply, to avoid puncturing the lung.

B-38 *(Gaohuangshu)* 膏肓俞 "Vital's Hollow"

Location
3 units lateral to the lower end of the spinous process of the 4th thoracic vertebra. (Dia. 2-20)

Anatomy
At the end of the medial border of the spine of the scapula, in the trapezius and rhomboid muscles; its deep position is in the iliocostalis muscle. Supplied by a posterior branch of the fourth intercostal artery and a descending branch of the transverse cervical artery. Supplied by a medial branch of the dorsal ramus of the second thoracic spinal nerve, and in its deep position by a lateral branch of the dorsal ramus of the third thoracic spinal nerve. In addition, there is the dorsal scapular nerve, and in its deepest position the trunk of the fourth intercostal nerve.

Traditional functions
Regulates the Lung Qi and strengthens Deficient conditions.

Indications
Bronchitis, asthma, pleurisy, pulmonary tuberculosis, neurasthenia, general weakness caused by prolonged illness.

Traditional indications
Consumptive Deficient diseases, coughing blood, hiccoughs, Deficient Spleen and Stomach, nocturnal emissions, absent-mindedness, pain along the spine.

Illustrative combinations
With B-13 *(Feishu)*, B-23 *(Shenshu)* for pulmonary tuberculosis (use moxibustion); with Co-22 *(Tiantu)*, M-BW-1 *(Dingchuan)* for asthma; with Co-4 *(Guanyuan)* and S-36 *(Zusanli)* for general weakness caused by prolonged illness (use moxibustion).

Classical combinations
With M-HN-30 *(Bailao)* for consumptive disorders. (Source: NPA)

Needling method
Slanted insertion away from the spine, 0.5-1 unit. Sensation: local distension and soreness, sometimes extending to shoulder. CAUTION: Care should be taken not to insert the needle too deeply, to avoid puncturing the lung.

B-15 *(Xinshu)* 心俞 "Heart's Hollow"

Location
1.5 units lateral to the lower end of the spinous process of the 5th thoracic vertebra. (Dia. 2-20)

Anatomy
In the trapezius and rhomboid muscles; in its deep position in the longissimus muscle. Supplied by medial, posterior branches of the fifth intercostal artery and vein, and by a medial branch of the dorsal ramus of the fifth thoracic spinal nerve; in its deep position by a lateral branch of that nerve.

Traditional functions
Calms the Heart and Spirit, regulates the Blood and Qi.

Indications
Neurasthenia, intercostal neuralgia, rheumatic heart disease, atrial fibrillation, tachycardia, psychosis, seizures, hysteria.

Traditional indications

Irritability and depressed feeling in the chest and heart, chest pain, coughing, coughing blood, vomiting without eating; tidal fevers, chills and fever, hot palms and soles of feet; spermatorrhea, night sweats, absent-mindedness.

Illustrative combinations

With Co-14 *(Juque)* for neurasthenia (injection therapy may be used); with B-14 *(Jueyinshu)* for rheumatic heart disease (injection therapy may be used); with H-7 *(Shenmen)*, P-6 *(Neiguan)* and join GB-34 *(Yanglingquan)* to Sp-9 *(Yinlingquan)* for cardiac arrhythmia; with H-7 *(Shenmen)*, S-40 *(Fenglong)* for pulmonary heart disease; with B-17 *(Geshu)*, Sp-10 *(Xuehai)*, Sp-6 *(Sanyinjiao)* for Buerger's disease (injection therapy may be used).

Classical combinations

With B-23 *(Shenmen)* for spermatorrhea. (Source: SJD)

Needling method

Same as B-12 *(Fengmen)* above. CAUTION: Care should be taken not to insert the needle too deeply, to avoid puncturing a lung.

Remarks

Associated point of the Heart.

Gv-10 *(Lingtai)*　灵治　"Spirit's Platform"

Location

Between the spinous processes of the 6th and 7th thoracic vertebrae. (Dia. 2-20)

Anatomy

In the supraspinal and interspinal ligaments. Supplied by a posterior branch of the sixth intercostal artery and the vertebral venous plexus, and by a medial branch of the dorsal ramus of the sixth thoracic spinal nerve.

Indications

Asthma, bronchitis, round worm in the bile duct, malaria, boils, stomach-ache.

Traditional indications

Hot or Cold common cold, stiffness in the neck and soreness along the spine, prolonged cough and asthma, Hot condition in the Spleen, carbuncles, boils.

Illustrative combinations

With GB-34 *(Yanglingquan)* for round worm in the bile duct; with Gv-13 *(Taodao)*, P-6 *(Neiguan)* for tertian malaria.

Needling method

Slanted insertion, pointed slightly upward, 0.5-1 unit. Sensation: distension and soreness, sometimes extending to the lower back or chest.

B-16 *(Dushu)*　督俞　"Governing Hollow"

Location

1.5 units lateral to the lower end of the spinous process of the 6th thoracic vertebra. (Dia. 2-20)

Anatomy

In the trapezius, latissimus dorsi and longissimus muscles. Supplied by a medial, posterior branch of the sixth intercostal artery and vein and a descending branch of the transverse cervical artery; by the dorsal scapular nerve, and a medial branch of the dorsal ramus of the sixth thoracic spinal nerve; in its deepest position supplied by a lateral branch of that nerve.

Indications

Endocarditis and pericarditis, abdominal pain, intestinal noises, spasms of the diaphragm, mastitis, alopecia, pruritis, psoriasis.

Traditional indications

Hot or Cold chest pain, abdominal pain, intestinal noises, rebellious Qi.

Illustrative combinations

B-13 *(Feishu)*, B-17 *(Geshu)*, LI-11 *(Quchi)*, Sp-10 *(Xuehai)* for psoriasis; with Gv-14 *(Dazhui)*, B-15 *(Xinshu)*, B-17 *(Geshu)* for furuncle, abcess, folliculitis.

Needling method

Slanted insertion toward the spine, 0.7-1 unit. Sensation: local distension and soreness, sometimes extending to ribs and chest.

Gv-9 *(Zhiyang)* 至陽 "Reaching Yang"

Location

Between the spinous processes of the 7th and 8th thoracic vertebrae. (Dia. 2-20)

Anatomy

In the supraspinal and interspinal ligaments. Supplied by a posterior branch of the seventh intercostal artery and the vertebral venous plexus, and by a medial branch of the dorsal ramus of the seventh thoracic spinal nerve.

Traditional functions

Regulates the Qi functions, transforms Damp Heat, expands the chest and diaphragm.

Indications

Hepatitis, cholecystitis, malaria, bronchial asthma, pleurisy, round worm in the bile duct, stomach-ache, intercostal neuralgia, back pain.

Traditional indications

Cough, panting, chest and back pain, jaundice, body curled up and lethargic, fullness in the chest, Cold Stomach, intestinal noises.

Illustrative combinations

With B-18 *(Ganshu)*, B-20 *(Pishu)*, S-36 *(Zusanli)*, GB-34 *(Yanglingquan)* for infectious hepatitis; with GB-34 *(Yanglingquan)*, TB-6 *(Zhigou)* for psoriasis; with P-6 *(Neiguan)* for cardiac arrhythmia.

Needling method

Slanted insertion, 0.7-1 unit. Sensation: distension and soreness extending to the lower back and chest.

B-17 *(Geshu)* 膈俞 "Diaphragm's Hollow"

Location
1.5 units lateral to the lower end of the spinous process of the 7th thoracic vertebra. (Dia. 2-20)

Anatomy
At the inferior margin of the trapezius muscle, and in the latissimus dorsi and longissimus muscles. Supplied by medial, posterior branches of the seventh intercostal artery and vein, and by a medial branch of the dorsal ramus of the seventh thoracic spinal nerve; in its deep position supplied by a lateral branch of that nerve.

Traditional functions
Regulates the Blood, transforms Congealed Blood, expands the chest and diaphragm, strengthens Deficient conditions.

Indications
Anemia, chronic hemorrhagic disorders, spasms of the diaphragm, nervous vomiting, urticaria, tuberculosis of the lymph glands, stomach cancer, constriction of the esophagus.

Traditional indications
Chills and fever, hot sensation in the bones (associated with Deficient Yin conditions) and night sweats, coughing or spitting blood, abdominal distension or lumps, lassitude, hypersomnia, hemorrhage.

Illustrative combinations
With Co-22 *(Tiantu)*, Co-17 *(Shanzhong)*, Co-14 *(Juque)*, S-36 *(Zusanli)* for spasm of the diaphragm; with Gv-14 *(Dazhui)*, B-21 *(Weishu)*, Sp-10 *(Xuehai)*, S-36 *(Zusanli)* for anemia.

Classical combinations
With L-8 *(Jingqu)* for swollen and painful throat. (Source: CNLAM)

Needling method
Same as B-12 *(Fengmen)* above.

B-18 *(Ganshu)* 肝俞 "Liver's Hollow"

Location
1.5 units lateral to the lower end of the spinous process of the 9th thoracic vertebra. (Dia. 2-20)

Anatomy
In the latissimus dorsi muscle, and between the longissimus and iliocostalis muscles. Supplied by medial posterior branches of the ninth intercostal artery and vein, by a medial branch of the dorsal ramus of the ninth thoracic spinal nerve, and in its deep position by a lateral branch of that nerve.

Traditional functions
Benefits the Liver and Gall Bladder, cools Damp Heat, moves stagnant Qi, benefits the eyes.

Indications
Chronic and acute hepatitis, cholecystitis, stomach diseases, eye diseases, intercostal neuralgia, neurasthenia, irregular menstruation.

Traditional indications
Nosebleed, spitting blood, eye diseases, jaundice, pain of lumps in the chest and abdomen.

Illustrative combinations

With M-HN-13 *(Yiming)*, Li-4 *(Zhongfeng)* for acute or chronic hepatitis; with Co-6 *(Qihai)*, Sp-6 *(Sanyinjiao)* for amenorrhea; with B-23 *(Shenshu)*, GB-39 *(Xuanzhong)* for acute leukemia; with B-30 *(Pishu)*, Li-14 *(Qimen)*, B-16 *(Dushu)*, Sp-10 *(Xuehai)*, Sp-6 *(Sanyinjiao)*, GB-34 *(Yanglingquan)* for cirrhosis of the liver.

Classical combinations

With Gv-4 *(Mingmen)* to clear dull eyes (Source:OSM); with B-20 *(Pishu)* and B-47 *(Zhishi)* for acute pain in the flanks. (Source: CNLAM)

Needling method

Same as B-12 *(Fengmen)* above.

Remarks

Associated point of the Liver.

B-19 *(Danshu)*   胆俞   "Gall Bladder's Hollow"

Location

1.5 units lateral to the lower end of the spinous process of the 10th thoracic vertebra. (Dia. 2-20)

Anatomy

In the latissimus dorsi muscle, and between the longissimus and iliocostalis muscles. Supplied by medial, posterior branches of the tenth intercostal artery and vein, and by a medial branch of the dorsal ramus of the tenth thoracic spinal nerve; in its deep position supplied by a lateral branch of that nerve.

Traditional functions

Cools and drains Heat from the Liver and Gall Bladder, calms the Stomach, regulates the Qi and expands the diaphragm.

Indications

Hepatitis, cholecystitis, gastritis, round worm in the bile duct, tuberculosis of the lymph glands, abdominal distension, soreness in chest and ribs, sciatica.

Traditional indications

Headache and chills, bitter taste in mouth, dry vomiting, sore throat, distension and fullness in the abdomen and chest, pain in the flanks, yellowish eyes, jaundice, hot sensation in the bones and fever (associated with Deficient Yin, consumptive diseases), sperm in the urine (associated with Deficient Yin diseases), swelling of the axillary lymph glands.

Illustrative combinations

With Gv-9 *(Zhiyang)*, S-36 *(Zusanli)*, Li-3 *(Taichong)* for acute infectious hepatitis; with GB-34 *(Yanglingquan)*, P-6 *(Neiguan)* for round worm in the bile duct; with M-LE-23 *(Dannangxue)* for cholecystitis.

Classical combinations

With Li-13 *(Zhangmen)* for rib pain preventing sleep. (Source: CNLAM)

Needling method

Same as B-12 *(Fengmen)* above.

Remarks

Associated point of the Gall Bladder.

B-20 *(Pishu)*　脾俞　"Spleen Hollow"

Location
1.5 units lateral to the lower end of the spinous process of the 11th thoracic vertebra. (Dia. 2-21)

Anatomy
In the latissimus dorsi muscle, and between the longissimus and iliocostalis muscles. Supplied by medial posterior branches of the eleventh intercostal artery and vein, and by a medial branch of the dorsal ramus of the eleventh thoracic spinal nerve; in its deep position supplied by the lateral branch of that nerve.

Traditional functions
Regulates the Qi of the Spleen and assists its transportive and transformative functions, eliminates Dampness, harmonizes the Blood and Nourishing Qi.

Indications
Gastritis, ulcers, prolapsed stomach, nervous vomiting, indigestion, hepatitis, enteritis, edema, anemia, enlargement of liver and spleen, chronic hemorrhagic diseases, prolapsed uterus, urticaria, weakness in the limbs.

Traditional indications
Constriction of esophagus inhibiting swallowing, diarrhea, dysentery, edema, abdominal distension, lumps in the chest and abdomen, jaundice.

Illustrative combinations
With B-17 *(Geshu),* M-BW-12 *(Yishu),* B-23 *(Shenshu),* N-BW-10 *(Pirexue)* for diabetes; with Gv-14 *(Dazhui),* S-36 *(Zusanli),* Sp-6 *(Sanyinjiao)* for leukopenia (use moxibustion).

Classical combinations
With B-28 *(Pangguangshu)* for poor digestion due to Deficient Spleen (Source: OHS); with B-18 *(Ganshu)* and Co-13 *(Shangwan)* for nosebleed with spitting of blood. (Source: GCAM)

Needling method
Straight insertion, pointed slightly toward spine, 1-1.5 units. Sensation: local distension, soreness and numbness extending into the lumbar region. CAUTION: Care should be taken not to insert needle too deeply, to avoid puncturing the kidneys or liver.

Remarks
Associated point of the Spleen.

B-21 *(Weishu)*　胃俞　"Stomach's Hollow"

Location
1.5 units lateral to the lower end of the spinous process of the 12th thoracic vertebra. (Dia. 2-21)

Anatomy
In the lumbodorsal fascia, between the longissimus and iliocostalis muscles. Supplied by medial posterior branches of the subcostal artery and vein, and by a medial branch of the dorsal ramus of the twelfth thoracic spinal nerve; in its deep position supplied by a lateral branch of that nerve.

Traditional functions
Regulates Stomach Qi, transforms Dampness, and eliminates stagnation.

Indications
Stomach-ache, gastritis, gastric distension, prolapsed stomach, ulcer, pancreatitis, hepatitis, enteritis, loss of appetite, insomnia, pain along the spine.

Traditional indications
Difficulty swallowing, regurgitant vomiting, infant vomiting milk, abdominal pain from Cold condition in Stomach, diarrhea, edema ('like a drum').

Illustrative combinations
With B-20 *(Pishu)*, Co-12 *(Zhongwan)*, S-36 *(Zusanli)* for chronic gastritis; or join this point to B-20 *(Pishu)*, and Co-12 *(Zhongwan)* to Co-13 *(Shangwan)*. ('Burying the thread' method may be used).

Classical combinations
With B-23 *(Shenshu)* for Cold and distended stomach. (Source: CNLAM)

Needling method
Same as B-20 *(Pishu)* above.

Remarks
Associated point of the Stomach.

B-22 *(Sanjiaoshu)*   三焦俞   "Triple Burner's Hollow"

Location
1.5 units lateral to the lower end of the spinous process of the 1st lumbar vertebra. (Dia. 2-21)

Anatomy
In the lumbodorsal fascia, between the longissimus and iliocostalis muscles. Supplied by medial posterior branches of the first lumbar artery and vein, by a lateral branch of the dorsal ramus of the tenth thoracic spinal nerve, and in its deep position by a lateral branch of the dorsal ramus of the first lumbar spinal nerve.

Traditional functions
Regulates the transforming function of Qi, eliminates Dampness.

Indications
Gastritis, enteritis, nephritis, ascites, urinary retention, enuresis, neurasthenia, low back pain.

Traditional indications
Dizziness and headache, vomiting, indigestion, abdominal distension and intestinal noises, diarrhea, edema, jaundice.

Illustrative combinations
With B-24 *(Qihaishu)*, B-25 *(Dachangshu)*, S-36 *(Zusanli)* for acute or chronic nephritis.

Needling method
Straight insertion, 1-1.5 units. Sensation: distension and soreness as far as the waist. CAUTION: Care should be taken not to insert needle too deeply, to avoid puncturing the kidneys.

Remarks
Associated point of the Triple Burner.

Gv-4 *(Mingmen)* 命门 "Life's Door"

Location

Between the spinous processes of the 2nd and 3rd lumbar vertebrae. (Dia. 2-21)

Anatomy

In the lumbodorsal fascia, and the supraspinal and interspinal ligaments. Supplied by a posterior branch of the lumbar artery and the vertebral venous plexus, by a medial branch of the dorsal ramus of a lumbar spinal nerve.

Traditional functions

Nourishes the Source Qi and strengthens the Kidneys, benefits the lumbar vertebrae.

Indications

Low back pain or sprain, enuresis, spermatorrhea, impotence, leukorrhea, endometritis, peritonitis, spinal myelitis, sciatica, nephritis, sequelae of infantile paralysis.

Traditional indications

Headache, tidal fevers, infantile convulsions, related pain in lower back and abdomen, pain of intestinal colic, loss of sperm, vaginal discharge with blood, uterine bleeding, prolapsed anus.

Illustrative combinations

With Gv-14 *(Dazhui)*, B-17 *(Geshu)*, LI-11 *(Quchi)*, S-36 *(Zusanli)* for iron defiency anemia; with Gv-20 *(Baihui)*, Co-4 *(Guanyuan)*, Sp-6 *(Sanyinjiao)*, B-33 *(Zhongliao)* for enuresis (use moxibustion).

Classical combinations

With B-23 *(Shenshu)* for copious urine in the elderly. (Source: SJD)

Needling method

Straight insertion, pointed slightly toward the spine, 1-1.5 units. Sensation: local distension; if the needle is inserted deeply, there is an electric, numb sensation extending into the lower limb.

B-23 *(Shenshu)* 肾俞 "Kidney's Hollow"

Location

1.5 units lateral to the lower end of the spinous process of the 2nd lumbar vertebra. (Dia. 2-21)

Anatomy

In the lumbodorsal fascia, between the longissimus and iliocostalis muscles. Supplied by medial posterior branches of the second lumbar artery and vein, by a medial branch of the dorsal ramus of the first lumbar spinal nerve, and in its deep position by a lateral branch of that nerve.

Traditional functions

Regulates the Kidney Qi, strengthens the lumbar vertebrae, benefits the ears and eyes.

Indications

Nephritis, nephroptosis, renal colic, low back pain, spermatorrhea, impotence, irregular menstruation, bronchial asthma, tinnitus, deafness, alopecia, anemia, injury to soft tissues of lower back, sequelae of infantile paralysis.

Traditional indications

Deafness, Deficient Kidneys, loss of sperm, impotence, blood in urine, edema, emaciation and thirst, seizures, tidal fevers, low back pain and cold knees.

Illustrative combinations

With Co-3 *(Zhongji)*, Sp-6 *(Sanyinjiao)*, K-7 *(Fuliu)*, B-58 *(Feiyang)*, M-CA-18 *(Zigong)* for nephritis; with B-28 *(Pangguangshu)*, Co-3 *(Zhongji)*, Sp-6 *(Sanyinjiao)* for urinary tract infection; with Co-4 *(Guanyuan)*, S-36 *(Zusanli)* for diabetes.

Classical combinations

With S-3 *(Juliao)* for Congealed Blood in the chest and abdomen (Source: OHS); with Li-13 *(Zhangmen)* for Cold diarrhea with undigested particles. (Source: CNLAM)

Needling method

Straight insertion, pointed slightly toward the spine, 1.5-2 units. Sensation: distension in the lower back, or an electric, numb sensation extending to the buttocks and lower extremity. CAUTION: Care should be taken not to insert needle too deeply, or away from the spine, to avoid puncturing the kidneys.

Remarks

Associated point of the Kidneys.

B-47 *(Zhishi)*   志室   "Will's Dwelling"

Location

3 units lateral to the lower end of the spinous process of the 2nd lumbar vertebra. (Dia. 2-21)

Anatomy

In the latissimus dorsi and iliocostalis muscles. Supplied by dorsal branches of the second lumbar artery and vein, by a lateral branch of the dorsal ramus of the twelfth thoracic spinal nerve, and a lateral branch of the first lumbar spinal nerve.

Indications

Nephritis, low back pain, spermatorrhea, impotence, prostatitis, eczema of the scrotum, painful urination, edema, paralysis of lower limb.

Traditional indications

Vomiting, indigestion; incontinence, swelling and pain in the genitals, nocturnal emissions; edema.

Illustrative combinations

With B-28 *(Pangguangshu)*, K-3 *(Taixi)* for nephroptosis; with B-23 *(Guanyuanshu)*, B-51 *(Yinmen)* for injury to the soft tissues of the lower back; with B-23 *(Shenshu)*, Sp-6 *(Sanyinjiao)* for renal colic.

Classical combinations

With B-48 *(Baoyu)* for pain and swelling in the genital region. (Source: CNLAM)

Needling method

(1) Straight insertion, 1.5-2 units. (2) Transverse insertion, for injury to the soft tissues of the lower back, or nephroptosis, pointed toward B-23 *(Shenshu)* 2-3 units. Sensation: local distension and soreness, sometimes extending to the buttocks. CAUTION: Care should be taken not to insert needle too deeply, to avoid puncturing the kidneys.

B-24 *(Qihaishu)*　气海俞　"Sea of Qi Hollow"

Location

1.5 units lateral to the lower end of the spinous process of the 3rd lumbar vertebra. (Dia. 2-21)

Anatomy

In the lumbodorsal fascia, between the longissimus and iliocostalis muscles. Supplied by posterior branches of the third lumbar artery and vein, by a medial branch of the dorsal ramus of the second lumbar spinal nerve, and in its deep position by a lateral branch of that nerve.

Traditional functions

Regulates the Qi and Blood, strengthens the lower back and knees.

Indications

Pain in the lumbar vertebrae, hemorrhoids, irregular menstruation, functional uterine bleeding, paralysis of lower limbs.

Traditional indications

Low back pain, bleeding hemorrhoids.

Illustrative combinations

With M-BW-25 *(Shiqizhuixia)*, Sp-6 *(Sanyinjiao)* for functional uterine bleeding.

Needling method

Same as B-23 *(Shenshu)* above.

Gv-3 *(Yaoyangguan)*　腰陽关　"Lumbar Yang's Hinge"

Location

Between the spinous processes of the 4th and 5th lumbar vertebrae. (Dia. 2-21)

Anatomy

In the lumbodorsal fascia, and the supraspinal and interspinal ligaments. Supplied by posterior branches of the lumbar artery and vein and the vertebral venous plexus, and by a medial branch of the dorsal ramus of a lumbar spinal nerve.

Traditional functions

Regulates the Kidney Qi, benefits the lower back and knees, eliminates Cold Dampness.

Indications

Low back pain, paralysis of the lower limbs, irregular menstruation, spermatorrhea, impotence, chronic enteritis.

Traditional indications

Irregular menstruation, vaginal discharge with blood, loss of sperm; diarrhea, lower abdominal distension, continuous vomiting; low back pain, pain in the knees, numb and stiff lower limbs; scrofula.

Illustrative combinations

With Gv-4 *(Mingmen)* and Gv-5 *(Xuanshu)* for multiple neuritis (injection therapy may be used).

Needling method

Same as Gv-4 *(Mingmen)* above.

①	Gv-4 *(Mingmen)*	⑩	Gv-1 *(Changqiang)*
②	B-47 *(Zhishi)*	⑪	B-20 *(Pishu)*
③	B-23 *(Shenshu)*	⑫	B-21 *(Weishu)*
④	M-BW-24 *(Yaoyan)*	⑬	B-22 *(Sanjiaoshu)*
⑤	B-25 *(Dachangshu)*	⑭	B-24 *(Qihaishu)*
⑥	B-26 *(Guanyuanshu)*	⑮	Gv-3 *(Yaoyangguan)*
⑦	B-27 *(Xiaochangshu)*	⑯	M-BW-25 *(Shiqizhuixia)*
⑧	B-28 *(Pangguangshu)*	⑰	B-31—34 *(Baliao)*
⑨	B-49 *(Zhibian)*	⑱	B-30 *(Baihuanshu)*

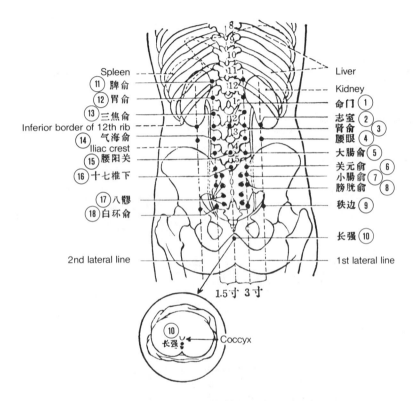

Dia. 2-21 Lumbosacral Points

B-25 *(Dachangshu)*　大腸俞　"Large Intestine's Hollow"

Location
1.5 units lateral to the lower end of the spinous process of the 4th lumbar vertebra. (Dia. 2-21)

Anatomy
In the lumbodorsal fascia, between the longissimus and iliocostalis muscles. Supplied by posterior branches of the fourth lumbar artery and vein, and by the dorsal ramus of the third lumbar spinal nerve.

Traditional functions
Regulates the Intestines and Stomach, benefits the lower back and knees.

211

Indications
Low back pain or sprain, pain in sacroiliac joint, enteritis, dysentery, constipation.

Traditional indications
Abdominal distension and intestinal noises, diarrhea, 'cutting' pain around navel, difficult or painful defecation or urination.

Illustrative combinations
With B-30 *(Baihuanshu)*, Gv-4 *(Mingmen)*, join S-38 *(Tiaokou)* to B-57 *(Chengshan)*, join GB-34 *(Yanglingquan)* to Sp-9 *(Yinlingquan)* for progressive muscular dystrophy.

Classical combinations
With B-32 *(Ciliao)* for bowel and urinary incontinence. (Source: CNLAM)

Needling method
(1) Straight insertion, for most indications, 1-2 units. Sensation: distension and soreness in lower back. (2) Slanted insertion, for sciatica, needle pointed slightly away from spine, 2-3 units. Sensation: electric, numb sensation possibly extending to leg. (3) Transverse insertion, for arthritis of the sacroiliac, join to B-27 *(Xiaochangshu)*. Sensation: distension and soreness, possibly reaching sacroiliac joint.

Remarks
Associated point of the Large Intestine.

M-BW-24 *(Yaoyan)*   腰眼   "Waist's Eye"

Location
In the depression, 3-4 units lateral to the lower end of the spinous process of the 3rd lumbar vertebra. (Dia. 2-21)

Anatomy
Above the iliac crest, at the lateral margin of the sacrospinalis muscle, directly on the superior clunial nerve. Below is the tendon of the latissimus dorsi, and the lateral margin of the sacrospinalis muscle. In its deep position are the lateral margin of the quadratus lumborum, the lumbar (spinal) nerve plexus, and branches of the lumbar artery and vein.

Indications
Injury to the soft tissues of the lumbar region, nephroptosis, orchitis, gynecological diseases.

Illustrative combinations
With B-23 *(Shenshu)*, B-54 *(Weizhong)* for low back pain; with B-20 *(Pishu)*, N-BW-15 *(Shenji)* for nephroptosis.

Needling method
Straight or transverse insertion, 1.5-2.5 units. Sensation: distension and soreness in the lumbar region, sometimes extending to the buttocks.

Remarks
The position of this point is listed elsewhere as being 3.8 units lateral to the lower end of the 4th lumbar vertebra.

212

M-BW-25 *(Shiqizhuixia)* 十七椎下 "Below 17 Vertebrae"

Location

In the depression below the spinous process of the 5th lumbar vertebra. (Dia. 2-21)

Anatomy

Below the spinous process of the fifth lumbar vertebra, in the supraspinal and interspinal ligaments. Supplied by a medial branch of the dorsal ramus of the fifth lumbar spinal nerve and accompanying arterial and venous branches. In its deep position, in the subflavous ligament, the dura mater and arachnoid membranes, the subarachnoid space, and cauda equina.

Indications

Pain in lumbosacral region, sciatica, functional uterine bleeding, dysmenorrhea, anal diseases, sequelae of infantile paralysis, traumatic paraplegia.

Illustrative combinations

With M-BW-35 *(Jiaji)* for paralysis of lower limb; with B-49 *(Zhibian)*, B-26 *(Guanyuanshu)* for pain in the lumbosacral region; with Co-3 *(Zhongji)*, Sp-6 *(Sanyinjiao)*, K-3 *(Taixi)* for dysmenorrhea.

Needling method

Straight insertion, 1.5-2 units. Sensation: local distension and numbness extending to the buttocks; if the insertion is deep, an electric, numb sensation extending down the leg.

B-26 *(Guanyuanshu)* 关元俞 "Hollow at the Hinge of the Source"

Location

1.5 units lateral to the lower end of the spinous process of the 5th lumbar vertebra. (Dia. 2-21)

Anatomy

In the sacrospinalis muscle. Supplied by posterior branches of the fifth lumbar artery and vein, and by the dorsal ramus of the fifth lumbar spinal nerve.

Traditional functions

Regulates the Lower Burner, strengthens the lower back and knees, transforms Damp stagnation.

Indications

Chronic enteritis, low back pain, diabetes, anemia, chronic peritonitis, cystitis.

Traditional indications

Emaciation and thirst, low back pain, frequent or painful urination, enuresis.

Illustrative combinations

With B-20 *(Pishu)*, B-23 *(Shenshu)* for chronic enteritis; with M-BW-12 *(Yishu)*, B-20 *(Pishu)*, B-22 *(Sanjiaoshu)*, B-23 *(Shenshu)* for diabetes; with B-18 *(Ganshu)*, B-20 *(Pishu)* for dysmenorrhea; with S-25 *(Tianshu)*, B-23 *(Shenshu)*, Sp-6 *(Sanyinjiao)* for acute or chronic nephritis.

Classical combinations

With B-28 *(Pangguangshu)* for Wind consumption with low back pain. (Source: CNLAM)

Needling method

Straight insertion, 1.5-2 units. Sensation: local distension and soreness, sometimes extending to the leg.

B-27 *(Xiaochangshu)* 小腸俞 "Small Intestine's Hollow"

Location

1.5 units lateral to the midline of the spine, level with the 1st posterior sacral foramen. (Dia. 2-21)

Anatomy

Between the origins of the sacrospinalis and gluteus maximus muscles. Supplied by lateral, posterior branches of the lateral sacral artery and vein, and by a lateral branch of the dorsal ramus of the first sacral nerve.

Traditional functions

Opens and regulates the Small Intestine, eliminates Dampness and cools Heat.

Indications

Low back pain, pain in the sacroiliac and diseases of the sacroiliac joint, spermatorrhea, enuresis, enteritis, constipation, peritonitis.

Traditional indications

Incontinence, blood in urine, dark or red urine, dry mouth, emaciation and thirst, colic, vaginal discharge.

Illustrative combinations

With Gv-14 *(Dazhui)*, B-20 *(Pishu)*, B-23 *(Shenshu)* and appropriate M-BW-35 *(Jiaji)* points for rheumatoid arthritis of vertebrae.

Needling method

(1) Straight insertion, 1-1.5 units. Sensation: distension and soreness. (2) Slanted insertion, for arthritis of sacroiliac or peritonitis, 2-3 units. Sensation: distension and soreness extending throughout the sacroiliac joint.

B-28 *(Pangguangshu)* 膀胱俞 "Bladder's Hollow"

Location

1.5 units lateral to the midline of the spine, level with the 2nd posterior sacral foramen. (Dia. 2-21)

Anatomy

Between the origins of the sacrospinalis and gluteus maximus muscles. Supplied by lateral, posterior branches of the posterior sacral artery and vein, by medial branches of the dorsal rami of the first and second sacral nerves, and a communicating branch of the first sacral nerve.

Traditional functions

Regulates the Bladder and benefits the lumbar vertebrae.

Indications

Pain in the lumbosacral region, sciatica, diarrhea, constipation, diabetes, diseases of the urogenital system.

Traditional indications

Pain in the lumbar vertebrae, loss of sperm, incontinence, dark and rough-flowing urine, swelling and pain in the genitals.

Illustrative combinations

With B-23 *(Shenshu)*, Sp-9 *(Yinlingquan)*, Sp-6 *(Sanyinjiao)* for urinary tract infection; with B-23 *(Shenshu)*, Co-2 *(Qugu)*, Sp-6 *(Sanyinjiao)* for prostatitis.

Needling method

Straight insertion, 1-1.5 units. Sensation: local distension and soreness, sometimes extending to the buttocks.

B-30 *(Baihuanshu)* 白环俞 "White Circle's Hollow"

Location

1.5 units lateral to the midline of the spine, level with the 4th posterior sacral foramen. (Dia. 2-21)

Anatomy

In the gluteus maximus muscle and the inferior, medial margin of the sacrotuberous ligament. Supplied by the inferior gluteal artery and vein, and in its deep position by the internal pudendal artery and vein. Supplied by the inferior clunial nerve, and in its deep position situated directly on the pudendal nerve.

Indications

Sciatica, pain in the lumbosacral region, endometritis, anal diseases, sequelae of infantile paralysis.

Traditional indications

Acute pain in the lumbar vertebrae, debility of the leg and knee, loss of sperm, excessive uterine bleeding, vaginal discharge, colic, painful defecation or urination.

Illustrative combinations

With M-CA-18 *(Zigong)*, Sp-10 *(Xuehai)*, Sp-6 *(Sanyinjiao)* for chronic peritonitis; with Gv-1 *(Changqiang)*, B-57 *(Chengshan)* for prolapsed anus.

Classical combinations

With B-54 *(Weizhong)* for back pain extending to the waist. (Source: OHS)

Needling method

Straight insertion, 1-2 units. Sensation: local distension and numbness extending to buttocks.

B-49 *(Zhibian)* 秩边 "Order's Edge"

Location

3 units lateral to the spinous process of the 4th sacral vertebra. (Dia. 2-21)

Anatomy

In the gluteus maximus muscle and the inferior margin of the piriformis muscle. Directly above the inferior gluteal artery and vein. In its deep position supplied by the inferior gluteal and the posterior femoral cutaneous nerve. Lateral to the point is the sciatic nerve.

Indications

Sciatica, strained muscles of the buttocks, paralysis of the lower limbs, diseases of the reproductive organs and anus.

Traditional indications

Pain in the lumbosacral region, painful urination, genital pain, hemorrhoids, difficult defecation.

Illustrative combinations

With B-51 *(Yinmen)*, GB-34 *(Yanglingquan)* for sciatica extending to the legs.

Needling method

(1) Straight insertion, for sciatica, 2-3 units. Sensation: local distension and soreness, deep insertion accompanied by a numb, electric sensation reaching the leg. (2) Slanted insertion, for diseases of the reproductive organs, needle slanted 45° toward the spine, 2-3 units. Sensation: local distension and soreness, sometimes an electric numb sensation reaching the genitals or anus. (3) Slanted insertion, for anal diseases, needle slanted 45° downward toward spine, 2-3 units. Sensation: distension and soreness reaching anus. (4) Straight insertion, for strained muscles of the buttocks, pointed away from the spine and joined to either GB-30 *(Huantiao)* or N-BW-16 *(Tiaoyue)*.

Gv-1 *(Changqiang)*　长强　"Long Strength"

Location

Midway between the tip of the coccyx and the anus. (Dia. 2-21)

Anatomy

Supplied by branches of the anal artery and vein, the vertebral venous plexus, and the coccygeal and anal nerves.

Traditional functions

Opens the Conception and Governing channels and regulates the Intestines.

Indications

Hemorrhoids, prolapsed anus, eczema of the scrotum, diarrhea, inducing labor, impotence, psychosis.

Traditional indications

Diarrhea, prolapsed anus, loss of sperm, cloudy and turbid urine, infantile convulsions, madness.

Illustrative combinations

With LI-4 *(Hegu)*, Sp-9 *(Yinlingquan)*, Sp-6 *(Sanyinjiao)* for inducing of labor; with M-BW-29 *(Yaoqi)*, M-BW-36 *(Dianxian)* for seizures (use a pyramid needle at Gv-1 *(Changqiang)* and prick around the circumference of this point, about 0.5-1 unit in depth, drawing a small amount of blood); with B-25 *(Dachangshu)*, B-57 *(Chengshan)*, Gv-20 *(Baihui)* for prolapsed anus.

Classical combinations

With B-57 *(Chengshan)* for Wind in the intestines with bleeding. (Source: OHS)

Needling method

Straight insertion, between the coccyx and rectum, 0.5-1 unit. Sensation: local distension and soreness, possibly extending to the anus.

Remarks

Connecting point of the Governing channel with the Conception channel.

B-31 thru 34 *(Baliao)*　八髎　"Eight Seams"
B-31 *(Shangliao)*, B-32 *(Ciliao)*, B-33 *(Zhongliao)*, B-34 *(Xialiao)*

Location

These points are located in the 1st through 4th posterior sacral foramen, respectively, 4 on the left side and 4 on the right. (Dia. 2-21)

Anatomy

In the sacrospinalis and the origin of the gluteus maximus muscles. In the first through fourth posterior sacral foramen. Supplied by posterior branches of the first through fourth sacral nerves.

Traditional functions

Regulates the Lower Burner, strengthens the lower back and legs.

Indications

Diseases of the lumbosacral joint, sciatica, irregular menstruation, inducing labor, leukorrhea, peritonitis, orchitis, paralysis of lower limb, sequelae of infantile paralysis.

Illustrative combinations

With Sp-6 *(Sanyinjiao)*, join Co-4 *(Guanyuan)* to Co-3 *(Zhongji)* for dysmenorrhea; with S-36 *(Zusanli)*, Sp-6 *(Sanyinjiao)*, Sp-10 *(Xuehai)*, M-CA-18 *(Zigong)*, Co-6 *(Qihai)*, Co-4 *(Guanyuan)* for functional uterine bleeding; with Gv-1 *(Changqiang)*, B-57 *(Chengshan)* for anal fissures; B-31 *(Shangliao)* and B-32 *(Ciliao)* with LI-4 *(Hegu)*, Sp-6 *(Sanyinjiao)* for inducing labor.

Needling method

Straight insertion, 1-2 units. Sensation: distension and soreness in the sacral region, sometimes extending to the legs. When locating the foramen, the fingers can be used to find the 'hole', whereafter the needle is inserted. If the foramen cannot be found, withdraw the needle slightly and try a different angle.

M-BW-35 *(Jiaji)*　夹脊　"Lining the Spine"

Location

Altogether 48 points distributed on both sides of each of the 24 cervical, thoracic and lumbar vertebrae, 0.5-1 unit lateral to the median line of the spine, at the lower end of the spinous process of each vertebra. (Dia. 2-22)

Anatomy

In the muscle between the spinous and transverse processes of the vertebrae. Although the position of each point varies somewhat from the others, the arrangement of muscles can be generally divided into three layers: superficailly, there are the trapezius, latissimus dorsi and rhomboid; in the middle layer are the superior and inferior posterior serratus; and in the deep layer are the sacrospinalis and intertransversarii muscles, etc. Each point is supplied by a medial branch of the dorsal ramus of its corresponding spinal nerve, and accompanying artery and vein.

Indications

See Table II-4 below.

Needling method

(1) Straight insertion, for needling the nerve root, pointed slightly toward the spine, 1.5 units deep for the cervical and thoracic points, 2.5 units deep for the lumbar points. Sensation: local distension and soreness, or an electric, numb sensation extending to the limbs and between the ribs. (2) Slanted insertion for arthritis of the vertebral joints, pointed into the interspinal ligament, 1-1.5 units; or transverse insertion, joining to another vertebral point below, 2-3 units. Sensation: distension and soreness extending around the point.

Remarks

In other books, these "Hua Tuo Lining the Spine Points" are situated 0.5 unit from the spinous processes of the 1st thoracic to the 5th lumbar vertebrae (17 on a side).

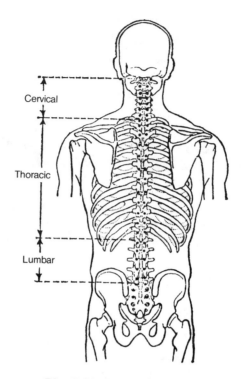

Cervical

Thoracic

Lumbar

Dia. 2-22 Vertebral Points
M-BW-35 *(Jiaji)*

Table II-4
Indications of Vertebral Points M-BW-35 *(Jiaji)*

Vertebral Points

Indications

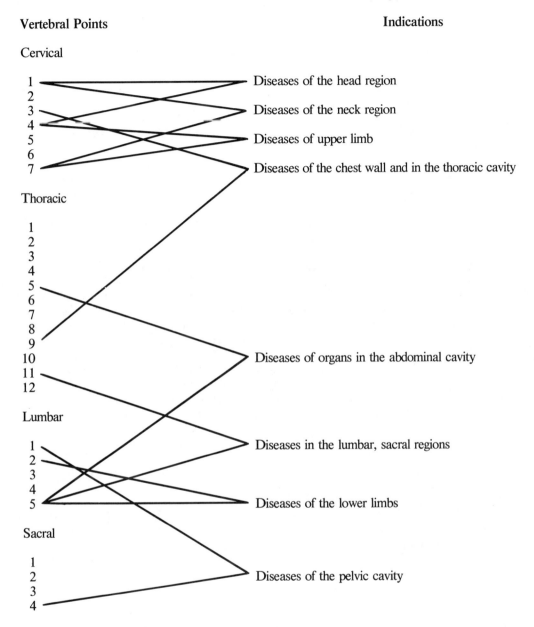

Cervical

1
2
3
4
5
6
7

Diseases of the head region

Diseases of the neck region

Diseases of upper limb

Diseases of the chest wall and in the thoracic cavity

Thoracic

1
2
3
4
5
6
7
8
9
10
11
12

Diseases of organs in the abdominal cavity

Lumbar

1
2
3
4
5

Diseases in the lumbar, sacral regions

Diseases of the lower limbs

Sacral

1
2
3
4

Diseases of the pelvic cavity

219

SUMMARY OF COMMON POINTS OF BACK

Region	Points	Common Characteristics	Particular Characteristics
From 7th cervical to 8th thoracic vertebra	Gv-14 (Dazhui), Gv-13 (Taodao), Gv-12 (Shenzhu), Gv-10 (Lingtai), Gv-9 (Zhiyang)	Diseases of Heart, Pericardium and Lungs; diseases of vertebrae, fever, malaria, mental illness	Gv-14 (Dazhui): anemia, eczema; Gv-10 (Lingtai): boils, round worm in bile duct; Gv-9 (Zhiyang): hepatitis
	M-BW-1 (Dingchuan), S-27 (Daju), B-12 (Fengmen), B-13 (Feishu), B-14 (Jueyinshu), B-38 (Gaohuangshu), B-15 (Xinshu), B-16 (Dushu), B-17 (Geshu)	Diseases of Heart, Pericardium and Lungs; local diseases of soft tissues	M-BW-1 (Dingchuan): asthma; B-12 (Fengmen): common cold; B-13 (Feishu): respiratory diseases; B-38 (Gaohuangshu): various chronic illnesses; B-15 (Xinshu): mental illness, heart disease; B-17 (Geshu): chronic hemorrhagic diseases, spasm of diaphragm
From 9th thoracic to 1st lumbar vertebra	B-18 (Ganshu), B-19 (Danshu), B-20 (Pishu), B-21 (Weishu), B-22 (Sanjiaoshu)	Diseases of Liver, Gall Bladder, Spleen, Stomach and local soft tissues	B-18 (Ganshu): eye diseases; B-19 (Danshu): round worm in bile duct, anemia; B-20 (Pishu) and B-21 (Weishu): chronic hemorrhagic diseases, ulcers; B-22 (Sanjiaoshu): nephritis, ascites, retention of urine
From 2nd lumbar to 4th sacral vertebra	Gv-4 (Mingmen), Gv-3 (Yaoyangguan), M-BW-25 (Shiqizhuixia), Gv-1 (Changqiang)	Diseases of Kidneys, Intestines and urogenital system; diseases of vertebrae	Gv-4 (Mingmen): male genital diseases; Gv-3 (Yaoyangguan): paralysis of lower limb; M-BW-25 (Shiqizhuixia): abnormal uterine bleeding; Gv-1 (Changqiang): induce labor, anal diseases
	B-23 (Shenshu), B-47 (Zhishi), B-24 (Qihaishu), B-25 (Dachangshu), M-BW-24 (Yaoyan), B-26 (Guanyuanshu), B-27 (Xiaochangshu), B-28 (Pangguangshu), B-30 (Baihuanshu), B-31 to 34 (Baliao), B-49 (Zhibian)	Diseases of Kidneys, Intestines and urogenital system; local diseases of soft tissues	B-23 (Shenshu), B-47 (Zhishi), B-24 (Qihaishu): urogenital diseases; B-25 (Dachangshu), B-26 (Guanyuanshu), B-27 (Xiaochangshu): enteritis, diseases of sacro-iliac joint; B-31 to 34 (Baliao): urogenital diseases; B-30 (Baihuanshu), B-49 (Zhibian): sciatica, paralysis of lower limb, anal diseases
Scapula	GB-21 (Jianjing), SI-15 (Jianzhongshu), SI-13 (Quyuan), SI-11 (Tianzong)	Diseases of shoulder and upper limb	GB-21 (Jianjing): mastitis, scrofula; SI-11 (Tianzong): mastitis, insufficient lactation
Other	M-BW-35 (Jiaji)		M-BW-35 (Jiaji): diseases of spine, head, neck, limbs and various internal organ systems

① SI-15 (Jianzhongshu)
② GB-21 (Jianjing)
③ B-12 (Fengmen)
④ SI-13 (Quyuan)
⑤ Gv-12 (Shenzhu)
⑥ SI-11 (Tianzong)
⑦ B-38 (Gaohuangshu)
⑧ B-16 (Dushu)
⑨ Gv-9 (Zhiyang)
⑩ B-19 (Danshu)
⑪ B-21 (Weishu)
⑫ Gv-4 (Mingmen)
⑬ B-23 (Shenshu)
⑭ B-25 (Dachangshu)
⑮ Gv-3 (Yaoyangguan)
⑯ M-BW-25 (Shiqizhuixia)
⑰ B-31—34 (Baliao)
⑱ B-30 (Baihuanshu)
⑲ Gv-1 (Changqiang)

⑳ Gv-14 (Dazhui)
㉑ M-BW-1 (Dingchuan)
㉒ B-11 (Dashu)
㉓ Gv-13 (Taodao)
㉔ B-13 (Feishu)
㉕ B-14 (Jueyinshu)
㉖ B-15 (Xinshu)
㉗ Gv-10 (Lingtai)
㉘ B-17 (Geshu)
㉙ B-18 (Ganshu)
㉚ B-20 (Pishu)
㉛ B-22 (Sanjiaoshu)
㉜ B-47 (Zhishi)
㉝ M-BW-24 (Yaoyan)
㉞ B-24 (Qihaishu)
㉟ B-26 (Guanyuanshu)
㊱ B-27 (Xiaochangshu)
㊲ B-28 (Pangguangshu)
㊳ B-49 (Zhibian)

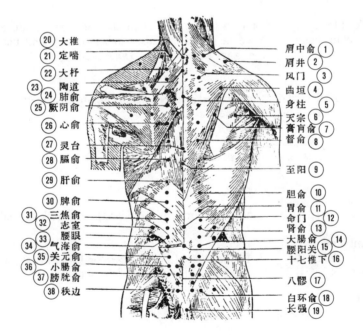

**Dia. 2-23 Points and Musculature
on Back and Waist**

Chapter 5

Common Points of the Upper Limb

LI-15 *(Jianyu)*　肩髃　"Shoulder Bone"

Location

In the middle of the upper part of the deltoid muscle at the shoulder, between the acromion and greater tubercle of the humerus. When the arm is abducted parallel to the ground, this point can be found in a distinct depression just in front of the shoulder. (Dia. 2-24)

Anatomy

In the middle of the deltoid muscle. Supplied by the posterior circumflex humeral artery and vein, and the supraclavicular and axillary nerves.

Indications

Hemiplegia, hypertension, pain in shoulder joint, perifocal inflammation of shoulder joint, excessive sweating.

Traditional indications

Wind Dampness in shoulder, hemiplegia, Wind rash (urticaria), arms lack strength, goiter.

Illustrative combinations

With M-UE-48 *(Jianneiling)*, TB-14 *(Jianliao)*, LI-11 *(Quchi)* for diseases of the shoulder joint; with TB-14 *(Jianliao)*, GB-34 *(Yanglingquan)* for bursitis of the shoulder.

Classical combinations

With LI-5 *(Yangxi)* for Wind rash. (Source: OHS)

Needling method

(1) Straight insertion, with the arm raised, needle pointed toward H-1 *(Jiquan)* in the armpit, 2-3 units. For supraspinatus tendinitis, with arm hanging freely at the side, insert needle between the acromion of the shoulder and the greater tubercle of the humerus, 0.7-1 unit. Sensation: local distension and soreness, sometimes extending to the forearm. (2) Slanted insertion, for perifocal inflammation of the shoulder joint, join to M-UE-48 *(Jianneiling)*, then to TB-14 *(Jianliao)* and finally along the deltoid muscle, 2-3 units. Sensation: distension and soreness spreading through the shoulder, or an electric sensation extending toward the forearm. (3) Transverse insertion, for limited

abduction of shoulder, needle pointed downward along the deltoid muscle, 2-3 units. Sensation: distension and soreness in the upper arm.

Remarks
Point of intersection of Yang Heel channel on the Large Intestine channel.

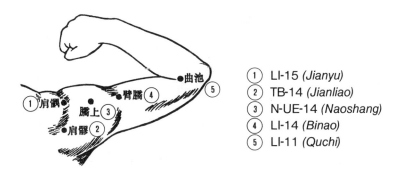

① LI-15 *(Jianyu)*
② TB-14 *(Jianliao)*
③ N-UE-14 *(Naoshang)*
④ LI-14 *(Binao)*
⑤ LI-11 *(Quchi)*

Dia. 2-24 Points on Shoulder

M-UE-48 *(Jianneiling)* 肩内陵 "Shoulder's Inner Tomb"

Location
With arm hanging freely at the side, this point is found mid-way between top of the anterior axillary crease and LI-15 *(Jianyu)* on the shoulder. (Dia. 2-25)

Anatomy
In the anterior part of the deltoid muscle. Supplied by the posterior branch of the supraclavicular nerve, and in its deep position situated on the axillary nerve. Supplied by anterior and posterior branches of the circumflex humeral artery and vein.

Indications
Same as LI-15 *(Jianyu)* above.

Illustrative combinations
With LI-15 *(Jianyu)*, TB-14 *(Jianliao)* and point of pain for perifocal inflammation of the shoulder joint or pain in the shoulder joint.

Needling method
(1) Straight insertion, for most conditions, needle pointed toward the back of the shoulder, 1-1.5 units. Sensation: local distension and soreness, or an electric, numb sensation in the upper arm extending as far as the fingertips. (2) Slanted insertion, for tendosynovitis of the long head of the biceps brachii muscle, 2-3 units. Sensation: local distension and soreness.

TB-14 *(Jianliao)* 肩髎 "Shoulder Seam"

Location
In the depression just posterior and inferior to the acromion of the shoulder. (Dia. 2-24)

Anatomy
In the deltoid muscle. Supplied by a branch of the posterior circumflex humeral artery and a muscle branch of the axillary nerve.

223

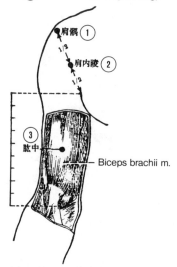

① LI-15 *(Jianyu)*
② M-UE-48 *(Jianneiling)*
③ N-UE-9 *(Gongzhong)*

肩髃 ①

肩内陵 ②

③
肱中

Biceps brachii m.

**Dia. 2-25 Points on Anterior
Aspect of Arm**

Indications
Same as LI-15 *(Jianyu)* above.

Illustrative combinations
Join to H-1 *(Jiquan)*, and join S-38 *(Tiaokou)* to B-57 *(Chengshan)* for perifocal inflammation of the shoulder joint.

Classical combinations
With SI-11 *(Tianzong)* and SI-5 *(Yanggu)* for arm pain. (Source: CNLAM)

Needling method
(1) Straight insertion, for arthritis of the shoulder, with arm abducted, needle pointed toward H-1 *(Jiquan)* in the armpit between the acromion of the shoulder and the greater tubercle of the humerus, 1.5-2 units; or join to H-1 *(Jiquan)*. (See Dia. 2-26.) Sensation: distension and soreness throughout the shoulder. (2) Slanted insertion, for perifocal inflammation, of shoulder joint, point needle downward, 2-3 units. Sensation: distension and soreness throughout shoulder, or a numb, electric sensation extending toward the fingers.

LI-16 *(Jugu)*　巨骨　"Great Bone"

Location
In the hollow between the acromial end of the clavicle and the shoulder blade, slightly posterior to the top of the shoulder. (Dia. 2-27)

Anatomy
In the trapezius and supraspinatus muscles. In its deep position supplied by the suprascapular

① TB-14 *(Jianliao)*
② LI-15 *(Jianyu)*
③ H-1 *(Jiquan)*

Acromion

① 肩髎

肩髃 ②

Trapezius m.

Pectoralis major m.

Trapezius m.

Shoulder joint capsule

Infraspinatus m.

极泉 ③

**Dia. 2-26 Cross Section of TB-14 *(Jianliao)*
Joined to H-1 *(Jiquan)***

artery and vein. Supplied by branches of the supraclavicular and accessory nerves, and in its deep position by the suprascapular nerve.

Traditional functions
Disperses Congealed Blood and clears the channels.

Indications
Diseases of the shoulder joint and soft tissues of the shoulder, spitting blood, scrofula.

Traditional indications
Pain in the arm and shoulder inhibiting movement, 'frightened convulsions', spitting blood, scrofula, nodular growths on the neck.

Illustrative combinations
With TB-14 *(Jianliao)* joined to H-1 *(Jiquan)*, and GB-34 *(Yanglingquan)* for perifocal inflammation of shoulder joint; with L-6 *(Kongzui)*, L-5 *(Chize)*, L-10 *(Yuji)* for coughing blood.

Classical combinations
With SI-2 *(Qiangu)* for inability to raise the arm. (Source: CNLAM)

Needling method
Straight insertion, slanted slightly toward the outside, 1-1.5 units. Sensation: distension and soreness around shoulder joint.

Remarks
Point of intersection of the Yang Heel channel with the Large Intestine channel.

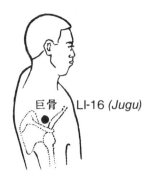

Dia. 2-27   LI-16 *(Jugu)*

SI-10 *(Naoshu)*   臑俞   "Scapula's Hollow"

Location
Directly above SI-9 *(Jianzhen)* at the inferior margin of the spine of the scapula. (Dia. 2-28)

Anatomy
In the deltoid muscle posterior to the glenoid fossa of the scapula, and in its deep position in the infraspinatus muscle. Supplied by the circumflex humeral artery and vein and in its deep position by the suprascapular artery and vein. Supplied by the axillary nerve, and in its deep position by the suprascapular nerve.

Indications
Same as LI-15 *(Jianyu)* above.

Traditional indications
Chills and fever, inability to raise the arm, soreness and lack of strength in the arm.

Illustrative combinations
With LI-15 *(Jianyu)*, SI-9 *(Jianzhen)*, M-HN-41 *(Jingbi)* for paralysis of upper limb.

Needling method
Straight insertion, pointed slightly downward, 1-2 units. Sensation: local distension and soreness, sometimes extending throughout the shoulder.

Remarks
Point of intersection of the Yang Linking and Yang Heel channels on the Small Intestine channel.

SI-9 *(Jianzhen)*   肩贞   "Shoulder Chastity"

Location
With arm hanging freely at the side, this point is found 1 unit directly above the posterior axillary crease. (Dia. 2-28)

Anatomy
At the lateral margin of the scapula below the infraglenoid tubercle. In the posterior margin of the deltoid muscle, and in its deep position in the teres major muscle. Supplied by the circumflex artery and vein of the scapula, a branch of the axillary nerve, and above its deepest position by the radial nerve.

226

Indications
Diseases of the shoulder and shoulder joint, paralysis of upper limb, excessive perspiration in the arm pits.

Traditional indications
Pain in shoulder blades, pain in arm inhibiting movement, tinnitus, deafness, toothache, swelling of the mandible.

Illustrative combinations
With LI-15 *(Jianyu),* TB-14 *(Jianliao)* for arthritis of the shoulder; with LI-11 *(Quchi),* M-HN 41 *(Jingbi)* for paralysis of the upper limb.

Needling method
Straight insertion, 1.5-2 units. Sensation: local distension and soreness. When treating paralysis of the upper limb, there may be an electric, numb sensation extending into the shoulder and toward the fingertips.

① LI-16 *(Jugu)*
② TB-14 *(Jianliao)*
③ N-UE-14 *(Naoshang)*
④ LI-14 *(Binao)*
⑤ SI-10 *(Naoshu)*
⑥ SI-9 *(Jianzhen)*
⑦ N-UE-12 *(Yingshang)*

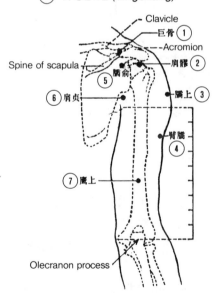

**Dia. 2-28 Points on Posterior
Aspect of Arm**

LI-14 *(Binao)* 臂臑   "Arm and Scapula"

Location
With arm hanging freely at the side and the elbow bent, this point may be found slightly anterior to the insertion of the deltoid muscle. (Dia. 2-24)

Anatomy

At the radial aspect of the humerus, in the posterior margin of the insertion of the deltoid muscle, and the anterior margin of the lateral head of the triceps muscle. Supplied by a branch of the posterior circumflex artery and the deep brachial artery, the lateral cutaneous nerve of the arm, and in its deep position by the radial nerve.

Traditional functions

Clears the channels and the vision.

Indications

Pain in the arm and shoulder, paralysis of upper limb, eye diseases.

Traditional indications

Chills and fever, pain in the shoulder and upper back inhibiting the lifting of the shoulder, scrofula.

Illustrative combinations

Join to N-UE-14 *(Naoshang),* and/or with LI-11 *(Quchi)* for pain in shoulder or upper arm; with B-1 *(Jingming),* S-1 *(Chengqi)* for eye diseases; join to LI-15 *(Jianyu)* to provide anesthesia for the thorax.

Needling method

(1) Straight insertion, 0.5-1 unit; or needle can penetrate the arm in front of or behind the humerus, 1-1.5 units. Sensation: local distension and soreness. (2) Slanted insertion, for eye diseases, needle slanted upward into the deltoid muscle, 1-2 units. Sensation: local distension and soreness.

N-UE-14 *(Naoshang)*　　臑上　　"Above the Scapula"

Location

In the middle of the deltoid muscle. (Dia. 2-24)

Anatomy

In the mid-section of the deltoid muscle. Supplied by the lateral cutaneous nerve of the arm, and in its deep position by the axillary nerve. Supplied by the circumflex artery and vein.

Indications

Hemiplegia in the upper limb, pain in the shoulder and arm.

Illustrative combinations

With LI-15 *(Jianyu),* SI-9 *(Jianzhen),* LI-11 *(Quchi)* for hemiplegia.

Needling method

Straight insertion, 1-2 units. Sensation: local distension and soreness.

H-1 *(Jiquan)*　　极泉　　"Summit's Spring"

Location

With the arm raised, this point can be found in the center of the armpit, medial to the axillary artery. (Dia. 2-26)

Anatomy

At the lateral, inferior margin of the pectoralis major muscle, and its deep position lies in the coracobrachialis muscle. The axillary artery is lateral to this point. Supplied by the ulnar and medial nerves, the medial cutaneous nerve of the forearm and the medial cutaneous nerve of the arm.

Indications
Arthritis of the shoulder, perifocal inflammation of the shoulder joint, angina pectoris, intercostal neuralgia.

Traditional indications
Chest pain and thirst, inability to raise arm, ribs 'full' and painful, jaundice, depression.

Illustrative combinations
With Co-7 (*Yinjiao*), Sp-7 (*Lougu*) for angina pectoris; with TB-5 (*Waiguan*), GB-34 (*Yanglingquan*) for intercostal neuralgia.

Classical combinations
With L-4 (*Xiabai*) for chest pain with dry vomiting, irritability, and a feeling of fullness. (Source: CNLAM)

Needling method
Straight insertion, 1-1.5 units. Sensation: local distension and soreness, or an electric, numb sensation extending toward the forearm.

N-UE-9 (*Gongzhong*)　　肱中　　"Middle of Humerus"

Location
2.5 units below P-2 (*Tianquan*) on the upper arm. (Dia. 2-25)

Anatomy
In the biceps and brachialis muscles, supplied by the medial cutaneous nerve of the arm. Its deep position is on the musculocutaneous nerve, and is supplied by muscle branches of the brachialis artery and vein.

Indications
Paralysis of upper limb, inability to raise arm, wrist drop, palpitations.

Illustrative combinations
With N-UE-10 (*Jubi*) for inability to bend arm at elbow.

Needling method
Straight insertion, 1-3 units. Sensation: local distension and soreness, sometimes numbness extending toward the shoulder and forearm.

N-UE-12 (*Yingshang*)　　鹰上　　"Above the Olecranon"

Location
4 units above the olecranon of the elbow. (Dia. 2-28)

Anatomy
In the triceps muscle. Supplied by the posterior cutaneous nerve of the arm. Its deep position is on a muscle branch of the radial nerve, and is supplied by the middle collateral artery and vein.

Indications
Sequelae of infantile paralysis, palpitations.

Illustrative combinations
With TB-14 (*Jianliao*), TB-13 (*Naohui*) for weakness in flexion of the elbow.

229

Needling method
Straight insertion, 1-2 units. Sensation: local distension and soreness, sometimes extending to the forearm.

LI-12 *(Zhouliao)*　肘髎　"Elbow Seam"

Location
With the arm flexed at the elbow, this point can be found approximately 1 unit above and lateral to LI-11 *(Quchi),* at the margin of the humerus. (Dia. 2-29)

Anatomy
At the superior margin of the lateral epicondyle of the humerus, at the origin of the anconeus muscle and the lateral margin of the triceps muscle. Supplied by the radial collateral artery, the posterior cutaneous nerve of the arm, and the radial nerve.

Indications
Pain in the elbow and arm, inflammation of the lateral epicondyle of the humerus.

Traditional indications
Pain in the elbow and arm, spasm or numbness (arm), lassitude.

Illustrative combinations
With LI-11 *(Quchi),* LI-10 *(Shousanli)* for inflammation of lateral epicondyle of the humerus.

Needling method
Slanted insertion, along the anterior margin of the humerus, 1-1.5 units. Sensation: local distension and soreness.

LI-11 *(Quchi)*　曲池　"Crooked Pool"

Location
With the arm flexed at the elbow, this point can be found midway between the end of the transverse crease of the elbow and the lateral epicondyle of the humerus. (Dia. 2-29)

Anatomy
On the radial aspect of the elbow at the origin of the extensor carpi radialis muscle and the radial side of the brachioradialis muscle. Supplied by a branch of the radial recurrent artery, the posterior cutaneous nerve of the forearm, and in its deep position by the radial nerve trunk.

Traditional functions
Eliminates Wind and Exterior conditions; cools Heat and alleviates Dampness; regulates the Blood.

Indications
Arthritic pain in the upper limb, paralysis, hemiplegia, hypertension, high fever, measles, anemia, allergies, goiter, skin diseases.

Traditional indications
Eyes red and painful, toothache, throat blockage, nodular growths in the neck, goiter, hives, Wind rash, dry and parched skin, little menstrual flow, hemiplegia.

Illustrative combinations
With LI-4 *(Hegu),* M-HN-3 *(Yintang),* L-11 *(Shaoshang)* for measles; with S-36 *(Zusanli),* S-9

(Renying) for hypertension; with Gv-14 *(Dazhui)*, M-UE-1 *(Shixuan)* for high fever; with Gv-14 *(Dazhui)*, Li-3 *(Taichong)*, S-36 *(Zusanli)*, LI-4 *(Hegu)* for idiopathic thrombocytopenic pupura.

Classical combinations

With LI-4 *(Hegu)* and LI-15 *(Jianyu)* for soreness and pain in the hand and arm (Source: SGJ); with H-7 *(Shenmen)* and L-10 *(Yuji)* for vomiting blood. (Source: GCAM)

Needling method

(1) Straight insertion, join to H-3 *(Shaohai)* if desired, 2-2.5 units. Sensation: local distension and soreness, sometimes an electric, numb sensation extending to the shoulder or fingers. (2) Straight insertion, slanted slightly toward hand, 1.5-2.5 units. Sensation: if, after 'obtaining Qi', the needle is twirled rapidly, this sensation can be perceived along the forearm and sometimes to the shoulder. (3) With the arm flexed at the elbow, needle may be inserted straight with a slight slant in the direction of the elbow joint, 0.5-1 unit, for paralysis of the upper limb. Sensation: numb, electric sensation extending to the fingertips.

Remarks

Uniting point of the Large Intestine channel.

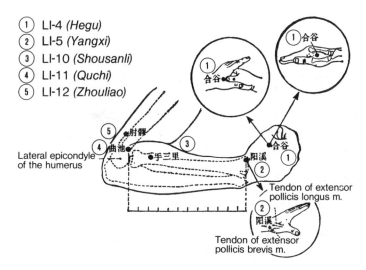

1. LI-4 *(Hegu)*
2. LI-5 *(Yangxi)*
3. LI-10 *(Shousanli)*
4. LI-11 *(Quchi)*
5. LI-12 *(Zhouliao)*

Dia. 2-29 Points on Lateral Aspect of Forearm

LI-10 *(Shousanli)* 手三里 "Arm's Three Measures"

Location

2 units distal to LI-11 *(Quchi)* on the forearm. (Dia. 2-29)

Anatomy

On the radial aspect of the radius, in the extensor carpi radialis brevis and longus muscles, and in its deep position in the supinator muscle. Supplied by a branch of the radial recurrent artery, by the posterior cutaneous nerve of the forearm, and a deep branch of the radial nerve.

Indications

Pain in shoulder and arm, paralysis of upper limb, ulcer, stomach-ache, abdominal pain, diarrhea, indigestion.

231

Traditional indications

Toothache, loss of voice, swelling of the mandible and cheek, scrofula, vomiting with diarrhea, hemiplegia.

Illustrative combinations

With Co-12 *(Zhongwan)* and S-36 *(Zusanli)* for ulcer.

Classical combinations

With S-36 *(Zusanli)* for lumps in the abdomen due to stagnation of food. (Source: OXH)

Needling method

Straight insertion, 1-2 units. Sensation: local distension and soreness, sometimes extending along the forearm.

LI-5 *(Yangxi)*   陽溪   "Yang Creek"

Location

With the thumb extended, this point can be found in the center of the hollow formed between the extensor pollicis longus and extensor pollicis brevis. (Dia. 2-29)

Anatomy

On the radial aspect of the wrist, between the extensor pollicis longus and brevis. Supplied by branches of the cephalic vein, a branch of the radial artery on the dorsal aspect of the wrist, and a superficial branch of the radial nerve.

Indications

Disease of the soft tissues of the wrist joint, headache, ophthalmalgia, tinnitus, toothache, deafness, infantile indigestion.

Traditional indications

Headache, eyes red and painful, membrane on the eye, deafness, throat blockage, toothache, pain in the root of the tongue, pain in the wrist, inability to flex the arm at the elbow.

Illustrative combinations

With L-7 *(Lieque)* for tenosynovitis of the wrist.

Classical combinations

With SI-5 *(Yanggu)* for red and painful eyes. (Source: CNLAM)

Needling method

Straight insertion, 0.3-1 unit. Sensation: local distension and soreness.

LI-4 *(Hegu)*   合谷   "Adjoining Valleys"

Location

With the thumb and index finger extended and stretched apart, this point can be found slightly to the index finger side of the area between the 1st and 2nd metacarpal bones. (Dia. 2-29)

Anatomy

In the dorsal interroseus muscle, between the first and second metacarpal bones; its deep position is in the transverse head of the adductor pollicis muscle. Supplied by the cephalic vein in the dorsal venous network, and near the site at which the radial artery passes from the dorsal to the palmar side of the hand. Supplied by a dorsal digital superficial branch of the radial nerve, and in its deep position by a palmar digital branch of the median nerve.

Traditional functions
Disperses Wind, relieves Exterior conditions, suppresses pain and clears the channels.

Indications
Common cold, headache, diseases of the sensory organs, facial paralysis, hemiplegia, neurasthenia, pain in general.

Trraditional indications
Headache, pain in the eyes, membrane on the eye, nosebleed, deafness, toothache, facial edema, throat blockage; mouth and face awry, 'locked jaw' due to stroke; tidal fevers, Wind rash; scabies, aborting dead fetus, abortion.

Illustrative combinations
With GB-20 *(Fengchi)* for common cold; with P-6 *(Neiguan)* for various anesthetic purposes.

Classical combinations
With K-7 *(Fuliu)* for insufficient sweating (Source: GCAM); with LI-11 *(Quchi)* for unilateral Wind rash. (Source: CNLAM)

Needling method
(1) Straight insertion, 0.5-1 unit. Sensation: local distension and soreness. (2) Join to P-8 *(Laogong)* or SI-3 *(Houxi)*, 2-3 units, for muscle spasm or muscle paralysis of fingers. Sensation: numb, distended sensation extending to fingertips. (3) Slanted insertion, along the surface of the 2nd metacarpus, 1-1.5 units, for diseases affecting the head. Sensation: distension and soreness, possibly extending upward to the elbow or shoulder. CAUTION: Needling this point on pregnant women who have histories of miscarriage is discouraged.

Remarks
Source point of the Large Intestine channel.

TB-10 *(Tianjing)*   天井   "Heaven's Well"

Location
With the elbow flexed, this point can be found approximately 1 unit above the olecranon of the elbow in a slight depression. (Dia. 2-30)

Anatomy
In the cavity above the olecranon at the posterior aspect of the lower end of the humerus; at the superior margin of the olecranon prominence of the ulna, in the tendon of the triceps muscle. Supplied by the arteriovenous network of the elbow, the dorsal cutaneous nerve of the arm and a muscle branch of the radial nerve.

Indications
Diseases of the soft tissues of the elbow, migraine headache, tonsillitis, urticaria, scrofula (use moxibustion).

Traditional indications
Pain in neck, shoulder and back; pain in the eyes, headache, deafness, throat blockage; tidal fevers, insanity.

233

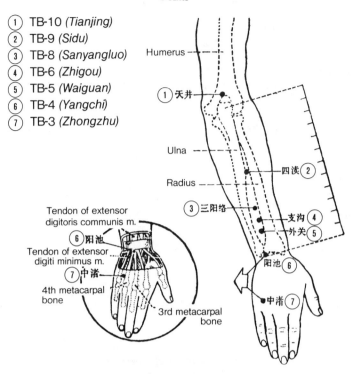

① TB-10 *(Tianjing)*
② TB-9 *(Sidu)*
③ TB-8 *(Sanyangluo)*
④ TB-6 *(Zhigou)*
⑤ TB-5 *(Waiguan)*
⑥ TB-4 *(Yangchi)*
⑦ TB-3 *(Zhongzhu)*

**Dia. 2-30 Points of Triple Burner
Channel on Hand and Forearm**

Illustrative combinations
With LI-11 *(Quchi)* joined to H-3 *(Shaohai)* for diseases of the elbow joint.

Classical combinations
With H-3 *(Shaohai)* for nodular growths in the neck. (Source: SGJ)

Needling method
Straight insertion, 0.5-1 unit. Sensation: local distension and soreness.

Remarks
Uniting point of the Triple Burner channel.

TB-9 *(Sidu)* 四渎 "Four Ditch"

Location
With the hand in a supine position, this point can be found 5 units below the elbow between the ulna and radius. (Dia. 2-30)

Anatomy
Between the ulna and radius, and the extensor digitorum and extensor carpi ulnaris muscles of the forearm. Its deep position is supplied by the anterior and posterior interosseus nerves of the forearm.

Indications
Headache, deafness, toothache, pain in forearm, paralysis of upper limb, neurasthenia, vertigo, nephritis.

Traditional indications
'Sudden deafness', toothache in the lower jaw, loss of voice, obstructed pharynx, pain in forearm.

Illustrative combinations
With GB-20 *(Fengchi)* on left joined to GB-20 *(Fengchi)* on right, and join M-HN-9 *(Taiyang)* to GB-8 *(Shuaigu)* for headache.

Classical combinations
With TB-16 *(Tianyou)* for sudden deafness. (Source: CNLAM)

Needling method
Straight insertion, 1-2 units. Sensation: distension and soreness, possibly extending to the elbow and hand.

TB-8 *(Sanyangluo)*　三陽络　"Three Yang Connection"

Location
1 unit above TB-6 *(Zhigou)* between the ulna and radius. (Dia. 2-30)

Anatomy
Between the ulna and radius, and between the exterior digitorum and origin of the abductor pollicis longus muscles. Supplied by the posterior interosseus artery and vein, a dorsal branch of the cutaneous nerve of the forearm and the posterior and anterior interosseus nerves of the forearm.

Traditional functions
Clears the channels and sensory orifices.

Indications
Deafness, pain in the arm, aphasia, post-operative pain associated with pneumonectomy.

Traditional indications
Deafness, sudden muteness, pain in forearm inhibiting movement, lassitude.

Illustrative combinations
Joined to P-4 *(Ximen)* for pain associated with pneumonectomy; with GB-20 *(Fengchi)* for headache.

Classical combinations
With TB-6 *(Zhigou)* and B-66 *(Tonggu)* for sudden muteness. (Source: CNLAM)

Needling method
(1) Straight insertion, 1-1.5 units. Sensation: distension and soreness extending toward elbow. (2) Slanted insertion, join to P-4 *(Ximen),* about 2-3 units. Sensation: distension and numbness possibly extending to fingertips or elbow.

TB-6 *(Zhigou)*　支沟　"Branch Ditch"

Location
3 units above the transverse crease on the dorsal side of the wrist; 1 unit above TB-5 *(Waiguan).* (Dia. 2-30)

Anatomy

Between the radius and ulna, and the extensor digitorum and extensor pollicis longus muscles. With the hand in a supine position, this point can be found on the radial side of the extensor digitorum muscle. Supplied in its deep position by the main trunk of the anterior and posterior interosseus arteries and veins. Supplied by the posterior cutaneous nerve of the forearm, and in its deep position by the anterior and posterior interosseus nerves.

Traditional functions

Spreads the Qi, disperses obstruction, opens the Intestines.

Indications

Pain in shoulder and arm, angina pectoris, intercostal neuralgia, pleurisy, insufficient lactation, habitual constipation.

Traditional indications

Soreness and heaviness in the shoulder and arm, chest pain, belching, swollen throat, acute pain in the ribs and axilla, vomiting and diarrhea, constipation.

Illustrative combinations

With GB-34 *(Yanglingquan)* for intercostal neuralgia; with S-36 *(Zusanli)* and Sp-15 *(Daheng)* joined to S-25 *(Tianshu)* for habitual constipation; with S-36 *(Zusanli)*, Co-17 *(Shanzhong)*, S-18 *(Rugen)* for insufficient lactation.

Classical combinations

With K-6 *(Zhaohai)* for constipation (Source: SJD); with Li-13 *(Zhangmen)* and TB-5 *(Waiguan)* for rib pain. (Source: GCAM)

Needling method

Straight insertion, 1-1.5 units. Sensation: local distension and soreness, possibly reaching the elbow,and sometimes an electric, numb sensation extending to the fingertips.

Remarks

Traversing point of the Triple Burner channel.

TB-5 *(Waiguan)*　外关　"Outer Gate"

Location

2 units above the transverse crease on the dorsal surface of the wrist, between the ulna and radius. (Dia. 2-30)

Anatomy

Same as TB-6 *(Zhigou)* above.

Traditional functions

Relieves Exterior and Hot conditions, facilitates the circulation of stagnant Qi in the channels.

Indications

Common cold, high fever, pneumonia, parotitis, deafness, tinnitus, migraine headache, enuresis, stiff neck, hemiplegia, pain in joints of upper limb, paralysis.

Traditional indications

Pain in fingers inhibiting grasp, hand tremors, swollen throat, tinnitus, deafness, febrile diseases, pain in the ribs, constipation, headache.

Illustrative combinations

Join through the arm to P-6 *(Neiguan),* also needle SI-6 *(Yanglao)* for lumbar pain; with Gv-20 *(Baihui),* LI-4 *(Hegu),* and L-7 *(Lieque)* for common cold.

Classical combinations

With GB-2 *(Tinghui)* for deafness. (Source: CNLAM)

Needling method

(1) Straight insertion, 1-1.5 units, or join through the arm to P-6 *(Neiguan).* Sensation: local distension and soreness, sometimes extending to the fingertips. (2) Slanted insertion, needle pointed up the arm 1.5-2 units, for diseases of the trunk. Sensation: distension and soreness extending up the arm.

Remarks

Connecting point between the Triple Burner and Pericardium channels; Meeting point of the Yang Linking channel on the Triple Burner channel.

TB-4 *(Yangchi)* 陽池 "Pool of Yang"

Location

With the hand supine, this point can be found directly above the transverse crease on the dorsal surface of the wrist, in a hollow above the 3rd and 4th metacarpal bones, between the tendon of the extensor digitorum and tendon of the extensor digiti minimi manus muscles. (Dia. 2-30)

Anatomy

In the region of the joint between the ulna and wrist, between the tendon of the extensor digitorum muscle and the tendon of the extensor digiti minimi manus muscle. Below are the dorsal arteriovenous network of the wrist and a branch of the radial artery. Supplied by a dorsal branch of the ulnar nerve and a branch of the dorsal cutaneous nerve of the forearm.

Traditional functions

Relaxes the sinews, clears the channels, relieves Heat.

Indications

Pain and diseases of the soft tissues of the wrist, common cold, tonsillitis, malaria.

Traditional indications

Thirst and dryness in mouth, eyes red and swollen, throat blockage, deafness, tidal fevers, pain and weakness of the wrist.

Illustrative combinations

With P-7 *(Daling),* M-UE-50 *(Shangbaxie),* M-UE-9 *(Sifeng)* for arthritis of wrist, fingers and bones of the hand; with B-12 *(Fengmen),* B-10 *(Tianzhu),* Gv-14 *(Dazhui)* for Hot or Cold headache without sweating.

Needling method

(1) Straight insertion, 0.3-0.5 unit. Sensation: local distension and soreness, sometimes extending to the middle finger. (2) Transverse insertion, needle pointed across the wrist, 0.5-1 unit, for diseases of the wrist. Sensation: distension and soreness possibly throughout wrist.

Remarks

Source point on the Triple Burner channel.

TB-3 *(Zhongzhu)*　中渚　"Middle Island"

Location
With the hand lying prone, this point can be found between the 4th and 5th metacarpal bones, in the hollow behind the metacarpophalangeal joints. (Dia. 2-31)

Anatomy
Behind the heads of the fourth and fifth metacarpal bones of the hand, in the fourth interosseous muscle. Supplied by the dorsal arteriovenous network of the hand, the fourth dorsal metacarpal artery, and by a dorsal branch of the ulnar nerve.

Traditional functions
Facilitates the circulation of Qi, benefits the ear.

Indications
Deaf-mutism, tinnitus, deafness, headache, pain in the shoulder and back, intercostal neuralgia.

Traditional indications
Pain in shoulder, back, elbow and arm, inability to bend fingers, headache, tinnitus, blurred vision.

Illustrative combinations
With TB-21 *(Ermen)*, TB-17 *(Yifeng)* for tinnitus and deafness.

Classical combinations
With TB-2 *(Yemen)* for red and swollen hand and arm (Source: SJD); with LI-1 *(Shangyang)* and GB-40 *(Qiuxu)* for chronic tidal fevers (Source: GCAM); with K-3 *(Taixi)* for swollen throat. (Source: GCAM)

Needling method
Straight insertion, or slanted toward the wrist, 1-1.5 units. Sensation: local distension and soreness, sometimes extending to the fingertips or forearm, or an electric, numb sensation reaching the fingertips.

Remarks
Transporting point of the Triple Burner channel.

SI-6 *(Yanglao)*　养老　"Nourish the Old"

Location
With the palm facing the chest, this point can be found in a seam slightly above the head of the ulna on its radial side. (Dia. 2-31)

Anatomy
On the dorsal aspect of the ulna, above the head of the ulna at the wrist, between the tendons of the extensor carpi ulnaris and the extensor digiti minimi manus muscles. Supplied by a branch of the anterior interosseus artery and the dorsal venous network of the wrist. Near the anastomosis of the dorsal cutaneous nerve of the forearm and a dorsal branch of the ulnar nerve.

Traditional functions
Relaxes the sinews, clears the channels and the vision.

238

Indications
Arthritis of the upper limb, pain in the shoulder and back, hemiplegia, stiff neck, eye diseases, low back pain, pain of hernia.

Traditional indications
Pain in shoulders and arm, blurred vision, restriction of movement in the lumbar area.

Illustrative combinations
With M-UE-30 *(Bizhong)* for wrist drop; with P-6 *(Neiguan)* for belching; joined to P-6 *(Neiguan)*, and SI-9 *(Jianzhen)* joined to H-1 *(Jiquan)* for perifocal inflammation of the shoulder joint.

Needling method
Slanted insertion, toward P-6 *(Neiguan)*, 1-1.5 units. Sensation: soreness and numbness in hand and wrist, possibly extending to elbow or shoulder.

Remarks
Accumulating point of the Small Intestine channel.

SI-4 *(Wangu)* 腕骨 "Wrist Bone"

Location
When the hand is clenched in a fist, this point can be found on the dorsal side of the hand at the ulnar aspect, in the hollow between the 5th metacarpus and the hamate and pisiform bones of the hand. (Dia. 2-31)

Anatomy
Between the base of the fifth metacarpus and the pisiform bone, lateral to the origin of the abductor digiti minimi manus. Supplied by the dorsal branch of the ulnar artery at the wrist and the dorsal venous network of the hand. Supplied by a dorsal branch of the ulnar nerve.

Indications
Arthritis of the wrist, elbow and fingers, headache, tinnitus, diabetes, gastritis, cholecystitis.

Traditional indications
Headache, Hot condition without sweating, throat blockage, emaciation and thirst, pain in ribs, jaundice, inhibited movement of fingers.

Illustrative combinations
With M-BW-12 *(Yishu)* and B-20 *(Pishu)* for diabetes.

Classical combinations
With B-62 *(Shenmai)*, TB-5 *(Waiguan)*, and K-1 *(Yongquan)* for jaundice from Cold-induced disease. (Source: GCAM)

Needling method
Straight insertion, 0.5-1 unit. Sensation: local distension and soreness, possibly extending to palm.

Remarks
Source point of the Small Intestine channel.

Points

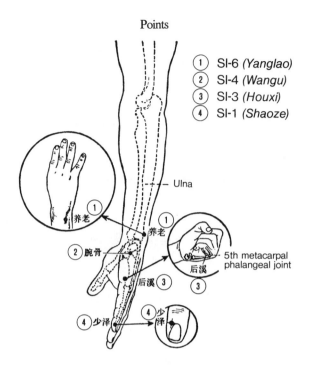

① SI-6 *(Yanglao)*
② SI-4 *(Wangu)*
③ SI-3 *(Houxi)*
④ SI-1 *(Shaoze)*

Ulna

养老 ①

① 养老

② 腕骨

后溪 ③

后溪 ③

5th metacarpal phalangeal joint

④ 少泽

④ 少泽

**Dia. 2-31 Points of Small Intestine
Channel on Hand and Forearm**

SI-3 *(Houxi)*　后溪　"Back Creek"

Location
When the hand is clenched in a fist, this point can be found behind and lateral to the head of the 5th metacarpus, at the top of the transverse crease formed by the clenched fist. (Dia. 2-31)

Anatomy
At the ulnar aspect of the fifth metacarpus, posterior to its head, and lateral to the abductor digiti minimi manus. Supplied by the dorsal digital artery and vein, the dorsal venous network of the hand, and by a dorsal branch of the ulnar nerve.

Traditional functions
Relaxes the Muscle channels, opens the Governing channel, clears the Spirit.

Indications
Malaria, seizures, psychosis, hysteria, intercostal neuralgia, night sweats, stiff neck, deaf-mutism, low back pain.

Traditional indications
Eyes red and painful, membrane on the eye, tinnitus, deafness, jaundice, madness, tidal fevers, finger spasm.

Illustrative combinations
With Gv-14 *(Dazhui)*, P-5 *(Jianshi)* for tertian malaria; with B-51 *(Yinmen)*, points of pain and other local points for lower back sprain.

Classical combinations
With P-8 *(Laogong)* for jaundice (Source: OHS); with GB-30 *(Huantiao)* for painful legs (Source:

240

OHS); with M-HN-30 *(Bailao),* LI-11 *(Quchi)* for tidal fevers with more chills than fevers. (Source: GCAM)

Needling method
Straight insertion, with fist clenched, along the metacarpus in a medial direction, 0.5-1 unit. For finger spasm, join to LI-4 *(Hegu),* 1.5-2 units. Sensation: local distension and soreness possibly extending throughout hand.

Remarks
Transporting point of the Small Intestine channel. Meeting point of the Governing channel on the Small Intestine channel.

SI-1 *(Shaoze)* 少泽 "Lesser Marsh"

Location
On the ulnar aspect of the little finger, about 0.1 unit outside the corner of the cuticle. (Dia. 2-31)

Anatomy
At the base of the vallum unguis on the ulnar aspect of the little finger, in the arterial network formed by the palmar proper digital artery and dorsal digital artery of the hand. Supplied by a palmar digital nerve of the ulnar and dorsal digital nerves.

Traditional functions
Disperses Wind and Heat, facilitates the flow of milk.

Indications
Headache, mastitis, insufficient lactation, pterygium.

Traditional indications
Fever and chills with no sweating, headache, chest pain, shortness of breath, pain in ribs, jaundice, swollen breast, membrane on the eye, deafness.

Illustrative combinations
With B-1 *(Jingming),* M-HN-9 *(Taiyang),* LI-4 *(Hegu)* for pterygium.

Classical combinations
With M-HN-9 *(Taiyang)* for swollen breasts (Source: SJD); with LI-4 *(Hegu),* Co-17 *(Shanzhong)* for lack of milk. (Source: GCAM)

Needling method
Slanted insertion, pointed slightly toward the wrist, 0.1 unit, or prick with the pyramid needle. Sensation: local distension and soreness.

Remarks
Well point of the Small Intestine channel.

L-5 *(Chize)* 尺泽 "Cubit Marsh"

Location
With the arm bent slightly at the elbow, this point can be found on the transverse crease of the elbow, just lateral to the tendon of the biceps muscle. (Dia. 2-32)

Anatomy

Lateral to the tendon of the biceps muscle at the elbow and at the origin of the brachioradialis muscle. Supplied by branches of the radial recurrent artery and vein, and the cephalic vein. Supplied by the lateral cutaneous nerve of the forearm, and directly below is the main trunk of the radial nerve.

Traditional functions

Drains the Heat in the Lungs, suppresses rebellious Qi.

Indications

Coughing, asthma, pneumonia, bronchitis, pleurisy, spitting blood, swelling and pain in the throat, swelling and pain in the elbow and arm, erysipelas.

Traditional indications

Asthma, spitting blood, chest pain, throat blockage, fullness in chest.

Illustrative combinations

With Gv-14 *(Dazhui)* joined to N-BW-6 *(Jiehexue)*, and Co-20 *(Huagai)* joined to Co-21 *(Xuanji)* for pulmonary tuberculosis; prick B-54 *(Weizhong)* for erysipelas.

Classical combinations

With LI-11 *(Quchi)* for spasms and pain in the elbow (Source: SJD); with SI-1 *(Shaoze)* for irritability. (Source: CNLAM)

Needling method

Straight insertion, 0.5-1 unit. Sensation: local distension and soreness, or an electric, numb sensation extending toward the forearm.

Remarks

Uniting point of the Lung channel.

L-6 *(Kongzui)*　孔最　"Opening Maximum"

Location

On the radial aspect of the forearm, 7 units above the transverse crease of the wrist. (Dia. 2-32)

Anatomy

In the brachioradialis muscle, in the lateral margin at the upper extremity of the pronator teres muscle and the medial margin of the extensor carpi radialis brevis and longus muscles. Supplied by the cephalic vein and the radial artery and vein, the lateral cutaneous nerve of the forearm and a superficial branch of the radial nerve.

Traditional functions

Regulates and suppresses rebellious Lung Qi, cools Heat and stops bleeding.

Indications

Coughing, asthma, pneumonia, tonsillitis, hemoptysis, pain in elbow and arm.

Traditional indications

Headache, absence of sweating, spitting blood, loss of voice, sore throat, belching, pain in elbow and arm, difficulty bending the arm.

Illustrative combinations

With Gv-14 *(Dazhui)*, B-13 *(Feishu)* for pneumonia.

Classical combinations
With LI-11 *(Quchi)* and B-13 *(Feishu)* for coughing blood. (Source: CNLAM)

Needling method
Straight insertion, 1-1.5 units. Sensation: local distension and soreness, sometimes extending through the forearm.

Remarks
Accumulating point of the Lung channel.

L-7 *(Lieque)* 列缺 "Broken Sequence"

Location
Proximal to the styloid process of the radius, 1.5 units above the transverse crease of the wrist, in a small hollow. (Dia. 2-32)

Anatomy
Between the tendons of the brachioradialis and abductor pollicis longus muscles. Supplied by the cephalic vein and branches of the radial artery and vein, by a branch of the lateral cutaneous nerve of the forearm and a superficial branch of the radial nerve.

Traditional functions
Opens up the Lungs, disperses Wind, clears and regulates the Conception channel.

Indications
Headache, coughing, asthma, urticaria, facial paralysis, stiff neck, diseases of the wrist joint.

Traditional indications
Headache, panting, swelling of the pharynx, hemiplegia, mouth awry, Wind rash, blood in the urine, acute edema of the limbs.

Illustrative combinations
With LI-5 *(Yangxi)* and the point of pain for stenosans tenosynovitis.

Classical combinations
With L-8 *(Jingqu)* and L-9 *(Taiyuan)* for a burning sensation in the hand. (Source: GCAM)

Needling method
(1) Slanted insertion pointed toward the elbow, 0.5-1 unit. Sensation: local distension and soreness extending toward the elbow. (2) For stenosans tenosynovitis, point needle laterally 0.5-1 unit. Sensation: local distension and soreness.

Remarks
Connecting point of the Lung channel. Meeting point of the Lung channel with the Conception channel.

L-9 *(Taiyuan)* 太渊 "Great Abyss"

Location
With the palm facing up, this point can be found in a slight depression at the radial end of the transverse crease of the wrist. (Dia. 2-32)

243

① L-5 (Chize)
② L-6 (Kongzui)
③ L-7 (Lieque)
④ L-9 (Taiyuan)
⑤ L-10 (Yuji)
⑥ L-11 (Shaoshang)

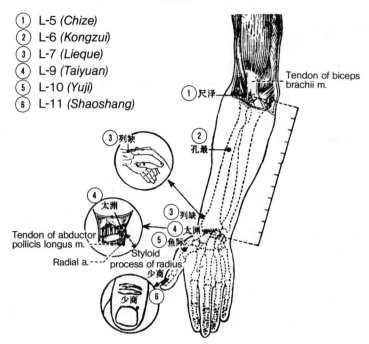

Dia. 2-32 Points of Lung Channel on Hand and Forearm

Anatomy

At the lateral aspect of the tendon of the flexor carpi radialis muscle and the medial aspect of the tendon of the abductor pollicis longus muscle. Supplied by the radial vein and artery, by the lateral cutaneous nerve of the forearm and a superficial branch of the radial nerve.

Traditional functions

Eliminates Wind and transforms Phlegm, regulates the Lungs and stops coughing.

Indications

Bronchitis, pertussis, influenza, asthma, pulmonary tuberculosis, pain in the chest, diseases affecting the radial side of the wrist joint.

Traditional indications

Headache, toothache, pain in the eyes, membrane on the eye, coughing blood, chest pain, pain and debility of the wrist.

Illustrative combinations

With P-6 (Neiguan), M-UE-9 (Sifeng) for pertussis.

Classical combinations

With L-7 (Lieque) for Wind Phlegm cough (Source: SJD); with L-10 (Yuji) for dry throat. (Source: GCAM)

Needling method

Straight insertion, 0.3-0.5 unit, causing local distension and soreness.

Remarks

Transporting point and Source point of the Lung channel. Meeting point of the Blood vessels.

L-10 *(Yuji)*　鱼际　"Fish Border"

Location

With the palm facing up, this point can be found at the midpoint on the thenar surface of the 1st metacarpus, at the 'border' separating the light colored skin of the palm from the darker colored skin of the back of the hand. (Dia. 2-32)

Anatomy

In the lateral abductor pollicis brevis and opponens pollicis muscles. Supplied by a branch of the cephalic vein in the thumb, by the lateral cutaneous nerve of the forearm and a superficial branch of the radial nerve.

Traditional functions

Cools Heat in the Lungs, benefits the throat.

Indications

Coughing, laryngopharyngitis, tonsillitis, hoarseness, asthma, hemoptysis, fever, infantile malnutrition syndrome.

Traditional indications

Coughing, throat blockage, spitting blood, loss of voice, emotional disturbance, tidal fevers, abdominal pain, pain in the chest and back.

Illustrative combinations

With LI-16 *(Jugu)*, L-5 *(Chize)* for hemoptysis.

Classical combinations

With TB-2 *(Yemen)* for sore throat. (Source: OHS)

Needling method

Straight insertion, 0.5-1 unit, causing local distension and soreness.

Remarks

Gushing point of the Lung channel.

L-11 *(Shaoshang)*　少商　"Lesser Merchant"

Location

Approximately 0.1 unit from the base of the cuticle on the inside of the thumb. (Dia. 2-32)

Anatomy

Supplied by the arteriovenous network formed by the proper palmar digital artery and vein, by the lateral cutaneous nerve of the forearm and a superficial branch of the radial nerve, as well as the distal network of the proper palmar digital nerves of the median nerve.

Traditional functions

Cools the Lungs, benefits the pharynx and revives from fainting.

Indications

Tonsillitis, parotitis, common cold, coughing, pneumonia, stroke, fainting, infantile indigestion, psychosis.

245

Traditional indications

Apoplectic delirium, coughing, cervical swelling with throat blockage, mumps, swollen patchy tonsils.

Illustrative combinations

With LI-4 *(Hegu)*, and prick L-11 *(Shaoshang)* for acute tonsillitis.

Classical combinations

With LI-11 *(Quchi)* for thirst with Deficient Blood (Source: OHS); with Co-22 *(Tiantu)* and LI-4 *(Hegu)* for swollen painful throat. (Source: GCAM)

Needling method

(1) Slanted insertion, needle pointed in proximal direction 0.1 unit, causing local pain. (2) Prick the point, drawing a few drops of blood.

Remarks

Well point of the Lung channel.

P-3 *(Quze)*　　曲泽　　"Crooked Marsh"

Location

With the arm bent slightly at the elbow, this point can be found just medial to the tendon of the biceps muscle at the transverse crease of the elbow. (Dia. 2-33)

Anatomy

At the medial aspect of the tendon of the biceps muscle. Supplied by the brachialis artery and vein, and by the trunk of the median nerve.

Traditional functions

Opens up the Heart Qi, drains Heat from the Blood, regulates the Intestines.

Indications

Acute gastroenteritis, enteritis, rheumatic heart disease, myocarditis, bronchitis, heat exhaustion, pain in the elbow and arm.

Traditional indications

Chest pain and easily frightened, heat exhaustion, diarrhea with vomiting (acute gastroenteritis), fever, irritability and fullness.

Illustrative combinations

With B-54 *(Weizhong)*, prick the point to draw blood for acute gastroenteritis; with P-6 *(Neiguan)*, P-5 *(Jianshi)*, H-8 *(Shaofu)* for rheumatic heart disease.

Classical combinations

With L-11 *(Shaoshang)* for thirst with Deficient Blood; with P-6 *(Neiguan)* and P-7 *(Daling)* for chest pain (Source: GCAM); with B-23 *(Shenshu)* and B-17 *(Geshu)* for chest pain. (Source: CNLAM)

Needling method

(1) Straight insertion, 0.5-1 unit, causing local distension and soreness and sometimes causing a numb, sore sensation extending as far as the middle finger. (2) For acute gastritis or enteritis, or heat exhaustion accompanied by high fever, the point may be pricked for a few drops of blood.

Remarks

Uniting point of the Pericardium channel.

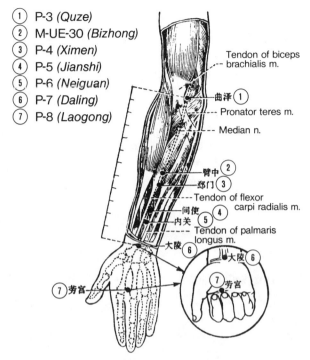

① P-3 *(Quze)*
② M-UE-30 *(Bizhong)*
③ P-4 *(Ximen)*
④ P-5 *(Jianshi)*
⑤ P-6 *(Neiguan)*
⑥ P-7 *(Daling)*
⑦ P-8 *(Laogong)*

Tendon of biceps brachialis m.

曲澤 ①

Pronator teres m.

Median n.

臂中 ②

郄门 ③

Tendon of flexor carpi radialis m.

间使 ④

内关 ⑤

Tendon of palmaris longus m.

大陵 ⑥

川 大陵 ⑥

⑦ 劳宫

⑦ 劳宫

Dia. 2-33 Points of Pericardium Channel on Hand and Forearm

M-UE-30 *(Bizhong)*　臂中　"Middle of Arm"

Location

At the midpoint between the transverse creases of the wrist and elbow, between the ulna and radius on the forearm. (Dia. 2-33)

Anatomy

In the flexor carpi radialis and the flexor digitorum superficialis manus muscles. In its deep position, this point lies between the flexor digitorum subliminis and flexor pollicis longus muscles; after penetrating the interosseous membrane, there are the abductor pollicis longus, the extensor pollicis brevis and the extensor digitorum manus muscles. Situated directly on the median nerve. Supplied by the median artery and vein as well as the anterior and posterior interosseous nerves, veins and arteries of the forearm.

Indications

Hemiplegia of the upper limb, spasms of the upper limb, neuralgia of the forearm, hysteria.

Illustrative combinations

With LI-11 *(Quchi),* LI-4 *(Hegu)* for hemiplegia of the upper limb or neuralgia of the forearm.

247

Needling method

Straight insertion through the arm but not penetrating the skin on the opposite side (i.e., through the interosseous membrane). This will cause a distended, numb sensation that may extend throughout the forearm or to the elbow.

P-4 *(Ximen)* 郄门 "Gate of the Crevice"

Location

5 units directly above the midpoint of the transverse crease of the wrist, between two tendons. (Dia. 2-33)

Anatomy

Between the tendons of the flexor carpi radialis and palmaris longus muscles, in the flexor digitorum superficialis manus muscle, and in its deep position in the flexor digitorum sublimis muscle. Supplied by the median artery and vein of the forearm, and by the median cutaneous nerve of the forearm. Below the point is the median nerve, and in its deep position is the anterior interosseous nerve of the forearm.

Traditional functions

Pacifies the Heart and calms the Spirit, regulates the Qi and expands the diaphragm.

Indications

Rheumatic heart disease, myocarditis, angina pectoris, palpitations, mastitis, pleurisy, spasm of the diaphragm, hysteria.

Traditional indications

Irritability and pain in the chest, depression, chest pain with vomiting, fear of strangers.

Illustrative combinations

With P-6 *(Neiguan)*, P-3 *(Quze)* for rheumatic heart disease; with LI-11 *(Quchi)*, TB-8 *(Sanyangluo)* for hemoptysis.

Needling method

Straight insertion, 1-1.5 units, causing local distension and soreness, or a distended, numb sensation reaching to the fingertips.

Remarks

Accumulating point of the Pericardium channel.

P-5 *(Jianshi)* 间使 "Intermediary"

Location

With the hand supine, this point can be found 1 unit above P-6 *(Neiguan)*, or 3 units above the transverse crease of the wrist, between the two tendons. (Dia. 2-33)

Anatomy

Between the tendons of the flexor carpi radialis and the palmar longus muscles, in the flexor digitorum superficialis manus muscle, and in its deep position in the flexor digitorum sublimis muscle. Supplied by the median artery and vein, and in its deep position by the anterior interosseous artery and vein of the forearm. Supplied by the medial cutaneous nerve of the forearm, the lateral cutaneous nerve of the forearm, and below which is a branch of the median nerve. In its deep position, supplied by the anterior interosseus nerve of the forearm.

248

Traditional functions

Calms the Spirit, harmonizes the Stomach, and eliminates Phlegm.

Indications

Rheumatic heart disease, stomach-ache, malaria, seizures, hysteria, psychosis.

Traditional indications

Chest pain, palpitations, stomach-ache and vomiting, tidal fevers, yellow eyes, insanity, generalized scabies, irregular menstruation.

Illustrative combinations

With P-6 *(Neiguan)*, H-8 *(Shaofu)*, P-4 *(Ximen)*, P-3 *(Quze)* for rheumatic heart disease; with N-HN-43 *(Qiying)*, Sp-6 *(Sanyinjiao)* for hyperthyroidism.

Classical combinations

With B-11 *(Dazhu)* for tidal fevers (Source: SGJ); with SI-3 *(Houxi)* and LI-4 *(Hegu)* for madness. (Source: GCAM)

Needling method

(1) Straight insertion, 0.5-1.5 units, causing local distension and soreness, or a numb, distended sensation extending toward the fingertips. (2) Slanted insertion, in a proximal direction slightly toward the radial side, 1.5-2 units, for diseases of the trunk. With strong needle stimulation, the Qi sensation may extend to the elbow or axilla.

Remarks

Traversing point of the Pericardium channel.

P-6 *(Neiguan)*   内关   "Inner Gate"

Location

With the hand supine, this point can be found 2 units directly above the midpoint of the transverse crease of the wrist, between the two tendons. (Dia. 2-33)

Anatomy

Between the tendons of the flexor carpi radialis and the palmaris longus muscles, in the flexor digitorum superficialis manus muscle, and in its deep position in the flexor digitorum sublimis muscle. Supplied by the median artery and vein and the anterior interosseous artery and vein of the forearm. Supplied by the medial and lateral cutaneous nerves of the forearm. Below the point is the median nerve, and in its deep position the anterior interosseous nerve of the forearm.

Traditional functions

Calms the Heart and Spirit, regulates the Qi, and suppresses pain.

Indications

Rheumatic heart disease, shock, angina pectoris, palpitations, vomiting, chest pain, stomach-ache, abdominal pain, spasm of the diaphragm, migraine headache, hyperthyroidism, seizures, hysteria, asthma, swollen and painful throat, pain associated with surgery.

Traditional indications

Chest pain, diseases of the chest, vomiting, disharmony between the Stomach and Spleen, tidal fever, jaundice, apoplexy, prolapsed rectum.

Illustrative combinations

With P-5 *(Jianshi)*, H-8 *(Shaofu)* for rheumatic heart disease; with P-5 *(Jianshi)*, S-36 *(Zusanli)* for angina pectoris; with Gv-25 *(Suliao)* for low blood pressure; with K-1 *(Yongquan)*, S-36 *(Zusanli)* for septic shock.

Classical combinations
With K-6 *(Zhaohai)* for pain and lumps in the abdomen. (Source: SJD)

Needling method
(1) Straight insertion, 0.5-1.5 units, reaching as far as TB-5 *(Waiguan)* on the opposite side of the forearm. Sensation: local distension, soreness and numbness possibly extending to fingertips. (2) Slanted insertion, needle pointed in a proximal direction, 1-2 units, for diseases of the trunk. Sensation: a numb, distended sensation possibly extending to the elbow, axilla or chest. (3) For numbness in fingers, point needle slightly toward the radial side of the arm, 0.3-0.5 unit. Sensation: a numb, electric sensation extending toward the fingertips.

Remarks
Connecting point of the Pericardium channel with the Divergent channel of the Triple Burner; Meeting point of the Yin Linking channel on the Pericardium channel.

P-7 *(Daling)*　大陵　"Big Tomb"

Location
With the hand supine, this point can be found at the midpoint of the transverse crease of the wrist. (Dia. 2-33)

Anatomy
Between the tendons of the flexor carpi radialis and palmaris longus muscles, in the flexor pollicis longus muscle and the tendon of the flexor digitorum sublimis muscle. Supplied by the arteriovenous network of the palmar side of the wrist. Situated directly above the trunk of the median nerve, and also supplied by the medial cutaneous nerve of the forearm and a palmar cutaneous branch of the median nerve.

Traditional functions
Clears the Heart and calms the Spirit, harmonizes the Stomach and expands the chest.

Indications
Myocarditis, palpitations, gastritis, tonsillitis, insomnia, intercostal neuralgia, mental illness, diseases and pain of the wrist joint.

Traditional indications
Seizures, throat blockage, swelling of the axilla, spitting blood, scabies, pain at the root of the tongue, Damp skin disease of upper extremities.

Illustrative combinations
With P-6 *(Neiguan)*, P-4 *(Ximen)*, H-8 *(Shaofu)* for premature contractions associated with rheumatic heart disease; with Gv-20 *(Baihui)*, M-HN-3 *(Yintang)*, K-3 *(Taixi)* for insomnia.

Classical combinations
With Co-4 *(Guanyuan)* for blood in the urine (Source: GCAM); with P-6 *(Neiguan)* and P-3 *(Quze)* for chest pain. (Source: GCAM)

Needling method
(1) Straight insertion, 0.3-0.5 unit, causing local distension and soreness or a numb, electric sensation extending toward the fingertips. (2) Slanted insertion, needle pointed into the blood vessels

250

of the wrist, for vascular syndrome of the wrist, causing local distension and pain, or possibly a numb, electric sensation extending toward the fingertips.

Remarks
Transporting and Source point of the Pericardium channel.

P-8 *(Laogong)*   劳宫   "Labor's Palace"

Location
With the fingers cupped in the palm in a half fist, this point can be found in front of the tip of the middle finger between the 2nd and 3rd metacarpal bones. (Dia. 2-33)

Anatomy
Between the second and third metacarpal bones. Below the point are the palmar aponeurosis, the second lumbrical and the superficial and deep tendons of the flexor digitorum muscles; in its deep position are the origin of the transverse head of the adductor pollicis muscle and the interossei muscle. Supplied by the common palmar digital artery and by the second palmar digital branch of the median nerve.

Traditional functions
Cools the Heart and drains Heat.

Indications
Coma from stroke, heat exhaustion, angina pectoris, stomatitis, frightened fainting among infants, hysteria, mental illness, excessive sweating of the palms, numb fingers.

Traditional indications
Chest pain, inability to swallow food, jaundice, hand tremors, "swan hand," madness, ulcerated oral cavity.

Illustrative combinations
With Gv-26 *(Renzhong)*, and LI-4 *(Hegu)* joined to P-8 *(Laogong)* for hysteria.

Classical combinations
With P-7 *(Daling)* for stuffy Heart [mild depression]. (Source: SJD)

Needling method
Straight insertion, about 0.5 unit, causing local distension and pain.

Remarks
Gushing point of the Pericardium channel.

H-3 *(Shaohai)*   少海   "Lesser Sea"

Location
With the arm bent at the elbow, this point can be found in the depression between the end of the transverse crease on the ulnar side of the elbow and the medial condyle of the humerus. (Dia. 2-39)

Anatomy
In the pronator teres and brachialis muscles. Supplied by the basilic vein, the inferior ulnar collateral artery and the ulnar recurrent artery. Supplied by the medial cutaneous nerve of the forearm.

Traditional functions
Calms the Spirit, clears the Vessels.

Indications
Neurasthenia, psychosis, intercostal neuralgia, ulnar nerve neuralgia, lymphadenitis, numbness of the forearm, diseases of the elbow.

Traditional indications
Headache and dizziness, stiff neck, toothache, chest pain, vomiting, nodular growths in the neck, pain in the axilla, absent-mindedness, madness, debility of the limbs.

Illustrative combinations
With N-HN-54 *(Anmian),* Sp-6 *(Sanyinjiao)* for neurasthenia.

Classical combinations
With LI-10 *(Shousanli)* for numbness in arm (Source: OHS); with S-33 *(Yinshi)* for chest pain with tremors of the hand. (Source: OXH)

Needling method
Straight insertion, 0.5-1.5 units, causing local distension and soreness, or an electric, numb sensation extending through the forearm.

Remarks
Uniting point of the Heart channel.

H-5 *(Tongli)*　通里　"Reaching the Measure"

Location
With the hand supine, this point can be found 1 unit above H-7 *(Shenmen),* on the ulnar aspect of the wrist. (Dia. 2-39)

Anatomy
Between the tendon of the flexor carpi ulnaris muscle and the flexor digitorum superficialis manus muscle, its deep position being in the flexor digitorum sublimis muscle. Supplied by the ulnar artery, and by the medial cutaneous nerve of the forearm. In its deep position, supplied by the ulnar nerve.

Traditional functions
Calms the Spirit, regulates the Heart Qi.

Indications
Palpitations, chest pain, bradycardia, neurasthenia, hysterical aphasia, psychosis, cough, asthma.

Traditional indications
Headache and dizziness, stiffness of the tongue, throat blockage; palpitations due to nervous fright, abnormal uterine bleeding, incontinence.

Illustrative combinations
With Gv-25 *(Suliao),* N-HN-23 *(Xingfen)* for bradycardia; with B-15 *(Xinshu)* for cardiac arrhythmia.

Classical combinations
With K-4 *(Dazhong)* for disinterest in talking and desire to sleep (Source: OHS); with Li-2 *(Xingjian)* and Sp-6 *(Sanyinjiao)* for excessive uterine bleeding. (Source: GCAM)

Needling method

Straight insertion, 0.5-1 unit, causing local distension and soreness, possibly extending along the ulnar side of forearm.

Remarks

Connecting point of the Heart channel with the Divergent channel of the Small Intestine channel.

H-7 *(Shenmen)* 神门 "Spirit's Door"

Location

With the hand supine, this point can be found in the small hollow on the ulnar aspect at the end of the transverse crease of the wrist. (Dia. 2-39)

Anatomy

Between the tendon of the flexor carpi ulnaris muscle and the flexor digitorum superficialis manus muscle, its deep position being in the flexor digitorum sublimis muscle. Supplied by the ulnar artery, and by the medial cutaneous nerve of the forearm. In its deep position, supplied by the ulnar nerve.

Traditional functions

Calms the Spirit, pacifies the Heart, clears the channels.

Indications

Neurasthenia, palpitations, absent-mindedness, insomnia, excessive dreaming, heart disease, angina pectoris, mental illness, hysteria, paralysis of the hyoglossus muscle.

Traditional indications

Idiocy and seizures, irritability and insomnia, vomiting blood, jaundice, pain in the ribs, loss of voice, panting.

Illustrative combinations

With B-15 *(Xinshu)*, P-6 *(Neiguan)* and GB-34 *(Yanglingquan)* joined to Sp-9 *(Yinlingquan)* for cardiac arrythmia.

Classical combinations

With Co-13 *(Shangwan)* for madly running around. (Source: OHS)

Needling method

Straight insertion, 0.3-0.5 unit, pointed slightly toward the ulnar side, causing local distension and soreness, possibly a numb, electric sensation extending toward the fingertips.

Remarks

Source and Transporting point of the Heart channel.

H-8 *(Shaofu)* 少府 "Lesser Residence"

Location

With the hand supine and the fingers cupped in a half fist, this point can be found on the palm just below the tip of the little finger. (Dia. 2-39)

Anatomy

Between the fourth and fifth metacarpal bones, in the fourth lumbrical muscle and the tendon of the flexor digitorum sublimis muscle, its deep position being in the interosseous muscle. Supplied by the common palmar digital artery and vein, and by the fourth common palmar digital branch of the ulnar nerve.

Traditional functions
Calms the Spirit and regulates the Heart Qi.

Indications
Rheumatic heart disease, palpitations, cardiac arrhythmia, angina pectoris, dysuria, enuresis, hysteria.

Traditional indications
Palpitations, chest pain, spasms of the little finger, itching of the groin, difficult urination, incontinence.

Illustrative combinations
With H-5 *(Tongli)*, P-6 *(Neiguan)*, P-7 *(Daling)* for cardiac arrhythmia; with P-3 *(Quze)*, P-4 *(Ximen)*, P-5 *(Jianshi)* for rheumatic heart disease.

Classical combinations
With S-36 *(Zusanli)* for lack of urine. (Source: CNLAM)

Needling method
Straight insertion, about 0.5 unit, causing local distension and pain.

Remarks
Gushing point of the Heart channel.

M-UE-22 *(Baxie)*   八邪   "Eight Evils"

Location
With the hand in a clenched fist, these points can be found between the heads of each of the metacarpal bones, four on each hand for a total of eight. (Dia. 2-34)

Anatomy
In the dorsal interossei muscles. Supplied by the intercapital veins, and by the dorsal digital arteries, veins and nerves as well as branches of the common palmar digital arteries, veins and nerves.

Indications
Diseases of the finger joints, numbness of the fingers, headache, stiff neck, toothache, sore throat, snake bite.

Illustrative combinations
With TB-5 *(Waiguan)* for numbness in the fingers.

Needling method
With the hand making a fist (so as to stretch the skin tight between the knuckles), straight insertion along the metacarpal bone, up to 1 unit, causing local distension and soreness, and possibly a numb, electric sensation extending toward the fingertips.

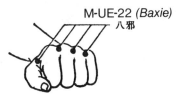

Dia. 2-34 M-UE-22 (Baxie)

M-UE-50 *(Shangbaxie)* 上八邪 "Upper Eight Evils"

Location
Eight points (four on each hand) located in the small depression just behind and between the metacarpophalangeal joints on the back of the hand. (Dia. 2-35)

Anatomy
In the interossei muscles on the dorsal aspect of the hand. Directly above the dorsal digital and the common palmar digital arteries, veins and nerves.

Indications
Same as M-UE-22 *(Baxie)* above.

Illustrative combinations
With LI-11 *(Quchi),* TB-5 *(Waiguan)* for pain and swelling of the finger joints.

Needling method
Straight insertion, 0.3-0.5 unit, causing local distension and soreness, or an electric, numb sensation extending toward the fingertips.

Remarks
The point between the 1st and 2nd metacarpal bones is more commonly called LI-4 *(Hegu),* between the 2nd and 3rd metacarpal bones is called M-UE-24 *(Luozhen),* and between the 4th and 5th metacarpal bones is called TB-3 *(Zhongzhu).*

① M-UE-50 *(Shangbaxie)*
② M-UE-24 *(Luozhen)*

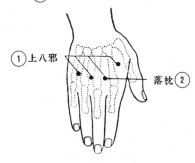

**Dia. 2-35   M-UE-50 *(Shangbaxie)*
and M-UE-24 *(Luozhen)***

M-UE-24 *(Luozhen)*   落枕   "Stiff Neck"

Location

Approximately 0.5 unit proximal to and between the metacarpophalangeal joints of the 2nd and 3rd metacarpal bones on the back of the hand. (Dia. 2-35)

Anatomy

In the interossei muscle of the second metacarpus. Directly above the dorsal digital and common palmar arteries, veins and nerves, as well as branches of the deep palmar arch and the deep terminal branch of the ulnar nerve.

Indications

Stiff neck, migraine headache, stomach-ache, sore throat, pain in the shoulder and arm.

Illustrative combinations

With M-HN-29 *(Xinshi)* for stiff neck.

Needling method

Straight or slanted insertion, 0.5-1 unit, causing local distension and soreness and sometimes a numb sensation extending to the fingertips.

M-UE-9 *(Sifeng)*   四缝   "Four Seams"

Location

On the palmar surface of the four fingers (excluding the thumb), at the midpoint on the transverse crease of each proximal phalangeal joint. (Dia. 2-36)

Anatomy

In the fibrous sheaths, synovial sheaths, and tendons of the flexor digitorum sublimis muscles. The deep position is within the joint cavity. Supplied by branches of the proper palmar digital arteries, veins and nerves.

Indications

Pertussis, infantile indigestion, infantile malnutrition syndrome, arthritis of the fingers, round worm in the intestines.

Illustrative combinations

With P-6 *(Neiguan)*, LI-4 *(Hegu)* for pertussis; with S-36 *(Zusanli)* for infantile indigestion.

Needling method

Prick the skin over the points, drawing a small amount of yellow/white fluid.

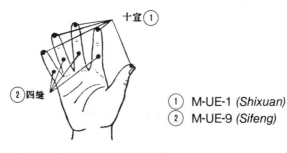

十宣 ①

② 四缝

① M-UE-1 *(Shixuan)*
② M-UE-9 *(Sifeng)*

**Dia. 2-36   M-UE-1 *(Shixuan)*
and M-UE-9 *(Sifeng)***

256

M-UE-1 *(Shixuan)*　　十宣　　"Ten Spreadings"

Location
Ten points, one on the middle of the tip of each finger, about 0.1 unit from the fingernail. (Dia. 2-36)

Anatomy
In the thick skin are pain and touch sensory receptors. Supplied by the nerve and blood vessel network formed by the proper palmar digital arteries, veins and nerves. The deep position is on the unguicular tuberosity.

Indications
Shock, fainting, high fever, heat exhaustion, seizures, hysteria, infantile fainting due to fright, numbness of the fingertips.

Illustrative combinations
With Gv-14 *(Dazhui)*, M-HN-10 *(Erjian)* for heat exhaustion or high fever.

Needling method
Either shallow insertion of needle, or prick the skin to draw a little blood.

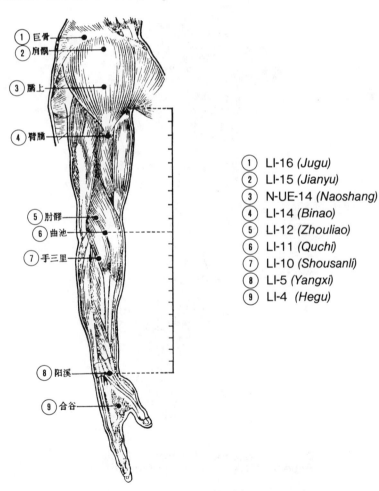

1　巨骨
2　肩髃
3　臑上
4　臂臑
5　肘髎
6　曲池
7　手三里
8　阳溪
9　合谷

1 LI-16 *(Jugu)*
2 LI-15 *(Jianyu)*
3 N-UE-14 *(Naoshang)*
4 LI-14 *(Binao)*
5 LI-12 *(Zhouliao)*
6 LI-11 *(Quchi)*
7 LI-10 *(Shousanli)*
8 LI-5 *(Yangxi)*
9 LI-4 *(Hegu)*

Dia. 2-37 Relation of Points on Lateral Aspect of Upper Limb with Musculature

① LI-16 (Jugu)
② TB-14 (Jianliao)
③ SI-10 (Naoshu)
④ N-UE-14 (Naoshang)
⑤ SI-9 (Jianzhen)
⑥ LI-14 (Binao)
⑦ N-UE-12 (Yingshang)
⑧ TB-10 (Tianjing)
⑨ LI-12 (Zhouliao)
⑩ LI-11 (Quchi)
⑪ LI-10 (Shousanli)
⑫ TB-9 (Sidu)

⑬ TB-8 (Sanyangluo)
⑭ TB-5 (Waiguan)
⑮ TB-6 (Zhigou)
⑯ SI-6 (Yanglao)
⑰ LI-5 (Yangxi)
⑱ M-UE-50 (Shangbaxie)
⑲ LI-4 (Hegu)
⑳ M-UE-22 (Baxie)
㉑ TB-4 (Yangchi)
㉒ SI-4 (Wangu)
㉓ TB-3 (Zhongzhu)
㉔ SI-3 (Houxi)
㉕ SI-1 (Shaoze)

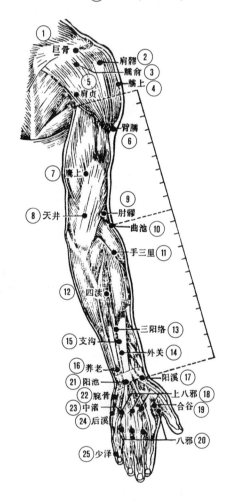

**Dia. 2-38 Relation of Points on Posterior
Aspect of Upper Limb with Musculature**

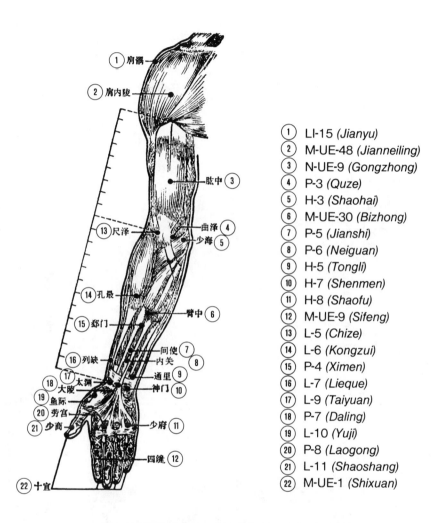

① 肩髃
② 肩内陵
③ 肱中
⑬ 尺泽
④ 曲泽
⑤ 少海
⑭ 孔最
⑮ 郄门
⑥ 臂中
⑦ 间使
⑧ 内关
⑯ 列缺
⑨ 通里
⑰ 太渊
⑩ 神门
⑱ 大陵
⑲ 鱼际
⑳ 劳宫
㉑ 少商
⑪ 少府
⑫ 四缝
㉒ 十宣

① LI-15 *(Jianyu)*
② M-UE-48 *(Jianneiling)*
③ N-UE-9 *(Gongzhong)*
④ P-3 *(Quze)*
⑤ H-3 *(Shaohai)*
⑥ M-UE-30 *(Bizhong)*
⑦ P-5 *(Jianshi)*
⑧ P-6 *(Neiguan)*
⑨ H-5 *(Tongli)*
⑩ H-7 *(Shenmen)*
⑪ H-8 *(Shaofu)*
⑫ M-UE-9 *(Sifeng)*
⑬ L-5 *(Chize)*
⑭ L-6 *(Kongzui)*
⑮ P-4 *(Ximen)*
⑯ L-7 *(Lieque)*
⑰ L-9 *(Taiyuan)*
⑱ P-7 *(Daling)*
⑲ L-10 *(Yuji)*
⑳ P-8 *(Laogong)*
㉑ L-11 *(Shaoshang)*
㉒ M-UE-1 *(Shixuan)*

Dia. 2-39 Relation of Points on Anterior Aspect of Upper Limb with Musculature

SUMMARY OF COMMON POINTS OF THE UPPER LIMB

Region	Points	Common Characteristics	Particular Characteristics
Shoulder	LI-15 (*Jianyu*), M-UE-48 (*Jianneiling*), TB-14 (*Jianliao*), LI-16 (*Jugu*), SI-10 (*Naoshu*), SI-9 (*Jianzhen*), LI-14 (*Binao*), H-1 (*Jiquan*)	Diseases of the shoulder joint and surrounding soft tissues	LI-15 (*Jianyu*) and SI-9 (*Jianzhen*): paralysis of upper limb; LI-16 (*Jugu*): coughing blood; LI-14 (*Binao*): eye diseases
Upper Arm	N-UE-12 (*Yingshang*), N-UE-9 (*Gongzhong*)	Paralysis of upper limb, palpitations	
Elbow, Forearm and Hand	Large Intestine channel: LI-12 (*Zhouliao*), LI-11 (*Quchi*), LI-10 (*Shousanli*), LI-5 (*Yangxi*), LI-4 (*Hegu*)	Diseases of the head and throat, fever	LI-12 (*Zhouliao*): tendinitis of elbow; LI-11 (*Quchi*): hypertension, allergies; LI-10 (*Shousanli*): gastro-intestinal diseases; LI-5 (*Yangxi*): diseases of wrist; LI-4 (*Hegu*): surgical analgesia, induce labor, deafness, tinnitus, excessive sweating.
	Triple Burner channel: TB-10 (*Tianjing*), TB-9 (*Sidu*), TB-8 (*Sanyangluo*), TB-6 (*Zhigou*), TB-5 (*Waiguan*), TB-4 (*Yangchi*), TB-3 (*Zhongzhu*)	Diseases of the head and throat, fever; diseases of the temporal region, eyes, ears, chest and ribs	TB-10 (*Tianjing*): scrofula; TB-9 (*Sidu*): lateral headaches; TB-6 (*Zhigou*): intercostal neuralgia, constipation; TB-5 (*Waiguan*): high fevers, numbness in hand and fingers; TB-4 (*Yangchi*): diseases of wrist
	Small Intestine channel: SI-6 (*Yanglao*), SI-4 (*Wangu*), SI-3 (*Houxi*), SI-1 (*Shaoze*)	Diseases of the head and throat, fever; diseases of the neck, eyes, ears, nose; mental illness	SI-6 (*Yanglao*): eye diseases; SI-3 (*Houxi*): seizures, night sweats, spasm of hand and fingers; SI-1 (*Shaoze*): diseases of breast, pterygium

Region	Points	Common Characteristics	Particular Characteristics
Elbow, Forearm and Hand (cont)	Lung channel: L-5 (Chize), L-6 (Kongzui), L-7 (Lieque), L-9 (Taiyuan), L-10 (Yuji), L-11 (Shaoshang)	Diseases of the chest; diseases of Lungs and upper respiratory tract	L-5 (Chize), L-6 (Kongzui): coughing blood, pneumonia; L-7 (Lieque): diseases affecting radial aspect of wrist, pain in head and neck; L-9 (Taiyuan): diseases affecting radial aspect of wrist; L-10 (Yuji): coughing blood, asthma, infantile malnutrition syndrome; L-11 (Shaoshang): fainting
	Pericardium channel: P-3 (Quze), M-UE-33 (Bizhong), P-4 (Ximen), P-5 (Jianshi), P-6 (Neiguan), P-7 (Daling), P-8 (Laogong)	Diseases of the chest; diseases of Heart, Pericardium, and mental illness	M-UE-33 (Bizhong): paralysis of upper limb, palpitations; P-3 (Quze): gastro-intestinal inflammation; P-5 (Jianshi): malaria, seizures; P-6 (Neiguan): rheumatic heart disease, gastro-intestinal diseases; P-8 (Laogong): diseases of mouth, hiccoughs, itching hands
	Heart channel: H-3 (Shaohai), H-5 (Tongli), H-7 (Shenmen), H-8 (Shaofu)	Diseases of the chest; diseases of Heart, Pericardium, and mental illness	H-3 (Shaohai): diseases of elbow, H-8 (Shaofu): rheumatic heart disease
Other	M-UE-22 (Baxie), M-UE-50 (Shangbaxie), M-UE-24 (Luozhen)	Diseases of the metacarpal joints	M-UE-22 (Baxie): snake bite; M-UE-24 (Luozhen): stiff neck, stomach-ache
	M-UE-9 (Sifeng), M-UE-1 (Shixuan)		M-UE-9 (Sifeng): pertussis, infantile indigestion; M-UE-1 (Shixuan): high fever, revive from faint

Chapter 6

Common Points of the Lower Limb

GB-29 *(Juliao)*   居髎   "Stationary Seam"

Location
At the mid-point on a line connecting the anterior, superior iliac spine with the greater trochanter of the femur. (Dia. 2-40)

Anatomy
At the anterior margin of the tensor fascia lata, and its deep position in the vastus lateralis muscle. Supplied by superficial branches of the circumflex iliac artery and vein and ascending branches of the lateral circumflex femoral artery and vein, and by the lateral cutaneous nerve of the thigh.

Indications
Stomach-ache, lower abdominal pain, orchitis, endometritis, cystitis, disease of the hip joint and surrounding soft tissues, pain in the lower back and leg.

Traditional indications
Low back pain and associated pain in lower abdomen, paralysis or atrophy of the leg, diarrhea.

Illustrative combinations
With B-17 *(Geshu)*, B-18 *(Ganshu)*, B-20 *(Pishu)* for gastric or duodenal ulcer.

Classical combinations
With GB-30 *(Huantiao)* and B-54 *(Weizhong)* for Wind Dampness pain in the leg. (Source: SJD)

Needling method
Slanted insertion, pointed toward hip joint 2-3 units, causing distension and soreness extending to the hip joint.

GB-30 *(Huantiao)*   环跳   "Encircling Leap"

Location
At a point situated one third the distance on a line drawn from the greater trochanter of the femur to the sacral hiatus. (Dia. 2-41)

Anatomy
In the gluteus maximus and inferior margin of the piriformis muscles. Supplied on its medial aspect

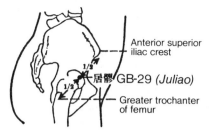

Dia. 2-40   GB-29 (Juliao)

by the inferior gluteal artery and vein. Supplied by the inferior gluteal cutaneous and inferior gluteal nerves, and in its deep position directly on the sciatic nerve.

Traditional functions
Benefits the lower back and leg, clears the channels.

Indications
Sciatica, pain in the lower back and leg, numbness and paralysis of the lower extremity, diseases of the hip joint and surrounding soft tissues.

Traditional indications
Hemiplegia, pain of the lower back and groin, leg Qi*, edema, Wind rash.

Illustrative combinations
With GB-34 *(Yanglingquan)* and GB-39 *(Xuanzhong)* for paralysis of the lower limb.

Classical combinations
With GB-39 *(Xuanzhong)* for leg pain and drop foot (Source: OSM); with B-67 *(Zhiyin)* for pain in the chest that changes location with corresponding acute pain in the waist and legs. (Source: CNLAM)

Needling method
(1) Straight insertion, for sciatica, pointed toward genitals 2-3.5 units, causing local distension and soreness or an electric numb sensation extending down the leg. (2) Straight insertion, or probe by inserting the needle on both sides of the point, 2-3 units in depth, for diseases of the hip joint or surrounding soft tissues. Sensation: distension and soreness, possibly extending to the hip joint.

Remarks
Point of intersection of the Bladder channel on the Gall Bladder channel.

N-BW-17 *(Zuogu)*   坐骨   "Ischium"

Location
1 unit below the mid-point between the greater trochanter and the coccyx. (Dia. 2-42)

---

*Leg Qi, also known as edema of the leg, is characterized in the beginning by swollen legs that are numb, painful, and weak. Spasms, atrophy, fever, palpitations, vomiting, etc., will develop if it attacks the Heart. It is caused by improper eating habits, Dampness, etc. (Western medicine: beriberi).—*Editors*

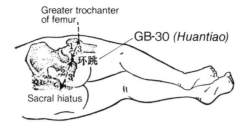

Dia. 2-41 GB-30 *(Huantiao)*

Anatomy
    Posterior and lateral to the ischial tuberosity, in the gluteus maximus muscle. Supplied by the inferior clunial nerve and in its deep position by branches of the inferior gluteal nerve, artery and vein, the root of the posterior cutaneous nerve of the thigh and situated lateral to the sciatic nerve. Below the point is the quadratus femoris muscle, and deeper are the tendon of the obturator externus muscle, muscle branches of nerves in the quadratus femoris muscle, and deep branches of the medial circumflex femoral artery and vein.

Indications
    Sciatica, paralysis of lower limb.

Illustrative combinations
    With B-51 *(Yinmen),* GB-34 *(Yanglingquan)* for sciatica.

Needling method
    Straight insertion, 2-3 units. Sensation: local distension and soreness, sometimes an electric, numb sensation reaching the lower leg.

B-50 *(Chengfu)*   承扶   "Receive Support"

Location
    On the posterior aspect of the thigh, at the midpoint of the transverse crease below the buttock. (Dia. 2-42)

Anatomy
    At the inferior margin of the gluteus maximus muscle. Supplied by the comitans artery and vein of the sciatic nerve, by the posterior cutaneous nerve of the thigh and in its deep position by the sciatic nerve.

Indications
    Low back pain, sciatica, paralysis of lower extremity, hemorrhoids, retention of urine, constipation.

Traditional indications
    Pain in lower back and leg, hemorrhoids, pain in the genitals, difficulty in urination, swelling of the coccyx.

Illustrative combinations
    With B-26 *(Guanyuanshu),* N-BW-17 *(Zuogu),* B-54 *(Weizhong)* for pain in lower back and leg.

264

Needling method

Straight insertion, 2-3 units, causing local distension and soreness or an electric numb sensation extending down the leg.

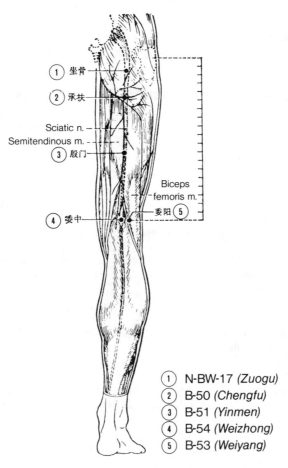

Dia. 2-42 Points on Posterior
Aspect of Thigh

1. N-BW-17 (Zuogu)
2. B-50 (Chengfu)
3. B-51 (Yinmen)
4. B-54 (Weizhong)
5. B-53 (Weiyang)

B-51 *(Yinmen)*   殷门   "Door of Abundance"

Location

With patient lying prone, this point can be found on the back of the thigh, 6 units directly below B-50 *(Chengfu)*. (Dia. 2-42)

Anatomy

In the semitendinosus muscle, lateral to which are the third perforating branches of the deep femoral artery and vein. Supplied by the posterior cutaneous nerve of the thigh, and in its deep position situated directly on the sciatic nerve.

Indications

Pain in lower back, herniated disc, sciatica, occipital headache, paralysis of lower limb, paralysis.

Traditional indications
Low back pain that inhibits flexion and extension, distension on the lateral side of thigh.

Illustrative combinations
With the vertebral points M-BW-35 *(Jiaji)* of the 4th and 5th lumbar vertebrae for vertebral disk abnormality of the lumbar vertebrae.

Classical combinations
With B-53 *(Weiyang)* for back pain inhibiting extension. (Source: CNLAM)

Needling method
Straight insertion, 2-3 units, causing a numb, electric sensation possibly extending to the buttock or foot.

GB-31 *(Fengshi)*　风市　"Wind's Market"

Location
At the median line on the lateral aspect of the thigh, 7 units above the kneecap; or directly below the tip of the middle finger when the arm is extended at the side of the leg. (Dia. 2-43)

Anatomy
Beneath the tensor fasciae latae, in the vastus lateralis muscle. Supplied by muscle branches of the lateral circumflex femoral artery and vein, by the lateral cutaneous nerve of the thigh and a muscle branch of the femoral nerve.

Indications
Paralysis of lower limb, pain in lower back and leg, neuritis of the lateral cutaneous nerve of the thigh and a muscle branch of the femoral nerve.

Traditional indications
Soreness and pain in the lower back and leg, numbness and stiffness of the lower leg and foot, hemiplegia, itching on one side of the body, headache, eyes red and swollen.

Illustrative combinations
With S-33 *(Yinshi)*, GB-34 *(Yanglingquan)* for arthritis of the knee, or paralysis of lower limb.

Classical combinations
With S-33 *(Yinshi)* for weak legs (Source: SJD); with B-54 *(Weizhong)*, Li-2 *(Xingjian)* for low back pain with difficulty in movement. (Source: GCAM)

Needling method
Straight insertion, 1.5-2.5 units, causing local distension and soreness possibly extending downward.

GB-33 *(Xiyangguan)*　膝陽关　"Knee's Yang Hinge"

Location
In the hollow above the lateral condyle of the femur at the knee, between the bone and tendon. (Dia. 2-43)

Anatomy
At the posterior aspect of the iliotibial band and the anterior aspect of the biceps femoris tendon.

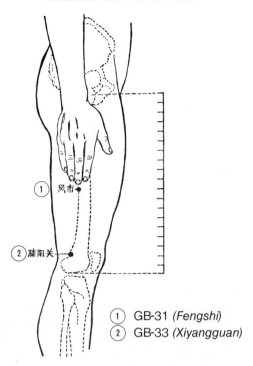

1 GB-31 *(Fengshi)*
2 GB-33 *(Xiyangguan)*

**Dia. 2-43 Points on Lateral
Aspect of Thigh**

Supplied by the lateral superior genicular artery and vein, and by a branch of the lateral cutaneous nerve of the thigh.

Indications
Diseases of the knee and surrounding soft tissues, paralysis of lower limb.

Traditional indications
Inability to flex or extend the knee, progressive swelling and pain of the knee, leg Qi.

Illustrative combinations
Join to Li-8 *(Ququan)* and join GB-34 *(Yanglingquan)* to Sp-9 *(Yinlingquan)* for arthritis of the knee.

Needling method
Straight insertion, 1.5-2.5 units, causing distension and soreness possibly extending to the medial aspect of the thigh.

N-LE-58 *(Waiyinlian)* 外阴廉 "Outer Yin's Modesty"

Location
With patient lying supine, this point can be found about 1 finger width below the inguinal ligament, lateral to the femoral artery at the place where its pulse can be felt. (Dia. 2-44)

Anatomy
Below the inguinal ligament, at the medial aspect above the origin of the sartorius muscle. Below the

267

point is a branch of the great saphenous vein, and to its medial side is the femoral artery. Supplied by a branch of the anterior cutaneous nerve of the thigh, and situated directly on the path of the femoral nerve.

Indications
Paralysis of lower limb, pain of lower back and leg, neuralgia of the femoral nerve.

Illustrative combinations
With N-LE-23 *(Maibu)*, N-LE-21 *(Xinfutu)*, N-LE-18 *(Jianxi)*, S-36 *(Zusanli)* for paralysis of lower limb.

Needling method
Straight insertion, needle pointed slightly laterally, 1-1.5 units, causing local distension and soreness or an electric, numb sensation extending toward the knee. CAUTION: Do not insert needle into the femoral artery.

N-LE-23 *(Maibu)*　迈步　"Stride"

Location
At the lateral margin of the rectus femoris muscle and the vastus lateralis muscle. Directly on the lateral cutaneous nerve of the thigh; in its deep position supplied by branches of the lateral circumflex femoral artery and vein, and a branch of the femoral nerve. (Dia. 2-44)

Indications
Sequelae of infantile paralysis, hemiplegia.

Illustrative combinations
With GB-30 *(Huantiao)*, B-51 *(Yinmen)*, N-LE-18 *(Jianxi)*, S-36 *(Zusanli)* for paralysis of lower limb.

Needling method
Straight insertion, 1-3 units, causing distension and soreness possibly extending to the knee.

S-31 *(Biguan)*　脾关　"Hip's Hinge"

Location
This point can be found directly below the anterior superior iliac spine, level with the perineum. (Dia. 2-44)

Anatomy
Inferior and medial to the greater trochanter of the femur, between the sartorius and tensor fascia lata muscles. In its deep position are branches of the lateral circumflex femoral artery and vein. Supplied by the lateral cutaneous nerve of the thigh.

Indications
Paralysis of lower limb, lymphadenitis of the inguinal lymph glands, arthritis of the knee, low back pain.

Traditional indications
Atrophy or blockage of muscles of the thigh and buttock, inhibited movement of the leg muscles due to sinew tension, low back pain and Cold in the knees, numbness of the leg.

① N-LE-58 *(Waiyinlian)*
② S-31 *(Biguan)*
③ N-LE-23 *(Maibu)*
④ S-32 *(Futu)*
⑤ S-34 *(Liangqiu)*

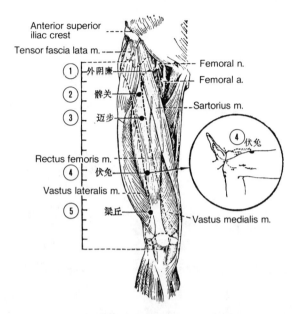

Dia. 2-44 Points on Anterior Aspect of Thigh

Illustrative combinations

With B-54 *(Weizhong),* B-50 *(Chengfu)* for arthritis of the hip joint.

Needling method

Straight or slanted insertion, 1.5-3 units, causing local distension and soreness possibly extending to the knee.

S-32 *(Futu)* 伏兔 "Hidden Rabbit"

Location

On the thigh, 6 units above the lateral margin of the kneecap. (Dia. 2-44)

Anatomy

At the lateral, anterior aspect of the femur, in the middle of the belly of the rectus femoris muscle. Supplied by a branch of the lateral circumflex femoral artery and vein, the anterior femoral cutaneous nerve, and situated on the lateral femoral cutaneous nerve.

Indications

Paralysis of lower limb, arthritis of the knee, urticaria.

Traditional indications

Pain in the waist and groin, numbness of the lower limb, leg Qi.

269

Illustrative combinations
With N-LE-23 *(Maibu)*, GB-31 *(Fengshi)*, M-LE-24 *(Linghou)* for paralysis or numbness of the lower limb.

Needling method
Straight insertion, 1.5-2.5 units, causing distension and soreness possibly extending to the knee.

S-34 *(Liangqiu)* 梁丘 "Ridge Mound"

Location
On the thigh, 2 units above the lateral, superior margin of the kneecap. (Dia. 2-44)

Anatomy
Between the rectus femoris and vastus lateralis muscles of the thigh. Supplied by a descending branch of the lateral circumflex femoral artery, the anterior femoral cutaneous nerve and situated directly on the lateral femoral cutaneous nerve.

Traditional functions
Pacifies the Stomach, clears the channels.

Indications
Gastritis, stomach-ache, diarrhea, mastitis, diseases of the knee and surrounding soft tissues.

Traditional indications
Pain of low back and leg, progressive swelling and pain of the knee, swelling and pain of the breast.

Illustrative combinations
With Co-12 *(Zhongwan)*, P-6 *(Neiguan)* for gastritis.

Classical combinations
With GB-42 *(Diwuhui)* for swelling of the breast. (Source: CNLAM)

Needling method
Straight insertion, 1-1.5 units, causing local distension and soreness possibly extending to the knee.

Remarks
Accumulating point of the Stomach channel.

M-LE-13 *(Lanweixue)* 阑尾穴 "Appendix Orifice"

Location
Approximately 2 units below S-36 *(Zusanli)* on the lower leg. (Dia. 2-45)

Anatomy
In the anterior tibial muscle. Supplied by the lateral cutaneous nerve of the calf, and in its deep position by the deep peroneal nerve and the anterior tibial artery and vein.

Indications
Acute and chronic appendicitis, paralysis of lower limb, drop foot, indigestion.

Illustrative combinations

With S-36 *(Zusanli)* and the 'point of pain' on the lower right side of the abdomen for uncomplicated appendicitis.

Needling method

Straight insertion, 1.5-2.5 units, causing distension and soreness possibly extending to the foot.

S-35 *(Xiyan)*　膝眼　"Eyes of Knee"

Locations

With the knee flexed, this point can be found below the kneecap in the hollow on either side of the patellar tendon, the 'eyes' of the knee. (Dia. 2-45)

Anatomy

One finger width on either side of the patellar tendon. Supplied by the arterio-venous network of the knee, by infrapatellar branches of the saphenous nerve and medial and lateral infrapatellar branches of the common peroneal nerve.

Indications

Diseases of the knee and surrounding soft tissue.

Traditional indications

Pain of the knee, leg Qi, paralysis of lower limb.

Illustrative combinations

With S-34 *(Liangqiu),* GB-34 *(Yanglingquan)* for arthritis of the knee.

Needling method

(1) Straight insertion, pointed medially or laterally, 1.5-2 units. Sensation: local distension, possibly extending downward. (2) Slanted insertion, through the patellar tendon joining the first 'eye' with the second, 2-2.5 units. Sensation: local distension and soreness.

Remarks

The lateral point is also listed as M-LE-16 *(Dubi),* 'calf's nose.'

S-36 *(Zusanli)*　足三里　"Three Measures on the Leg"

Location

On the lower leg, 3 units below the lateral 'eye' of the knee, approximately 1 finger width lateral to the tibia. (Dia. 2-45)

Anatomy

Between the tibialis anterior muscle and the tendon of the extensor digitorum longus pedis. Supplied by the anterior tibial artery and vein, the lateral cutaneous nerve of the calf, a cutaneous branch of the saphenous nerve and in its deep position by the deep peroneal nerve.

Traditional functions

Orders the Spleen and Stomach, regulates the Qi and Blood, and strengthens weak and Deficient conditions.

Indications

Acute and chronic gastritis, ulcers, acute and chronic enteritis, acute pancreatitis, indigestion and other disorders of the digestive system, hemiplegia, shock, general weakness, anemia, hypertension, allergies, jaundice, seizures, asthma, enuresis, diseases of the reproductive system, neurasthenia.

Traditional indications

Abdominal pain and distension, vomiting, constipation or diarrhea, paralysis, seizures, abcessed breast, swelling (edema) of the limbs, difficult urination, pain and distension of the lower abdomen, loss of urine.

Illustrative combinations

With S-39 *(Xiajuxu)*, GB-34 *(Yanglingquan)*, P-6 *(Neiguan)* for pancreatitis; with LI-4 *(Hegu)*, P-6 *(Neiguan)*, Co-12 *(Zhongwan)*, S-25 *(Tianshu)*, B-25 *(Dachangshu)*, B-32 *(Ciliao)* for acute intestinal obstruction; with LI-4 *(Hegu)*, S-25 *(Tianshu)*, Co-4 *(Guanyuan)* for indigestion.

Classical combinations

With Li-4 *(Zhongfeng)* and Li-3 *(Taichong)* for difficulty and pain on walking (Source: SJD); with S-19 *(Burong)* for accumulated Qi. (Source: CNLAM)

Needling method

(1) Straight insertion, pointed slightly toward the tibia, 1-2 units. Sensation: an electric, numb sensation extending toward the foot. (2) Slanted insertion downward, 2-3 units. Sensation: distension and soreness possibly extending to the foot below or knee above.

Remarks

Lower Uniting point of the Stomach.

S-37 *(Shangjuxu)*　上巨虚　"Upper Void"

Location

On the lower leg, 3 units below S-36 *(Zusanli)*. (Dia. 2-45)

Anatomy

In the tibialis anterior muscle. Supplied by the anterior tibial artery and vein, the lateral cutaneous nerve of the calf and a cutaneous branch of the saphenous nerve; in its deep position, situated directly on the deep peroneal nerve.

Traditional functions

Regulates the Intestines and Stomach, clears and cools Dampness and Heat, eliminates accumulations and stagnation.

Indications

Abdominal pain or distension, diarrhea, appendicitis, enteritis, dysentery, gastritis, hemiplegia, beriberi.

Traditional indications

Deficient, weak conditions of the Spleen and Stomach, indigestion, leg Qi, sharp pain in the intestines, diarrhea, hemiplegia.

Illustrative combinations

With S-25 *(Tianshu)* for enteritis or dysentery.

Classical combinations
With S-39 *(Xiajuxu)* for diarrhea due to indigestion. (Source: GCAM)

Needling method
Same as S-36 *(Zusanli)* above.

Remarks
Lower Uniting point of the Large Intestine.

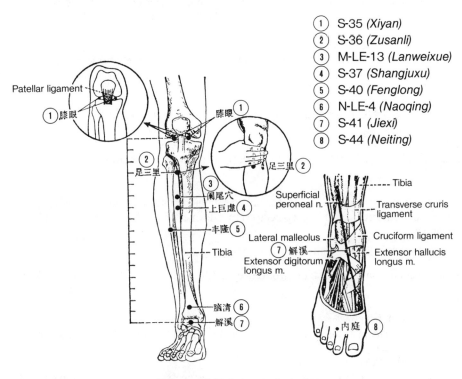

1. S-35 *(Xiyan)*
2. S-36 *(Zusanli)*
3. M-LE-13 *(Lanweixue)*
4. S-37 *(Shangjuxu)*
5. S-40 *(Fenglong)*
6. N-LE-4 *(Naoqing)*
7. S-41 *(Jiexi)*
8. S-44 *(Neiting)*

**Dia. 2-45 Points on Anterior
Aspect of Lower Limb**

S-40 *(Fenglong)* 丰隆 "Abundance and Prosperity"

Location
On the lower leg, 8 units above the lateral malleolus of the ankle and 1 unit lateral to S-38 *(Tiaokou)*. (Dia. 2-45)

Anatomy
Between the lateral side of the extensor digitorum longus pedis and the peroneus brevis muscles. Supplied by a branch of the anterior tibial artery. Situated on the superficial peroneal nerve.

Traditional functions
Transforms Phlegm and Dampness, calms the Spirit.

Indications
Coughing, abundant mucous, headache, vertigo, beriberi, swelling of the limbs, amenorrhea, abnormal uterine bleeding.

273

Illustrative combinations
With N-HN-54 *(Anmian)*, H-7 *(Shenmen)* for insomnia and vertigo.

Classical combinations
With B-13 *(Feishu)* for cough with abundant phlegm (Source: SJD); with GB-40 *(Qiuxu)* to treat stabbing pain in the chest. (Source: CNLAM)

Needling method
Straight insertion, pointed slightly toward the tibia, 1.5-3 units. Sensation: distension and soreness extending upward to the thigh and downward to the lateral malleolus.

Remarks
Connecting point of the Stomach channel with the Divergent channel of the Spleen.

N-LE-4 *(Naoqing)*　　脑清　　"Brain's Clearing"

Location
Approximately 2 finger widths above S-41 *(Jiexi)* at the lateral margin of the tibia. (Dia. 2-45)

Anatomy
Between the tibialis anterior and extensor hallucis longus muscles. Supplied by a branch of the superficial peroneal nerve, and in its deep position by the anterior tibial artery and vein and the deep peroneal nerve.

Indications
Lassitude, mental retardation resulting from encephalitis, vertigo, amnesia, drop foot resulting from infantile paralysis.

Illustrative combinations
With GB-20 *(Fengchi)*, Gv-14 *(Dazhui)* for mental retardation resulting from encephalitis.

Needling method
Straight insertion, 0.5-1 unit, causing distension and soreness extending to the top of the foot.

S-41 *(Jiexi)*　　解溪　　"Release Stream"

Location
At the midpoint of the transverse crease on the front of the ankle, between the two tendons and level with the lateral malleolus. (Dia. 2-45)

Anatomy
Between the tendons of the extensor hallucis longus and the extensor digitorum longus pedis muscles. Supplied by the anterior tibial artery and vein. Superficially, situated directly on the superficial peroneal nerve, and in its deep position on the deep peroneal nerve.

Indications
Headache, nephritis, enteritis, seizures, diseases of the ankle and surrounding soft tissues, drop foot.

Traditional indications
Headache, vertigo, eye diseases, pain in the mouth, seizures, distended abdomen, severe palpitations, pain in foot and ankle.

Illustrative combinations

With B-23 *(Shenshu)*, K-7 *(Fuliu)*, Sp-9 *(Yinlingquan)* for nephritis.

Classical combinations

With Co-22 *(Tiantu)* for fainting secondary to abdominal problems. (Source: GCAM)

Needling method

Straight insertion toward the ankle joint, 0.3-0.5 unit, then to either side of the joint, 1-1.5 units. Sensation: local distension and soreness possibly extending throughout the ankle.

Remarks

Traversing point of the Stomach channel.

S-44 *(Neiting)*　　内庭　　"Inner Court"

Location

At the proximal end of the web between the 2nd and 3rd toes. (Dia. 2-45)

Anatomy

In the dorsal venous network of the foot, directly at the point where the second branch of the medial dorsal cutaneous nerve of the foot divides into two digital nerves.

Traditional functions

Cools and drains Heat from the Stomach, regulates the Qi and suppresses pain.

Indications

Toothache, trigeminal neuralgia, tonsillitis, stomach-ache, acute and chronic enteritis, pain of intestinal hernia, beriberi.

Traditional indications

Toothache, nosebleed, eye pain, paralysis of the mouth, lock jaw, throat blockage, ringing in the ears, abdominal distension, diarrhea, red and white dysentery, blood in the urine, Wind rash.

Illustrative combinations

With LI-4 *(Hegu)* for toothache or tonsillitis.

Classical combinations

With GB-41 *(Zulinqi)* for distension of the lower abdomen (Source: SJD); with Gv-23 *(Shangxing)* for eyeball pain. (Source: GCAM)

Needling method

Slanted insertion toward the ankle, 0.3-0.8 unit, causing local distension and soreness.

Remarks

Gushing point of the Stomach channel.

GB-34 *(Yanglingquan)*　　陽陵泉　　"Yang Tomb Spring"

Location

With the leg bent at the knee, this point can be found in the hollow anterior to and slightly below the head of the fibula. (Dia. 2-46)

Anatomy

Anterior to the capitulum of the fibula, between the peroneus longus and extensor digitorum longus pedis muscles. Supplied by the lateral, inferior genicular artery and vein. Situated at the point where the common peroneal nerve divides into the superficial and deep peroneal nerves.

Traditional functions

Benefits the Liver and Gall Bladder, clears and cools Dampness and Heat, strengthens sinews and bones.

Indications

Hepatitis, cholecystitis, round worm in the bile duct, hypertension, intercostal neuralgia, perifocal inflammation of the shoulder, pain in the knee, paralysis of lower limb, numbness of lower limb, habitual constipation.

Traditional indications

Distension of the mouth, tongue, throat, face and head, fullness of the chest and ribs, distension of the Gall Bladder, loss of urine, constipation, leg Qi.

Illustrative combinations

With Sp-9 *(Yinlingquan)* for malaria; with M-LE-23 *(Dannangxue)*, P-6 *(Neiguan)*, and the vertebral points M-BW-35 *(Jiaji)* of the 8th and 9th thoracic vertebrae for cholecystitis.

Classical combinations

With LI-11 *(Quchi)* for hemiplegia (Source: OHS); use moxibustion at GB-34 *(Yanglingquan)* for incontinence of urine (Source: GCAM); with S-36 *(Zusanli)* and LI-9 *(Shanglian)* for fullness in the flanks and abdomen. (Source: GCAM)

Needling method

Straight insertion, pointed slightly downward toward the back of the tibia, 1-3 units. Sensation: distension and soreness extending downward.

Remarks

Uniting point of the Gall Bladder channel; Meeting point of the sinews.

M-LE-23 *(Dannangxue)*　胆囊穴　"Gall Bladder Orifice"

Locations

On the lower leg, 1-2 units below GB-34 *(Yanglingquan)*. (Dia. 2-46)

Anatomy

Between the peroneus longus and the extensor digitorum longus pedis muscles. Supplied by a branch of the lateral cutaneous nerve of the calf. In its deep position situated directly on the peroneal nerve.

Indications

Diseases of the bile duct, paralysis of lower limb.

Illustrative combinations

With P-6 *(Neiguan)*, GB-40 *(Qiuxu)* for cholecystitis.

Needling method

Straight insertion, 1-2 units, causing distension and soreness extending downward.

GB-37 *(Guangming)* 光明 "Bright Light"

Location
Five units above the lateral malleolus of the ankle, at the anterior margin of the fibula. (Dia. 2-46)

Anatomy
Between the extensor digitorum longus pedis and peroneus brevis muscles. Supplied by branches of the anterior tibial artery and vein, and situated directly on the superficial peroneal nerve.

Traditional functions
Regulates the Liver, clears the vision.

Indications
Night blindness, atrophy of optic nerve, cataract, migraine headache, pain along lateral aspect of calf.

Traditional indications
Chills and fever without sweating, soreness of the leg and knee, atrophy, blockage and numbness of the leg, seizures, pain and itching of the eye.

Illustrative combinations
With M-HN-5 *(Touguangming)*, S-1 *(Chengqi)*, GB-20 *(Fengchi)* for early stage of cataracts.

Needling method
Straight insertion, 1-1.5 units. Sensation: soreness extending upward to the knee and downward to the top of the foot.

Remarks
Connecting point of the Gall Bladder channel with a Divergent channel of the Liver.

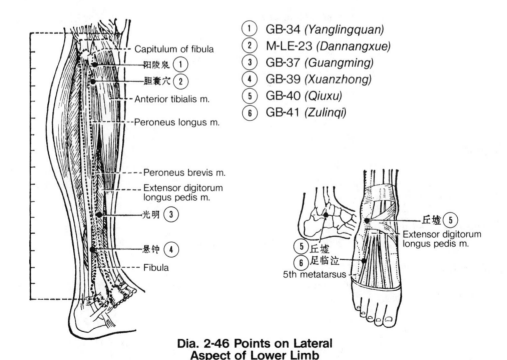

1. GB-34 *(Yanglingquan)*
2. M-LE-23 *(Dannangxue)*
3. GB-37 *(Guangming)*
4. GB-39 *(Xuanzhong)*
5. GB-40 *(Qiuxu)*
6. GB-41 *(Zulinqi)*

Capitulum of fibula
阳陵泉 (1)
胆囊穴 (2)
Anterior tibialis m.
Peroneus longus m.
Peroneus brevis m.
Extensor digitorum longus pedis m.
光明 (3)
悬钟 (4)
Fibula

丘墟 (5)
Extensor digitorum longus pedis m.
(5) 丘墟
(6) 足临泣
5th metatarsus

Dia. 2-46 Points on Lateral Aspect of Lower Limb

277

GB-39 *(Xuanzhong)*　悬钟　"Suspended Time"

Location
Three units directly above the lateral malleolus of the ankle, between the posterior margin of the fibula and the tendon of the peroneus longus muscle. (Dia. 2-46)

Anatomy
Between the posterior margin of the fibula and the tendon of the peroneus longus muscle. Supplied by branches of the peroneal artery and vein, and situated directly on the superficial peroneal nerve.

Indications
Stiff neck, migraine headache, hemiplegia, scrofula, sciatica, diseases of the knee and ankle joints and surrounding soft tissues.

Traditional indications
Nosebleed, throat blockage, coughing, fullness in the chest and abdomen, stiff neck, hemiplegia due to stroke, leg Qi.

Illustrative combinations
With GB-43 *(Xiaxi)*, GB-20 *(Fengchi)* for migraine headache.

Classical combinations
With S-36 *(Zusanli)* and Sp-6 *(Sanyinjiao)* for leg Qi (Source: SJD); with S-44 *(Neiting)* for swollen and distended chest and abdomen. (Source: GCAM)

Needling method
Straight insertion, 1-2 units, may be joined to Sp-6 *(Sanyinjiao)*. Sensation: local distension and soreness possibly extending to the sole of the foot.

Remarks
Meeting point of the marrow; point of intersection of the three Primary Yang channels of the Leg.

GB-40 *(Qiuxu)*　丘墟　"Mound of Ruins"

Location
In the hollow just below and slightly anterior to the lateral malleolus of the ankle. (Dia. 2-46)

Anatomy
At the origin of the extensor digitorum brevis pedis muscle. Supplied by a branch of the lateral anterior malleolar artery, a branch of the lateral dorsal cutaneous nerve of the foot and a branch of the superficial peroneal nerve.

Traditional functions
Spreads the Liver Qi and benefits the Gall Bladder. Clears the channels.

Indications
Pain in the chest and ribs, cholecystitis, axillary lymphadenitis, sciatica, diseases of the ankle and surrounding soft tissues.

Traditional indications
Rib pain, soreness of the leg due to twisted muscles, tidal fevers, distension of the lower abdomen, colic.

Illustrative combinations
  With TB-8 *(Sanyangluo)* for intercostal neuralgia.

Classicl combinations
  With GB-32 *(Zhongdu)* for rib pain. (Source:GCAM)

Needling method
  Straight insertion toward the inferior margin of the medial malleolus, 1-1.5 units. Sensation: local distension and soreness.

Remarks
  Source point of the Gall Bladder channel.

GB-41 *(Zulinqi)* 足临泣 "Near Tears on the Foot"

Location
  In the hollow just in front of the union of the 4th and 5th metatarsal bones. (Dia. 2-46)

Anatomy
  Supplied by the arteriovenous network in the dorsum of the foot, the fourth dorsal metatarsal artery and vein, and by the dorsal digital nerve of the fourth metatarsus.

Traditional functions
  Spreads and drains the Liver and Gall Bladder, clears and regulates of the Girdle channel.

Indications
  Headache, vertigo, conjunctivitis, mastitis, scrofula, rib pain, abscessed breast, irregular menstruation, Dampness and swelling of the foot.

Illustrative combinations
  With GB-20 *(Fengchi)*, S-40 *(Fenglong)* for headache and vertigo.

Classical combinations
  With Sp-6 *(Sanyinjiao)* and Co-3 *(Zhongji)* for difficult menstruation. (Source: GCAM)

Needling method
  Straight insertion, 0.3-0.5 unit, causing local distension and soreness possibly extending to the tip of the 4th toe.

Remarks
  Transporting point of the Gall Bladder; Meeting point with the Girdle channel.

B-53 *(Weiyang)* 委陽 "Commission the Yang"

Location
  With the patient lying prone, this point can be found on the back of the knee, 1 unit lateral to B-54 *(Weizhong)*. (Dia. 2-47)

Anatomy
  At the medial aspect of the biceps femoris tendon. Supplied by the lateral superior genicular artery and vein, by the posterior femoral cutaneous nerve, and situated directly on the common peroneal nerve.

279

Traditional functions
Regulates the water pathways, benefits the Bladder.

Indications
Low back pain, nephritis, cystitis, chyluria, spasm of the gastrocnemius muscle.

Traditional indications
Fullness in the chest or abdomen, low back pain extending to the abdomen, loss or retention of urine, hemorrhoids, constipation.

Illustrative combinations
With B-22 *(Sanjiaoshu)*, B-28 *(Pangguangshu)*, Co-3 *(Zhongji)*, Sp-6 *(Sanyinjiao)* for chyluria.

Classical combinations
With B-47 *(Zhishi)* and B-33 *(Zhongliao)* for incontinence. (Source: CNLAM)

Needling method
Straight insertion, 1-1.5 units, causing distension and soreness extending to the thigh.

Remarks
Lower Uniting point of the Triple Burner.

B-54 *(Weizhong)* 委中 "Commission the Middle"

Location
At the middle of the transverse crease on the back of the knee. (Dia. 2-47)

Anatomy
In the fascia of the popliteal fossa. Supplied by the femoro-popliteal vein; in its deep position, medial to the point, by the popliteal vein, and in its deepest position by the popliteal artery. Supplied by the posterior femoral cutaneous nerve, and situated directly on the tibial nerve.

Traditional functions
Drains Summer Heat, benefits the lower back and knees.

Indications
Heat exhaustion, acute gastroenteritis, low back pain, sciatica, arthritis of the knee, paralysis of lower limb, spasm of the gastrocnemius muscle.

Traditional indications
Coma due to stroke, hemiplegia, stiffness and pain of the lumbar spine, seizures, leprosy, tidal fevers, carbuncles, twisting pain in the chest and abdomen.

Illustrative combinations
With M-UE-1 *(Shixuan)*, Gv-26 *(Renzhong)* for heat exhaustion; with Gv-28 *(Yinjiao)* and point of pain for acute sprain of lower back.

Classical combinations
With K-7 *(Fuliu)* for back pain (Source:GCAM); with B-23 *(Shenshu)* and B-60 *(Kunlun)* for low back pain. (Source: GCAM)

Needling method
(1) Straight insertion, 0.5-1 unit, causing local distension and soreness, or an electric numb

sensation extending to the bottom of the foot. (2) For acute sprain of the lower back, prick the point to draw a few drops of blood.

Remarks
Lower Uniting point of the Bladder.

B-57 *(Chengshan)*   承山   "Support the Mountain"

Location
With the patient lying prone, the point can be found by stretching the foot as if standing on tip-toe. This will reveal a triangular shaped hollow in the middle of the calf, midway between the transverse crease at the back of the knee and the heel. The point is at the top of this triangle. (Dia. 2-47)

Anatomy
At the bottom of the border separating the two bellies of the gastrocnemius muscle. Supplied by the lesser saphenous vein, and in its deep position by the posterior tibial artery and vein; by the medial cutaneous nerve of the calf, and in its deep position by the tibial nerve.

Traditional functions
Relaxes the Muscle channels, regulates the Qi in the Yang Organs, benefits hemorrhoids.

Indications
Pain of lower back and leg, sciatica, hemorrhoids, spasm of the gastrocnemius muscle, paralysis of lower limb, prolapsed anus.

Traditional indications
Sore throat, leg Qi, hemorrhoids, vomiting and diarrhea, twisted muscles of the calf, pain of the lumbar spine.

Illustrative combinations
With M-UE-29 *(Erbai)* for hemorrhoids.

Classicl combinations
With K-7 *(Fuliu)*, Li-3 *(Taichong)* and Sp-3 *(Taibai)* for hemorrhoids (Source: CNLAM); with K-3 *(Taixi)* for difficult defecation. (Source:CNLAM)

Needling method
Straight insertion, 1-2.5 units. Sensation: local distension and soreness, possibly extending to the back of the knee; when inserting the needle deeply for sciatica, there may be an electric, numb sensation extending to the bottom of the foot.

B-58 *(Feiyang)*   飞扬   "Soaring"

Location
At the posterior margin of the fibula, 7 units directly above B-60 *(Kunlun)* and approximately 1 unit below and lateral to B-57 *(Chengshan)*. (Dia. 2-47)

Anatomy
In the gastrocnemius and soleus muscles. Supplied by the lateral cutaneous nerve of the calf.

Indications
Rheumatoid arthritis, nephritis, cystitis, beriberi, hemorrhoids, seizures, pain of the lower back and leg.

Traditional indications

Vertigo, nasal congestion, back and head pain, pain and weakness of the lower back and knee, pain in the calf, insanity, progressive painful joints.

Illustrative combinations

With Co-3 *(Zhongji),* B-28 *(Pangguangshu),* Sp-9 *(Yinlingquan)* for cystitis.

Classical combinations

With SI-5 *(Yanggu)* for dizziness and eye pain. (Source: CNLAM)

Needling method

Straight insertion, 1.5-2.5 units, causing local distension, numbness and soreness, possibly extending downward.

Remarks

Connecting point of the Bladder channel with the Kidney Divergent channel.

B-60 *(Kunlun)*   昆仑   "Kunlun Mountains"

Location

In the depression midway between the lateral malleolus and the Achilles' tendon. (Dia. 2-47)

Anatomy

In the peroneus brevis muscle. Supplied by the lesser saphenous vein and the lateral posterior malleolar artery and vein. Situated directly on the sural nerve.

Traditional functions

Disperses Wind and clears the channels, relaxes the sinews and muscles and benefits the lower back.

Indications

Headache, stiff neck, goiter, low back pain, sciatica, paralysis of lower limb, diseases of the ankle joint and surrounding soft tissues.

Traditional indications

Headache and stiffness along the cervical vertebrae, tidal fevers, pain of the lower back and buttocks, difficult delivery, retained placenta, infantile fright.

Illustrative combinations

With B-61 *(Pushen)* for laryngeal tuberculosis.

Classical combinations

With GB-39 *(Xuanzhong)* and GB-40 *(Qiuxu)* for ankle pain (Source: SGJ); with GB-41 *(Zulinqi),* Sp-9 *(Yinlingquan),* and H-7 *(Shenmen)* for wheezing. (Source: GCAM)

Needling method

(1) Straight insertion, either joined to K-3 *(Taixi)* or inclined slightly toward the lateral malleolus, 0.5-1 unit. Sensation: local distension and soreness extending toward the little toe. (2) Slanted insertion, needle directed upward or joined to B-59 *(Fuyang),* for treating goiter. Sensation: local distension and soreness possibly extending to the heel or toe.

Remarks

Traversing point of the Bladder channel.

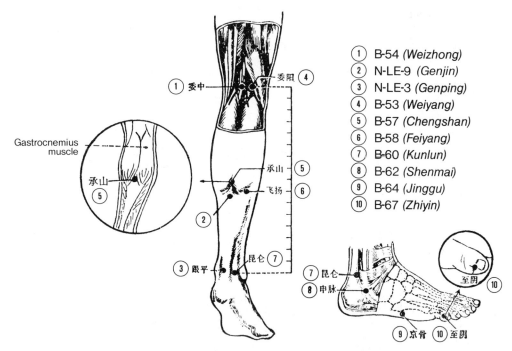

1. B-54 (Weizhong)
2. N-LE-9 (Genjin)
3. N-LE-3 (Genping)
4. B-53 (Weiyang)
5. B-57 (Chengshan)
6. B-58 (Feiyang)
7. B-60 (Kunlun)
8. B-62 (Shenmai)
9. B-64 (Jinggu)
10. B-67 (Zhiyin)

**Dia. 2-47 Points on Posterior Aspect of
Lower Leg, Lateral Aspect of Foot**

B-62 *(Shenmai)*　申脉　"Extending Vessel"

Location

In the depression at the inferior margin of the lateral malleolus of the ankle. (Dia. 2-47)

Anatomy

Supplied by the arterial network of the lateral malleolus, and by a branch of the sural nerve.

Traditional functions

Clears the Spirit, relaxes the Muscle channels, opens the Yang Heel channel.

Indications

Headache, meningitis, Meniere's disease, seizures, psychosis, arthritis of the ankle, pain of the lower back and leg.

Traditional indications

Lateral and midline headache, dizziness, ringing in the ears, palpitations, loss of speech due to stroke, hemiplegia, mouth and eyes awry, insanity.

Illustrative combinations

With TB-17 *(Yifeng)*, N-HN-54 *(Anmian)*, Li-3 *(Taichong)* for Meniere's disease.

Classical combinations

With B-63 *(Jinmen)* for severe headache (Source: OSM); with SI-3 *(Houxi)* and SI-2 *(Qiangu)* for seizures. (Source: CNLAM)

Needling method

Slanted insertion pointed downward, 0.3-0.5 unit, causing local distension and soreness.

Remarks

One of the Meeting points of the eight Miscellaneous channels, joining the Bladder channel with the Yang Heel channel.

B-64 *(Jinggu)*   京骨   "Capital Bone"

Location

In the depression on the lateral side of the tuberosity of the 5th metatarsus. (Dia. 2-47)

Anatomy

At the inferior margin of the lateral abductor digiti minimi pedis. Supplied by the lateral plantar artery and vein, by the lateral dorsal cutaneous nerve of the foot, and in its deep position by the lateral plantar nerve.

Traditional functions

Disperses Wind, calms the Spirit, clears the brain.

Indications

Headache, stiff neck, myocarditis, meningitis, seizures, pain of the lower back and leg.

Traditional indications

Membrane over the eye, heaviness in the head and Cold in the legs, stiff neck, palpitations, seizures, insanity, tidal fevers.

Illustrative combinations

With N-UE-5 *(Xishang)*, P-6 *(Neiguan)*, H-5 *(Tongli)*, H-8 *(Shaofu)* for myocarditis.

Needling method

Slanted insertion pointed downward and medially, 0.5-1 unit. Sensation: local distension and soreness.

Remarks

Source point of the Bladder channel.

B-67 *(Zhiyin)*   至阴   "End of Yin"

Location

On the little toe, 0.1 unit from the lower lateral corner of the cuticle of the toenail. (Dia. 2-47)

Anatomy

Supplied by the arterial network formed by the dorsal digital artery and the dorsal metatarsal and digital arteries, by the dorsal digital and metatarsal nerves and the lateral dorsal cutaneous nerve of the foot.

Traditional functions

Clears the brain (above) and regulates pregnancy and childbirth (below).

Indications
Headache, stroke, malposition of fetus, difficult labor.

Traditional indications
Occipital headache, membrane and pain of the eye, nosebleed, clear nasal discharge, itching over the entire body, infantile convulsions, failure to discharge placenta, difficult labor.

Illustrative combinations
With GB-20 *(Fengchi),* M-HN-9 *(Taiyang)* for occipital headache.

Needling method
Slanted insertion pointed upward, 0.1-0.2 unit, causing local pain; or prick the point to draw a few drops of blood.

Remarks
Well point of the Bladder channel.

Sp-10 *(Xuehai)*   血海   "Sea of Blood"

Location
With knee flexed, this point can be found 2 units above the superior medial border of the kneecap, in the medial margin of the vastus medialis muscle of the thigh. (Dia. 2-48)

Anatomy
At the superior margin of the medial condyle of the femur, in the medial margin of the vastus medialis muscle. Supplied by muscle branches of the femoral artery and vein, by the anterior femoral cutaneous nerve and a muscle branch of the femoral nerve.

Traditional functions
Harmonizes Nourishing Qi and cools Heat.

Indications
Irregular menstruation, abnormal uterine bleeding, urticaria, pruritus, neurodermatitis, anemia.

Traditional indications
Irregular menstruation, lack of menstruation, continuous uterine bleeding, dripping urine, distended abdomen due to rebellious Qi.

Illustrative combinations
With LI-11 *(Quchi),* L-7 *(Lieque),* S-36 *(Zusanli),* Sp-6 *(Sanyinjiao)* for urticaria.

Needling method
Straight insertion, 1-2 units, causing local distension and soreness possibly extending into the knee.

Sp-9 *(Yinlingquan)*   阴陵泉   "Yin Tomb Spring"

Location
With knee flexed, this point can be found at the inferior margin of the medial condyle of the tibia, in the depression between the posterior margin of the tibia and the gastrocnemius muscle. (Dia. 2-48)

285

Anatomy

Between the posterior margin of the tibia and the gastrocnemius muscle, in the upper part at the origin of the soleus muscle. Supplied by the great saphenous vein and the arteria genu suprema, and in its deep position by the posterior tibial artery and vein; by a cutaneous branch of the saphenous nerve, and in its deep position by the tibial nerve.

Traditional functions

Transforms Damp stagnation, benefits the Lower Burner.

Indications

Distension of the abdomen, ascites, retention of urine, incontinence, urinary tract infection, irregular menstruation, nocturnal emissions, impotence, nephritis, beriberi, enteritis, dysentery, knee pain.

Traditional indications

Distension of the abdomen, edema, diarrhea with undigested food, abdominal pain, retention or incontinence of urine, pain of the genitals, nocturnal emissions, pain of the lower back and leg.

Illustrative combinations

With Co-4 *(Guanyuan)*, Co-9 *(Shuifen)*, S-36 *(Zusanli)*, Sp-6 *(Sanyinjiao)* for retention of urine or ascites.

Classical combinations

With GB-34 *(Yanglingquan)* for swollen, painful leg (Source: SJD); with Co-9 *(Shuifen)* for edema (Source: OHS); with Sp-8 *(Diji)* and Co-10 *(Xiawan)* for splinted abdomen. (Source: CNLAM)

Needling method

Straight insertion, along the posterior border of the tibia, 1-3 units. Sensation: local distension and soreness possibly extending downward.

Remarks

Uniting point of the Spleen channel.

Sp-8 *(Diji)*　　地机　　"Earth's Mechanism"

Location

At the posterior margin of the tibia, 3 units below Sp-9 *(Yinlingquan)*. (Dia. 2-48)

Anatomy

Between the posterior margin of the tibia and the soleus muscle. Supplied by the great saphenous vein and a branch of the arteria genu suprema, and in its deep position by the posterior tibial artery and vein. Supplied by a cutaneous branch of the saphenous nerve, and in its deep position, posterior to the point, by the tibial nerve.

Traditional functions

Harmonizes the Blood, regulates the uterus.

Indications

Irregular menstruation, abnormal uterine bleeding, dysmenorrhea, edema, nocturnal emissions.

Traditional indications
Distension of the abdomen and flanks, edema, difficult urination, irregular menstruation, colic, hemorrhoids, nocturnal emissions.

Illustrative combinations
With K-13 *(Qixue)*, Sp-6 *(Sanyinjiao)* for irregular menstruation.

Classical combinations
With Sp-10 *(Xuehai)* for irregular menstruation. (Source: OHS)

Needling method
Straight insertion, 1.5-2.5 units, causing distension and soreness possibly extending throughout the lower leg.

Remarks
Accumulating point of the Spleen channel.

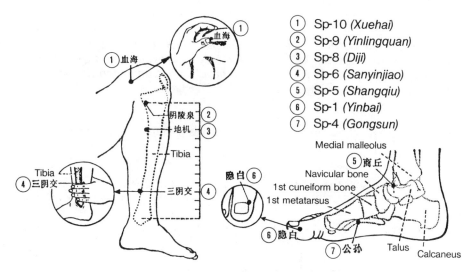

**Dia. 2-48 Points of Spleen Channel
on Lower Limb**

Sp-6 *(Sanyinjiao)* 三阴交 "Three Yin Junction"

Location
At the posterior margin of the tibia, 3 units directly above the medial malleolus of the ankle. (Dia. 2-48)

Anatomy
Between the posterior margin of the tibia and the soleus muscle, and in its deep position in the flexor digitorum longus pedis muscle. Supplied by the greater saphenous vein and the posterior tibial artery and vein, by a cutaneous branch of the saphenous nerve and, in its deep position posterior to the point, by the tibial nerve.

Traditional functions
Strengthens the Spleen and transforms Dampness, spreads the Liver Qi and benefits the Kidneys.

287

Indications
Incontinence, diseases of the reproductive system, distension or pain of the abdomen, diarrhea, hemiplegia, neurasthenia, neurodermatitis, eczema, urticaria.

Traditional indications
Distension and fullness of the upper abdomen, Deficient and weak condition of the Stomach and Spleen, intestinal noises and diarrhea, poor digestion, irregular menstruation, abnormal bleeding, vaginal discharge, lack of menstruation, sterility (of women), difficult labor, fetal death in uterus, failure to discharge placenta, nocturnal emissions, incontinence, difficult urination, cloudy urine, colic, vertigo from Deficient Blood.

Illustrative combinations
With Co-12 *(Zhongwan)*, P-6 *(Neiguan)*, S-36 *(Zusanli)* for Buerger's disease.

Classical combinations
With LI-4 *(Hegu)* and Li-3 *(Taichong)* for difficult labor. (Source: GCAM)

Needling method
(1) Straight insertion toward GB-39 *(Xuanzhong)*, 1.5-2 units, causing local distension and soreness. (2) Straight insertion pointed slightly posterior, 1-1.5 units, for diseases of the leg. Sensation: a numb, electric sensation possibly extending toward the bottom of the foot. (3) Slanted insertion pointed slightly upward, 1.5-2.5 units, for diseases of the trunk. After Qi has been obtained, a strong needling method should be used for a short time. Sensation: distension and soreness possibly extending to the knee or along the medial aspect of the thigh.

Remarks
Point of intersection of the Kidney and Liver channels with the Spleen channel.

Sp-5 *(Shangqiu)* 商丘 "Mound of Commerce"

Location
In the depression anterior to and slightly below the medial malleolus of the ankle. (Dia. 2-48)

Anatomy
Supplied by the medial dorsal artery and the greater saphenous vein, by the nerve branch plexus of the saphenous and superficial peroneal nerves.

Traditional functions
Strengthens the Spleen and Stomach, transforms Damp stagnation.

Indications
Gastritis, enteritis, indigestion, beriberi, edema, diseases of the ankle and surrounding soft tissues.

Traditional indications
Abdominal distension associated with Deficient Spleen, intestinal noises, diarrhea, constipation, stomach-ache, jaundice, breast pain, hemorrhoids, colic.

Illustrative combinations
With S-25 *(Tianshu)*, Sp-9 *(Yinlingquan)* for chronic enteritis.

Classical combinations
With K-21 *(Youmen)* and B-66 *(Tonggu)* for a predeliction towards vomiting (Source: CNLAM); with S-41 *(Jiexi)* and GB-40 *(Qiuxu)* for foot pain. (Source: SJD)

Needing method
Straight insertion, 0.3-0.5 unit, or transverse insertion joined to S-41 *(Jiexi)*, 1-1.5 units, causing distension and soreness in the ankle.

Remarks
Traversing point of the Spleen channel.

Sp-4 *(Gongsun)*   公孙   "Grandfather's Grandson"

Location
On the medial aspect of the foot at the anterior, inferior margin of the 1st metatarsus, one unit behind the joint of the big toe. (Dia. 2-48)

Anatomy
At the anterior, inferior margin of the base of the first metatarsus, in the abductor hallucis muscle. Supplied by the medial dorsal artery and the dorsal venous network of the foot, at the anastomosis of the saphenous nerve and a branch of the superficial peroneal nerve.

Traditional functions
Regulates the Spleen and Stomach, and regulates the Penetrating channel.

Indications
Stomach-ache, acute and chronic enteritis, vomiting, endometritis, irregular menstruation, foot and ankle pain.

Traditional indications
Stomach-ache, intestines (hard) 'like a drum' and abdominal pain, vomiting and diarrhea, tidal fevers, seizures.

Illustrative combinations
With S-36 *(Zusanli)*, P-6 *(Neiguan)*, S-44 *(Neiting)* for bleeding of the upper digestive tract; with P-6 *(Neiguan)*, M-CA-8 *(Jibiansixue)* for acute or chronic gastroenteritis; with K-1 *(Yongquan)*, K-2 *(Rangu)*, S-36 *(Zusanli)*, S-34 *(Liangqiu)* for leprosy.

Classical combinations
With S-42 *(Chongyang)* and use moxibustion at S-36 *(Zusanli)* for leg Qi. (Source: GCAM)

Needling method
Straight insertion toward K-1 *(Yongquan)*, 1.5-2 units, causing local distension and soreness possibly extending to the bottom of the foot.

Remarks
Connecting point of the Spleen channel with the Divergent channel of the Stomach; one of the Meeting points of the eight Miscellaneous channels, joining the Spleen channel with the Penetrating channel.

Sp-1 *(Yinbai)*   隐白   "Hidden White"

Location
At the medial aspect of the big toe, approximately 0.1 unit lateral to the lower corner of the cuticle. (Dia. 2-48)

289

Anatomy
Supplied by a dorsal digital artery. At the anastomosis of the dorsal digital branch of the superficial peroneal nerve and the plantar proper digital nerve.

Traditional functions
Benefits the Spleen, regulates the Blood.

Indications
Abnormal uterine bleeding, bleeding of the digestive tract, abdominal pain or distension, mental diseases.

Traditional indications
Continuous nosebleed, spitting blood, abnormal uterine bleeding, blood in urine or stool, chronic infantile convulsions.

Illustrative combinations
With Co-6 *(Qihai),* Sp-10 *(Xuehai),* Sp-6 *(Sanyinjiao)* for abnormal uterine bleeding.

Classical combinations
With S-36 *(Zusanli)* for uterine or rectal bleeding (Source: GCAM); with B-54 *(Weizhong)* for severe nosebleeds that will not stop. (Source: CNLAM)

Needling method
Slanted insertion in a proximal direction, 0.1-0.2 unit, causing local pain. Alternatively, prick the point to draw a few drops of blood.

Remarks
Well point of the Spleen channel.

Li-8 *(Ququan)*　曲泉　"Crooked Spring"

Location
With knee flexed, this point can be found in the depression at the medial end of the transverse crease on the posterior aspect of the knee. (Dia. 2-49)

Anatomy
At the posterior margin of the medial condyle of the femur, in the anterior part of the insertion of the semimembranosus and semitendinosus muscles, and at the posterior margin of the sartorius muscle. Anterior to the point is the great saphenous vein; also supplied by the arteria genu suprema and a branch of the saphenous nerve.

Traditional functions
Benefits the Bladder, clears and cools Damp Heat, relaxes the Muscle channels.

Indications
Prolapsed uterus, vaginitis, prostatitis, nephritis, pain of hernia, nocturnal emissions, impotence, diseases of the knee and surrounding soft tissues.

Traditional indications
Prolapsed uterus, itching and distension of the genitals, pain in the penis, painful and rough urination, dysentery, knee pain.

Illustrative combinations
    With Li-12 *(Jimai),* Sp-6 *(Sanyinjiao)* for pain of hernia.

Classical combinations
    With K-6 *(Zhaohai)* and Li-1 *(Dadun)* for severe prolapsed uterus (Source: GCAM); with Li-2 *(Xingjian)* for retained urine and penile pain. (Source: CNLAM)

Needling method
    Straight insertion, 1-1.5 units, causing local distension and soreness.

Remarks
    Uniting point of the Liver channel.

Li-5 *(Ligou)* 蠡沟 "Worm-eater's Groove"

Location
    Five units above the medial malleolus of the ankle in the trough between the posterior margin of the tibia and the gastrocnemius muscle. (Dia. 2-49)

Anatomy
    At the medial margin of the tibia, ⅓ of the bone's length from the ankle to the knee. Anterior to the point is the great saphenous vein; also supplied by an anterior branch of the saphenous nerve.

Traditional functions
    Spreads the Liver Qi, benefits the Qi, clears the channels.

Indications
    Irregular menstruation, endometritis, retention of urine, pain of hernia, orchitis, sexual dysfunction.

Traditional indications
    Irregular menstruation, abnormal uterine bleeding, vaginal discharge, swollen and painful testicles, prolapsed uterus, impotence, difficult urination, low back pain.

Illustrative combinations
    With Li-8 *(Ququan),* Li-3 *(Taichong)* for orchitis.

Needling method
    (1) Straight insertion along the posterior margin of the tibia, 0.5-1 unit, causing local distension and soreness. (2) Slanted insertion pointed upward along the posterior margin of the tibia, 1.5-2 units, for diseases of the trunk. After Qi has been obtained, use strong stimulation for a short time, causing distension and soreness possibly reaching the knee or genitals.

Remarks
    Connecting point of the Liver channel with the Divergent channel of the Gall Bladder.

Li-4 *(Zhongfeng)* 中封 "Middle Seal"

Location
    One unit anterior to the inferior margin of the medial malleolus of the ankle, midway between S-41 *(Jiexi)* and Sp-5 *(Shangqiu).* (Dia. 2-49)

Anatomy

Above the tubercle of the navicular, medial to the anterior tibialis tendon. Supplied by the dorsal venous network of the foot and the anterior malleolar artery, by a branch of the medial dorsal cutaneous nerve of the foot and the medial cutaneous nerve of the calf.

Traditional functions

Spreads the Liver Qi and clears the channels.

Indications

Hepatitis, retention of urine, nocturnal emissions, genital pain, pain of hernia, lower abdominal pain, diseases of the ankle and surrounding soft tissues.

Traditional indications

Nocturnal emissions, dripping urine, colic, jaundice with slight fever, low back pain, pain of the knee or ankle.

Illustrative combinations

With B-18 *(Ganshu)*, M-HN-13 *(Yiming)* for acute infectious hepatitis.

Classical combinations

With Li-3 *(Taichong)* for difficulty in walking (Source: SGJ); with K-14 *(Siman)* for drumlike abdomen. (Source: CNLAM)

Needling method

Slanted insertion, 0.5-1 unit, causing local distension and soreness.

Remarks

Traversing point of the Liver channel.

Li-3 *(Taichong)*　太冲　"Great Pouring"

Location

On the foot, 1.5-2 units above the web between the first and second toes. (Dia. 2-49)

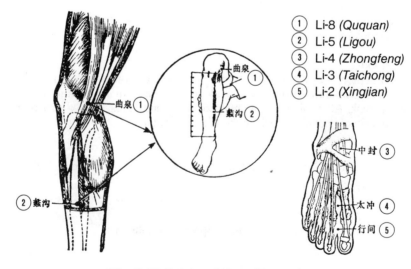

① Li-8 *(Ququan)*
② Li-5 *(Ligou)*
③ Li-4 *(Zhongfeng)*
④ Li-3 *(Taichong)*
⑤ Li-2 *(Xingjian)*

**Dia. 2-49 Points of Liver Channel
on Lower Limb**

Anatomy
Between the first and second metatarsal bones, at the lateral margin of the extensor hallucis longus tendon. Supplied by the dorsal venous network of the foot and the first dorsal metatarsal artery, and by a branch of the deep peroneal nerve on the dorsum of the metatarsus.

Traditional functions
Pacifies the Liver, regulates the Blood, opens the channels.

Indications
Headache, vertigo, hypertension, insomnia, hepatitis, mastitis, irregular menstruation, thrombocytopenia, soreness of the joints of the extremities.

Traditional indications
Sore throat, pain of the eyes, chest and rib pain, low back pain, abscessed breast, irregular menstruation, continuous sweating after childbirth, retention of urine.

Illustrative combinations
With LI-11 *(Quchi)*, LI-4 *(Hegu)*, S-36 *(Zusanli)* for soreness in the joints of the extemities.

Classical combinations
With Sp-6 *(Sanyinjiao)* for continuous uterine bleeding (Source: GCAM); with Co-8 *(Shenque)* and Sp-6 *(Sanyinjiao)* for watery diarrhea. (Source: GCAM)

Needling method
Slanted insertion toward K-1 *(Yongquan)* at the bottom of the foot, 1-1.5 units. Sensation: local distension and soreness or an electric, numb sensation extending toward the bottom of the foot.

Remarks
Transporting and Source point of the Liver channel.

Li-2 *(Xingjian)*   行间   " Walk Between"

Location
In the web between the 1st and 2nd toes. (Dia. 2-49)

Anatomy
Supplied by the dorsal venous network of the foot and the first dorsal metatarsal artery. Situated at the point where the medial branch of the deep peroneal nerve divides into dorsal digital branches.

Traditional functions
Drains Fire from the Liver, spreads the stagnant Qi.

Indications
Headache, vertigo, glaucoma, intercostal neuralgia, orchitis, pain of hernia, abnormal uterine bleeding, infantile convulsions, night sweats.

Traditional indications
Abnormal uterine bleeding, pain in the penis, cloudy urine or urethral discharge, loss of urine, eyes red and swollen, rib pain, seizures, insomnia, vomiting, distension of lower abdomen, colic.

Illustrative combinations
With GB-20 *(Fengchi)*, LI-4 *(Hegu)* for glaucoma.

293

Classical combinations
With K-1 *(Yongquan)* for thirst and emaciated condition (Source: OHS); with Li-3 *(Taichong)* for parched throat with thirst. (Source: CNLAM)

Needling method
Slanted insertion, 0.5-1 unit, causing distension and soreness extending through the foot.

Remarks
Gushing point of the Liver channel.

K-9 *(Zhubin)* 筑宾 "House Guest"

Location
About 5 units above K-3 *(Taixi)* and 2 units posterior to the medial margin of the tibia. (Dia. 2-50)

Anatomy
Below the medial belly of the gastrocnemius muscle where it forms the calcaneous tendon; underneath is the soleus muscle. Served in its deep position by the posterior tibial artery and vein. Supplied by the medial cutaneous nerve of the calf and a medial branch of the saphenous nerve of the calf, and in its deep position by the tibial nerve.

Indications
Nephritis, cystitis, orchitis, pelvic inflammatory disease, seizures, psychosis, spasm of the gastrocnemius muscle.

Traditional indications
Insanity, colic, pain along medial aspect of lower leg.

Illustrative combinations
With B-23 *(Shenshu),* K-7 *(Fuliu),* Sp-6 *(Sanyinjiao)* for nephritis; with Co-3 *(Zhongji),* S-29 *(Guilai),* B-58 *(Feiyang),* K-7 *(Fuliu)* for urinary tract infection.

Classical combinations
With H-3 *(Shaohai)* for foamy vomiting. (Source: CNLAM)

Needling method
Straight insertion, 1-2 units, causing soreness and numbness extending upward to the thigh and downward to the bottom of the foot.

Remarks
Accumulating point of the Yin Linking channel.

K-7 *(Fuliu)* 复溜 "Returning Column"

Location
On the medial aspect of the lower leg, 2 units above K-3 *(Taixi).* (Dia. 2-50)

Anatomy
Posterior to the tibia, at the inferior part of the soleus muscle and in the medial part of the calcaneous tendon. In its deep position supplied by the posterior tibial artery and vein. Supplied by a branch of the sural nerve and a medial cutaneous branch of the saphenous nerve; in its deep position, anterior to the point, is the tibial nerve.

Traditional functions
Regulates the Kidney Qi, clears and cools Damp Heat.

Indications
Nephritis, orchitis, functional uterine bleeding, urinary tract infection, leukorrhea, night sweats, low back pain.

Traditional indications
Edema, abdominal distension, pus and blood in the stool, urinary dysfunction, night sweats, absence of sweating, tidal fevers, insanity, pain of the lumbar vertebrae.

Illustrative combinations
With Co-9 *(Shuifen)*, K-9 *(Zhubin)*, S-36 *(Zusanli)*, M-HN-13 *(Yiming)* for cirrhosis of the liver.

Classical combinations
With Li-3 *(Taichong)* and B-35 *(Huiyang)* for blood in the stool (Source: CNLAM); with Co-8 *(Shenque)* for edema and Qi distension. (Source:GCAM)

Needling method
Straight insertion, 1-1.5 units. Sensation: local distension and soreness, possibly a numb sensation extending to the bottom of the foot.

Remarks
Traversing point of the Kidney channel.

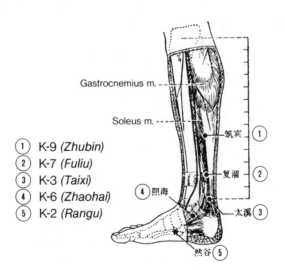

1. K-9 *(Zhubin)*
2. K-7 *(Fuliu)*
3. K-3 *(Taixi)*
4. K-6 *(Zhaohai)*
5. K-2 *(Rangu)*

Dia. 2-50 Points of Kidney Channel on Lower Limb

K-3 *(Taixi)*　太溪　"Great Creek"

Location
At the midpoint between the medial malleolus of the ankle and the Achilles' tendon. (Dia. 2-50)

295

Anatomy

Between the medial malleolus and the calcaneous tendon. Supplied anteriorly by the posterior tibial artery and vein. Supplied by a medial cutaneous branch of the saphenous nerve, and situated directly on the tibial nerve.

Traditional functions

Benefits the Kidneys, cools Heat, strengthens the lower back and knee.

Indications

Nephritis, cystitis, irregular menstruation, spermatorrhea, enuresis, toothache, chronic laryngitis, tinnitus, alopecia, emphysema, neurasthenia, low back pain, paralysis of lower limb (up-turned foot), pain in the sole of foot.

Traditional indications

Throat blockage, toothache, asthmatic wheezing, abcessed breast, thirst and emaciation, dark urine, irregular menstruation, impotence, nocturnal emissions, lumbar vertebrae pain, constipation.

Illustrative combinations

With N-HN-54 *(Anmian)*, Li-3 *(Taichong)* for aural vertigo.

Classical combinations

With B-60 *(Kunlun)* and B-62 *(Shenmai)* for swollen foot with difficulty walking (Source: SJD); with SI-1 *(Shaoze)* for parched throat. (Source: CNLAM)

Needling method

(1) Straight insertion, toward B-60 *(Kunlun)* 0.5-1 unit. Sensation: distension and soreness, possibly a numb sensation extending to the sole of the foot. (2) For pain in the sole of foot, point needle slightly toward the medial malleolus, 0.5-1 unit. Sensation: an electric, numb sensation extending to the sole of the foot.

Remarks

Transporting and Source point of the Kidney channel.

K-6 *(Zhaohai)*　照海　"Shining Sea"

Location

One unit directly below the medial malleolus of the ankle. (Dia. 2-50)

Anatomy

At the insertion of the abductor hallucis muscle below the medial malleolus. Posterior and inferior to the point are the posterior tibial artery and vein. Supplied by the medial, cutaneous branch of the saphenous nerve, and in its deep position by the main trunk of the tibial nerve.

Traditional functions

Cools Heat, calms the Spirit, benefits the throat.

Indication

Pharyngitis, tonsillitis, neurasthenia, seizures, psychosis, irregular menstruation, prolapsed uterus.

Traditional indications

Throat blockage, dry throat, eye pain, edema, irregular menstruation, vaginal discharge, prolapsed uterus, itching in the genital region, difficult labor, hemiplegia, seizures, insomnia.

Illustrative combinations
With Co-14 *(Juque)*, P-6 *(Neiguan)*, S-40 *(Fenglong)* for seizures.

Classical combinations
With TB-5 *(Waiguan)* for retained placenta. (Source: OSM)

Needling method
Straight insertion, 0.5-1 unit, causing soreness and numbness extending toward the calf and ankle.

Remarks
Meeting point of the Yin Heel channel at the Kidney channel.

K-2 *(Rangu)*　然谷　"Burning Valley"

Location
Below and anterior to the medial malleolus of the ankle in the depression below the tubercle of the navicular bone. (Dia. 2-50)

Anatomy
Anterior and inferior to the joint of the navicular, in the abductor hallucis muscle. Supplied by branches of the medial plantar and medial tarsal arteries and veins, by a medial cutaneous branch of the saphenous nerve of the calf and the medial plantar nerve.

Indications
Pharyngitis, cystitis, irregular menstruation, diabetes, tetanus.

Traditional indications
Congested throat, thirst and emaciation, jaundice, diarrhea with intestinal pain and noises, tidal fevers, sterility (of women), itching in the genital region, prolapsed uterus, irregular menstruation.

Illustrative combinations
With Li-3 *(Taichong)* joined to K-1 *(Yongquan)* for pain of the toes.

Classical combinations
With K-7 *(Fuliu)* for drooling (Source: CNLAM); with K-3 *(Taixi)* for swelling in the throat. (Source: CNLAM)

Needling method
Straight insertion, 0.5-1.5 units. Sensation: distension and soreness possibly extending to the sole of the foot.

Remarks
Gushing point of the Kidney channel.

K-1 *(Yongquan)*　涌泉　"Gushing Spring"

Location
On the sole of the foot, at a point ⅓ the distance from the base of the 2nd toe to the back of the heel. (Dia. 2-51)

Anatomy
Between the second and third metatarsal bones in the aponeurosis of the sole of the foot. Medial to

the point are the tendons of the flexor digitorum pedis, longus and brevis, and the second lubricalis pedis muscle; in its deep position in the interossei plantares muscle. Supplied by the anastomosis of the lateral plantar and anterior tibial arteries in the plantar arch. Supplied by a common digital plantar nerve.

Traditional functions
Opens the sensory orifices, calms the Spirit.

Indications
Shock, heat exhaustion, insomnia, stroke, hypertension, seizures, psychosis, mental illness, infantile convulsions, headache at the vertex, paralysis of the lower limbs.

Traditional indications
Vertigo, headache at the vertex, blurred vision, swollen throat, dry tongue, nosebleed, difficult urination and defecation, diarrhea, colic, edema, infantile convulsions, insanity, soles of feet hot, pain in the tips of toes.

Illustrative combinations
With S-36 *(Zusanli)* for septic shock.

Classical combinations
With Co-4 *(Guanyuan)*, S-40 *(Fenglong)* for consumptive coughing (Source: SJD); with K-4 *(Dazhong)* for swollen, painful throat with difficulty swallowing. (Source: CNLAM)

Needling method
Straight insertion, 0.5-1 unit, causing local pain and distension, possibly extending throughout the ankle.

Remarks
Well point of the Kidney channel.

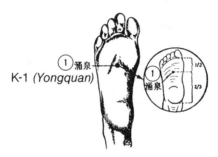

Dia. 2-51   K-1 *(Yongquan)*

M-LE-24 *(Linghou)*   陵后   "Behind the Tomb"

Location
Posterior to the head of the fibula below the knee, in a slight depression that feels sore and numb when pressed. (Dia. 2-52)

Anatomy
At the posterior, inferior margin of the capitulum of the fibula, between the peroneus longus muscle

and the lateral head of the gastrocnemius muscle. Situated directly on the common peroneal nerve. In its deep position supplied by a gastrocnemius muscle branch of the tibial nerve, and branches of the popliteal vein and artery.

Indications
Sciatica, arthritis of the knee, paralysis of the lower limb.

Illustrative combinations
With GB-30 *(Huantiao),* N-LE-18 *(Jianxi)* for sciatica or paralysis of the lower limb.

Needling method
Straight insertion, 0.5-1 unit. Sensation: an electric, numb sensation extending in the direction of the foot.

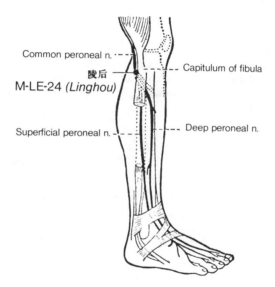

Dia. 2-52   M-LE-24 *(Linghou)*

M-LE-8 *(Bafeng)*   八风   "Eight Winds"

Location
In the web between each of the toes, four on each foot. (Dia. 2-53)

Anatomy
Anterior to and between the heads of each of the metatarsal bones. Supplied by the deep peroneal nerve (between the first and second metatarsals) and the superficial peroneal nerve (between the second to fifth metatarsals), by branches of the dorsal metatarsal artery and vein, and in its deep position by metatarsophalangeal common nerves, and branches of the metatarsal plantar artery and vein.

Indications
Headache, toothache, stomach-ache, irregular menstruation, malaria, snake bite, inflammation of the dorsum of the foot and toes, peripheral neuritis.

Illustrative combinations

With M-LE-24 *(Linghou)*, S-36 *(Zusanli)* for numbness of the lower limb or toes.

Needling method

Slanted insertion, 0.5-1.5 units. Sensation: local distension, soreness and a numb sensation, possibly extending to the tips of the toes.

Remarks

Three of these points are listed separately under the names Li-2 *(Xingjian)*, S-44 *(Neiting)* and GB-43 *(Xiaxi)*.

M-LE-41 *(Shangbafeng)* 上八风 "Upper Eight Winds"

Location

Posterior to the metatarsophalangeal joints of the foot, between all of the metatarsal bones. (Dia. 2-53)

Anatomy

Situated directly on terminal branches of the deep peroneal nerve (between the first and second metatarsals) and branches of the superficial peroneal nerve (between each of the second through fifth metatarsals). Supplied by the dorsal metatarsal arteries and veins. In their deep positions, in the interossei plantares muscles. Supplied by metatarsophalangeal common nerves, and branches of the metatarsal plantar artery and vein.

Indications

Same as M-LE-8 *(Bafeng)* above.

Illustrative combinations

With S-36 *(Zusanli)*, GB-34 *(Yanglingquan)* for inflammation of the dorsum of the foot.

Needling method

Straight insertion, 0.5-1 unit. Sensation: local distension and soreness, possibly extending to the tips of the toes.

Remarks

Three of these points are listed separately as Li-3 *(Taichong)*, S-43 *(Xiangu)* and GB-42 *(Diwuhui)*.

① M-LE-41 *(Shangbafeng)*
② M-LE-8 *(Bafeng)*

上八风①

②八风

**Dia. 2-53   M-LE-41 *(Shangbafeng)*
and M-LE-8 *(Bafeng)***

N-LE-9 *(Genjin)* 跟紧 "Rigid Heel"

Location

9.5 units directly below the middle of the transverse crease at the back of the knee. (Dia. 2-47)

Anatomy

In the gastrocnemius and soleus muscles. Situated directly on the sural nerve. Supplied by the lesser saphenous vein, and in its deep position by the tibial nerve and posterior tibial artery and vein.

Indications

'Hoof foot' due to infantile paralysis.

Illustrative combinations

With B-53 *(Weiyang)*, M-LE-24 *(Linghou)*, N-LE-3 *(Genping)* for 'hoof foot.'

Needling method

Straight insertion, 1-2 units. Sensation: local distension and soreness, possibly extending to the ankle.

N-LE-3 *(Genping)* 跟平 "Level with the Heel"

Location

At the Achilles' tendon, on a line connecting the medial and lateral malleoli of the ankle. (Dia. 2-47)

Anatomy

In the calcaneous tendon, supplied by a branch of the sural nerve. In its deep position, in the flexor pollicis longus tendon, supplied by a branch of the tibial nerve and communicating branches of the posterior tibial and peroneal arteries and veins.

Indications

'Hoof foot' due to infantile paralysis.

Illustrative combinations

With GB-30 *(Huantiao)*, N-LE-18 *(Jianxi)*, M-LE-24 *(Linghou)*, N-LE-9 *(Genjin)* for 'hoof foot.'

Needling method

Straight insertion, 0.5-0.8 unit, causing local distension and soreness.

① N-LE-58 (Waiyinlian)
② S-31 (Biguan)
③ N-LE-23 (Maibu)
④ S-32 (Futu)
⑤ S-34 (Liangqiu)
⑥ S-35 (Xiyan)
⑦ S-36 (Zusanli)
⑧ M-LE-13 (Lanweixue)
⑨ S-37 (Shangjuxu)
⑩ S-40 (Fenglong)
⑪ N-LE-4 (Naoqing)
⑫ Li-4 (Zhongfeng)
⑬ S-41 (Jiexi)
⑭ Li-2 (Xingjian)
⑮ Li-3 (Taichong)
⑯ S-44 (Neiting)

① GB-29 (Juliao)
② GB-30 (Huantiao)
③ GB-31 (Fengshi)
④ GB-33 (Xiyangguan)
⑤ M-LE-24 (Linghou)
⑥ GB-34 (Yanglingquan)
⑦ M-LE-23 (Dannangxue)
⑧ B-58 (Feiyang)
⑨ GB-37 (Guangming)
⑩ GB-39 (Xuanzhong)
⑪ GB-40 (Qiuxu)
⑫ GB-41 (Zulinqi)
⑬ B-67 (Zhiyin)
⑭ B-64 (Jinggu)
⑮ B-62 (Shenmai)
⑯ B-60 (Kunlun)

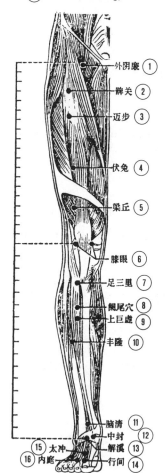

Dia. 2-54 Relation of Points on Anterior Aspect of Lower Limb with Musculature

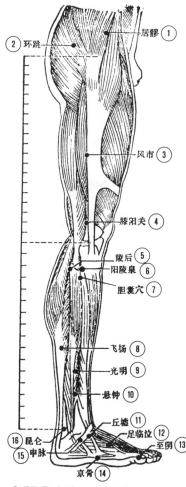

Dia. 2-55 Relation of Points on Lateral Aspect of Lower Limb with Musculature

302

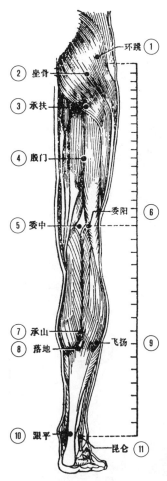

① 环跳 ① GB-30 (Huantiao)
② 坐骨 ② N-BW-17 (Zuogu)
③ 承扶 ③ B-50 (Chengfu)
④ 殷门 ④ B-51 (Yinmen)
⑤ 委中 ⑤ B-54 (Weizhong)
   委阳 ⑥ B-53 (Weiyang)
⑦ 承山 ⑦ B-57 (Chengshan)
⑧ 落地 ⑧ N-LE-9 (Luodi)
   飞扬 ⑨ B-58 (Feiyang)
⑩ 跟平 ⑩ N-LE-3 (Genping)
   昆仑 ⑪ B-60 (Kunlun)

**Dia. 2-56 Relation of Points on Posterior
Aspect of Lower Limb with Musculature**

① Sp-10 (Xuehai)
② Li-8 (Ququan)
③ Sp-9 (Yinlingquan)
④ Sp-8 (Diji)
⑤ Li-5 (Ligou)
⑥ Sp-6 (Sanyinjiao)
⑦ K-9 (Zhubin)
⑧ K-7 (Fuliu)
⑨ Sp-5 (Shangqiu)
⑩ Sp-1 (Yinbai)
⑪ Sp-4 (Gongsun)
⑫ K-2 (Rangu)
⑬ K-6 (Zhaohai)
⑭ K-3 (Taixi)

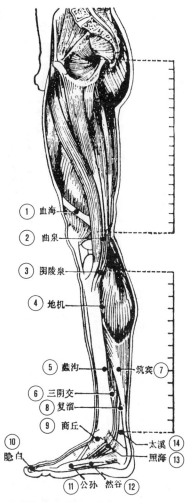

① 血海
② 曲泉
③ 阴陵泉
④ 地机
⑤ 蠡沟   筑宾 ⑦
⑥ 三阴交
⑧ 复溜
⑨ 商丘
⑩   太溪 ⑭
   隐白   照海 ⑬
⑪ 公孙 然谷 ⑫

**Dia. 2-57 Relation of Points on Medial
Aspect of Lower Limb with Musculature**

303

SUMMARY OF COMMON POINTS OF LOWER LIMB

Region	Points	Common Characteristics	Particular Characteristics
Buttock	GB-29 (*Juliao*), GB-30 (*Huantiao*), N-BW-17 (*Zuogu*)	Diseases of hip joint	GB-30 (*Huantiao*) and N-BW-17 (*Zuogu*): sciatica, paralysis of lower limb
	B-50 (*Chengfu*), B-51 (*Yinmen*)	Diseases of abdomen, paralysis of lower limb; sciatica, diseases of soft tissues on posterior aspect of thigh	B-50 (*Chengfu*): anal diseases, ischuria; B-51 (*Yinmen*): low back pain
	GB-31 (*Fengshi*), GB-33 (*Xiyangguan*)	Diseases of abdomen, paralysis of lower limb; diseases of soft tissues on lateral aspect of thigh	GB-31 (*Fengshi*): neuritis of lateral cutaneous nerve of thigh
	N-LE-58 (*Waiyinlian*), S-31 (*Biguan*), N-LE-23 (*Maibu*), S-32 (*Futu*), S-34 (*Liangqiu*)	Diseases of abdomen, paralysis of lower limb; diseases of soft tissues on anterior aspect of thigh	N-LE-58 (*Waiyinlian*): paralysis of quadriceps femoris muscle; S-34 (*Liangqiu*): stomach-ache
Knee	S-35 (*Xiyan*)		Diseases of the soft tissues of the knee
Lower Leg	Stomach channel: S-36 (*Zusanli*), S-37 (*Shangjuxu*), M-LE-13 (*Lanweixue*), S-40 (*Fenglong*), N-LE-4 (*Naoqing*), S-41 (*Jiexi*), S-44 (*Neiting*)	Diseases of head, febrile diseases, paralysis of lower limb and local diseases; diseases of face, mouth, eyes, nose, teeth and gastro-intestinal tract	S-36 (*Zusanli*): hypertension, anemia, Deficient conditions; M-LE-13 (*Lanweixue*): acute, chronic appendicitis; S-37 (*Shangjuxu*): enteritis, dysentery; N-LE-4 (*Naoqing*): sequela of encephalitis, drop foot; S-44 (*Neiting*): toothache, tonsillitis
	Gall Bladder channel: GB-34 (*Yanglingquan*), M-LE-23 (*Dannangxue*), GB-37 (*Guangming*), GB-39 (*Xuanzhong*), GB-40 (*Qiuxu*), GB-41 (*Zulinqi*)	Diseases of head, Febrile diseases, paralysis of lower limb and local diseases; diseases of eyes, ears, chest and ribs, bile duct	GB-34 (*Yanglingquan*) and M-LE-23 (*Dannangxue*): diseases of Liver and Gall Bladder; GB-37 (*Guangming*): eye diseases; GB-39 (*Xuanzhong*): stiff neck, scrofula; GB40 GB-40 (*Qiuxu*): costalgia, diseases of ankle; GB-41 (*Zulinqi*): insufficient lactation, foot pain

Region	Points	Common Characteristics	Particular Characteristics
Lower Leg (cont.)	Bladder channel: B-54 (*Weizhong*), B-53 (*Weiyang*), B-57 (*Chengshan*), B-58 (*Feiyang*), B-60 (*Kunlun*), B-62 (*Shenmai*), B-64 (*Jinggu*), B-67 (*Zhiyin*)	Diseases of head, febrile diseases, paralysis of lower limb and local diseases; diseases of nape of neck, eyes, nose; low back pain, sciatica	B-54 (*Weizhong*): pain or sprain of lower back, acute gastro-intestinal inflammation; B-53 (*Weiyang*): paralysis of lower limb, ischuria, edema; B-57 (*Chengshan*): spasm of calf muscles, diseases of anus; B-60 (*Kunlun*): pain along channel in head, neck, back, thigh; B-62 (*Shenmai*): seizures; B-67 (*Zhiyin*): headache, induce labor, correct foetal position
	Spleen channel: Sp-10 (*Xuehai*), Sp-9 (*Yinlingquan*), Sp-8 (*Diji*), Sp-6 (*Sanyinjiao*), Sp-5 (*Shangqiu*), Sp-4 (*Gongsun*), Sp-1 (*Yinbai*)	Diseases of abdomen, urogenital system, paralysis of lower limb and local diseases; gastro-intestinal diseases	Sp-10 (*Xuehai*): skin diseases, allergies, menstrual disorders; Sp-9 (*Yinlingquan*): abdominal distension, edema, ischuria; Sp-6 (*Sanyinjiao*): neurasthenia, diseases of reproductive system; Sp-4 (*Gongsun*): gastro-intestinal diseases; Sp-1 (*Yinbai*): menstrual disorders, chronic hemorrhaging of internal organs
	Liver channel: Li-8 (*Ququan*), Li-5 (*Ligou*), Li-4 (*Zhongfeng*), Li-3 (*Taichong*), Li-2 (*Xingjian*)	Diseases of abdomen, urogenital system, paralysis of lower limb and local diseases; diseases of Liver, genitals	Li-8 (*Ququan*): diseases of knee, hernia, prostatitis; Li-5 (*Ligou*): ischuria, spermatorrhea, impotence; Li-3 (*Taichong*): hypertension, headache, vertigo; Li-2 (*Xingjian*): glaucoma, intercostal neuralgia
	Kidney channel: K-9 (*Zhubin*), K-7 (*Fuliu*), K-3 (*Taixi*), K-6 (*Zhaohai*), K-2 (*Rangu*), K-1 (*Yongquan*)	Diseases of abdomen, urogenital system, paralysis of lower limb and local diseases; Kidney diseases	K-9 (*Zhubin*): nephritis, cystitis; K-7 (*Fuliu*): excessive sweating, edema; K-3 (*Taixi*): low back pain, sole of foot pain; K-6 (*Zhaohai*): seizures, brain diseases; K-1 (*Yongquan*): shock, hypertension, neurasthenia
Other	M-LE-24 (*Linghou*), M-LE-8 (*Bafeng*), M-LE-41 (*Shangbafeng*), N-LE-9 (*Genjin*), N-LE-3 (*Genping*)		M-LE-8 (*Bafeng*), M-LE-41 (*Shangbafeng*): pain in feet, toes; M-LE-24 (*Linghou*): sciatica; N-LE-9 (*Genjin*), N-LE-3 (*Genping*): 'hoof foot' (sequela of infantile paralysis)

Chapter 7

*Other Channel Points**

LUNG CHANNEL (ARM GREATER YIN)

L-2 *(Yunmen)* 云门 "Cloud's Door"

Location: At the inferior margin of the clavicle, between the pectoralis major and deltoid muscles.
Indications: Cough, chest painful or depressed, asthma, perifocal inflammation of the shoulder joint.
Method: Slanted insertion, 0.5-1 unit.

L-3 *(Tianfu)* 天府 "Heaven's Residence"

Location: 3 units below the anterior end of the axillary crease at the lateral margin of the biceps brachii.
Indications: Bronchitis, asthma, nosebleed, pain along medial side of the upper arm.
Method: Straight insertion, 1-1.5 units.

L-4 *(Xiabai)* 侠白 "Gallantry"

Location: At the anterior, lateral aspect of the humerus, 1 unit directly below L-3 *(Tianfu)*.
Indications: Same as L-3 *(Tianfu)* above.
Method: Straight insertion, 1-1.5 units.

L-8 *(Jingqu)* 经渠 "Across the Ditch"

Location: 1 unit directly above the transverse crease of the wrist, at the medial margin of the radius.
Indications: Bronchitis, chest pain, asthma.
Method: Slanted insertion, 0.5-0.7 unit.

---

*Points in this chapter are illustrated on the fold-out chart only.—*Editors*

HEART CHANNEL (ARM LESSER YIN)

H-2 *(Qingling)*　青灵　"Youthful Spirit"

Location: 3 units above H-3 *(Shaohai)*.
Indications: Costalgia, icteric sclera, pain in shoulder and arm.
Method: Straight insertion, 0.5-1 unit.

H-4 *(Lingdao)*　灵道　"Spirit's Path"

Location: On the ulnar side of the wrist, 1.5 units above H-7 *(Shenmen)*.
Indications: Chest pain, psychosis, hysteria, neuralgia of the ulnar nerve.
Method: Straight insertion, 0.5-0.8 unit.
Other: Traversing point of the Heart channel.

H-6 *(Yinxi)*　阴郄　"Yin Xi"

Location: 0.5 unit above H-7 *(Shenmen)*.
Indications: Neurasthenia, night sweats, palpitations, pulmonary tuberculosis.
Method: Straight insertion, 0.5-1 unit.
Other: Accumulating point of the Heart channel.

H-9 *(Shaochong)*　少冲　"Lesser Pouring"

Location: About 0.1 unit from the base of the little fingernail at the radial side.
Indications: High fever, apoplectic coma, palpitations, hysteria, infantile convulsions.
Method: Straight insertion, 0.1-0.2 unit, or prick to let blood.
Other: Well point of the Heart channel.

PERICARDIUM CHANNEL (ARM ABSOLUTE YIN)

P-1 *(Tianchi)*　天池　"Heaven's Pool"

Location: 1 unit lateral to the nipple, in the 4th intercostal space.
Indications: Angina pectoris, intercostal neuralgia, pain and swelling below the axilla.
Method: Slanted insertion, toward outside, 0.3-0.5 unit.

P-2 *(Tianquan)*　天泉　"Heaven's Spring"

Location: 2 units below the level of the axilla, between the two heads of the biceps brachii muscle.
Indications: Cough, angina pectoris, palpitation, pain in the chest and flank, pain along the medial aspect of the upper arm.
Method: Straight insertion, 1-2 units.

P-9 *(Zhongchong)*　中冲　"Middle Pouring"

Location: About 0.1 unit from the base of the middle fingernail at the radial side.
Indications: Shock, apoplectic coma, heat exhaustion, high fever, angina pectoris.
Method: Straight insertion, 0.1 unit, or prick to let blood.
Other: Another source says this point is located at the middle of the fingertip. Well point of the Pericardium channel.

LARGE INTESTINE CHANNEL (ARM YANG BRIGHTNESS)

LI-1 *(Shangyang)*　商陽　"Trade Yang"

Location: About 0.1 unit from the base of the index fingernail at the radial side.
Indications: Apoplectic coma, high fever, toothache, sore throat, deafness, finger numb.
Method: Straight insertion, 0.2-0.3 unit, or prick to let blood.
Other: Well point of the Large Intestine channel.

LI-2 *(Erjian)*　二间　"Between Two"

Location: In the depression anterior to the metacarpophalangeal joint of the index finger at the radial side.
Indications: Toothache, sore throat, nosebleed, facial paralysis, trigeminal neuralgia, fever.
Method: Straight insertion, 0.3 unit.
Other: Gushing point of the Large Intestine channel.

LI-3 *(Sanjian)*　三间　"Between Three"

Location: In the depression behind the capitulum of the 2nd metacarpal bone, at the radial side of the index finger.
Indications: Toothache, sore throat, trigeminal neuralgia, eyes painful, malaria, inflammation of the dorsum of the hand.
Method: Straight insertion, 0.3 unit.
Other: Transporting point of the Large Intestine channel.

LI-6 *(Pianli)*　偏历　"Partial Order"

Location: 3 units above LI-5 *(Yangxi)* on the forearm.
Indications: Nosebleed, facial paralysis, tonsillitis, neuralgia of forearm.
Method: Straight or slanted insertion, 0.5-1 unit.
Other: Connecting point of the Large Intestine channel.

LI-7 *(Wenliu)*　温溜　"Warm Slide"

Location: 5 units above LI-5 *(Yangxi)* on the forearm.
Indications: Stomatitis, parotitis, glossitis, facial paralysis, sore throat.
Method: Straight insertion, 1-1.5 units.
Other: Accumulating point of the Large Intestine channel.

LI-8 *(Xialian)* 下廉 "Lower Integrity"

Location: 4 units below LI-11 *(Quchi)* on the forearm.
Indications: Headache, painful eyes, vertigo, abdominal pain, mastitis, pain of the elbow and arm.
Method: Straight insertion, 1-2 units.

LI-9 *(Shanglian)* 上廉 "Upper Integrity"

Location: 3 units below LI-11 *(Quchi)* on the forearm.
Indications: Hemiplegia, sprain, numbness of the arms and legs, intestinal noises and abdominal pain.
Method: Straight insertion, 1-2 units.

LI-13 *(Shouwuli)* 手五里 "Five Measures on the Arm"

Location: 3 units above LI-11 *(Quchi)* on the upper arm.
Indications: Coughing blood, pneumonia, peritonitis, scrofula, pain of the elbow and arm.
Method: Straight insertion, 1-2 units. CAUTION: Exercise care to avoid the artery.

LI-17 *(Tianding)* 天鼎 "Heaven's Vessel"

Location: Midway between LI-18 *(Futu)* and S-12 *(Quepen),* at the posterior margin of the sternocleidomastoid muscle.
Indications: Tonsillitis, laryngitis, scrofula, paralysis of the hyoglossus muscle.
Method: Straight insertion, 0.5-1 unit.

SMALL INTESTINE CHANNEL (ARM GREATER YANG)

SI-2 *(Qiangu)* 前谷 "Forward Valley"

Location: On the ulnar aspect of the metacarpophalangeal joint of the little finger, at the end of the skin crease.
Indications: Pannus, tinnitus, congested throat, mastitis, numb finger.
Method: Straight insertion, 0.3-0.5 unit.
Other: Gushing point of the Small Intestine channel.

SI-5 *(Yanggu)* 陽谷 "Valley of Yang"

Location: In the depression at the ulnar end of the transverse crease on the dorsum of the wrist, between the styloid process of the ulna and triquetral bone.
Indications: Wrist pain, parotitis, fever, insanity, deafness, tinnitus.
Method: Straight or slanted insertion, 0.3-0.5 unit.
Other: Traversing point of the Small Intestine channel.

SI-7 *(Zhizheng)*　支正　"Branch of Uprightness"

Location: On a line connecting SI-5 *(Yanggu)* and SI-8 *(Xiaohai)*, 5 units above SI-5 *(Yanggu)*, at the posterior margin of the ulna.
Indications: Neurasthenia, insanity, stiff neck, pain of the elbow or arm.
Method: Straight insertion, 0.5-0.8 unit.
Other: Connecting point of the Small Intestine channel.

SI-8 *(Xiaohai)*　小海　"Small Sea"

Location: With the arm bent at the elbow, between the olecranon of the ulna and the medial epicondyle of the humerus.
Indications: Neuralgia or paralysis of the ulnar nerve, seizures, psychosis, chorea (St. Vitus' Dance), pain of the back of the shoulder.
Method: Straight insertion, 0.5-0.8 unit.
Other: Uniting point of the Small Intestine channel.

SI-12 *(Bingfeng)*　秉风　"Holding Wind"

Location: In the middle of the supraspinatus fossa, between SI-13 *(Quyuan)* and LI-16 *(Jugu)*.
Indications: Inflammation of the supraspinatus tendon, soreness and pain of the back of the shoulder.
Method: Straight insertion, 0.5-1 unit.

SI-14 *(Jianwaishu)*　肩外俞　"Shoulder's Outer Hollow"

Location: 3 units lateral to the bottom of the spinous process of the 1st thoracic vertebra.
Indications: Soreness and pain of the back of the shoulder.
Method: Slanted insertion, 0.5-1 unit.

SI-16 *(Tianchuang)*　天窗　"Heaven's Window"

Location: 3.5 units lateral to the laryngeal prominence, at the posterior margin of the sternocleidomastoid muscle, 0.5 unit behind LI-18 *(Futu)*.
Indications: Sore throat, goiter, tinnitus, deafness, stiff neck.
Method: Straight insertion, 0.5-1 unit.

SI-18 *(Quanliao)*　颧髎　"Cheek Seam"

Location: At the middle of the inferior margin of the zygomatic bone, level with LI-20 *(Yingxiang)*, directly below the outer canthus of the eye.
Indications: Trigeminal neuralgia, facial paralysis, spasm of the facial muscles.
Method: Slanted insertion, 1-1.5 units.

TRIPLE BURNER CHANNEL (ARM LESSER YANG)

TB-1 *(Guanchong)*　关冲　"Gate's Pouring"

Location: About 0.1 unit from the base of the 4th fingernail on the ulnar side.
Indications: Fever, laryngitis, conjunctivitis, headache.
Method: Straight insertion, 0.1-0.3 unit, or prick to let blood.
Other: Well point of the Triple Burner channel.

TB-2 *(Yemen)*　液门　"Fluid's Door"

Location: In the web between the 4th and 5th fingers.
Indications: Headache, laryngopharyngitis, deafness, malaria, pain of the hand and arm, pain and swelling of the fingers.
Method: Straight insertion, 0.3-0.5 unit.
Other: Gushing point of the Triple Burner channel.

TB-7 *(Huizong)*　会宗　"Meeting of the Clan"

Location: One finger width to the ulnar side of TB-6 *(Zhigou)* on the forearm.
Indications: Deafness, pain of the arm, seizures.
Method: Straight insertion, 0.3-0.5 unit.
Other: Accumulating point of the Triple Burner channel.

TB-11 *(Qinglengyuan)*　清冷渊　"Cooling Gulf"

Location: With the arm bent at the elbow, 1 unit above TB-10 *(Tianjing)*.
Indications: Headache, pain of the eyes, pain of the shoulder and arm.
Method: Straight insertion, 1-1.5 units.

TB-12 *(Xiaoluo)*　消濼　"Melting Luo River"

Location: Midway between TB-11 *(Qinglengyuan)* and TB-13 *(Naohui)* on the upper arm.
Indications: Headache, stiff neck, toothache, pain of the arm, seizures.
Method: Straight insertion, 1-1.5 units.
Other: Another source locates this point 6 units above the tip of the elbow.

TB-13 *(Naohui)*　臑会　"Shoulder's Meeting"

Location: 3 units directly below TB-14 *(Jianliao)* at the posterior margin of the deltoid muscle.
Indications: Pain of the arm and shoulder, goiter.
Method: Straight insertion, 1-1.5 units.

TB-15 *(Tianliao)*　天髎　"Heaven's Seam"

Location: Midway between GB-21 *(Jianjing)* and SI-13 *(Quyuan)* above the shoulder blade.
Indications: Inflammation of the supraspinatus tendon, pain or soreness in the region of the scapula and back of neck, fever.
Method: Straight insertion toward the spine of the scapula, 0.5-1 unit.

TB-18 *(Qimai)*　瘈脉　　"Feeding the Vessels"

Location: 1/3 of the distance from TB-17 *(Yifeng)* to TB-20 *(Jiaosun)* at the root of the auricle.
Indications: Tinnitus, deafness, headache, infantile convulsions.
Method: Slanted insertion, 0.5-1 unit.

TB-19 *(Luxi)*　颅息　　"Skull's Rest"

Location: 1 unit above TB-18 *(Qimai)* behind the ear.
Indications: Headache, tinnitus, ear ache, otitis media, vomiting.
Method: Slanted insertion, 0.1-0.3 unit.

TB-20 *(Jiaosun)*　角孙　　"Angle of Regeneration"

Location: Above the tip of the ear at the natural hairline.
Indications: Parotitis, toothache, pannus, red and swollen earlobe.
Method: Slanted insertion, 0.3-0.5 unit.

TB-22 *(Heliao)*　和髎　　"Harmony's Seam"

Location: Above and anterior to TB-21 *(Ermen)* at the natural hairline.
Indications: Headache, tinnitus, "lockjaw", facial paralysis.
Method: Slanted insertion, 0.3-0.5 unit.

STOMACH CHANNEL (LEG YANG BRIGHTNESS)

S-3 *(Juliao)*　巨髎　　"Great Seam"

Location: Directly below the pupil of the eye and level with the bottom of the nostrils.
Indications: Rhinitis, trigeminal neuralgia, facial paralysis.
Method: Slanted insertion, 0.3-0.5 unit.

S-5 *(Daying)*　大迎　　"Big Welcome"

Location: 0.5 unit anterior to S-6 *(Jiache)*, in a trough on the border of the mandible formed when the mouth is closed tightly.
Indications: Parotitis, "lockjaw," facial paralysis, toothache.
Method: Slanted insertion, 0.5-0.8 unit.

S-10 *(Shuitu)*　水突　　"Water Prominence"

Location: At the anterior margin of the sternocleidomastoid muscle, midway between S-9 *(Renying)* and S-11 *(Qishe)*.
Indications: Sore throat, diseases of the vocal cords, goiter, asthma.
Method: Straight insertion, pointed in a medial direction, 0.5-1 unit.

S-11 *(Qishe)*　气舍　"Qi's Residence"

Location: In the depression between the two heads of the sternocleidomastoid muscle at the medial end of the clavicle, directly below S-9 *(Renying)*.
Indications: Pharyngitis, asthma, goiter, scrofula.
Method: Straight insertion, 0.3-0.5 unit.

S-12 *(Quepen)*　缺盆　"Empty Basin"

Location: In the depression at the middle of the superior border of the clavicle and directly above the nipple, 4 units from the median line of the chest.
Indications: Asthma, hiccoughs, intercostal neuralgia, scrofula.
Method: Straight insertion, 0.3-0.5 unit. CAUTION: Care must be taken to avoid the blood vessel.

S-13 *(Qihu)*　乞户　"Qi's Household"

Location: At the middle of the inferior border of the clavicle, 4 units lateral to Co-21 *(Xuanji)*.
Indications: Bronchitis, asthma, hiccoughs, intercostal neuralgia.
Method: Slanted insertion, 0.5-0.8 unit. CAUTION: Avoid deep insertion.

S-14 *(Kufang)*　库房　"Storehouse"

Location: On the mammillary line in the 1st intercostal space, 4 units lateral to Co-20 *(Huagai)*.
Indications: Bronchitis, intercostal neuralgia.
Method: Slanted insertion, 0.5-0.8 unit.

S-15 *(Wuyi)*　屋翳　"Room Screen"

Location: On the mammillary line, in the 2nd intercostal space, 4 units lateral to Co-19 *(Zigong)*.
Indications: Bronchitis, mastitis, intercostal neuralgia.
Method: Slanted insertion, 0.5-0.8 unit.

S-16 *(Yingchuang)*　膺窗　"Breast's Window"

Location: In the 3rd intercostal space on the mammillary line, 4 units lateral to Co-18 *(Yutang)*.
Indications: Bronchitis, mastitis, asthma, intercostal neuralgia, intestinal noises and diarrhea.
Method: Slanted insertion, 0.5-0.8 unit.

S-17 *(Ruzhong)*　乳中　"Middle of Breast"

Location: In middle of nipple, on mammillary line in the 4th intercostal space.
Indications: This point is used primarily as a physical mark in finding other points.
Method: *Systematic Classic of Acupuncture and Moxibustion* prohibits acupuncture and moxibustion at this point. *Emergency Prescriptions to Keep Up One's Sleeve, Thousand Ducat Prescriptions,* and *Necessities of a Frontier Official* permit moxibustion alone.

S-18 *(Rugen)* 乳根 "Breast's Root"

Location: Directly below the nipple in the 5th intercostal space.
Indications: Insufficient lactation, mastitis, bronchitis.
Method: Transverse insertion, 0.5-1 unit.

S-19 *(Burong)* 不容 "Uncontainable"

Location: 6 units above navel, 2 units lateral to Co-14 *(Juque)*.
Indications: Stomach-ache, vomiting, gastrectasis, intercostal neuralgia.
Method: Straight insertion, 0.5-0.8 unit.

S-20 *(Chengman)* 承满 "Support Fullness"

Location: 5 units above navel and 2 units lateral to Co-13 *(Shangwan)*.
Indications: Stomach-ache, acute and chronic gastritis, intestinal noises, colic, indigestion.
Method: Straight insertion, 0.5-0.8 unit.

S-22 *(Guanmen)* 关门 "Gate"

Location: 3 units above navel, 2 units lateral to Co-11 *(Jianli)*.
Indications: Abdominal distension, lack of appetite, intestinal noises, diarrhea, edema.
Method: Straight insertion, 1-2 units.

S-23 *(Taiyi)* 太乙 "Great Yi"

Location: 2 units above navel and 2 units lateral to Co-10 *(Xiawan)*.
Indications: Stomach-ache, intestinal pain, hernia, beriberi, enuresis, insanity.
Method: Straight insertion, 1-2 units.

S-24 *(Huaroumen)* 滑肉门 "Door of Slippery Flesh"

Location: 1 unit above navel and 2 units lateral to Co-9 *(Shuifen)*.
Indications: Chronic and acute gastritis, insanity.
Method: Straight insertion, 1-2 units.

S-26 *(Wailing)* 外陵 "Outer Tomb"

Location: 1 unit below navel and 2 units lateral to Co-7 *(Yinjiao)*.
Indications: Abdominal pain, hernia, painful menstruation.
Method: Straight insertion, 1-2 units.

S-27 *(Daju)* 大巨 "The Great"

Location: 2 units below navel and 2 units lateral to Co-5 *(Shimen)*.
Indications: Abdominal pain, intestinal obstruction, retention of urine, cystitis, spermatorrhea.
Method: Straight insertion, 1-2 units.

S-33 *(Yinshi)*　阴市　"Yin's Market"

Location: 3 units above superior, lateral margin of the patella, between the rectus femoris and vastus lateralis muscles.
Indications: Arthritis of knee, paralysis of lower limb.
Method: Straight insertion, 1-3 units.

S-38 *(Tiaokou)*　条口　"Line's Opening"

Location: 2 units below S-37 *(Shangjuxu),* or 8 units below the knee.
Indications: Arthritis of the knee, paralysis of lower limb, stomach-ache, enteritis, perifocal inflammation of shoulder.
Method: Straight insertion, 1.5-2.5 units.

S-39 *(Xiajuxu)*　下巨虚　"Lower Void"

Location: 3 units below S-37 *(Shangjuxu),* or 9 units below the knee.
Indications: Acute or chronic enteritis, hepatitis, paralysis of the lower limb.
Method: Straight insertion, 1-2 units.
Other: Lower Uniting point of Small Intestine channel.

S-42 *(Chongyang)*　冲陽　"Pouring Yang"

Location: 1.5 units below S-41 *(Jiexi)* at the hump on the dorsum of foot and to the side of the dorsalis pedis artery.
Indications: Headache, facial paralysis, toothache, pain on dorsum of foot, malaria, insanity, fever, no strength in arms or legs.
Method: Straight insertion, 0.3-0.5 unit.
Other: Source point of Stomach channel. CAUTION: Avoid blood vessel.

S-43 *(Xiangu)*　陷谷　"Sinking Valley"

Location: Between the 2nd and 3rd metatarsal bones, directly above the lateral side of the 2nd toe.
Indications: Facial edema, conjunctivitis, edema, intestinal noises, abdominal pain, hysteria.
Method: Slanted insertion, 0.5-1 unit.

S-45 *(Lidui)*　历兑　"Strict Exchange"

Location: About 0.1 unit from the lateral corner of the second toenail.
Indications: Ischemia of the brain, neurasthenia, tonsillitis, hepatitis, indigestion, hysteria.
Method: Straight insertion, 0.1-0.3 unit.
Other: Well point of Stomach channel.

BLADDER CHANNEL (LEG GREATER YANG)

B-3 *(Meichong)*　眉冲　"Eyebrow's Pouring"

Location: On natural hairline directly above medial end of eyebrow, between Gv-24 *(Shenting)*

315

and B-4 *(Quchai).*
  Indications: Headache, occluded nose, vertigo, seizures.
  Method: Slanted insertion, 0.3-0.5 unit.

B-4 *(Quchai)* 曲差 "Discrepancy"

  Location: On natural hairline, 1.5 units lateral to Gv-24 *(Shenting).*
  Indications: Headache, occluded nose, nosebleed, eye diseases.
  Method: Slanted insertion, 0.3-0.5 unit.

B-5 *(Wuchu)* 五处 "Five Places"

  Location: 1.5 units lateral to Gv-23 *(Shangxing),* and 1 unit above natural hairline.
  Indications: Headache, vertigo, rhinitis, seizures.
  Method: Slanted insertion, 0.3-0.5 unit.

B-6 *(Chengguang)* 承光 "Support Light"

  Location: 1.5 units behind B-5 *(Wuchu),* and about 2.5 units above natural hairline.
  Indications: Headache, common cold, pannus, rhinitis, vertigo.
  Method: Slanted insertion, 0.3-0.5 unit.

B-8 *(Luoque)* 络却 "Decline"

  Location: 1.5 units behind B-7 *(Tongtian)* on the top of the head.
  Indications: Vertigo, facial paralysis, rhinitis, goiter, vomiting.
  Method: Slanted insertion, 0.3-0.5 unit.

B-9 *(Yuzhen)* 玉枕 "Jade Pillow"

  Location: 1.3 units lateral to Gv-17 *(Naohu),* on the lateral part of upper margin of external occipital protuberance.
  Indications: Headache, vertigo, myopia.
  Method: Slanted insertion, 0.3-0.5 unit.

B-29 *(Zhonglushu)* 中膂俞 "Mid-Spine Hollow"

  Location: 1.5 units from median line of back, level with the 3rd posterior sacral foramen.
  Indications: Enteritis, lumbosacral pain, sciatica.
  Method: Straight insertion, 1-1.5 units.

B-35 *(Huiyang)* 会阳 "Meeting of Yang"

  Location: 0.5 unit from median line of back, level with the tip of coccyx.
  Indications: Pain in lower back during menstruation, leukorrhea, impotence, diarrhea, hemorrhoids.
  Method: Straight insertion, 1-1.5 units.

B-36 *(Fufen)*   附分   "Appended Part"

Location: 3 units lateral to lower end of spinous process of 2nd thoracic vertebra.
Indications: Soreness and pain of the shoulder, neck and back regions, numbness in elbow and arm.
Method: Slanted insertion, 0.5-0.8 unit.

B-37 *(Pohu)*   魄戶   "Soul's Household"

Location: 3 units lateral to lower end of spinous process of 3rd thoracic vertebra.
Indications: Bronchitis, asthma, pleurisy, pulmonary tuberculosis, atelectasis.
Method: Slanted insertion, 0.5-0.8 unit.

B-39 *(Shentang)*   神堂   "Spirit's Hall"

Location: 3 units lateral to lower end of spinous process of 5th thoracic vertebra.
Indications: Bronchitis, asthma, intercostal neuralgia, heart disease.
Method: Slanted insertion, 0.5-0.8 unit.

B-40 *(Yixi)*   噫嘻   "Surprise"

Location: 3 units lateral to lower end of spinous process of 6th thoracic vertebra.
Indications: Pericarditis, asthma, malaria, intercostal neuralgia, hiccoughs.
Method: Slanted insertion, 0.5-0.8 unit.

B-41 *(Geguan)*   膈关   "Diaphragm's Hinge"

Location: 3 units lateral to lower end of spinous process of 7th thoracic vertebra.
Indications: Intercostal neuralgia, spasms of esophagus, gastric hemorrhage.
Method: Slanted insertion, 0.5-0.8 unit.

B-42 *(Hunmen)*   魂门   "Soul's Door"

Location: 3 units lateral to lower end of spinous process of 9th thoracic vertebra.
Indications: Neurasthenia, diseases of liver and gall bladder, pleurisy, stomach-ache.
Method: Slanted insertion, 0.5-0.8 unit.

B-43 *(Yanggang)*   陽纲   "Yang's Parameter"

Location: 3 units lateral to lower end of spinous process of 10th thoracic vertebra.
Indications: Hepatitis, cholecystitis, gastritis.
Method: Slanted insertion, 0.5-0.8 unit.

B-44 *(Yishe)*   意舍   "Will's Residence"

Location: 3 units lateral to lower end of spinous process of 11th thoracic vertebra.
Indications: Hepatitis, cholecystitis, gastritis.
Method: Slanted insertion, 0.5-0.8 unit.

B-45 *(Weicang)*   胃仓   "Stomach's Storehouse"

Location: 3 units lateral to lower end of spinous process of 12th thoracic vertebra.
Indications: Stomach-ache, gastritis, abdominal pain, back pain.
Method: Slanted insertion, 0.5-0.8 unit.

B-46 *(Huangmen)*   肓门   "Vitals' Door"

Location: 3 units lateral to the lower end of spinous process of 1st lumbar vertebra.
Indications: Mastitis, pain in upper abdomen, low back pain, paralysis of lower limb.
Method: Straight insertion, 1-1.5 units. CAUTION: Avoid deep insertion which may penetrate kidney.

B-48 *(Baohuang)*   胞肓   "Placenta and Vitals"

Location: 3 units from median line of back, level with 2nd sacral foramen.
Indications: Low back pain, retention of urine, intestinal noises and abdominal pain, sciatica.
Method: Straight insertion, 1-2 units.

B-52 *(Fuxi)*   浮郄   "Floating Xi"

Location: 1 unit above B-53 *(Weiyang)*.
Indications: Acute gastroenteritis, cystitis, constipation, paralysis along lateral aspect of lower extremities.
Method: Straight insertion, 1-2 units.

B-55 *(Heyang)*   合陽   "Confluence of Yang"

Location: 2 units below B-54 *(Weizhong)*, between the two heads of the gastrocnemius muscle.
Indications: Soreness from lower back to knee, abnormal uterine bleeding.
Method: Straight insertion, 1-2 units.

B-56 *(Chengjin)*   承筋   "Support Sinews"

Location: In the center of the belly of the gastrocnemius muscle, midway between B-55 *(Heyang)* and B-57 *(Chengshan)*.
Indications: Headache, low back pain, pain in calf, paralysis of lower limb, hemorrhoids.
Method: Straight insertion, 1-2 units.

B-59 *(Fuyang)*   跗陽   "Tarsal Yang"

Location: 3 units directly above B-60 *(Kunlun)*, at the lateral aspect of gastrocnemius muscle.
Indications: Headache, low back pain, paralysis of lower limb, inflammation of ankle joint.
Method: Straight insertion, 1-2 units.
Other: Accumulating point of Yang Heel channel.

B-61 *(Pushen)*   仆参   "Serve and Consult"

Location: 1.5 units below B-60 *(Kunlun)*.
Indications: Low back pain, pain in ankle and foot, paralysis of lower limb, beriberi.
Method: Straight insertion, 0.3-0.5 unit.

B-63 *(Jinmen)*   金门   "Golden Door"

Location: Anterior to and below the lateral malleolus, in the depression behind the tuberosity of the 5th metatarsal bone.
Indications: Pain in lower back and legs, pain at bottom of foot, seizures, infantile convulsions.
Method: Straight insertion, 0.3-0.5 unit.

B-65 *(Shugu)*   束骨   "Restraining Bone"

Location: In depression posterior and lateral to the head of the 5th metatarsal bone.
Indications: Headache and stiff neck, malaria, pannus, seizures, mental illness.
Method: Straight insertion, 0.3-0.5 unit.

B-66 *(Zutonggu)*   足通谷   "Connecting Valley of the Foot"

Location: In depression anterior and lateral to the 5th metatarsophalangeal joint.
Indications: Headache, vertigo, asthma, nosebleed, mental illness.
Method: Straight insertion, 0.2-0.3 unit.

GALL BLADDER CHANNEL (LEG LESSER YANG)

GB-3 *(Shangguan)*   上关   "Upper Hinge"

Location: On the superior margin of the zygomatic arch, directly above S-7 *(Xiaguan)*.
Indications: Tinnitus, deafness, otitis media, toothache, "lockjaw", facial paralysis.
Method: Straight insertion, 0.7-1 unit.

GB-4 *(Hanyan)*   颔厌   "Jaw's Dislike"

Location: On the temple, 1/4 the distance from S-8 *(Touwei)* to GB-7 *(Qubin)*.
Indications: Migraine headache, tinnitus, rhinitis, seizures, convulsions.
Method: Slanted insertion, 1-1.5 units.

GB-5 *(Xuanlu)*   悬颅   "Suspended Skull"

Location: On the temple, midway between S-8 *(Touwei)* and GB-7 *(Qubin)*.
Indications: Migraine headache, toothache, facial swelling, neurasthenia.
Method: Slanted insertion, 1-1.5 units.

319

GB-6 *(Xuanli)*　悬厘　"Suspended Millimeter"

Location: Below the temple, 3/4 distance from S-8 *(Touwei)* to GB-7 *(Qubin)*.
Indications: Migraine headache, toothache, facial swelling, neurasthenia.
Method: Slanted insertion, 1-1.5 units.

GB-7 *(Qubin)*　曲鬓　"Crook of the Temple"

Location: On the temple level with the apex of the ear, roughly 1 unit anterior to TB-20 *(Jiaosun)*.
Indications: Migraine headache, trigeminal neuralgia, spasms of temporalis muscle.
Method: Slanted insertion, 1-1.5 units.

GB-8 *(Shuaigu)*　率谷　"Leading to Valley"

Location: Directly above the apex of ear and 1.5 units above natural hairline.
Indications: Migraine headache, vertigo, eye diseases.
Method: Transverse insertion, 1-2 units.

GB-9 *(Tianchong)*　天冲　"Heaven's Pouring"

Location: About 0.5 unit posterior to GB-8 *(Shuaigu)* behind the ear.
Indications: Headache, gingivitis, seizures, goiter.
Method: Slanted insertion, 0.5-1 unit.

GB-10 *(Fubai)*　浮白　"Floating White"

Location: About 1 unit below and posterior to GB-9 *(Tianchong)* on the superior part of the mastoid process.
Indications: Headache, toothache, tinnitus, deafness, bronchitis.
Method: Slanted insertion, 0.5-1 unit.

GB-11 *(Touqiaoyin)*　头窍阴　"Yin Cavity on the Head"

Location: At the base of the mastoid process, 1 unit below GB-10 *(Fubai)*.
Indications: Headache and stiff neck, ear ache, tinnitus, deafness, bronchitis.
Method: Slanted insertion, 0.5-1 unit.

GB-12 *(Wangu)*　完骨　"Finished Bone"

Location: At the posterior border of the mastoid process, 0.7 unit below GB-11 *(Qiaoyin)*, and level with Gv-16 *(Fengfu)*.
Indications: Headache, facial swelling, toothache, seizures, facial paralysis, parotitis.
Method: Slanted insertion, 0.5-1 unit.

GB-13 *(Benshen)*　本神　"Original Spirit"

Location: 3 units lateral to Gv-24 *(Shenting)*, at the side of the forehead.

320

Indications: Headache, vertigo, stiff neck, costalgia, seizures, hemiplegia.
Method: Slanted insertion, 0.5-1 unit.

GB-15 *(Toulinqi)*　头临泣　"Near Tears on the Head"

Location: Directly above GB-14 *(Yangbai)* and midway between Gv-24 *(Shenting)* and S-8 *(Touwei)*, 0.5 unit above natural hairline.
Indications: Vertigo, occluded nose, pannus, apoplectic coma, malaria, seizures, acute and chronic conjunctivitis.
Method: Slanted insertion, 0.5-1 unit.

GB-16 *(Muchuang)*　目窗　"Vision's Window"

Location: 1.5 units above GB-15 *(Toulinqi)*.
Indications: Headache, vertigo, facial edema, conjunctivitis, toothache, apoplectic coma.
Method: Slanted insertion, 0.5-1 unit.

GB-17 *(Zhengying)*　正营　"Upright Encampment"

Location: 1.5 units above GB-16 *(Muchuang)*.
Indications: Headache and stiff neck, vertigo, toothache, vomiting.
Method: Slanted insertion, 0.5-1 unit.

GB-18 *(Chengling)*　承灵　"Support the Spirit"

Location: 1.5 units behind GB-17 *(Zhengying)*.
Indications: Headache, common cold, bronchitis, eye diseases, nosebleed, occluded nose.
Method: Slanted insertion, 0.5-1 unit.

GB-19 *(Naokong)*　脑空　"Brain Cavity"

Location: Directly above GB-20 *(Fengchi)* and level with Gv-17 *(Naohu)* on the back of the head.
Indications: Headache, common cold, asthma, seizures, mental illness, palpitations, tinnitus.
Method: Slanted insertion, 0.5-1 unit.

GB-22 *(Yuanye)*　渊液　"Gulf's Fluids"

Location: On the mid-axillary line 3 units below the middle of axilla and in the 5th intercostal space.
Indications: Pleurisy, intercostal neuralgia, axillary lymphadenitis, pain of shoulders and arm.
Method: Slanted insertion, 0.5-0.8 unit. CAUTION: Avoid deep insertion.

GB-23 *(Zhejin)*　辄筋　"Flank's Sinews"

Location: 1 unit anterior to GB-22 *(Yuanye)* in the 5th intercostal space.
Indications: Pleurisy, asthma, vomiting, acidic belching.
Method: Slanted insertion, 0.5-0.8 unit.

GB-24 *(Riyue)* 日月 "Sun Moon"

Location: One rib below Li-14 *(Qimen)* in the 7th intercostal space.
Indications: Intercostal neuralgia, cholecystitis, acute and chronic hepatitis, peptic ulcer, hiccoughs.
Method: Slanted insertion, 0.5-1 unit.
Other: Alarm point of the Gall Bladder.

GB-25 *(Jingmen)* 京门 "Capitol's Door"

Location: At the side, just below the end of the 12th rib.
Indications: Nephritis, pain of intestinal hernia, intercostal neuralgia, lumbago.
Method: Straight insertion, 0.7-1 unit.
Other: Alarm point of the Kidneys.

GB-28 *(Weidao)* 维道 "Maintain the Way"

Location: 0.5 unit below GB-27 *(Wushu)*, anterior to and slightly below the anterior superior iliac spine.
Indications: Adnexitis, endometritis, prolapsed uterus, pain of intestinal hernia, chronic constipation.
Method: Straight insertion, 1-2 units.

GB-32 *(Zhongdu)* 中渎 "Middle Ditch"

Location: 2 units below GB-31 *(Fengshi)* and 5 units above the knee.
Indications: Beriberi, paralysis of lower limb, sciatica.
Method: Straight insertion, 1.5-3 units.

GB-35 *(Yangjiao)* 陽交 "Yang's Intersection"

Location: 7 units directly above lateral malleolus at the posterior margin of the fibula.
Indications: Pain on lateral aspect of leg, sciatica, asthma.
Method: Straight insertion, 1-2 units.
Other: Accumulating point of Yang Linking channel.

GB-36 *(Waiqiu)* 外丘 "Outer Mound"

Location: Midway between GB-34 *(Yanglingquan)* and the lateral malleolus, in front of GB-35 *(Yangjiao)* at the anterior margin of fibula.
Indications: Headache, hepatitis, paralysis of lower limb.
Method: Straight insertion, 1-1.5 units.
Other: Accumulating point of the Gall Bladder channel.

GB-38 *(Yangfu)* 陽辅 "Yang's Help"

Location: 4 units above the lateral malleolus at the anterior margin of the fibula.
Indications: Migraine headache, scrofula, hemiplegia, paralysis of lower limb, arthritis of knee.
Method: Straight insertion, 1-2 units.
Other: Traversing point of the Gall Bladder channel.

GB-42 *(Diwuhui)*　地五会　"Earth's Fifth Meeting"

Location: Between the 4th and 5th metatarsal bones, 1 unit above GB-43 *(Xiaxi)*.
Indications: Tinnitus, mastitis, low back pain, inflammation of the dorsum of the foot.
Method: Straight insertion, 0.3-0.5 unit.

GB-43 *(Xiaxi)*　侠溪　"Gallantry's Stream"

Location: 0.5 unit posterior to the web between the 4th and 5th toes.
Indications: Migraine headache, hypertension, tinnitus, intercostal neuralgia.
Method: Straight insertion, 0.3-0.5 unit.
Other: Gushing point of the Gall Bladder channel.

GB-44 *(Zuqiaoyin)*　足窍阴　"Yin Cavity on the Foot"

Location: About 0.1 unit from the lateral corner of the 4th toenail.
Indications: Headache, hypertension, conjunctivitis, intercostal neuralgia, asthma, pleurisy.
Method: Straight insertion, 0.1-0.2 unit.
Other: Well point of the Gall Bladder channel.

SPLEEN CHANNEL (LEG GREATER YIN)

Sp-2 *(Dadu)*　大都　"Big Metropolis"

Location: On the medial aspect of the big toe, slightly anterior to the metatarsophalangeal joint, at the border of the light and dark skin.
Indications: Fever, abdominal distension or diarrhea, stomach-ache, edema of the limbs, apoplectic coma.
Method: Straight insertion, 0.5-1 unit.
Other: Gushing point of the Spleen channel.

Sp-3 *(Taibai)*　太白　"Most White"

Location: On the posterior, inferior aspect at the head of the 1st metatarsal bone.
Indications: Headache, stomach-ache, abdominal distension, edema, dysentery, acute gastro-enteritis, constipation.
Method: Straight insertion, 0.5-1 unit.
Other: Transporting and Source point of the Spleen channel.

Sp-7 *(Lougu)*　漏谷　"Seeping Valley"

Location: At the posterior margin of the tibia, 3 units directly above Sp-6 *(Sanyinjiao)*.
Indications: Abdominal distension, intestinal noises, urinary tract infection, paralysis of lower limb.
Method: Straight insertion, 1-1.5 units.

Sp-11 *(Jimen)*　箕门　"Basket's Door"

Location: 6 units above Sp-10 *(Xuehai)* at the medial aspect of the sartorius muscle.
Indications: Urethritis, enuresis, inguinal lymphadenitis.
Method: Straight insertion, 1-2 units.

Sp-12 *(Chongmen)*　冲门　"Pouring Door"

Location: At the superior margin of the pubic symphysis in the groin, 3.5 units lateral to Co-2 *(Qugu)*.
Indications: Pain of hernia, retention of urine, endometritis, orchitis.
Method: Straight insertion, 1-1.5 units. CAUTION: Avoid blood vessel.

Sp-13 *(Fushe)*　府舍　"Dwelling"

Location: 0.7 unit above Sp-12 *(Chongmen)*, 3.5 units lateral to the median line of the abdomen.
Indications: Pain of hernia, inguinal lymphadenitis, adnexitis, pain of lower abdomen, appendicitis.
Method: Straight insertion, 1-1.5 units.

Sp-14 *(Fujie)*　腹结　"Abdomen's Knot"

Location: 3 units above Sp-13 *(Fushe)*, and 3.5 units lateral to the median line of the abdomen.
Indications: Pain in the region of the umbilicus, diarrhea, pain of hernia.
Method: Straight insertion, 1.5 units.

Sp-16 *(Fuai)*　腹哀　"Abdomen's Sorrow"

Location: 3 units above Sp-15 *(Daheng)*, and 3.5 units lateral to the midsternal line.
Indications: Pain in the region of the umbilicus, indigestion, dysentery, constipation.
Method: Straight insertion, 1-1.5 units.

Sp-17 *(Shidou)*　食窦　"Food's Cavity"

Location: In the 5th intercostal space, 6 units lateral to the midsternal line.
Indications: Intercostal neuralgia, ascites, retention of urine, gastritis.
Method: Slanted insertion, 0.5-0.8 unit. CAUTION: Avoid deep insertion.

Sp-18 *(Tianxi)*　天溪　"Heaven's Stream"

Location: In the 4th intercostal space, 6 units lateral to the midsternal line.
Indications: Bronchitis, asthma, hiccough, mastitis.
Method: Slanted insertion, 0.5-0.8 unit. CAUTION: Avoid deep insertion.

Sp-19 *(Xiongxiang)*　胸乡　"Chest Home"

Location: In the 3rd intercostal space, 6 units lateral to the midsternal line.
Indications: Intercostal neuralgia.

Method: Slanted insertion, 0.5-0.8 unit. CAUTION: Avoid deep insertion.

Sp-20 *(Zhourong)*　周荣　"Encircling Glory"

Location: In the 2nd intercostal space, 6 units lateral to the midsternal line.
Indications: Intercostal neuralgia, pleurisy, pulmonary empyema, bronchiectasis.
Method: Slanted insertion, 0.5-0.8 unit. CAUTION: Avoid deep insertion.

Sp-21 *(Dabao)*　大包　"Big Wrapping"

Location: On midaxillary line, 6 units below middle of the axilla in the 7th intercostal space.
Indications: Asthma, intercostal neuralgia, general body soreness.
Method: Slanted insertion, 0.5-0.8 unit.
Other: Connecting point of the Great Connecting channel of the Spleen.

KIDNEY CHANNEL (LEG LESSER YIN)

K-4 *(Dazhong)*　大钟　"Big Goblet"

Location: 0.5 unit below and slightly posterior to K-3 *(Taixi)*, between the medial margin of the calcaneous tendon and the calcaneous bone.
Indications: Asthma, malaria, neurasthenia, hysteria, retention of urine, soreness in pharynx, pain in heel.
Method: Slanted insertion, 0.3-0.5 unit.
Other: Connecting point of the Kidney channel.

K-5 *(Shuiquan)*　水泉　"Spring"

Location: 1 unit directly below K-3 *(Taixi)*, above the calcaneous bone.
Indications: Amenorrhea, prolapsed uterus, myopia.
Method: Slanted insertion, 0.3-0.5 unit.
Other: Accumulating point of the Kidney channel.

K-8 *(Jiaoxin)*　交信　"Communicate Belief"

Location: At the medial margin of the tibia, 2 units above the medial malleolus.
Indications: Irregular menstruation, abnormal uterine bleeding, retention of urine, diarrhea, constipation, pain on medial aspect of lower limb.
Method: Straight insertion, 0.5-1 unit.

K-10 *(Yingu)*　阴谷　"Yin's Valley"

Location: On the medial apsect at the back of the knee, between the semitendinosus muscle and lower end of semimembranosus muscle.
Indications: Diseases of urogenital system, arthritis of knee.
Method: Straight insertion, 1-2 units.
Other: Uniting point of the Kidney channel.

K-11 *(Henggu)*　横骨　"Horizontal Bone"

Location: 0.5 unit lateral to Co-2 *(Qugu)*, on the lower abdomen.
Indications: Hernia, urethritis, incontinence of urine, spermatorrhea, impotence.
Method: Straight insertion, 1-1.5 units.

K-12 *(Dahe)*　大赫　"Great Clarity"

Location: 0.5 unit lateral to Co-3 *(Zhongji)*, on the lower abdomen.
Indications: Spermatorrhea, leukorrhea, neuralgia of the spermatic cord.
Method: Straight insertion, 1-1.5 units.

K-13 *(Qixue)*　气穴　"Qi's Orifice"

Location: 0.5 unit lateral to Co-4 *(Guanyuan)*, on the lower abdomen.
Indications: Irregular menstruation, leukorrhea, sterility, urinary tract infection, diarrhea.
Method: Straight insertion, 1-1.5 units.

K-14 *(Siman)*　四满　"Four Full"

Location: 0.5 unit lateral to Co-5 *(Shimen)*, on the lower abdomen.
Indications: Irregular menstruation, leukorrhea, sterility, urinary tract infection, diarrhea.
Method: Straight insertion, 1-1.5 units.

K-15 *(Zhongzhu)*　中注　"Middle Flow"

Location: 0.5 unit lateral to Co-7 *(Yinjiao)*, on the lower abdomen.
Indications: Irregular menstruation, low back pain, abdominal pain, constipation.
Method: Straight insertion, 1-1.5 units.

K-16 *(Huangshu)*　肓俞　"Vitals' Hollow"

Location: 0.5 unit lateral to the navel.
Indications: Stomach spasms, pain of hernia, enteritis, habitual constipation, hiccough.
Method: Straight insertion, 1-1.5 units.

K-17 *(Shangqu)*　商曲　"Trade's Bend"

Location: 0.5 unit lateral to Co-10 *(Xiawan)*, on the abdomen.
Indications: Stomach-ache, colic, peritonitis.
Method: Straight insertion, 1-1.5 units.

K-18 *(Shiguan)*　石关　"Stone Hinge"

Location: 0.5 unit lateral to Co-11 *(Jianli)*, on the abdomen.
Indications: Stomach-ache, hiccoughs, constipation, spasms of esophagus.
Method: Straight insertion, 1-1.5 units.

K-19 *(Yindu)*　　阴都　　"Yin's Metropolis"

Location: 0.5 unit lateral to Co-12 *(Zhongwan)*, on the abdomen.
Indications: Emphysema, pleurisy, malaria, abdominal distension or pain.
Method: Straight insertion, 1-1.5 units.

K-20 *(Futonggu)*　　腹通谷　　"Connecting Valley on the Abdomen"

Location: 0.5 unit lateral to Co-13 *(Shangwan)*, on the abdomen.
Indications; Stiff neck, seizures, palpitations, intercostal neuralgia, vomiting, diarrhea.
Method: Straight insertion, 1-1.5 units.

K-21 *(Youmen)*　　幽门　　"Secluded Door (Pylorus)"

Location: 0.5 unit lateral to Co-14 *(Juque)*, on the abdomen.
Indications: Intercostal neuralgia, distended stomach, stomach spasms, chronic gastritis.
Method: Straight insertion, 0.7-1 unit. CAUTION: Avoid deep insertion which might puncture the liver.

K-22 *(Bulang)*　　步廊　　"Stepping Corridor"

Location: 2 units beside Co-16 *(Zhongting)*, in the 5th intercostal space.
Indications: Pleurisy, intercostal neuralgia, rhinitis, gastritis, bronchitis.
Method: Slanted insertion, 0.5-0.8 unit. CAUTION: Avoid deep insertion.

K-23 *(Shenfeng)*　　神封　　"Spirit's Seal"

Location: 2 units lateral to Co-17 *(Shanzhong)*, in the 4th intercostal space.
Indications: Pleurisy, intercostal neuralgia, mastitis, bronchitis.
Method: Slanted insertion, 0.5-0.8 unit. CAUTION: Avoid deep insertion.

K-24 *(Lingxu)*　　灵墟　　"Spirit's Ruins"

Location: 2 units lateral to Co-18 *(Yutang)*, in the 3rd intercostal space.
Indications: Intercostal neuralgia, bronchitis, vomiting, mastitis.
Method: Slanted insertion, 0.5-0.8 unit. CAUTION: Avoid deep insertion.

K-25 *(Shencang)*　　神藏　　"Spirit's Storage"

Location: 2 units lateral to Co-19 *(Zigong)*, in the 2nd intercostal space.
Indications: Bronchitis, vomiting, intercostal neuralgia.
Method: Slanted insertion, 0.5-0.8 unit. CAUTION: Avoid deep insertion.

K-26 *(Yuzhong)*　　彧中　　"Amid Elegance"

Location: 2 units lateral to Co-20 *(Huagai)*, in the first intercostal space.
Indications: Bronchitis, vomiting, intercostal neuralgia.
Method: Slanted insertion, 0.5-0.8 unit. CAUTION: Avoid deep insertion.

K-27 *(Shufu)*　俞府　　"Hollow Residence"

Location: 2 units lateral to Co-21 *(Xuanji),* in the depression beneath the inferior margin at the medial end of the clavicle.
Indication: Bronchitis, asthma, chest pain, vomiting, abdominal distension.
Method: Slanted insertion, 0.5-0.8 unit.

LIVER CHANNEL (LEG ABSOLUTE YIN)

Li-1 *(Dadun)*　大敦　　"Great Honesty"

Location: On the lateral aspect of the big toe, about 0.1 unit from the corner of the toenail.
Indications: Irregular menstruation, pain of hernia, prolapsed uterus, incontinence of urine, orchitis, hematuria, abnormal uterine bleeding.
Method: Straight insertion, 0.1-0.2 unit.

Li-6 *(Zhongdu)*　中都　　"Middle Metropolis"

Location: 7 units above the medial malleolus on the posterior margin of the tibia, 2 units directly above Li-5 *(Ligou).*
Indications: Abnormal uterine bleeding, acute hepatitis, paralysis of lower limb.
Method: Slanted insertion, 1-1.5 units.

Li-7 *(Xiguan)*　膝关　　"Knee's Hinge"

Location: 1 unit posterior to Sp-9 *(Yinlingquan),* on the lower leg.
Indications: Strong recurrent headache, arthritis of the knee.
Method: Straight insertion, 1.5-2 units.

Li-9 *(Yinbao)*　阴包　　"Yin's Wrapping"

Location: 4 units above Li-8 *(Ququan),* on the medial aspect of the thigh.
Indications: Irregular menstruation, enuresis, retention of urine, low back pain.
Method: Straight insertion, 1.5-3 units.

Li-10 *(Zuwuli)*　足五里　　"Five Measures on the Foot"

Location: On the medial aspect of the thigh, 1 unit below Li-11 *(Yinlian).*
Indications: Retention of urine, lassitude, incontinence, eczema of scrotum, pain on medial side of thigh.
Method: Straight insertion, 1.5-3 units.

Li-11 *(Yinlian)*　阴廉　　"Yin's Modesty"

Location: 2 units below S-30 *(Qichong),* on the medial aspect of the thigh.
Indications: Irregular menstruation, pain of the thigh, pain of hernia.
Method: Straight insertion, 1-1.5 units.

Li-12 *(Jimai)*　急脉　"Urgent Pulse"

Location: Below the pubic symphysis and lateral to the median line 2.5 units.
Indications: Prolapsed uterus, pain of hernia, penial pain.
Method: Straight insertion, 1-1.5 units. CAUTION: Avoid the artery.

GOVERNING CHANNEL

Gv-2 *(Yuoshu)*　腰俞　"Lower Back's Hollow"

Location: In the sacral hiatus, below the 4th sacral vertebra.
Indications: Seizures, irregular menstruation, hemorrhoids, low back pain, enuresis, paralysis of lower limb, incontinence due to paraplegia.
Method: Slanted insertion into the sacral hiatus, 0.7-1.5 units.

Gv-5 *(Xuanshu)*　悬枢　"Suspended Axis"

Location: Below the spinous process of the 1st lumbar vertebra.
Indications: Dysentery, abdominal pain, diarrhea, prolapsed anus, stiffness and pain of lumbar vertebrae.
Method: Slanted insertion, 0.5-1 unit.

Gv-6 *(Jizhong)*　脊中　"Middle of Spine"

Location: Below the spinous process of the 11th thoracic vertebra.
Indications: Hepatitis, seizures, low back pain, paralysis of lower limb.
Method: Slanted insertion, 0.5-1 unit.

Gv-7 *(Zhongshu)*　中枢　"Middle Axis"

Location: Below the spinous process of the 10th thoracic vertebra.
Indications: Stomach-ache, cholecystitis, diminishing vision, low back pain.
Method: Slanted insertion, 0.5-1 unit.

Gv-8 *(Jinsuo)*　筋缩　"Sinew's Shrinking"

Location: Below the spinous process of the 9th thoracic vertebra.
Indications: Hepatitis, cholecystitis, pleurisy, seizures, hysteria, intercostal neuralgia.
Method: Slanted insertion, 0.5-1 unit.

Gv-11 *(Shendao)*　神道　"Spirit's Path"

Location: Below the spinous process of the 5th thoracic vertebra.
Indications: Fever, heart disease, malaria, seizures, intercostal neuralgia.
Method: Slanted insertion, 0.5-1 unit.

Gv-16 *(Fengfu)* 风府 "Wind's Dwelling"

Location: 1 unit above the middle of the natural hairline at the back of the head, in the depression directly below the occipital protuberance.
Indications: Stiff neck, numbness of the limbs, common cold, headache, stroke, mental illness.
Method: Straight insertion, 0.5-1 unit. CAUTION: Avoid deep insertion.

Gv-17 *(Naohu)* 脑户 "Brain's Household"

Location: At the superior margin of the occipital protuberance, 1.5 units directly above Gv-16 *(Fengfu)*.
Indications: Headache, stiff neck, insomnia, seizures.
Method: Slanted insertion, 0.5-1 unit.

Gv-18 *(Qiangjian)* 强间 "Between Strength"

Location: 1.5 unit above Gv-17 *(Naohu)*, on the back of the head.
Indications: Headache, stiff neck, insomnia, seizures.
Method: Slanted insertion, 0.5-1 unit.

Gv-19 *(Houding)* 后顶 "Behind Top"

Location: 1.5 units behind Gv-20 *(Baihui)*, near the vertex.
Indications: Migraine headache, common cold, insomnia, seizures.
Method: Slanted insertion, 0.5-1 unit.

Gv-21 *(Qianding)* 前顶 "Before Top"

Location: 1.5 units anterior to Gv-20 *(Baihui)*, near the vertex.
Indications: Headache, vertigo, rhinitis, rhinopolypus, infantile convulsions.
Method: Slanted insertion, 0.5-1 unit.

Gv-22 *(Xinhui)* 囟会 "Fontanel's Meeting"

Location: 3 units in front of Gv-20 *(Baihui)*.
Indications: Headache, vertigo, rhinitis, rhinopolypus, infantile convulsions.
Method: Slanted insertion, 0.5-1 unit.

Gv-24 *(Shenting)* 神庭 "Spirit's Hall"

Location: 0.5 unit posterior to the middle of the natural hairline at the forehead.
Indications: Headache, vertigo, rhinitis, rhinopolypus, seizures, stomatitis.
Method: Slanted insertion, 0.5-0.8 unit.

Gv-27 *(Duiduan)* 兑端 "Exchange Terminus"

Location: At the lower tip of the philtrum.
Indications: Vomiting, occluded nose, rhinopolypus, seizures, stomatitis.

Method: Slanted insertion, 0.2-0.3 unit.

Gv-28 *(Yinjiao)*   龈交   "Gum's Junction"

Location: Midpoint between the inside of the upper lip and the upper gum, slightly above the incisive suture when the upper lip is rolled back.
Indications: Acute wrist sprain, rhinopolypus, pain and bleeding around the teeth, mental illness.
Method: Slanted insertion upward, 0.2-0.3 unit.

CONCEPTION CHANNEL

Co-1 *(Huiyin)*   会阴   "Perineum"

Location: Midway between the anus and the scrotum (men), or between the anus and the commissura labiorum (women).
Indications: Revive from drowning, urethritis, irregular menstruation, prostatitis.
Method: Straight insertion, 1-1.5 units.

Co-2 *(Qugu)*   曲骨   "Crooked Bone"

Location: 5 units directly below the navel, at the superior aspect of the pubic symphysis.
Indications: Irregular menstruation, prolapsed uterus, cystitis, orchitis.
Method: Straight insertion, 1-1.5 units.

Co-5 *(Shimen)*   石门   "Stone Door"

Location: 2 units directly below the navel.
Indications: Abnormal uterine bleeding, amenorrhea, edema, retention of urine, mastitis.
Method: Straight insertion, 1-1.5 units.
Other: Alarm point of the Triple Burner channel.

Co-7 *(Yinjiao)*   阴交   "Yin's Junction"

Location: 1 unit directly below the navel.
Indications: Irregular menstruation, abnormal uterine bleeding, leukorrhea, edema, pain of hernia, prolapsed uterus.
Method: Straight insertion, 1-1.5 units.

Co-9 *(Shuifen)*   水分   "Water Part"

Location: 1 unit directly above the navel.
Indications: Ascites, vomiting, diarrhea, nephritis.
Method: Straight insertion, 1-1.5 units.

Co-10 *(Xiawan)*   下脘   "Lower Cavity"

Location: 2 units directly above the navel.

Indications: Indigestion, stomach-ache, prolapsed stomach, diarrhea.
Method: Straight insertion, 1-1.5 units.

Co-11 *(Jianli)*　建里　"Establish Measure"

Location: 3 units directly above the navel.
Indications: Acute and chronic gastritis, angina pectoris, ascites, intestinal noises and abdominal pain.
Method: Straight insertion, 1-1.5 units.

Co-15 *(Jiuwei)*　鸠尾　"Wild Pigeon's Tail"

Location: 7 units directly above the navel, 0.5 unit below the xiphoid process.
Indications: Angina pectoris, seizures, hiccoughs, mental illness, asthma.
Method: Slanted insertion pointed slightly downward, 1 unit.

Co-16 *(Zhongting)*　中庭　"Middle Hall"

Location: 1.6 units below Co-17 *(Shanzhong)*, level with the 5th intercostal space.
Indications: Asthma, vomiting, food stuck in throat.
Method: Slanted insertion, 0.5-1 unit.

Co-18 *(Yutang)*　玉堂　"Jade Court"

Location: 1.6 units above Co-17 *(Shanzhong)*, level with the 3rd intercostal space.
Indications: Bronchitis, asthma, vomiting, emphysema, intercostal neuralgia.
Method: Slanted insertion, 0.5-1 unit.

Co-19 *(Zigong)*　紫宫　"Purple Palace"

Location: 1.6 units above Co-18 *(Yutang)*, level with the 2nd intercostal space.
Indications: Bronchiectasis, asthma, pulmonary tuberculosis.
Method: Slanted insertion, 0.5-1 unit.

Co-20 *(Huagai)*　华盖　"Lustrous Cover"

Location: 1 unit below Co-21 *(Xuanji)*, level with the 1st intercostal space.
Indications: Bronchitis, asthma, intercostal neuralgia, pharyngitis.
Method: Slanted insertion, 0.5-1 unit.

Co-23 *(Lianquan)*　廉泉　"Modesty's Spring"

Location: In the depression between the pharyngeal prominence and the lower margin of hyoid bone.
Indications: Bronchitis, pharyngitis, tonsillitis, loss of voice, paralysis of hypoglossus muscle.
Method: Slanted insertion toward base of tongue, 1-1.5 units.

Chapter 8

Other New and Miscellaneous Points

NEW POINTS OF THE HEAD AND NECK

N-HN-1 *(Shangjingming)* 上睛明 "Upper Eyes Bright"

Location: Approximately 0.2 units above B-1 *(Jingming)*. (Dia. 2-61)
Indications: Atrophy of the optic nerve, keratoleukoma, strabismus, excessive lacrimation with wind, ametropia.
Method: Straight insertion, 1-1.5 units.

N-HN-2 *(Xiajingming)* 下睛明 "Lower Eyes Bright"

Location: Approximately 0.2 unit below B-1 *(Jingming)*. (Dia. 2-61)
Indications: Same as N-HN-1 *(Shangjingming)* above.
Method: Straight insertion, 1-1.5 units.

N-HN-3 *(Jianming)* 健明 "Strengthen Brightness"

Location: 0.2 unit below and slightly lateral to N-HN-2 *(Xiajingming)*, just inside the inferior margin of the orbit. (Dia. 2-61)
Indications: Retinitis, retinitis pigmentosa, cataract, atrophy of the optic nerve, strabismus, ametropia, dacryocystitis.
Method: Insert along the margin of the orbit slightly toward the inner canthus, 1-1.5 units.

N-HN-3(a) *(Jianming #1)* 健明₁ "Strengthen Brightness #1"

Location: Between N-HN-3 *(Jianming)* and S-1 *(Chengqi)*, on the medial side of the inferior margin of the orbit. (Dia. 2-61)
Indications: Ulcer of the cornea, nebula.
Method: Insert along the margin of the orbit slightly toward the inner canthus, 1-1.5 units.

N-HN-3(b) *(Jianming #2)*   健明₂   "Strengthen Brightness #2"

Location: Between S-1 *(Chengqi)* and M-HN-8 *(Qiuhou)*, inside the inferior margin of the orbit. (Dia. 2-61)
Indications: Atrophy of the optic nerve, nebula, dacryocystitis, retinochoroiditis, macula corneae.
Method: Insert along the margin of the orbit slightly toward the inner canthus, 1-1.5 units.

N-HN-3(c) *(Jianming #3)*   健明₃   "Strengthen Brightness #3"

Location: 0.3 unit lateral and superior to M-HN-8 *(Qiuhou)*, just inside the lateral margin of the orbit. (Dia. 2-61)
Indications: Atrophy of the optic nerve, strabismus.
Method: Insert along the margin of the orbit slightly toward the inner canthus, 1-1.5 units.

N-HN-3(d) *(Jianming #4)*   健明₄   "Strengthen Brightness #4"

Location: 0.3 unit above N-HN-1 *(Shangjingming)*, just inside the superior medial corner of the orbit. (Dia. 2-61)
Indications: Glaucoma, ametropia, cataract.
Method: Insert along the margin of the orbit slightly toward the inner canthus, 1-1.5 units.

N-HN-5(a) *(Zengming #1)*   增明₁   "Increase Brightness #1"

Location: 0.2 unit medial to N-HN-4 *(Shangming)*. (Dia. 2-61)
Indications: Nebula, opacity of cornea, ametropia.
Method: Insert along the margin of the orbit slightly toward the inner canthus, 1-1.5 units.

H-HN-5(b) *(Zengming #2)*   增明₂   "Increase Brightness #2"

Location: 0.2 unit lateral to N-HN-4 *(Shangming)*. (Dia. 2-61)
Indications: Nebula, opacity of cornea, ametropia.
Method: Insert along the margin of the orbit slightly toward the inner canthus, 1-1.5 units.

N-HN-8 *(Tingxue)*   听穴   "Hearing Orifice"

Location: Midway between SI-19 *(Tinggong)* and GB-2 *(Tinghui)* in front of the ear. (Dia. 2-62)
Indications: Deaf-mutism.
Method: With mouth open slightly, straight insertion, 1-2 units.

N-HN-9 *(Tingling)*   听灵   "Hearing's Inspiration"

Location: Midway between N-HN-8 *(Tingxue)* and GB-2 *(Tinghui)*. (Dia. 2-62)
Indications: Tinnitus, deafness, deaf-mutism.
Method: With mouth slightly open, straight insertion, 1.5-2 units.

N-HN-10 *(Tingcong)* 听聪 "Hearing"

Location: 0.2 unit below GB-2 *(Tinghui)* in front of the ear. (Dia. 2-62)
Indications: Deafness.
Method: Straight insertion, 1.5-2 units.

N-HN-11 *(Tingmin)* 听敏 "Hearing Sensitivity"

Location: At the lower root of the earlobe. (Dia. 2-62)
Indications: Deafness.
Method: Straight insertion, 1.5 units.

N-HN-12 *(Shangergen)* 上耳根 "Upper Ear Root"

Location: At the middle of the upper root of the auricle. (Dia. 2-63)
Indications: Hemiplegia, lateral sclerosis.
Method: Slanted insertion, 0.5-1 unit.

N-HN-13 *(Houtinggong)* 后听宫 "Posterior Palace of Hearing"

Location: At the root of the auricle, behind the ear, level with SI-19 *(Tinggong)*. (Dia. 2-63)
Indications: Deafness.
Method: Slanted insertion, 0.5-1 unit.

N-HN-14 *(Houtingxue)* 后听穴 "Posterior Hearing Point"

Location: Midway between SI-19 *(Tinggong)* and N-HN-15 *(Yilong)*. (Dia. 2-63)
Indications: Deafness.
Method: Slanted insertion, 0.5-1 unit.

N-HN-16 *(Houcong)* 后聪 "Posterior Hearing"

Location: Midway between the root of the auricle and the natural hairline on the back of the head. (Dia. 2-63)
Indications: Deafness.
Method: Slanted insertion, 0.3-0.5 unit.

N-HN-17 *(Chiqian)* 池前 "Before the Pool"

Location: 0.5 unit anterior to GB-20 *(Fengchi)*. (Dia. 2-64)
Indications: Deafness, cataract.
Method: Slanted insertion toward TB-17 *(Yifeng)*, 1-2 units.

N-HN-18 *(Yimingxia)* 翳明下 "Below Dim Light"

Location: 0.5 unit below M-HN-13 *(Yiming)*. (Dia. 2-64)
Indications: Deafness.
Method: Straight insertion, 1.5 units.

N-HN-19 *(Tianting)*　　天听　　"Heaven's Hearing"

Location: 0.5 unit below N-HN-22(b) *(Anmian #2)*. (Dia. 2-64)
Indications: Deafness.
Method: Straight insertion, 1.5 units.

N-HN-21 *(Yanchi)*　　岩池　　"Cliff's Pool"

Location: At the intersection of a line level with the highest point of the mastoid process with the natural hairline. (Dia. 2-64)
Indications: Glaucoma, vertigo, hypertension.
Method: Straight insertion, pointed backward slightly, 1-1.5 units.

N-HN-22(a) *Anmian #1)*　　安眠₁　　"Peaceful Sleep #1"

Location: Midway between TB-17 *(Yifeng)* and M-HN-13 *(Yiming)*. (Dia. 2-64)
Indications: Migraine, vertigo, insomnia, tinnitus, psychosis.
Method: Straight insertion, 1-1.5 units.

N-HN-22(b) *(Anmian #2)*　　安眠₂　　"Peaceful Sleep #2"

Location: Midway between GB-20 *(Fengchi)* and M-HN-13 *(Yiming)*. (Dia. 2-64)
Indications: Insomnia, palpitations, hypertension, hysteria, psychosis.
Method: Straight insertion, 1-1.5 units.

N-HN-23 *(Xingfen)*　　兴奋　　"Excitement"

Location: About 0.5 unit in a slanted direction above N-HN-22(b) *(Anmian #2)*, just posterior to the margin of the mastoid process. (Dia. 2-64)
Indications: Bradycardia, idiocy resulting from brain disease, hypersomnia.
Method: Straight insertion, 1-1.5 units.

N-HN-24 *(Ronghou)*　　客后　　"Behind (Heaven's) Contents"

Location: 1.5 units below TB-17 *(Yifeng)*, just posterior to SI-17 *(Tianrong)*. (Dia. 2-59)
Indications: Deafness, toothache, headache.
Method: Straight insertion, 0.5-1 unit.

N-HN-25 *(Qiangyin)*　　强音　　"Strong Sound"

Location: 2 units lateral to the laryngeal prominence, behind and above S-9 *(Renying)*. (Dia. 2-59)
Indications: Aphasia due to diseases of the vocal cords.
Method: Insert toward the root of the tongue, 0.5-1 unit.

N-HN-26 *(Zengyin)*　　增音　　"Increase Sound"

Location: Midway between the laryngeal prominence and the angle of the mandible. (Dia. 2-59)

Indications: Same as N-HN-25 (Qiangyin) above.
Method: Insert toward laryngopharynx, 0.5-1 unit. CAUTION: Avoid the carotid artery.

N-HN-27 (Xiafutu)　下扶突　"Lower Support Prominence"

Location: 0.5 unit below S-32 (Futu). (Dia. 2-59)
Indications: Goiter, tremor, paralysis of upper limb.
Method: Slanted insertion, directed upward, 0.3-1.5 units.

N-HN-28 (Jingzhong)　颈中　"Middle of Neck"

Location: 2 units below N-HN-22(b) (Anmian #2), at the posterior margin of the sternocleidomastoid muscle. (Dia. 2-59)
Indications: Stiff and painful neck, hemiplegia.
Method: Straight insertion, or slanted upward, 0.5-1 unit.

N-HN-29 (Jianei)　頬内　"Inside Cheek"

Location: At the buccal mucosa in the mouth, level with the 1st molar. (Dia. 2-65)
Indications: Facial paralysis, deafness, ulceration of the mouth or gums.
Method: Slanted insertion toward the ear, 0.5-1 unit, or prick the point to let a few drops of blood.

N-HN-30 (Sizhong)　四中　"Four at the Middle"

Location: 2-3 units from Gv-20 (Baihui), on each of its four sides. (Dia. 2-58)
Indications: Hydrocephalus.
Method: Transverse insertion, 1-2 units. CAUTION: For patients whose fontanels protrude from the skull, care must be taken to avoid penetrating these when inserting the needle transversely.

N-HN-31 (Tounie)　头顳　"Temple"

Location: 1 unit posterior to M-HN-9 (Taiyang), level with the tip of the ear. When the teeth are clenched, at a prominence in the temporal region. (Dia. 2-59)
Indications: Psychosis, seizures, progressive loss of memory.
Method: Slanted insertion, 1.5-2 units.

N-HN-32 (Dingshen)　定神　"Settle Spirit"

Location: In the philtrum, ⅓ the distance from the top of the lip to the base of the nose. (Dia. 2-60)
Indications: Psychosis, seizures, dysmenorrhea.
Method: Slanted insertion directed upward, 1-1.5 units.

N-HN-33 (Guangcai)　光彩　"Luster"

Location: In a small depression 0.2 unit above and 0.1 unit anterior to the tip of the ear. (Dia. 2-59)
Indications: Infectious parotitis.
Method: Burning lamp wick grass touched to this point has shown good results.

N-HN-34 *(Xinzanzhu)*　新攒竹　"New Gathered Bamboo"

Location: 0.5 unit above and lateral to N-HN-1 *(Shangjingming)*. (Dia. 2-61)
Indications: Supraorbital neuralgia, rhinitis.
Method: Straight insertion, 0.5-0.8 unit.

N-HN-35 *(Tongming)*　瞳明　"Pupil's Brightness"

Location: 0.5 unit below GB-1 *(Tongziliao)*. (Dia. 2-61)
Indications: Ametropia.
Method: Slanted insertion, 1-1.5 units.

N-HN-36 *(Tingxiang)*　听响　"Hear Sound"

Location: 0.1 unit above TB-21 *(Ermen)* in a small hollow. (Dia. 2-62)
Indications: Deafness.
Method: Straight insertion, 1-1.5 units.

N-HN-37 *(Shanglong)*　上聋　"Upper Deafness"

Location: Midway between TB-21 *(Ermen)* and SI-19 *(Tinggong)*. (Dia. 2-62)
Indications: Deafness, deaf-mutism.
Method: With the mouth open slightly, straight insertion, 1-2 units.

N-HN-38 *(Tinglongjian)*　听聋间　"Between Hearing and Deafness"

Location: Midway between SI-19 *(Tinggong)* and N-HN-8 *(Tingxue)*. (Dia. 2-62)
Indications: Deafness.
Method: With the mouth slightly open, straight insertion, 1-2 units.

N-HN-39 *(Yaming)*　哑鸣　"Mute Call"

Location: 1 unit anterior to GB-20 *(Fengchi)*. (Dia. 2-64)
Indications: Deaf-mutism, pharyngolaryngitis.
Method: Slanted insertion toward the tip of the nose, 1-1.5 units.

N-HN-40 *(Chixia)*　池下　"Below the Pool"

Location: 0.5 unit below GB-20 *(Fengchi)*. (Dia. 2-64)
Indications: Occipital headache, glaucoma, retinitis pigmentosa.
Method: Straight insertion, 1.5-2 units.

N-HN-41 *(Tongerdao)*　通耳道　"Through the Ear Canal"

Location: 1 unit below M-HN-13 *(Yiming)*. (Dia. 2-64)
Indications: Tinnitus, deaf-mutism.
Method: Slanted insertion toward eardrum, 1-2 units.

N-HN-42 *(Waierdaokou)*   外耳道口   "Opening of the External Ear Canal"

Location: At the top of the opening of the external ear canal. (Dia. 2-62)
Indications: Tinnitus, deafness.
Method: Straight insertion, 0.3-0.5 unit.

N-HN-43 *(Qiying)*   气瘿   "Cervical Lump of Qi"

Location: Near S-10 *(Shuitu),* on the lateral superior side of the swelling associated with goiter. (Dia. 2-59)
Indications: Simple goiter, hyperthyroidism.
Method: Straight insertion, 1-1.5 units.

N-HN-45 *(Xiayamen)*   下哑门   "Lower Door of Muteness"

Location: 1 unit below Gv-15 *(Yamen).* (Dia. 2-66)
Indications: Sequelae of brain disease.
Method: Straight insertion, 0.5-1 unit.

N-HN-46 *(Fuyamen)*   副哑门   "Secondary Door of Muteness"

Location: 1 unit below and 0.5 unit lateral to Gv-15 *(Yamen).* (Dia. 2-66)
Indications: Sequelae of brain disease.
Method: Straight insertion, 0.51 unit.

N-HN-47 *(Xinyi)*   新一   "New One"

Location: Between the spinous processes of the 5th and 6th cervical vertebrae. (Dia. 2-66)
Indications: Incomplete maturation of the cerebral cortex, seizures, psychosis.
Method: Slightly slanted, 0.5-1 unit.

N-HN-48 *(Xiaxinshi)*   下新识   "Lower New Recognition"

Location: 0.5 unit below M-HN-29 *(Xinshi).* (Dia. 2-66)
Indications: Pituitary adenoma.
Method: Straight insertion, 1-1.5 units.

N-HN-49 *(Zhongjie)*   中接   "Middle Connection"

Location: 0.7 unit above Gv-16 *(Fengfu).* (Dia. 2-66)
Indications: Hydrocephalus.
Method: Slanted insertion, either toward right or left, 0.5 unit.

N-HN-50(a) *(Dijia #1)*   地甲₁   "Endemic Goiter #1"

Location: 0.5 unit above and one finger width lateral to Gv-14 *(Dazhui).* (Dia. 2-66)
Indications: Endemic goiter.

Method: Straight insertion, 1 unit.

N-HN-50(b) *(Dijia #2)* 地甲₂ "Endemic Goiter #2"

Location: 1 unit lateral to the posterior margin at the middle of the sternocleidomastoid muscle. (Dia. 2-59)
Indications Endemic goiter.
Method: Straight insertion, 0.5 unit.

N-HN-51(a-e) *(Zhinao #1-5)* 治脑₁₋₅ "Heal Brain #1-5"

Location: 5 points, one on the midline between each of the 2nd to 7th cervical vertebrae, numbered 1 through 5 respectively. (Diagram not shown.)
Indications: Brain diseases.
Method: Straight insertion, 1-1.5 units. CAUTION: If the patient feels an electric shock-like sensation, withdraw the needle immediately.

N-HN-52 *(Huxi)* 呼吸 "Breathing"

Location: About 0.3 unit below the intersection of the jugular vein with the lateral margin of the sternocleidomastoid muscle. (Dia. 2-59)
Indications: Apnea, paralysis of respiratory muscles, spasms of the diaphragm.
Method: Straight insertion, 0.5-1 unit.

N-HN-53 *(Zhiou)* 止呕 "Stop Vomiting"

Location: Midway between Co-23 *(Lianquan)* and Co-22 *(Tiantu).* (Dia. 2-59)
Indications: Vomiting, excessive phlegm.
Method: Slanted insertion toward Co-22 *(Tiantu),* 0.5-1 unit.

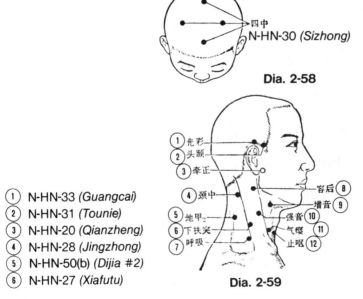

四中
N-HN-30 *(Sizhong)*

Dia. 2-58

1 光彩
2 头颞
3 牵正
4 颈中
5 地甲₂
6 下扶突
7 呼吸

容后 8
增音 9
强音 10
气瘿 11
止呕 12

① N-HN-33 *(Guangcai)*	⑦ N-HN-52 *(Huxi)*
② N-HN-31 *(Tounie)*	⑧ N-HN-24 *(Ronghou)*
③ N-HN-20 *(Qianzheng)*	⑨ N-HN-26 *(Zengyin)*
④ N-HN-28 *(Jingzhong)*	⑩ N-HN-25 *(Qiangyin)*
⑤ N-HN-50(b) *(Dijia #2)*	⑪ N-HN-43 *(Qiying)*
⑥ N-HN-27 *(Xiafutu)*	⑫ N-HN-53 *(Zhiou)*

Dia. 2-59

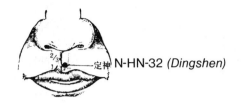

定神 N-HN-32 *(Dingshen)*

Dia. 2-60

① N-HN-5(a) *(Zengming #1)*
② N-HN-34 *(Xinzanzhu)*
③ N-HN-3(d) *(Jianming #4)*
④ N-HN-1 *(Shangjingming)*
⑤ N-HN-2 *(Xiajingming)*
⑥ N-HN-3 *(Jianming)*
⑦ N-HN-3(a) *(Jianming #1)*
⑧ N-HN-3(b) *(Jianming #2)*
⑨ N-HN-35 *(Tongming)*
⑩ N-HN-3(c) *(Jianming #3)*
⑪ N-HN-6 *(Waiming)*
⑫ N-HN-5(b) *(Zengming #2)*
⑬ N-HN-4 *(Shangming)*

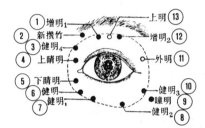

Dia. 2-61

Note: ● signifies less commonly used New points
○ signifies more commonly used New points

① N-HN-36 *(Tingxiang)*
② N-HN-42 *(Waierdaokou)*
③ N-HN-37 *(Shanglong)*
④ N-HN-38 *(Tinglongjian)*
⑤ N-HN-8 *(Tingxue)*
⑥ N-HN-9 *(Tingling)*
⑦ N-HN-10 *(Tingcong)*
⑧ N-HN-11 *(Tingmin)*

① N-HN-12 *(Shangergen)*
② N-HN-16 *(Houcong)*
③ N-HN-13 *(Houtinggong)*
④ N-HN-14 *(Houtingxue)*
⑤ N-HN-15 *(Yilong)*

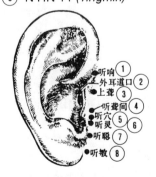

Dia. 2-62

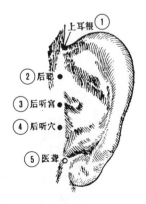

Dia. 2-63

① N-HN-23 *(Xingfen)*
② N-HN-39 *(Yaming)*
③ N-HN-17 *(Chiqian)*
④ N-HN-40 *(Chixia)*
⑤ N-HN-19 *(Tianting)*
⑥ N-HN-18 *(Yimingxia)*
⑦ N-HN-21 *(Yanchi)*
⑧ N-HN-22(b) *(Anmian #2)*
⑨ N-HN-22(a) *(Anmian #1)*
⑩ N-HN-54 *(Anmian)*
⑪ N-HN-41 *(Tongerdao)*

① N-HN-44 *(Shangtianzhu)*
② N-HN-45 *(Xiayamen)*
③ N-BW-48 *(Xiaxinshi)*
④ N-HN-50(a) *(Dijia #1)*
⑤ N-HN-49 *(Zhongjie)*
⑥ N-HN-46 *(Fuyamen)*
⑦ N-HN-47 *(Xinyi)*

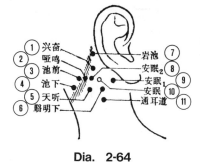

Dia. 2-64

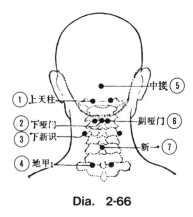

Dia. 2-66

頬内
N-HN-29 *(Jianei)*

Dia. 2-65

NEW POINTS OF THE CHEST AND ABDOMEN

N-CA-1 *(Shuishang)* 水上 "Above Water"

Location: 0.5 unit above Co-9 *(Shuifen)*. (Dia. 2-67)
Indications: Diarrhea, abdominal distension, abdominal pain, gastric hyperacidity.
Method: Straight insertion, 1-1.5 units.

N-CA-2 *(Weile)*　胃乐　"Stomach's Happiness"

Location: 0.2 unit above and 4 units lateral to Co-9 *(Shuifen).* (Dia. 2-67)
Indications: Stomach-ache, prolapsed stomach.
Method: Straight insertion, 1-1.5 units.

N-CA-3 *(Zhixie)*　止泻　"Stop Diarrhea"

Location: 2.5 units below the navel on the median line of the abdomen. (Dia. 2-67)
Indications: Enteritis, round worm in intestinal tract, retention of urine, enuresis.
Method: Straight insertion, 1 1.5 units.

N-CA-5 *(Chongjian)*　冲间　"Pour Between"

Location: 3 units lateral to Co-2 *(Qugu).* (Dia. 2-67)
Indications: Prolapsed uterus, paralysis of legs.
Method: Straight insertion, 1-2 units.

N-CA-6 *(Shuxi)*　鼠蹊　"Mouse Path"

Location: At a point ⅓ of the length of the inguinal ligament from its lateral end, 0.5 unit lateral to the femoral artery. (Dia. 2-67)
Indications: Tuberculosis of the inguinal lymph glands, weakness of leg adductors.
Method: Straight insertion, 1.5-2.5 units.

N-CA-7 *(Xiongdaji)*　胸大肌　"Pectoralis Major"

Location: 2 finger widths lateral to the nipple. (Dia. 2-67)
Indications: Atrophy of pectoralis major muscle.
Method: Slanted insertion, 0.5-0.8 unit.

N-CA-8 *(Ganshi)*　肝室　"Liver's Dwelling"

Location: Directly below the nipple between the 6th and 7th ribs. (Dia. 2-67)
Indications: Enlargement of the liver, pain in the region of the liver.
Method: Slanted insertion, 0.3-0.5 unit.

N-CA-9 *(Chuangxinmen)*　创新门　"Create New Door"

Location: In the triangular cavity at the medial, superior side of the angle of the 9th rib. (Dia. 2-67)
Indications: Chronic schistosomiasis.
Method: Slanted insertion, 0.5-0.8 unit.

N-CA-10 *(Tiwei)*　提胃　"Lift Stomach"

Location: 4 units lateral to Co-12 *(Zhongwan).* (Dia. 2-67)
Indications: Prolapsed stomach, indigestion.
Method: Slanted insertion toward S-25 *(Tianshu),* 3-4 units.

N-CA-11 *(Tongbian)* 通便 "Bowel Movement"

Location: 3 units lateral to the navel. (Dia. 2-67)
Indications: Constipation due to paraplegia.
Method: Straight insertion, 1-2 units.

N-CA-12 *(Xinqixue)* 新气穴 "New Qi Orifice"

Location: With the navel as the apex of an equilateral triangle, each side 3 units in length, this point is located at either end of the base line. (Dia. 2-67)
Indications: Infertility, pelvic inflammatory diseases.
Method: Straight insertion, 0.5-1 unit.

N-CA-13 *(Xiazhongji)* 下中极 "Below Middle Summit"

Location: 0.5 unit below Co-3 *(Zhongji).* (Dia. 2-67)
Indications: Incontinence due to paraplegia.
Method: Slanted insertion toward pubis, 2-2.5 units.

N-CA-14 *(Yeniao)* 夜尿 "Night Urine"

Location: 1 unit lateral to N-CA-13 *(Xiazhongji).* (Dia. 2-67)
Indications: Bed wetting.
Method: Slanted insertion, 1-1.5 units.

N-CA-15 *(Zigongjing)* 子宫颈 "Cervix Uteri"

Location: At the 3:00 and 9:00 positions at the opening of the cervix uteri. (Diagram not shown.)
Indications: Chronic cervicitis.
Method: Straight insertion, 0.5 unit. Do not retain or rotate the needle.

N-CA-16 *(Tigangjixue)* 提肛肌穴 "Levator Ani Orifice"

Location: At both sides of the vaginal opening. (Diagram not shown.)
Indications: Prolapsed uterus.
Method: Straight insertion into the levator ani muscle, 2-3 units.

N-CA-17 *(Yinbian)* 阴边 "Beside Genitals"

Location: On the lower border of the pubic symphysis, 0.5 unit lateral to M-CA-24 *(Longmen).* (Dia. 2-67)
Indications: Bladder dysfunction due to paraplegia.
Method: Slanted insertion toward the median line of the abdomen, 0.5-1 unit.

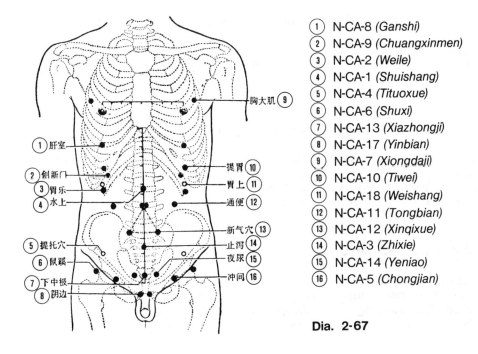

1. N-CA-8 *(Ganshi)*
2. N-CA-9 *(Chuangxinmen)*
3. N-CA-2 *(Weile)*
4. N-CA-1 *(Shuishang)*
5. N-CA-4 *(Tituoxue)*
6. N-CA-6 *(Shuxi)*
7. N-CA-13 *(Xiazhongji)*
8. N-CA-17 *(Yinbian)*
9. N-CA-7 *(Xiongdaji)*
10. N-CA-10 *(Tiwei)*
11. N-CA-18 *(Weishang)*
12. N-CA-11 *(Tongbian)*
13. N-CA-12 *(Xinqixue)*
14. N-CA-3 *(Zhixie)*
15. N-CA-14 *(Yeniao)*
16. N-CA-5 *(Chongjian)*

Dia. 2-67

NEW POINTS OF THE BACK

N-BW-1 *(Liujingzhuipang)*   六颈椎旁   "Beside the 6th Cervical Vertebra"

Location: 0.5 unit lateral to the spinous process of the 6th cervical vertebra. (Dia. 2-68)
Indications: Rhinitis, diminished sense of smell.
Method: Straight insertion, 0.5-1 unit.

N-BW-2 *(Xueyadian)*   血压点   "Blood Pressure Point"

Location: 2 units lateral to the spinous process of the 6th cervical vertebra. (Dia. 2-68)
Indications: High or low blood pressure.
Method: Straight insertion, 0.5-1 unit.

N-BW-3 *(Qijingzhuipang)*   七颈椎旁   "Beside the 7th Cervical Vertebra"

Location: 0.5 unit lateral to the spinous process of the 7th cervical vertebra. (Dia. 2-68)
Indications: Tonsillitis, pharyngitis.
Method: Straight insertion, 0.5-1 unit.

N-BW-5 *(Waidingchuan)*   外定喘   "Outer Stop Wheezing"

Location: 1.5 units lateral to Gv-14 *(Dazhui)* on the upper back. (Dia. 2-68)
Indications: Bronchitis, asthma.
Method: Slanted insertion toward the spine, 0.5-0.8 unit.

N-BW-6 *(Jiehexue)*　结核穴　"Tuberculosis Orifice"

Location: 3.5 units lateral to Gv-14 *(Dazhui)* on the upper back. (Dia. 2-68)
Indications: Pulmonary tuberculosis, tuberculosis generally.
Method: Straight insertion, 0.5-0.8 unit.

N-BW-7 *(Weirexue)*　胃热穴　"Stomach Heat Orifice"

Location: 0.5 unit lateral to the spinous process of the 4th thoracic vertebra. (Dia. 2-68)
Indications: Vomiting, swollen and painful gums, stomach-ache.
Method: Slanted insertion toward the spine, 0.5-1 unit.
Other: This is one of the vertebral points, M-BW-35 *(Jiaji)*.

N-BW-8 *(Ganrexue)*　肝热穴　"Liver Heat Orifice"

Location: 0.5 unit lateral to 5th thoracic vertebra. (Dia. 2-68)
Indications: Bronchitis, hepatitis, cholecystitis, intercostal neuralgia.
Method: Slanted insertion toward the spine, 0.5-1 unit.
Other: This is one of the vertebral points, M-BW-35 *(Jiaji)*.

N-BW-9 *(Jiantongdian)*　肩痛点　"Shoulder Pain Point"

Location: At the midpoint of the lateral margin of the scapula. (Dia. 2-68)
Indications: Diseases of the shoulder joint and surrounding soft tissues, paralysis of the upper limb.
Method: Straight insertion, 0.5-0.8 unit.

N-BW-10 *(Pirexue)*　脾热穴　"Spleen Heat Orifice"

Location: 0.5 unit lateral to the spinous process of the 6th thoracic vertebra. (Dia. 2-68)
Indications: Hepatitis, pancreatitis, enlargement of the spleen, hyperfunction of the spleen.
Method: Slanted insertion toward the spine, 0.5-1 unit.
Other: This is one of the vertebral points, M-BW-35 *(Jiaji)*.

N-BW-11 *(Shenrexue)*　肾热穴　"Kidney Heat Point"

Location: 0.5 unit lateral to the spinous process of the 7th thoracic vertebra. (Dia. 2-68)
Indications: Urinary tract infection, nephritis.
Method: Slanted insertion toward the spine, 0.5-1 unit.
Other: This is one of the vertebral points, M-BW-35 *(Jiaji)*.

N-BW-12 *(Jianming #5)*　健明₅　"Strengthen Brightness #5"

Location: 1.5 unit lateral to the spinous process of the 9th thoracic vertebra, about 0.5 unit below B-18 *(Ganshu)*. (Dia. 2-68)
Indications: Atrophy of the optic nerve, retinitis.
Method: Not specified.

N-BW-13 *(Kuiyangxue)*　潰瘍穴　"Ulcer Orifice"

Location: 2 units lateral to B-45 *(Weicang)*. (Dia. 2-68)
Indications: Stomach and duodenal ulcer.
Method: Slanted insertion, 0.5-0.8 unit.

N-BW-14 *(Weishu)*　胃舒　"Stomach's Comfort"

Location: About 4.5 units lateral to the 2nd lumbar vertebra, at the intersection of the 12th rib with the sacrospinalis muscle. (Dia. 2-68)
Indications: Stomach spasm, ulcer, stomach pain.
Method: Straight insertion, 1-2 units.

N-BW-15 *(Shenji)*　肾脊　"Kidney Spine"

Location: 0.5 unit lateral to the lower end of the spinous process of the 2nd lumbar vertebra. (Dia. 2-68)
Indications: Spondylitis, inflammation of vertebral ligaments, paralysis of lower limb.
Method: Straight insertion, 1.5-2 units.
Other: This is one of the vertebral points, M-BW-35 *(Jiaji)*.

N-BW-16 *(Tiaoyue)*　跳跃　"Leap"

Location: 2 units posterior and inferior to the highest point of the iliac crest. (Dia. 2-68)
Indications: Sequelae of infantile paralysis.
Method: Straight insertion, 2-3 units.

N-BW-18 *(Pangqiang)*　旁强　"Beside Strength"

Location: 1.5 units lateral to Gv-1 *(Changqiang)*. (Dia. 2-68)
Indications: Prolapsed anus or uterus.
Method: Slanted insertion upward, 3-4 units.

N-BW-19 *(Juguxia)*　巨骨下　"Below Great Bone"

Location: 2 units below LI-16 *(Jugu)*. (Dia. 2-68)
Indications: Diseases of shoulder joint and surrounding soft tissues.

Method: Straight insertion, 1-2 units.

N-BW-20 *(Feirexue)*　肺热穴　"Lung Heat Orifice"

Location: 0.5 unit lateral to the spinous process of the 3rd thoracic vertebra. (Dia. 2-68)
Indications: Bronchitis, pleurisy, pneumonia, back pain.
Method: Slanted insertion toward the spine, 0.5-1 unit.
Other: This is one of the vertebral points, M-BW-35 *(Jiaji)*.

N-BW-21 *(Anmian #3)*   安眠₃   "Peaceful Sleep #3"

Location: 0.5 unit lateral to B-17 *(Geshu)*. (Diagram not shown.)
Indications: Insomnia, irritability.
Method: Slanted insertion, 0.5-1 unit.
Other: Approximately same location as M-BW-9 *(Qichuan)*.

N-BW-22 *(Zhongjiaoshu)*   中焦俞   "Middle Burner's Hollow"

Location: 2 units lateral to the 12th thoracic vertebra. (Dia. 2-68)
Indications: Chronic schistosomiasis.
Method: Slanted insertion, 75° angle, pointed slightly upward. For point on the left side of the body, insert 2-2.5 units; for the right side, superficial insertion only.

N-BW-23 *(Shenxin)*   肾新   "Kidney New"

Location: 0.3-0.5 unit lateral to B-23 *(Shenshu)*. (Dia. 2-68)
Indications: Rheumatic heart disease.
Method: Slanted insertion at 45° angle, pointed toward the spine, 1.5-2 units.

N-BW-24 *(Zhantan)*   战瘫   "Fight Paralysis"

Location: 2.5 units lateral to the lower end of the spinous process of the 2nd lumbar vertebra. (Dia. 2-68)
Indications: Paraplegia.
Method: Slanted insertion, 3-4 units.

N-BW-25 *(Xishang)*   溪上   "Above the Creek"

Location: 0.3-0.5 unit lateral to the interspinal process between the 4th and 5th lumbar vertebrae. (Dia. 2-68)
Indications: Chronic pain of the lower back and leg.
Other: This is one of the vertebral points, M-BW-35 *(Jiaji)*.

N-BW-26 *(Zhigao)*   制高   "Make High"

Location: At the mid-point above any vertebra, 2 vertebrae above the point of injury on the spine. (Diagram not shown.)
Indications: Paraplegia.
Method: Straight insertion, 1-2 units.

N-BW-27 *(Gaoweishu)*   高位俞   "High Position's Hollow"

Location: 1.5 units lateral to whichever N-BW-26 *(Zhigao)* point is selected. (Diagram not shown.)
Indications: Paraplegia.
Method: Slanted insertion toward spine, 1-1.5 units.

N-BW-28 *(Diwei)*   低位   "Low Position"

Location: At the mid-point below any vertebra, 2 vertebrae below the point of injury on the spine. (Diagram not shown.)
Indications: Paraplegia.
Method: Straight insertion, 1-2 units.

N-BW-29 *(Diweishu)*   低位俞   "Low Position's Hollow"

Location: 1.5 units lateral to whichever N-BW-28 *(Diwei)* point is selected. (Diagram not shown.)
Indications: Paraplegia.
Method: Slanted insertion toward spine, 1-1.5 units.

N-BW-30(a) *(Juejin #1)*   掘进₁   "Dig Forward #1"

Location: 2 units lateral to the mid-point between the 1st and 2nd lumbar vertebrae. (Diagram not shown.)
Indications: Paraplegia.
Method: Slanted insertion toward the spine, 2-2.5 units.

N-BW-30(b) *(Juejin #2)*   掘进₂   "Dig Forward #2"

Location: 2 units lateral to the mid-point between the 2nd and 3rd lumbar vertebrae. (Diagram not shown.)
Indications: Paraplegia.
Method: Same as #1 above.

N-BW-30(c) *(Juejin #3)*   掘进₃   "Dig Forward #3"

Location: 2 units lateral to the mid-point between the 3rd and 4th vertebrae. (Diagram not shown.)
Indications: Paraplegia.
Method: Same as #1 above.

N-BW-30(d) *(Juejin #4)*   掘进₄   "Dig Forward #4"

Location: 2 units lateral to the mid-point between the 4th and 5th lumbar vertebrae. (Diagram not shown.)
Indications: Paraplegia.
Method: Same as #1 above.

N-BW-31 *(Maigen)*   脉根   "Vessel's Root"

Location: 3 units lateral to, and 0.5 unit below the 2nd posterior sacral foramen. (Dia. 2-68)
Indications: Buerger's disease.
Method: Straight insertion, 3-5 units.

N-BW-32 *(Dayan)*   打眼   "Strike Eye"

Location: 2.5 units lateral and 0.5-1 unit posterior to Gv-2 *(Yaoshu)*. (Dia. 2-68)
Indications: Incontinence of urine and feces due to paraplegia.
Method: Straight insertion, 3-4 units.

N-BW-33 *(Libian)*   理便   "Regulate Excretion"

Location: 1 unit lateral to the tip of the coccyx. (Dia. 2-68)
Indications: Same as N-BW-32 *(Dayan)* above.
Method: Straight insertion, 2-3 units.

N-BW-34 *(Bikong)*   闭孔   "Close Hole"

Location: 2 units lateral to the tip of the coccyx. (Dia. 2-68)
Indications: Sciatica, paralysis of the lower limb.
Method: Straight insertion, 3-4 units.

N-BW-35 *(Weigupang)*   尾骨旁   "Beside the Coccyx"

Location: 0.5 unit below Co-1 *(Huiyin)*. (Dia. 2-68)
Indications: Same as N-BW-32 *(Dayan)* above.
Method: Straight insertion, 2-3 units.

N-BW-36 *(Qiahoushangji)*   髂后上棘   "Posterior Superior Iliac Spine"

Location: At the posterior superior iliac spine. (Dia. 2-68)
Indications: Paralysis of the lower limb.
Method: Straight insertion, 1-2 units.

N-BW-37 *(Huanyue)*   环跃   "Encircling"

Location: The point at which a line drawn from the greater trochanter of the femur to the spinous process of the 5th lumbar vertebra crosses a line drawn from the anterior superior iliac spine to the coccyx. (Dia. 2-68)
Indications: Paralysis of the lower limb.
Method: Straight insertion, 2-2.5 units.

N-BW-38 *(Xiajiaoshu)*   下焦俞   "Lower Burner's Hollow"

Location: At the mid-point between Gv-1 *(Changqiang)* and the anus. (Dia. 2-68)
Indications: Chronic schistosomiasis.
Method: Slanted insertion upward, 2-3 units.
Other: Stimulates nerves of the pelvic plexus.

N-BW-39 *(Gangmensixue)* 　　肛门四穴　　 "Four Anal Orifices"

Location: 0.5 unit above, below and on both sides of the anus, 4 points altogether. (Dia. 2-68)
Indications: Same as N-BW-32 *(Dayan)* above.
Method: Straight insertion, 1-2 units.

① N-BW-3 *(Qijingzhuipang)*	⑨ N-BW-24 *(Zhantan)*
② N-BW-2 *(Xueyadian)*	⑩ N-BW-36 *(Qiahoushangji)*
③ N-BW-5 *(Waidingchuan)*	⑪ N-BW-37 *(Huanyue)*
④ N-BW-7 *(Weirexue)*	⑫ N-BW-32 *(Dayan)*
⑤ N-BW-9 *(Jiantongdian)*	⑬ N-BW-33 *(Libian)*
⑥ N-BW-10 *(Pirexue)*	⑭ N-BW-35 *(Weigupang)*
⑦ N-BW-22 *(Zhongjiaoshu)*	⑮ N-BW-1 *(Liujingzhuipang)*
⑧ N-BW-15 *(Shenji)*	⑯ N-BW-6 *(Jiehexue)*
	⑰ N-BW-19 *(Juguxia)*
	⑱ N-BW-20 *(Feirexue)*
	⑲ N-BW-8 *(Ganrexue)*
	⑳ N-BW-11 *(Shenrexue)*
	㉑ N-BW-12 *(Jianming #5)*
	㉒ N-BW-13 *(Kuiyangxue)*
	㉓ N-BW-23 *(Shenxin)*
	㉔ N-BW-14 *(Weishu)*
	㉕ Same as M-BW-24 *(Yaoyan)*
	㉖ N-BW-25 *(Xishang)*
	㉗ N-BW-16 *(Tiaoyue)*
	㉘ N-BW-31 *(Maigen)*
	㉙ N-BW-34 *(Bikong)*
	㉚ N-BW-18 *(Pangqiang)*
	㉛ N-BW-39 *(Gangmensixue)*
	㉜ N-BW-38 *(Xiajiaoshu)*

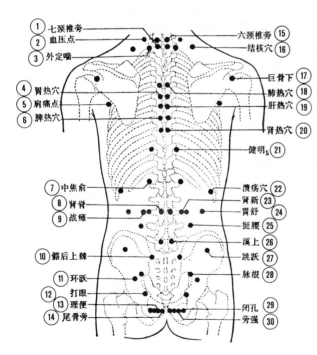

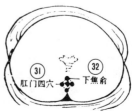

Dia. 2-68

NEW POINTS OF THE UPPER LIMB

N-UE-1 *(Yatong)*　牙痛　"Toothache"

Location: On the palmar surface, between the 3rd and 4th metacarpal bones, 1 unit below the metacarpophalangeal crease. (Dia. 2-70)
Indications: Toothache.
Method: Straight insertion, 0.5 unit.

N-UE-2 *(Nüemen)*　疟门　"Malaria's Door"

Location: On the dorsal surface, between the 3rd and 4th metacarpal bones, at the border between the light and dark skin. (Dia. 2-69)
Indications: Malaria, eye diseases, scabies.
Method: Slanted insertion, 1-1.5 units.

N-UE-3 *(Luolingwu)*　落零五　"Stiff (Neck) One Half"

Location: 0.5 unit above M-UE-24 *(Luozhen)* on the dorsum of the hand. (Dia. 2-69)
Indications: Stomach spasms, hypertension, stiff neck.
Method: Slanted insertion, 0.5-1 unit.

N-UE-4 *(Shanghouxi)*　上后溪　"Upper Back Creek"

Location: Between SI-3 *(Houxi)* and SI-4 *(Wangu)* on the dorsum of the hand, lateral aspect. (Dia. 2-69)
Indications: Deaf-mutism, numbness of the fingers.
Method: Straight insertion, 1-1.5 units.

N-UE-5 *(Xishang)*　郄上　"Above *Xi*"

Location: At the forearm, 3 units above P-4 *(Ximen)*. (Dia. 2-70)
Indications: Palpitations, cardiac valvular disease, mastitis.
Method: Straight insertion, 1-2 units.

N-UE-6 *(Luoshang)*　络上　"Above Connection"

Location: 3 units above TB-5 *(Waiguan)* on the forearm. (Dia. 2-69)
Indications: Paralysis of the upper limb, deafness.
Method: Straight insertion, 1-2 units.

N-UE-7 *(Yingxia)*　鹰下　"Below the Olecranon"

Location: Between the ulna and radius 3 units below the olecranon of the elbow. (Dia. 2-69)
Indications: Paralysis of upper limb, deafness.
Method: Straight insertion, 1-2 units.

352

N-UE-8 *(Niushangxue)*　扭伤穴　"Sprain's Orifice"

Location: ¼ of the distance from LI-11 *(Quchi)* to TB-4 *(Yangchi)* on the forearm. (Dia. 2-69)
Indications: Acute sprain of lower back.
Method: Straight insertion, 1-2 units.
Other: Approximately the same location as LI-9 *(Shanglian)*.

N-UE-10 *(Jubi)*　举臂　"Raise Arm"

Location: At the shoulder, 2 units below N-UE-11 *(Taijian)*. (Dia. 2-70)
Indications: Sequelae of infantile paralysis.
Method: Straight insertion, 1-3 units.

N-UE-11 *(Taijian)*　抬肩　"Lift Shoulder"

Location: 1.5 units below and anterior to the acromion of the shoulder. (Dia. 2-70)
Indications: Sequelae of infantile paaralysis.
Method: Straight insertion, 1-2 units.

N-UE-13 *(Jianming)*　见明　"See Brightness"

Location: About 0.5 unit posterior to the insertion of the deltoid muscle at the upper arm. (Dia. 2-69)
Indications: Eye diseases, paralysis of upper limb.
Method: Slanted insertion upward, 2-3 units.

N-UE-15 *(Hubian)*　虎边　"Beside the Tiger"

Location: On the dorsum of the hand, between LI-3 *(Sanjian)* and LI-4 *(Hegu)*. (Dia. 2-69)
Indications: Hysteria, seizures, psychosis.
Method: Slanted insertion, pointed toward SI-3 *(Houxi)*, 1.5-2.5 units.

N-UE-16 *(Zhizhang)*　指掌　"Finger Palm"

Location: On the palmar surface between the metacarpophalangeal joints of the middle and ring fingers, but closer to the middle finger. (Dia. 2-70)
Indications: Insomnia, progressive loss of memory, seizures, psychosis.
Method: Straight insertion, 1-1.5 units.

N-UE-17 *(Neihegu)*　内合谷　"Inner Adjoining Valleys"

Location: Slightly medial and proximal to the head of the 2nd metacarpal bone, palmar aspect. (Dia. 2-70)
Indications: Stiff neck.
Method: Slanted insertion toward LI-4 *(Hegu)*, 1-1.5 units.

N-UE-18 *(Tongling)*   痛灵   "Painful Spirit"

Location: On the dorsum of the hand between the 3rd and 4th metacarpal bones, 1 unit behind the knuckles. (Dia. 2-69)
Indications: Headache, toothache, stomach-ache.
Method: Slanted insertion toward the wrist, 1-1.5 units.

N-UE-19(a) *(Yaotong #1)*   腰痛₁   "Low Back Pain #1"

Location: On the dorsum of the hand at the articulation of the 2nd and 3rd metacarpal bones. (Dia. 2-69)
Indications: Pain from injury to the head, lower back and limbs.
Method: Slanted insertion toward the wrist, 1-1.5 units.
Other: Same location as M-UE-25 *(Weiling)*.

N-UE-19(b) *(Yaotong #2)*   腰痛₂   "Low Back Pain #2"

Location: On the dorsum of the hand at the articulation of the 3rd and 4th metacarpal bones. (Dia. 2-69)
Indications: Pain from injury to the chest or the limbs.
Method: Same as N-UE-19(a) *(Yaotong #1)* above.

N-UE-19(c) *(Yaotong #3)*   腰痛₃   "Low Back Pain #3"

Location: On the dorsum of the hand at the articulation of the 4th and 5th metacarpal bones. (Dia. 2-69)
Indications: Pain from injury to the lower back and limbs.
Method: Same as N-UE-19(a) *(Yaotong #1)* above.
Other: Same location as M-UE-26 *(Jingling)*.

N-UE-20 *(Sanliwai)*   三里外   "Outside Three Measures"

Location: On the forearm, 2 units below and one finger width lateral to LI-11 *(Quchi)*. (Dia. 2-69)
Indications: Paralysis of the upper limb, sprain.
Method: Straight insertion, 1-2 units.

N-UE-21 *(Xinquchi)*   新曲池   "New Crooked Pool"

Location: On the upper arm, 0.5 unit directly above LI-11 *(Quchi)*. (Dia. 2-69)
Indications: Hypertension.
Method: Straight insertion, 2-3 units.

N-UE-22 *(Shangquchi)*   上曲池   "Upper Crooked Pool"

Location: On the upper arm, 1.5 units above LI-11 *(Quchi)*. (Dia. 2-69)
Indications: Paralysis of upper limb.
Method: Straight insertion, 1.5-2 units.

① N-UE-13 *(Jianming)*
② N-UE-12 *(Yingshang)*
③ N-UE-22 *(Shangquchi)*
④ N-UE-8 *(Niushangxue)*
⑤ N-UE-19(b) *(Yaotong #2)*
⑥ N-UE-19(a) *(Yaotong #1)*
⑦ N-UE-15 *(Hubian)*
⑧ N-UE-3 *(Luolingwu)*
⑨ N-UE-2 *(Nüemen)*

⑩ N-UE-18 *(Tongling)*
⑪ N-UE-4 *(Shanghouxi)*
⑫ N-UE-19(c) *(Yaotong #3)*
⑬ N-UE-6 *(Luoshang)*
⑭ N-UE-7 *(Yingxia)*
⑮ N-UE-20 *(Sanliwai)*
⑯ N-UE-21 *(Xinquchi)*
⑰ N-UE-23 *(Zhiyang)*
⑱ N-UE-24 *(Shenzhou)*

① N-UE-27 *(Zhitan #1)*
② N-UE-11 *(Taijian)*
③ N-UE-26 *(Xiaokuai)*
④ N-UE-25 *(Xiaxiabai)*
⑤ N-UE-5 *(Xishang)*
⑥ N-UE-1 *(Yatong)*
⑦ N-UE-16 *(Zhizhang)*
⑧ N-UE-17 *(Neihegu)*
⑨ N-UE-9 *(Gongzhong)*
⑩ N-UE-10 *(Jubi)*

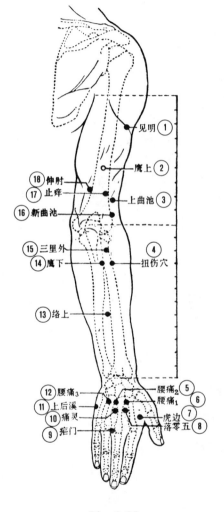

Dia. 2-69

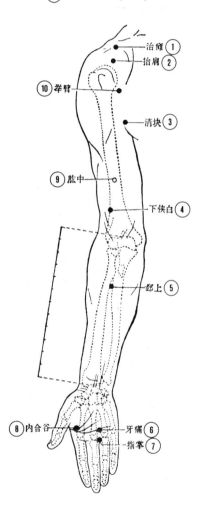

Dia. 2-70

N-UE-23 *(Zhiyang)* 止痒 "Stop Itching"

Location: On the upper arm, 1 unit above LI-12 *(Zhouliao)*. (Dia. 2-69)
Indications: Urticaria, allergic dermatitis, itching symptoms.
Method: Slanted insertion toward the shoulder, 2 units.

355

N-UE-24 *(Shenzhou)*   伸肘   "Extend Elbow"

Location: Three finger widths above the olecranon on the ulnar side. (Dia. 2-69)
Indications: Stiffness of the elbow joint after simple fracture of the arm.
Method: Straight insertion, 1-1.5 units.

N-UE-25 *(Xiaxiabai)*   下侠白   "Lower Gallantry"

Location: On the upper arm, 3 units below L-4 *(Xiabai)*. (Dia. 2-70)
Indications: Rheumatic heart disease, palpitations.
Method: Straight insertion, 1.5-2 units.

N-UE-26 *(Xiaokuai)*   消块   "Eliminate Lump"

Location: At the top of the anterior axillary crease. (Dia. 2-70)
Indications: Breast tumor.
Method: Slanted insertion upward, 1-1.5 units.

N-UE-27 *(Zhitan #1)*   治瘫₁   "Head Paralysis #1"

Location: In the hollow below the acromial end of the clavicle. (Dia. 2-70)
Indications: Hemiplegia due to stroke, diseases of the shoulder joint and surrounding soft tissues.
Method: Straight insertion, 2-3 units.
Other: Same location as M-UE-42 *(Jianshu)*.

NEW POINTS OF THE LOWER LIMB

N-LE-1 *(Zhiping)*   趾平   "Toe Level"

Location: At the midpoint of the transverse crease above the metatarsophalangeal joint on the dorsum of each toe. (Dia. 2-72)
Indications: Sequelae of infantile paralysis, paraplegia.
Method: Slanted insertion, 0.3-0.5 unit.

N-LE-2 *(Panggu)*   旁谷   "Neighboring Valley"

Location: On the dorsum of the foot, 1 unit proximal to the web between the 3rd and 4th toes. (Dia. 2-72)
Indications: Sequelae of infantile paralysis.
Method: Straight insertion, 0.3-0.5 unit.

N-LE-5 *(Jingxia)*   胫下   "Below the Tibia"

Location: 3 units above S-41 *(Jiexi)* and 1 unit from the lateral margin of the tibia. (Dia. 2-73)
Indications: Paralysis of the lower limb, drop foot.
Method: Straight insertion, 0.5-1.5 units.

N-LE-6 *(Wanli)*   万里   "Ten Thousand Measures"

Location: 0.5 unit below S-36 *(Zusanli)*. (Dia. 2-73)
Indications: Night blindness, atrophy of the optic nerve, ametropia, diseases of the gastro-intestinal tract.
Method: Straight insertion, 2-3 units.

N-LE-7 *(Liwai)*   里外   "Outside the Measure"

Location: 1 unit lateral to S-36 *(Zusanli)*. (Dia. 2-73)
Indications: Sequelae of infantile paralysis.
Method: Straight insertion, 1-2 units.

N-LE-8 *(Lishang)*   里上   "Above the Measure"

Location: 1 unit above S-36 *(Zusanli)*. (Dia. 2-73)
Indications: Sequelae of infantile paralysis.
Method: Straight insertion, 1.5-2 units.

N-LE-10(a) *(Jiuwaifan #1)*   纠外翻₁   "Correct Outward Turning #1"

Location: 0.5 unit below Sp-6 *(Sanyinjiao)*. (Dia. 2-75)
Indications: Sequelae of infantile paralysis where foot is turned outward (everted).
Method: Straight insertion, 1-1.5 units.

N-LE-10(b) *(Jiuwaifan #2)*   纠外翻₂   "Correct Outward Turning #2"

Location: 1 unit medial to B-57 *(Chengshan)*. (Dia. 2-74)
Location: 1 unit lateral to B-57 *(Chengshan)*. (Dia. 2-74)
Indications: Same as N-LE-10(a) *(Jiuwaifan #1)* above.

N-LE-11 *(Jiuneifan)*   纠内翻   "Correct Inward Turning"

Location: 1 unit lateral to B-57 *(Chengshan)*. (Dia. 2-74)
Indications: Sequelae of infantile paralysis where foot is turned inward (inverted).
Method: Straight insertion, 1-2 units.

N-LE-12 *(Chengjian)*   承间   "Between Supports"

Location: Between B-57 *(Chengshan)* and B-56 *(Chengjin)*. (Dia. 2-74)
Indications: Sequelae of infantile paralysis.
Method: Straight insertion, 2-3 units.

N-LE-13 *(Shangxi)*   上溪   "Upper Stream"

Location: 0.5 unit above K-3 *(Taixi)*. (Dia. 2-75)
Indications: Foot turned outward (everted).

Method: Straight insertion, 0.5-1 unit.

N-LE-14 *(Ganyandian)*　肝炎点　"Hepatitis Point"

Location: 2 units above the medial malleolus. (Dia. 2-75)
Indications: Hepatitis, enuresis, dysmenorrhea.
Method: Straight insertion, 1-3 units.

N-LE-15 *(Dijian)*　地健　"Ground Strength"

Location: 1 unit below Sp-8 *(Diji)*. (Dia. 2-75)
Indications: Foot turned outward (everted).
Method: Straight insertion, 1-3 units.

N-LE-16 *(Zuyicong)*　足益聪　"Leg Benefit Hearing"

Location: 3 units below the capitulum of the fibula. (Dia. 2-76)
Indications: Deafness, round worm in the bile duct.
Method: Straight or slanted insertion, 1.5-2 units.

N-LE-17 *(Lingxia)*　陵下　"Below the Tomb"

Location: 2 units below GB-34 *(Yanglingquan)*. (Dia. 2-76)
Indications: Deafness, cholecystitis, round worm in the bile duct.
Method: Straight insertion, 1-2 units.

N-LE-18 *(Jianxi)*　健膝　"Strengthen Knee"

Location: With the knee flexed, this point can be found 3 units above the superior margin of the patella. (Dia. 2-73)
Indications: Paralysis of the lower limb, arthritis of the knee.
Method: Straight or slanted insertion, 1-2 units.

N-LE-19 *(Siqiang)*　四强　"Four Strengths"

Method: 4.5 units above the midpoint at the superior margin of the patella. (Dia. 2-73)
Indications: Paralysis of the lower limb.
Method: Straight insertion, 2-2.5 units.

N-LE-20 *(Jixia)*　箕下　"Below the Basket"

Location: 2 units below Sp-11 *(Jimen)*. (Dia. 2-75)
Indications: Paralysis of lower limb, weakness of leg adductors.
Method: Straight insertion, 1-3 units.

N-LE-21 *(Xinfutu)*　新伏兔　"New Hidden Rabbit"

Location: 0.3 unit lateral to S-32 *(Futu)*. (Dia. 2-73)
Indications: Paralysis of the lower limb, arthritis of the knee.
Method: Straight insertion, 2-3 units.

N-LE-24 *(Jiaoling)*　矫灵　"Straightening's Inspiration"

Location: 3 units below Li-10 *(Wuli)*. (Dia. 2-73)
Indications: Sequelae of infantile paralysis, hemiplegia, cholecystitis.
Method: Straight insertion, 1-3 units.

N-LE-25 *(Weishang)*　委上　"Above the Commission"

Location: 2 units above B-54 *(Weizhong)*. (Dia. 2-74)
Indications: Sequelae of infantile paralysis, pain of the leg.
Method: Straight insertion, 1-3 units.
Other: Also said to be situated 3 units above B-54 *(Weizhong)*.

N-LE-26 *(Zhili)*　直立　"Stand Erect"

Location: 4.5 units above, and 0.5 unit medial to B-54 *(Weizhong)*. (Dia. 2-74)
Indications: Sequelae of infantile paralysis.
Method: Straight insertion, 1-3 units.

N-LE-27 *(Waizhili)*　外直立　"Outer Stand Erect"

Location: 4.5 units above, and 1.5 units lateral to B-54 *(Weizhong)*. (Dia. 2-74)
Indications: Same as N-LE-26 *(Zhili)* above.
Method: Straight insertion, 1-3 units.

N-LE-28 *(Yinshang)*　殷上　"Above the Abundance"

Location: 2 units above B-51 *(Yinmen)*. (Dia. 2-74)
Indications: Headache, low back pain, sciatica.
Method: Straight insertion, 1-3 units.

N-LE-29 *(Yinkang)*　阴亢　"Yin's Excess"

Location: 1.5 units medial to B-50 *(Chengfu)*. (Dia. 2-74)
Indications: Sequelae of infantile paralysis, sciatica.
Method: Straight insertion, 1-3 units.

NLE-30 *(Houxuehai)*　后血海　"Posterior Sea of Blood"

Location: 1.5 units posterior to Sp-10 *(Xuehai)*. (Dia. 2-75)
Indications: "Scissor's gait" due to cerebral palsy.
Method: Straight insertion, 1-3 units.

N-LE-31 *(Jiejian)*　解剪　"Open Scissors"

Location: 4 units above N-LE-30 *(Houxuehai)*. (Dia. 2-75)
Indications: Same as N-LE-30 *(Houxuehai)* above.
Method: Straight insertion, 1-3 units.

N-LE-32 *(Houyangguan)*　后陽关　"Posterior Hinge of Yang"

Location: 1 unit posterior to GB-33 *(Xiyangguan)*. (Dia. 2-76)
Indications: Pain of the knee, mental illness, paralysis of lower limb.
Method: Straight insertion, 1-2 units.

N-LE-33 *(Shangyangguan)*　上陽关　"Upper Hinge of Yang"

Location: 1 unit above GB-33 *(Xiyangguan)*. (Dia.2-76)
Indications: Paralysis of the lower limb, arthritis of the knee.
Method: Straight insertion, 1-2 units.

N-LE-34 *(Shangfengshi)*　上风市　"Upper Market of Wind"

Location: 2 units above GB-31 *(Fengshi)*. (Dia. 2-76)
Indications: Hemiplegia, sciatica, sequelae of infantile paralysis.
Method: Straight insertion, 1-2 units.

N-LE-35 *(Qianjin)*　前进　"Advance"

Location: 2.5 units above GB-31 *(Fengshi)*. (Dia. 2-76)
Indications: Sequelae of infantile paralysis, hemiplegia, paraplegia.
Method: Straight insertion, 1-3 units.

N-LE-36 *(Zhiwen)*　趾纹　"Toe's Crease"

Location: At the midpoint of the transverse crease between the big toe and the 1st metatarsal bone on the plantar aspect of the foot. (Dia. 2-71)
Indications: Curled big toe.
Method: Straight insertion, 0.2-0.3 unit, or prick the point to let blood.

N-LE-37 *(Sili)*　四里　"Four Measures"

Location: 1-1.5 units below S-36 *(Zusanli)*, 2 finger widths lateral to the tibia. (Dia. 2-73)
Indications: Infantile paralysis, other forms of paralysis.
Method: Straight insertion, 1.5-2 units.

N-LE-38 *(Zhitan #6)*　治瘫₆　"Treat Paralysis #6"

Location: 1.5 units below M-LE-13 *(Lanwei)*. (Dia. 2-73)
Indications: Paralysis of the lower limb.
Method: Straight insertion, 1-2 units.

N-LE-39 *(Tanfu)* 瘫复 "Paralysis Recovered"

Location: 3 finger widths above the superior, lateral margin of the patella. (Dia. 2-73)
Indications: Paralysis of the lower limb.
Method: Straight insertion, 1-2 units.

N-LE-40 *(Tanli)* 瘫立 "Paralysis Erect"

Location: 5 finger widths above the superior, lateral margin of the patella. (Dia. 2-73)
Indications: Paralysis of the lower limb.
Method: Straight insertion, 1.5-2.5 units.

N-LE-41 *(Tankang)* 瘫康 "Paralysis Health"

Location: 7 finger widths above the superior, lateral margin of the patella. (Dia. 2-73)
Indications: Paralysis of the lower limb.
Method: Straight insertion, 2-3 units.

N-LE-42 *(Qiabinzhong)* 髂髌中 "Between Ilium and Knee"

Location: 3 units above, and 1 unit lateral to S-32 *(Futu)*. (Dia. 2-73)
Indications: Arthritis of the knee, paralysis of the lower limb, low back pain.
Method: Straight insertion, 2-3 units.

N-LE-43 *(Xiachengshan)* 下承山 "Lower Support Mountain"

Location: 0.5 unit below B-57 *(Chengshan)*. (Dia. 2-74)
Indications: Tinea pedis.
Method: Straight insertion, 2-3 units.

N-LE-44 *(Weixia)* 委下 "Below the Commission"

Location: 4 units below, and 1.5 units lateral to B-54 *(Weizhong)*. (Dia. 2-74)
Indications: Sequelae of infantile paralysis, 'concave' hyperextended knee, atrophy of the gastrocnemius muscle.
Method: Straight insertion, 2-3 units.

N-LE-45 *(Yinxia)* 殷下 "Below Abundance"

Location: Midpoint on the line between B-50 *(Chengfu)* and B-54 *(Weizhong)*. (Dia. 2-74)
Indications: Sciatica, low back pain, paralysis of lower limb.
Method: Straight insertion, 1-3 units.

N-LE-46 *(Yangkang)* 陽亢 "Yang's Excess"

Location: 1.5 units lateral to B-50 *(Chengfu)*. (Dia. 2-74)
Indications: Sequelae of infantile paralysis, sciatica.
Method: Straight insertion, 1-3 units.

N-LE-47 *(Xinhuantiao)*　新环跳　"New Encircling Leap"

Location: 3 units lateral to the coccyx. (Dia. 2-74)
Indications: Sciatica, paralysis of the lower limb.
Method: Straight insertion, 3-4 units.

N-LE-48 *(Chuqixue)*　出气穴　"Vent Gas Orifice"

Location: 0.5 unit posterior to K-2 *(Rangu)*. (Dia. 2-75)
Indications: Distension along the gastrointestinal tract with gas in the later stage of cancer of the esophagus.
Method: Slanted insertion, 0.5-1 unit.

N-LE-49 *(Yiniao)*　遗尿　"Incontinence"

Location: 1 unit above Sp-6 *(Sanyinjiao)*. (Dia. 2-75)
Indications: Incontinence.
Method: Straight insertion, 1-1.5 units.

N-LE-50 *(Anmian #4)*　安眠₄　"Peaceful Sleep #4"

Location: 1.5 unit above Sp-6 *(Sanyinjiao)*. (Dia. 2-75)
Indications: Insomnia, irritability.
Method: Straight insertion, 1.5-2 units.

N-LE-51 *(Lijimingandian)*　痢疾敏感点　"Dysentery Sensitivity Point"

Location: 2/5 the distance from the medial malleolus to Sp-9 *(Yinlingquan)*, at the most tender point. (Dia. 2-75)
Indications: Dysentery, sequelae of infantile paralysis.
Method: Straight insertion, 1-2 units.

N-LE-52 *(Shangququan)*　上曲泉　"Upper Crooked Spring"

Location: At the inside of the thigh, 3 units above the medial end of the transverse crease of the knee, behind the femur. (Dia. 2-75)
Indications: Buerger's disease.
Method: Straight insertion, 3-5 units.

N-LE-53 *(Xinsheng)*　新生　"New Life"

Location: 3 units above N-LE-52 *(Shangququan)*. (Dia. 2-75)
Indications: Same as N-LE-52 *(Shangququan)* above.
Method: Straight insertion, 3-5 units.

N-LE-54 *(Shangxuehai)* 上血海 "Upper Sea of Blood"

Location: 3 units above Sp-10 *(Xuehai)*. (Dia. 2-75)
Indications: Paralysis of the lower limb, inability to raise the leg.
Method: Straight insertion, 1-3 units.

N-LE-55 *(Jiankua)* 健胯 "Strengthen Thigh"

Location: Midpoint between the crest of the ilium and the greater trochanter of the femur. (Dia. 2-76)
Indications: Hemiplegia, paraplegia.
Method: Straight insertion, 2-3 units.

N-LE-56 (Kuanjiu) 髋臼 "Acetabulum"

Location: 0.5 unit directly above the greater trochanter of the femur. (Dia. 2-76)
Indications: 'Relaxed' hip joint resulting from infantile paralysis.
Method: Straight insertion, 1.5-2 units.

N-LE-57 *(Qiangkua)* 强胯 "Strong Thigh"

Location: 2 units below the greater trochanter at the posterior margin of the femur. (Dia. 2-76)
Indications: Paraplegia.
Method: Straight insertion, 3-4 units.

N-LE-59 *(Erliban)* 二里半 "Two and a Half Measures"

Location: 0.5 unit above S-36 *(Zusanli)*. (Dia. 2-73)
Indications: Acute gastroenteritis.
Method: Straight insertion, 1.5-2.5 units.

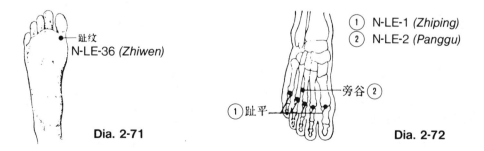

趾纹
N-LE-36 *(Zhiwen)*

Dia. 2-71

① N-LE-1 *(Zhiping)*
② N-LE-2 *(Panggu)*

旁谷②

①趾平

Dia. 2-72

363

①	N-LE-58 (Waiyinlian)	⑩	N-LE-6 (Wanli)	
②	N-LE-23 (Maibu)	⑪	N-LE-38 (Zhitan #6)	
③	N-LE-24 (Jiaoling)	⑫	N-LE-5 (Jingxia)	
④	N-LE-42 (Qiabinzhong)	⑬	N-LE-4 (Naoqing)	
⑤	N-LE-19 (Siqiang)	⑭	N-LE-37 (Sili)	
⑥	N-LE-40 (Tanli)	⑮	N-LE-7 (Liwai)	
⑦	N-LE-18 (Jianxi)	⑯	N-LE-39 (Tanfu)	
⑧	N-LE-8 (Lishang)	⑰	N-LE-41 (Tankang)	
⑨	N-LE-59 (Erliban)	⑱	N-LE-21 (Xinfutu)	

①	N-LE-47 (Xinhuantiao)
②	N-BW-17 (Zuogu)
③	N-LE-29 (Yinkang)
④	N-LE-28 (Yinshang)
⑤	N-LE-45 (Yinxia)
⑥	N-LE-26 (Zhili)
⑦	N-LE-25 (Weishang)
⑧	N-LE-12 (Chengjian)
⑨	N-LE-10(b) (Jiuwaifan #2)
⑩	N-LE-43 (Xiachengshan)
⑪	N-LE-3 (Genping)
⑫	N-LE-46 (Yangkang)
⑬	N-LE-27 (Waizhili)
⑭	N-LE-44 (Weixia)
⑮	N-LE-11 (Jiuneifan)
⑯	N-LE-9 (Luodi)

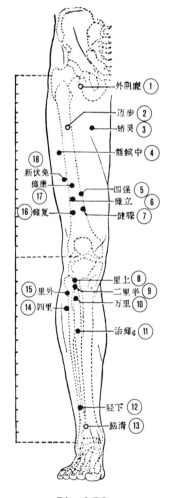

Dia. 2-73

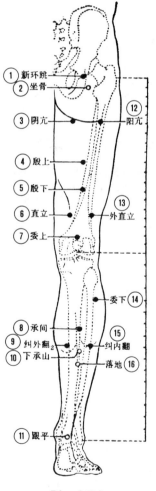

Dia. 2-74

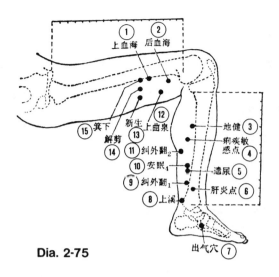

Dia. 2-75

① N-LE-54 (Shangxuehai)
② N-LE-30 (Houxuehai)
③ N-LE-15 (Dijian)
④ N-LE-51 (Lijimingandian)
⑤ N-LE-49 (Yiniao)
⑥ N-LE-14 (Ganyandian)
⑦ N-LE-48 (Chuqixue)
⑧ N-LE-13 (Shangxi)
⑨ N-LE-10(a) (Jiuwaifan #1)
⑩ N-LE-50 (Anmian #4)
⑪ N-LE-10(b) (Jiuwaifan #2)
⑫ N-LE-52 (Shangququan)
⑬ N-LE-53 (Xinsheng)
⑭ N-LE-31 (Jiejian)
⑮ N-LE-20 (Jixia)

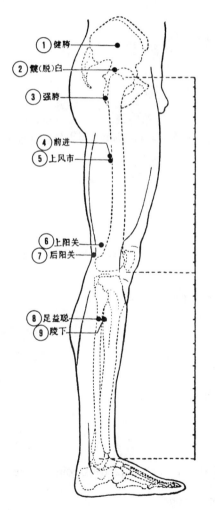

① N-LE-55 (Jiankua)
② N-LE-56 (Kuanjiu)
③ N-LE-57 (Qiangkua)
④ N-LE-35 (Qianjin)
⑤ N-LE-34 (Shangfengshi)
⑥ N-LE-33 (Shangyangguan)
⑦ N-LE-32 (Houyangguan)
⑧ N-LE-16 (Zuyicong)
⑨ N-LE-17 (Lingxia)

Dia. 2-76

Point Clusters (Not illustrated)

Three Needles at the Shoulder　肩三针

Location: Three points: LI-15 *(Jianyu)*, a point one unit above the anterior axillary crease, and a point one unit above the posterior axillary crease.
Indications: Diseases of the shoulder and surrounding soft tissues, paralysis of upper limb.
Method: Straight or slanted insertion, 1.5-2 units.

Four Ankle Points　踝四穴

Location: At the medial malleolus, lateral malleolus, below the Achilles' tendon, and S-41 *(Jiexi)*.
Indications: Spastic paraplegia.
Method: Straight insertion until patient responds.

Three Needles at the Ankle　踝三针

Location: B-60 *(Kunlun)*, S-41 *(Jiexi)*, K-3 *(Taixi)*.
Indications: Paraplegia.
Method: Straight insertion until patient responds.

Three Needles at the Knee　膝三针

Location: S-35 *(Xiyan)* both medial and lateral, and a needle joining GB-34 *(Yanglingquan)* to Sp-9 *(Yinlingquan)*.
Indications: Paraplegia, arthritis of knee.
Method: Straight insertion, 2-3 units.

Four Hand Points　手四穴

Location: About 0.1 unit from the tip of the fingernails on the radial aspect of the thumb and middle fingers of both hands.
Indications: Acute gastroenteritis, dysentery.
Method: Straight insertion, 0.1-0.2 unit, or prick point to let blood.

Four Abdomen Points　腹四穴

Location: On the four sides of the umbilicus.
Indications: Acute gastroenteritis, dysentery.
Method: Prick points with triangular needle, then apply cups.

Three Needles at the Liver　肝三针

Location: Point of tenderness on the back behind the liver region, and two points, one unit to the left and right of the point of tenderness.
Indications: Enlargement of liver, pain in liver region.
Method: Slanted insertion, 0.5-1 unit.

MISCELLANEOUS POINTS OF THE HEAD AND NECK

M-HN-1 *(Sishencong)*   四神聪   "Four Intelligence"

Location: 4 points, 1 unit from Gv-20 *(Baihui),* on each of the four sides. (Dia. 2-77)
Indications: Headache and swollen sensation at the vertex, vertigo, neurasthenia, seizures.
Method: Slanted insertion, 0.5-1 unit.

M-HN-2 *(Ezhong)*   额中   "Forehead's Middle"

Location: 1 unit above M-HN-3 *(Yintang).* (Dia. 2-78)
Indications: Sinusitis, insomnia, palpitations, vertigo.
Method: Slanted insertion, 0.5-1 unit.

M-HN-4 *(Shangen)*   山根   "Mountain's Base"

Location: On the bridge of the nose, midway between the inner canthi of the left and right eyes.
(Dia. 2-78)
Indications: Insomnia, sinusitis.
Method: Slanted insertion, 0.3-0.5 unit.

M-HN-5 *(Touguangming)*   头光明   "Brightness on the Head"

Location: 0.3 unit directly above M-HN-6 *(Yuyao).* (Dia. 2-78)
Indications: Ametropia, neuralgia of the supraorbital nerve, ptosis.
Method: Slanted insertion, 0.3-0.5 unit.

M-HN-7 *(Yuwei)*   鱼尾   "Fish Tail"

Location: Approximately 0.1 unit lateral to the outer canthus of the eye. (Dia. 2-78)
Indications: Migraine headache, facial paralysis or spasm.
Method: Slanted insertion, 0.3-0.5 unit.

M-HN-10 *(Erjian)*   耳尖   "Ear Tip"

Location: When the ear is bent forward, this point can be found at the tip of the auricle. (Dia. 2-82)
Indications: Conjunctivitis, high fever, pannus.
Method: Straight insertion, 0.1-0.2 unit, or prick to let blood.

M-HN-12 *(Erbeijingmaisantiao)*   "Three Branches of Vein on Dorsum of Ear"

耳背静脉三条

Location: On the 3 veins at the back of the auricle. (Dia. 2-83)
Indications: Conjunctivitis, hypertension, skin diseases.
Method: Prick to let blood.

M-HN-16 *(Biliu)*   鼻流   "Runny Nose"

Location: Between the septum nasi and the ala nasi at the outer nostril. (Dia. 2-78)
Indications: Rhinitis, trigeminal neuralgia, facial paralysis.
Method: Slanted insertion, 0.3-0.5 unit.

M-HN-17 *(Sanxiao)*   散笑   "Spread Smile"

Location: In the middle of the nasolabial sulcus, lateral and posterior to LI-20 *(Yingxiang)*. (Dia. 2-78)
Indications: Rhinitis, nasal furuncle, facial paralysis or spasm.
Method: Slanted insertion, 0.3-0.5 unit.

M-HN-19 *(Dihe)*   地合   "Earth's Union"

Location: The prominence at the middle of the mandible. (Dia. 2-78)
Indications: Toothache (lower jaw), facial paralysis.
Method: Slanted insertion, 0.3-0.5 unit.

M-HN-20 *(Jinjin, Yuye)*   金津、玉液   "Gold Fluid, Jade Fluid"

Location: At the veins on the 2 sides of the vinculum linguae, when the tongue is rolled back. Left side is *Jinjin,* right side is *Yuye.* (Dia. 2-81)
Indications: Stomatitis, glossitis, tonsillitis, acute gastritis, symptoms of emaciation and thirst, aphasia.
Method: Prick to let blood.

M-HN-22 *(Waijinjin, Yuye)*   外金津、玉液   "Outer Gold Fluid, Jade Fluid"

Location: With the head back, this point can be found 1 unit above the laryngeal prominence and 0.3 unit lateral to the midline of the neck. Left side is *Waijinjin,* on right is *Yuye.* (Dia. 2-84)
Indications: Aphasia due to stroke, paralysis of muscles of tongue, stomatitis.
Method: Slanted insertion toward root of tongue, 1-1.5 units.

M-HN-23 *(Hongyin)*   洪音   "Huge Sound"

Location: 0.5 unit lateral to laryngeal prominence. (Dia. 2-84)
Indications: Acute and chronic laryngitis, diseases of the vocal cords.
Method: Straight insertion, 0.3-0.5 unit.

M-HN-24 *(Panglianquan)*   旁廉泉   "Beside Spring of Integrity"

Location: 0.5 unit lateral to Co-23 *(Lianquan).* (Dia. 2-84)
Indications: Diseases of vocal cords, swollen tongue.
Method: Straight insertion, 0.5-1 unit.

M-HN-25 *(Yaxue)*   哑穴   "Mute Orifice"

Location: 4 points altogether. Two points are approximately 0.2 unit lateral to the midpoint between S-9 *(Renying)* and S-10 *(Shuitu)*. The other two points are on the back of the neck, about 0.4 unit above GB-20 *(Fengchi)*. (Dia. 2-82)
Indications: Deaf-mutism, diseases of vocal cords.
Method: Two points on front of neck, straight insertion, 1 unit. CAUTION: Avoid carotid artery. Two points on back of neck, straight insertion, 1-1.5 units.

M-HN-27 *(Luojing)*   落颈   "Stiff Neck"

Location: Below N-HN-24 *(Ronghou)* in the middle of the sternocleidomastoid muscle, about ⅓ the distance from the top of the muscle. (Dia. 2-82)
Indications: Stiff neck.
Method: Straight insertion, 1-1.5 units.

M-HN-28 *(Fengyan)*   风岩   "Wind's Cliff"

Location: About 0.5 unit in front of the midpoint between the inferior margin of the earlobe and Gv-15 *(Yamen)*. (Dia. 2-82)
Indications: Insanity, neurasthenia, hysteria, headache, sequelae of brain disease.
Method: Straight insertion, 1.5-2 units.

M-HN-29 *(Xinshi)*   新识   "New Recognition"

Location: 1.5 units lateral to the lower end of the spinous process of the 3rd cervical vertebra. (Dia. 2-85)
Indications: Stiff neck, occipital headache, sore throat.
Method: Straight insertion, 0.5-1 unit.

M-HN-30 *(Bailao)*   百劳   "Hundred Labors"

Location: 2 units above and 1 unit lateral to Gv-14 *(Dazhui)*. (Dia. 2-85)
Indications: Cough, stiff neck, scrofula.
Method: Straight insertion, 0.5-1 unit.

M-HN-31 *(Chonggu)*   崇骨   "Lofty Bone"

Location: Below the spinous process of the 6th cervical vertebra. (Dia. 2-85)
Indications: Common cold, malaria, stiff neck, bronchitis, seizures.
Method: Straight insertion, 0.5-1 unit.

M-HN-32 *(Muming)*   目明   "Vision Bright"

Location: On the border of the hairline at the forehead, directly above the pupil, 0.5 unit below GB-15 *(Linqi)*. (Dia. 2-78)
Indications: Headache, conjunctivitis, diminishing vision.
Method: Slanted insertion, 0.5-1 unit.

M-HN-33 *(Neijingming)*　内睛明　"Inner Eyes Bright"

Location: Just above the lacrimal caruncle at the inner canthus of the eye, medial to B-1 *(Jingming)*. (Dia. 2-78)
Indications: Bleeding of the retina, atrophy of optic nerve, conjunctivitis.
Method: Straight insertion, 1-1.5 units.

M-HN-34 *(Yankou)*　燕口　"Swallow's Mouth"

Location: At the corner of the mouth, on the border between the lip and cheek. (Dia. 2-78)
Indications: Facial paralysis, trigeminal neuralgia, infantile convulsions, retention of urine, constipation.
Method: Slanted insertion, 0.5-1 unit.

M-HN-35 *(Neiyingxiang)*　内迎香　"Inner Welcome Fragrance"

Location: In the mucous membrane of the nose, at the superior end near the opening of the nostril. (Dia. 2-79)
Indications: Conjunctivitis, laryngitis, heat exhaustion.
Method: Prick to let blood.

M-HN-36 *(Juquan)*　聚泉　"Gathering Spring"

Location: In the center of the dorsum of the tongue. (Dia. 2-80)
Indications: Paralysis of lingual muscles, asthma, symptoms of emaciation and thirst.
Method: Straight insertion, 0.3 unit.

M-HN-37 *(Haiquan)*　海泉　"Sea's Spring"

Location: In the center of the frenum linguae on the underside of the tongue. (Dia. 2-81)
Indications: Spasm of diaphragm, symptoms of emaciation and thirst, glossitis.
Method: Prick to let blood.

M-HN-38 *(Shezhu)*　舌柱　"Tongue's Pillar"

Location: At the intersection of the frenum linguae and the sublingual fold on the underside of the tongue. (Dia. 2-81)
Indications: Heavy tongue, symptoms of emaciation and thirst.
Method: Prick to let blood.

M-HN-39 *(Zhuding)*　珠顶　"Pearl's Top"

Location: At the tip of the tragus of the ear. (Dia. 2-82)
Indications: Toothache, diseases of the ear.
Method: Straight insertion, 0.3 unit.

M-HN-40 *(Damen)*　大门　"Big Door"

Location: On the median line at the vertex of the head, 0.5 unit behind Gv-18 *(Qiangjian)*. (Dia. 2-85)

Indications: Apoplectic hemiplegia.

Method: Not specified.

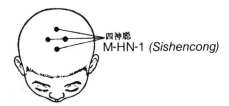

Dia. 2-77

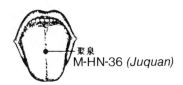

Dia. 2-80

① M-HN-32 *(Muming)*
② M-HN-3 *(Yintang)*
③ M-HN-6 *(Yuyao)*
④ M-HN-33 *(Neijingming)*
⑤ M-HN-14 *(Bitong)*
⑥ M-HN-17 *(Sanxiao)*
⑦ M-HN-18 *(Jiachengjiang)*
⑧ M-HN-19 *(Dihe)*
⑨ M-HN-2 *(Ezhong)*
⑩ M-HN-5 *(Touguangming)*
⑪ M-HN-7 *(Yuwei)*
⑫ M-HN-8 *(Qiuhou)*
⑬ M-HN-4 *(Shangen)*
⑭ M-HN-16 *(Biliu)*
⑮ M-HN-34 *(Yankou)*

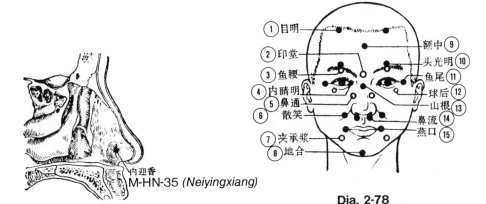

Dia. 2-79

Dia. 2-78

Note: ● signifies less commonly used Miscellaneous points
　　　○ signifies more commonly used Miscellaneous points

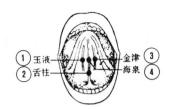

① M-HN-20 *(Yuye)*
② M-HN-38 *(Shezhu)*
③ M-HN-20 *(Jinjin)*
④ M-HN-37 *(Haiquan)*

Dia. 2-81

① M-HN-39 *(Zhuding)*   ⑤ M-HN-28 *(Fengyan)*
② M-HN-9 *(Taiyang)*   ⑥ M-HN-26 *(Biantao)*
③ M-HN-10 *(Erjian)*   ⑦ M-HN-27 *(Luojing)*
④ M-HN-25 *(Yaxue)*   ⑧ M-HN-25 *(Yaxue)*

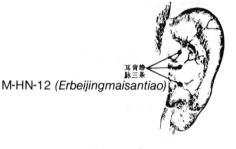

M-HN-12 *(Erbeijingmaisantiao)*

Dia. 2-83

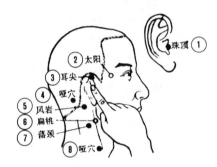

Dia. 2-82

① M-HN-40 *(Damen)*
② M-HN-30 *(Bailao)*
③ M-HN-29 *(Xinshi)*
④ M-HN-31 *(Chonggu)*

① M-HN-22 *(Waiyuye)*
② M-HN-24 *(Panglianquan)*
③ M-HN-21 *(Shanglianquan)*
④ M-HN-22 *(Waijinjin)*
⑤ M-HN-23 *(Hongyin)*

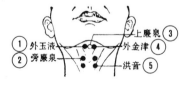

Dia. 2-84

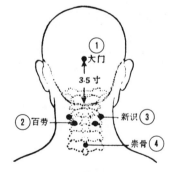

Dia. 2-85

MISCELLANEOUS POINTS OF THE CHEST AND ABDOMEN

M-CA-1 *(Chixue)*   赤穴   "Red Orifice"

Location: 1 unit lateral to Co-21 *(Xuanji)*. (Dia. 2-86)
Indications: Cough, asthma, intercostal neuralgia.
Method: Slanted insertion, 0.5-1 unit.

M-CA-2 *(Tanchuan)*   痰喘   "Phelgm and Wheezing"

Location: 1.8 units lateral to S-16 *(Yingchuang)*. (Dia. 2-86)
Indications: Chronic bronchitis, asthma.
Method: Slanted insertion, 0.5-1 unit.

M-CA-3 *(Longhan)*   龙颔   "Dragon Jaw"

Location: 1.5 units directly above Co-15 *(Jiuwei)*. (Dia. 2-86)
Indications: Chest pains, stomach-ache.
Method: Slanted insertion, 0.5-1 unit.

M-CA-4 *(Zuoyi, Youyi)*   左宜、右宜   "Right and Left Propriety"

Location: About 1 unit lateral to the base of each breast. (Dia. 2-86)
Indications: Mastitis, intercostal neuralgia, pleurisy, endocarditis.
Method: Slanted insertion, 0.3-0.5 unit.

M-CA-5 *(Meihua)*   梅花   "Plum Blossom"

Location: 5 points including Co-12 *(Zhongwan)* on the median line, and 0.5 unit above and below
K-19 *(Yindu)*, bilaterally. (Dia. 2-86)
Indications: Indigestion, gastric ulcer, gastritis.
Method: Straight insertion, 1-1.5 units.

M-CA-6 *(Shicang)*   食仓   "Grainery"

Location: 3 units lateral to Co-12 *(Zhongwan)*. (Dia. 2-86)
Indications: Stomach-ache, prolapsed stomach, ulcers.
Method: Straight insertion, 1-1.5 units.

M-CA-7 *(Shiguan)*   食关   "Food's Gate"

Location: 1 unit lateral to Co-11 *(Jianli)*. (Dia. 2-86)
Indications: Indigestion, gastritis, enteritis.
Method: Straight insertion, 1-1.5 units.

M-CA-8 *(Qisibian)* 脐四边 "Four Sides of Navel"

Location: 4 points altogether, about 1 unit above, below, and to the left and right of the navel. (Dia. 2-86)
Indications: Acute gastroenteritis, stomach spasm, edema, indigestion.
Method: Straight insertion, 1-1.5 units; moxibustion or cups may also be used.

M-CA-10 *(Qizhong)* 气中 "Middle of Qi"

Location: 1.5 units lateral to Co-6 *(Qihai)*. (Dia. 2-86)
Indications: Intestinal spasm, abdominal distension, intestinal noises, enteritis, anemia.
Method: Straight insertion, 1-1.5 units.

M-CA-11 *(Jingzhong)* 经中 "Middle of Channel"

Location: 3 units lateral to Co-6 *(Qihai)*. (Dia. 2-86)
Indications: Enteritis, irregular menstruation, retention of urine.
Method: Straight insertion, 1-1.5 units.

M-CA-12 *(Waisiman)* 外四满 "Outer Four Full"

Location: 1 unit lateral to K-14 *(Siman)*. (Dia. 2-86)
Indications: Irregular menstruation.
Method: Use moxibustion.

M-CA-13 *(Jueyun)* 绝孕 "Miscarriage"

Location: 0.3 unit below Co-5 *(Shimen)*. (Dia. 2-86)
Indications: Infantile diarrhea, miscarriage.
Method: Use moxibustion.

M-CA-14 *(Yijing)* 遗精 "Spermatorrhea"

Location: 1 unit lateral to Co-4 *(Guanyuan)*. (Dia. 2-86)
Indications: Spermatorrhea, permature ejaculation, impotence, eczema of scrotum.
Method: Straight insertion, 1-1.5 units.

M-CA-15 *(Qimen)* 气门 "Qi's Door"

Location: 3 units lateral to Co-4 *(Guanyuan)*. (Dia. 2-86)
Indications: Colic, abnormal uterine bleeding.
Method: Straight insertion, 1-1.5 units.

M-CA-17 *(Changyi)* 腸遗 "Intestinal Remnant"

Location: 2.5 units lateral to Co-3 *(Zhongji)*. (Dia. 2-86)
Indications: Penile pain, orchitis, irregular menstruation, adnexitis.
Method: Straight insertion, 1-1.5 units.

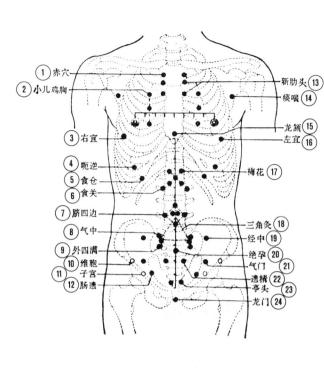

① M-CA-1 *(Chixue)*
② M-CA-22 *(Xiaoerjixiong)*
③ M-CA-4 *(Youyi)*
④ M-CA-21 *(Eni)*
⑤ M-CA-6 *(Shicang)*
⑥ M-CA-7 *(Shiguan)*
⑦ M-CA-8 *(Qisibian)*
⑧ M-CA-10 *(Qizhong)*
⑨ M-CA-12 *(Waisiman)*
⑩ M-CA-16 *(Weibao)*
⑪ M-CA-18 *(Zigong)*
⑫ M-CA-17 *(Changyi)*
⑬ M-CA-20 *(Xinleitou)*
⑭ M-CA-2 *(Tanchuan)*
⑮ M-CA-3 *(Longhan)*
⑯ M-CA-4 *(Zuoyi)*
⑰ M-CA-5 *(Meihua)*
⑱ M-CA-23 *(Sanjiaojiu)*
⑲ M-CA-11 *(Jingzhong)*
⑳ M-CA-13 *(Jueyun)*
㉑ M-CA-15 *(Qimen)*
㉒ M-CA-14 *(Yijing)*
㉓ M-CA-19 *(Tingtou)*
㉔ M-CA-24 *(Longmen)*

Dia. 2-86

M-CA-19 *(Tingtou)* 亭头 "Erect Head"

Location: 0.5 unit below K-12 *(Dahe)*. (Dia. 2-86)
Indications: Prolapsed uterus.
Method: Straight insertion, 1-1.5 units.

M-CA-20 *(Xinleitou)* 新肋头 "New Rib's Head"

Location: In the 1st and 2nd intercostal spaces, beside the sternum. (Dia. 2-86)
Indications: Intercostal neuralgia, bronchitis, asthma, costal chondritis.
Method: Slanted insertion, 0.3-0.5 unit.

M-CA-21 *(Eni)* 呃逆 "Hiccough"

Location: In the 7th intercostal space, directly below the nipple. (Dia. 2-86)
Indications: Hiccoughs.
Method: Slanted insertion, 0.3-0.5 unit; or use moxibustion.

M-CA-22 *(Xiaoerjixiong)* 小儿鸡胸 "Infantile Chicken Breast"

Location: In the 2nd, 3rd, and 4th intercostal spaces, about 2.5 units lateral to the median line of the thorax. (Dia. 2-86)

375

Indications: Chicken breast.
Method: Use moxibustion.

M-CA-23 *(Sanjiaojiu)*   三角灸   "Triangle Moxibustion"

Location: Construct an equilateral triangle whose apex is the navel, and whose sides are equal to the length of the patient's smile. These points are located at the three corners of the triangle. (Dia. 2-86)
Indications: Chronic enteritis, colic, stomach spasm, abdominal pain.
Method: Use moxibustion.

M-CA-24 *(Longmen)*   龙门   "Dragon's Gate"

Location: Inferior border of the pubic symphysis. (Dia. 2-86)
Indications: Abnormal uterine bleeding, incontinence, infertility (of women).
Method: Slanted insertion, 0.5-1 unit.

MISCELLANEOUS POINTS OF THE BACK

M-BW-2 *(Baizhongfeng)*   百种风   "Hundred Kinds of Wind"

Location: 2.3 units lateral to Gv-14 *(Dazhui)*. (Dia. 2-87)
Indications: Apoplexy, pain in back of shoulder, urticaria.
Method: Slanted insertion, 0.5-1 unit.

M-BW-3 *(Liuhua, Bahua)*   六华、八华   "Six Flowers, Eight Flowers"

Location: These are six or eight point configurations distributed 1 unit lateral to the spine, between the 2nd and 7th thoracic vertebrae. To find them, make an equilateral triangle 2 units on a side with its apex at Gv-14 *(Dazhui)*. The other two corners are the locations of the first two points. This process is then repeated with the apex of the triangle at the mid-point between the first two points, the other two corners being the third and fourth points. Repeated a third time, there are six points; and a fourth, eight points. (Dia. 2-87)
Indications: Bronchitis, asthma, pulmonary tuberculosis, anemia, general weakness due to chronic disease.
Method: Slanted insertion toward the spine, 0.5-1 unit; for chronic disease use moxibustion.

M-BW-5 *(Erzhuixia)*   二椎下   "Below Second Vertebra"

Location: Below the spinous process of the 2nd thoracic vertebra. (Dia. 2-87)
Indications: Mental disease, seizures, malaria.
Method: Slanted insertion, 0.5-1.5 units.

M-BW-6 *(Huanmen)*   患门   "Affliction's Door"

Location: Slightly above B-15 *(Xinshu)*. (Dia. 2-87)
Indications: Bronchitis, asthma, pulmonary tuberculosis, general weakness caused by chronic illness.
Method: Use moxibustion.

M-BW-7 *(Juqueshu)*　巨阙俞　"Great Palace Hollow"

Location: Below the spinous process of the 4th thoracic vertebra. (Dia. 2-87)
Indications: Bronchitis, asthma, heart disease, neurasthenia, stomach diseases.
Method: Slanted insertion, 0.5-1 unit.

M-BW-9 *(Qichuan)*　气喘　"Wheezing"

Location: 2 units lateral to the spinous process of the 7th thoracic vertebra. (Dia. 2-87)
Indications: Bronchitis, asthma, pleurisy.
Method: Slanted insertion toward the spine, 0.5-1 unit.

M-BW-10 *(Yinkou)*　银口　"Silver Mouth"

Location: At the inferior angle of the scapula. (Dia. 2-87)
Indications: Intercostal neuralgia, injury to soft tissues of the back.
Method: Slanted insertion toward the spine, 0.5-1 unit.

M-BW-11 *(Bazhuixia)*　八椎下　"Below Eighth Vertebra"

Location: Below the spinous process of the 8th thoracic vertebra. (Dia. 2-87)
Indications: Malaria, intercostal neuralgia, diabetes, hepatitis.
Method: Slanted insertion, 0.5-1 unit.

M-BW-12 *(Yishu)*　胰俞　"Pancreas Hollow"

Location: 1.5 units lateral to the spinous process of the 8th thoracic vertebra. (Dia. 2-87)
Indications: Diabetes, stomach diseases, intercostal neuralgia.
Method: Slanted insertion toward the spine, 0.5-1 unit.

M-BW-13 *(Shubian)*　枢边　"Beside the Axis"

Location: 1 unit lateral to the spinous process of the 10th thoracic vertebra. (Dia. 2-87)
Indications: Stomach diseases, diseases of the liver and gall bladder.
Method: Slanted insertion toward the spine, 0.5-1 unit.

M-BW-14 *(Zhuoyu)*　浊浴　"Bathing the Unclean"

Location: 2.5 units lateral to the spinous process of the 10th thoracic vertebra. (Dia. 2-87)
Indications: Anorexia, diseases of the liver and gall bladder.
Method: Slanted insertion toward the spine, 0.5-1 unit.

M-BW-15 *(Jiegu)*　接骨　"Connecting Bone"

Location: Below the spinous process of the 12th thoracic vertebra. (Dia. 2-87)
Indications: Stomach-ache, enteritis, lumbago, seizures.
Method: Slanted insertion, 0.5-1 unit.

M-BW-16 *(Pigen)* 痞根 "Lump's Root"

Location: 3.5 units lateral to the spinous process of the 1st lumbar vertebra. (Dia. 2-87)
Indications: Enlargement of the liver or spleen, gastritis, enteritis, prolapsed kidney.
Method: Straight insertion, 1-1.5 units.

M-BW-17 *(Xuechou)* 血愁 "Blood Worry"

Location: Above the spinous process of the 2nd lumbar vertebra. (Dia. 2-87)
Indications: Hemorrhagic diseases.
Method: Straight insertion, 1-1.5 units.

M-BW-18 *(Changfeng)* 腸风 "Intestinal Wind"

Location: 1 unit lateral to the spinous process of the 2nd lumbar vertebra. (Dia. 2-87)
Indications: Gastrointestinal diseases, enuresis, spermatorrhea.
Method: Straight insertion, 1-1.5 units.

M-BW-19 *(Xuefu)* 血府 "Blood's Residence"

Location: 4 units lateral to the spinous process of the 2nd lumbar vertebra. (Dia. 2-87)
Indications; Amenorrhea, swelling of the ovaries, spermatorrhea, enlargement of the spleen or liver.
Method: Straight insertion, 1-1.5 units.

M-BW-20 *(Zhuzhang)* 竹杖 "Bamboo Cane"

Location: Above the spinous process of the 3rd lumbar vertebra. (Dia. 2-87)
Indications: Enteritis, intestinal tuberculosis, prolapsed anus, hemorrhoids, sequelae of encephalitis or infantile paralysis.
Method: Use moxibustion.
Other: Location same as Gv-4 *(Mingmen)*.

M-BW-21 *(Xiajishu)* 下极俞 "Lower Level Hollow"

Location: Below the spinous process of the 3rd lumbar vertebra. (Dia. 2-87)
Indications: Low back pain, cystitis, paralysis of lower limb.
Method: Slanted insertion, 1-1.5 units.

M-BW-23 *(Yaoyi)* 腰宜 "Lower Back Propriety"

Location: 3 units lateral to the spinous process of the 4th lumbar vertebra. (Dia. 2-87)
Indications: Injury to the soft tissues of the lower back, gynecological diseases.
Method: Straight insertion, 1-2 units.

M-BW-26 *(Zhongkong)* 中空 "Middle Space"

Location: 3.5 units lateral to the spinous process of the 5th lumbar vertebra. (Dia. 2-87)
Indications: Injury to the soft tissues of the lower back.
Method: Straight insertion, 1.5-2 units.

M-BW-27 *(Yaogen)* 腰根 "Lower Back's Root"

Location: 3 units lateral to the 1st sacral spinous process. (Dia. 2-87)
Indications: Diseases of the sacro-iliac joint, diseases of the lower limbs.
Method: Straight insertion, 3 units.

M-BW-28 *(Jiuqi)* 鸠杞 "Wild Pigeon Willow"

Location: Below the spinous process of the 1st sacral vertebra. (Dia. 2-87)
Indications: Abnormal uterine bleeding, leukorrhagia.
Method: Use moxibustion.

M-BW-29 *(Yaoqi)* 腰奇 "Lower Back's Miscellany"

Location: Below the spinous process of the 2nd sacral vertebra. (Dia. 2-87)
Indications: Seizures.
Method: Slanted insertion upward, 2-2.5 units.

M-BW-30 *(Xiazhui)* 下椎 "Lower Vertebra"

Location: Below spinous process of the 3rd sacral vertebra. (Dia. 2-87)
Indications: Irregular menstruation, pelvic inflammatory diseases.
Method: Slanted insertion, 0.5-1 unit.

M-BW-31 *(Yutian)* 玉田 "Jade Field"

Location: Below the spinous process of the 4th sacral vertebra. (Dia. 2-87)
Indications: Low back pain, spasm of the gastrocnemius muscle, prolonged labor.
Method: Slanted insertion, 0.5-1 unit, or use moxibustion.

M-BW-32 *(Pinxueling)* 贫血灵 "Anemic's Inspiration"

Location: 0.3 unit below M-BW-31 *(Yutian).* (Dia 2-87)
Indications: Anemia.
Method: Use moxibustion.

M-BW-33 *(Tunzhong)* 臀中 "Middle of Buttock"

Location: This point is at the apex of an imaginary equilateral triangle whose base is a line drawn between the superior, posterior side of the greater trochanter of the femur to the ischial tuberosity. (Dia. 2-87)

Indications: Sciatica, paraplegia affecting lower limb.
Method: Straight insertion, 2-3 units.

M-BW-34 *(Huanzhong)*   环中   "Circle's Middle"

Location: At the mid-point between GB-30 *(Huantiao)* and Gv-2 *(Yaoshu)*. (Dia. 2-87)
Indications: Sciatica, low back pain, pain of the leg.
Method: Straight insertion, 2-3 units.

① M-BW-2 *(Baizhongfeng)*
② M-BW-3 *(Liuhua, Bahua)*
③ M-BW-9 *(Qichuan)*
④ M-BW-10 *(Yinkou)*
⑤ M-BW-12 *(Yishu)*
⑥ M-BW-11 *(Bazhuixia)*
⑦ M-BW-13 *(Shubian)*
⑧ M-BW-15 *(Jiegu)*
⑨ M-BW-16 *(Pigen)*
⑩ M-BW-19 *(Xuefu)*
⑪ M-BW-20 *(Zhuzhang)*
⑫ M-BW-24 *(Yaoyan)*
⑬ M-BW-25 *(Shiqizhuixia)*
⑭ M-BW-26 *(Zhongkong)*
⑮ M-BW-28 *(Jiuqi)*
⑯ M-BW-30 *(Xiazhui)*
⑰ M-BW-32 *(Pinxueling)*

⑱ M-BW-34 *(Huanzhong)*
⑲ M-BW-31 *(Yutian)*
⑳ M-BW-33 *(Tunzhong)*
㉑ M-BW-29 *(Yaoqi)*
㉒ M-BW-27 *(Yaogen)*
㉓ M-BW-23 *(Yaoyi)*
㉔ M-BW-21 *(Xiajishu)*
㉕ M-BW-18 *(Changfeng)*
㉖ M-BW-17 *(Xuechou)*
㉗ M-BW-36 *(Dianxian)*
㉘ M-BW-14 *(Zhuoyu)*
㉙ "Four Flowers"
㉚ M-BW-7 *(Juqueshu)*
㉛ M-BW-6 *(Huanmen)*
㉜ M-BW-5 *(Erzhuixia)*
㉝ M-BW-1 *(Dingchuan)*

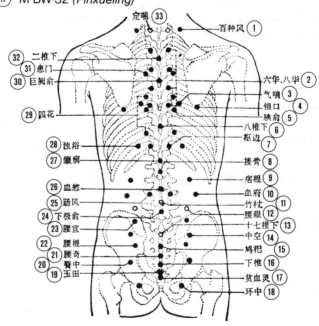

Dia. 2-87

380

M-BW-36 *(Dianxian)* 癲癇 "Epilepsy"

Location: At the mid-point of a line drawn from Gv-14 *(Dazhui)* to the end of the coccyx. This is (usually) the spinous process of the 11th thoracic vertebra. (Dia. 2-87)
Indications: Epilepsy (seizures).
Method: Use moxibustion.

M-BW-37 *(Jisanxue)* 脊三穴 "Three Vertebral Orifices"

Location: 1 unit below and 0.5 unit lateral to Gv-15 *(Yamen)*; 0.5 unit lateral to the 2nd thoracic vertebra; 0.5 unit lateral to the 2nd lumbar vertebra. (Diagram not shown.)
Indications: Spondylitis, myelitis, neuralgia of the back and other spinal and spinal cord disorders.
Method: Slanted insertion, 0.5-1 unit, or use moxibustion.

M-BW-38 *(Jifeng)* 脊縫 "Vertebral Seam"

Location: 4.5 units lateral to the interspinous spaces from the 1st thoracic to the 5th lumbar vertebra. (Diagram not shown.)
Indications: Spondylitis, myelitis.
Method: Slanted insertion, 0.3-0.7 unit. CAUTION: Piercing deeply may injure the internal organs.

MISCELLANEOUS POINTS OF THE UPPER LIMB

M-UE-6 *(Muzhijiehengwen)* 拇指节横纹 "Transverse Crease of Thumb Joint"

Location: At the middle of the transverse crease of the phalangeal joint of the thumb, palmar aspect. (Dia. 2-89)
Indications: Corneal nebula or pannus.
Method: Use moxibustion.

M-UE-7 *(Fengyan)* 凤眼 "Wind's Ear"

Location: At the radial end of the transverse crease of the phalangeal joint of the thumb. (Dia. 2-89)
Indications: Night blindness.
Method: Prick the point.

M-UE-8 *(Mingyan)* 明眼 "Bright Eyes"

Location: At the ulnar end of the transverse crease of the phalangeal joint of the thumb. (Dia. 2-88)
Indications: Night blindness, conjunctivitis, tonsillitis, infantile gastro-intestinal diseases.
Method: Prick the point.

M-UE-10 *(Shouzhongping)* 手中平 "Mid-Hand Level"

Location: At the middle of the transverse crease of the metacarpophalangeal joint of the middle finger, palmar aspect. (Dia. 2-89)

Indications: Stomatitis.
Method: Straight insertion, 0.2-0.3 unit.

M-UE-11 *(Panglaogong)* 旁劳宫 "Beside Labor's Palace"

Location: About 1 finger width to the ulnar side of P-8 *(Laogong)*. (Dia. 2-89)
Indications: Tonsillitis, numbness of the fingers, toothache.
Method: Straight insertion, 0.3-0.5 unit.

M-UE-12 *(Neiyangchi)* 内陽池 "Inner Yang's Pool"

Location: 1 unit distal to the middle of the transverse crease of the wrist, palmar aspect. (Dia. 2-89)
Indications: 'Swan palm' paralysis, stomatitis, infantile convulsions.
Method: Straight insertion, 0.3-0.5 unit.

M-UE-13 *(Banmen)* 板门 "Board's Door"

Location: 1 unit medial to the thenar eminence of the palm. (Dia. 2-89)
Indications: Asthma, tonsillitis.
Method: Straight insertion, 0.3-0.5 unit.

M-UE-14 *(Sanshang)* 三商 "Three Merchants"

Location: 3 points in a line at the tip of the thumb. (Dia. 2-88)
Indications: Influenza, tonsillitis, high fever, parotitis.
Method: Prick the points.

M-UE-15 *(Dagukong)* 大骨空 "Big Bone's Space"

Location: At the middle of the transverse crease of the phalangeal joint of the thumb, dorsal aspect. (Dia. 2-88)
Indications: Eye diseases, vomiting and diarrhea.
Method: Use moxibustion.

M-UE-16 *(Zhongkui)* 中魁 "Middle Eminence"

Location: At the tip of the bone on the proximal phalangeal joint of the middle finger, dorsal aspect. (Dia. 2-88)
Indications: Vomiting, hiccough, spasm of the esophagus, nosebleed.
Method: Use moxibustion.

M-UE-17 *(Xiaogukong)* 小骨空 "Little Bone's Space"

Location: At the middle of the transverse crease of the phalangeal joint of the little finger, dorsal aspect. (Dia. 2-88)
Indications: Eye diseases, sore throat, arthritis of the fingers.
Method: Use moxibustion.

M-UE-21 *(Quanjian)*　拳尖　"Fist's Tip"

Location: On the knuckle below the middle finger. (Dia. 2-88)
Indications: Eye diseases, sore throat.
Method: Use moxibustion or prick the point.

M-UE-27 *(Shoujinmen)*　手金门　"Hand's Golden Door"

Location: 3.5 units proximal to the middle of the transverse crease of the wrist, palmar aspect. (Dia. 2-89)
Indications: Scrofula.
Method: Straight insertion, 1-1.5 units.

M-UE-28 *(Dingshu)*　疔俞　"Carbuncle's Hollow"

Location: 4 units proximal to the ulnar end of the transverse crease of the wrist, palmar aspect. (Dia. 2-89)
Indications: Carbuncle.
Method: Use moxibustion.

M-UE-29 *(Erbai)*　二白　"Two Whites"

Location: 4 units proximal to the middle of the transverse crease of the wrist, palmar aspect. One point is between the two tendons and the second is on the radial side of the tendons. (Dia. 2-89)
Indications: Hemorrhoids, prolapsed anus, neuralgia of the forearm.
Method: Straight insertion, 0.5-1 unit.

M-UE-31 *(Zexia)*　泽下　"Below the Marsh"

Location: 2 units below L-5 *(Chize)*. (Dia. 2-89)
Indications: Toothache, hemorrhoids, pain of forearm.
Method: Straight insertion, 1-1.5 units.

M-UE-32 *(Zeqian)*　泽前　"Before the Marsh"

Location: 1 unit distal and slightly medial to L-5 *(Chize),* on a straight line from the middle finger. (Dia. 2-89)
Indications: Goiter, paralysis of uppper limb.
Method: Straight insertion, 1-1.5 units.

M-UE-33 *(Zhongquan)*　中泉　"Middle Spring"

Location: In the depression on the dorsum of the wrist between LI-5 *(Yangxi)* and TB-4 *(Yangchi)*. (Dia. 2-88)
Indications: Bronchitis, asthma, opacity of cornea, stomach-ache, diseases of the wrist and surrounding soft tissues.
Method: Straight insertion, 0.3-0.5 unit.

M-UE-34 *(Cunping)*　　寸平　　"Unit Level"

Location: 1 unit proximal to the middle of the transverse crease of the wrist, dorsal aspect, 0.4 unit toward the radial side. (Dia. 2-88)
Indications: Shock, heart failure.
Method: Straight insertion, 0.5-1 unit.

M-UE-35 *(Xiawenliu)*　　下温溜　　"Lower Warm Slide"

Location: 2 units proximal to the radial end of the transverse crease of the wrist, dorsal aspect. (Dia. 2-88)
Indications: Toothache of lower jaw.
Method: Straight insertion, 0.3-0.5 unit.

M-UE-36 *(Chirao)*　　尺桡　　"Ulna and Radius"

Location: 6 units proximal to the middle of the transverse crease of the wrist, dorsal aspect. (Dia. 2-88)
Indications: Mental illness, paralysis of upper limb.
Method: Straight insertion reaching to the other side of the arm (without breaking skin).

M-UE-38 *(Sanchi)*　　三池　　"Three Pools"

Location: 3 points: LI-11 *(Quchi)* and points 1 unit above and below. (Dia. 2-88)
Indications: Sinusitis, pain of elbow and arm.
Method: Straight insertion, 1-1.5 units.

M-UE-39 *(Zhoushu)*　　肘俞　　"Elbow's Hollow"

Location: On the dorsum of the elbow between the olecranon and the lateral epicondyle of the humerus. (Dia. 2-88)
Indications: Pain of elbow joint.
Method: With elbow flexed, straight insertion, 0.3 unit.

M-UE-40 *(Yeling)*　　腋灵　　"Axilla's Spirit"

Location: 0.5 unit above the anterior axillary fold. (Dia. 2-89)
Indications: Mental illness, shoulder pain.
Method: Straight insertion, 2-3 units.

M-UE-41 *(Tianling)*　　天灵　　"Heaven's Spirit"

Location: 1 unit above and 0.5 unit medial to the anterior axillary fold. (Dia. 2-89)
Indications: Same as M-UE-40 *(Yeling)* above.
Method: Slanted insertion in lateral direction, 2-3 units.

384

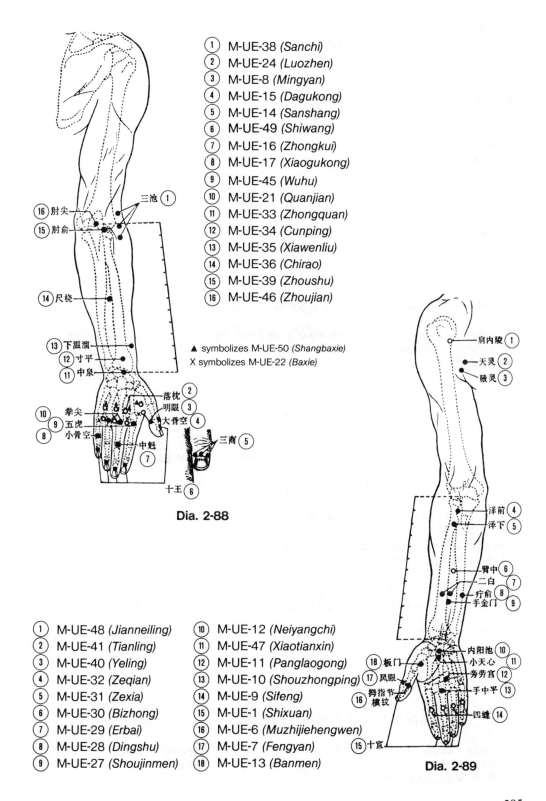

1. M-UE-38 (Sanchi)
2. M-UE-24 (Luozhen)
3. M-UE-8 (Mingyan)
4. M-UE-15 (Dagukong)
5. M-UE-14 (Sanshang)
6. M-UE-49 (Shiwang)
7. M-UE-16 (Zhongkui)
8. M-UE-17 (Xiaogukong)
9. M-UE-45 (Wuhu)
10. M-UE-21 (Quanjian)
11. M-UE-33 (Zhongquan)
12. M-UE-34 (Cunping)
13. M-UE-35 (Xiawenliu)
14. M-UE-36 (Chirao)
15. M-UE-39 (Zhoushu)
16. M-UE-46 (Zhoujian)

16 肘尖
15 肘俞
三池 1

14 尺桡

13 下温溜
12 寸平
11 中泉

▲ symbolizes M-UE-50 (Shangbaxie)
X symbolizes M-UE-22 (Baxie)

2 落枕
3 明眼
10 拳尖
9 五虎
8 小骨空
4 大骨空
三商 5
中魁 7
十王 6

Dia. 2-88

1. M-UE-48 (Jianneiling)
2. M-UE-41 (Tianling)
3. M-UE-40 (Yeling)
4. M-UE-32 (Zeqian)
5. M-UE-31 (Zexia)
6. M-UE-30 (Bizhong)
7. M-UE-29 (Erbai)
8. M-UE-28 (Dingshu)
9. M-UE-27 (Shoujinmen)
10. M-UE-12 (Neiyangchi)
11. M-UE-47 (Xiaotianxin)
12. M-UE-11 (Panglaogong)
13. M-UE-10 (Shouzhongping)
14. M-UE-9 (Sifeng)
15. M-UE-1 (Shixuan)
16. M-UE-6 (Muzhijiehengwen)
17. M-UE-7 (Fengyan)
18. M-UE-13 (Banmen)

肩内陵 1
天灵 2
腋灵 3

泽前 4
泽下 5

臂中 6
二白 7
疔俞 8
手金门 9

内阳池 10
小天心 11
旁劳宫 12
手中平 13
四缝 14

18 板门
17 凤眼
16 拇指节横纹
15 十宣

Dia. 2-89

385

M-UE-45 *(Wuhu)* 五虎 "Five Tigers"

Location: On the knuckles of the index and ring fingers. (Dia. 2-88)
Indications: Neck pain, sciatica, finger spasm.
Method: With hand in a fist, slanted insertion, 0.2-0.3 unit; or use moxibustion.

M-UE-46 *(Zhoujian)* 肘尖 "Elbow's Tip"

Location: At the prominence of the olecranon when the elbow is flexed. (Dia. 2-88)
Indications: Scrofula, abscessed carbuncle.
Method: Use moxibustion.

M-UE-47 *(Xiaotianxin)* 小天心 "Little Heaven's Heart"

Location: 1.5 units distal to the transverse crease of the wrist, palmar aspect. (Dia. 2-89)
Indications: Rheumatic heart disease, palpitations.
Method: Straight insertion, 0.3-0.5 unit.

M-UE-49 *(Shiwang)* 十王 "Ten Kings"

Location: At the middle of the fingertip of each finger, 10 points altogether. (Dia. 2-88)
Indications: Heat exhaustion, acute gastroenteritis, common cold.
Method: Prick the points.

MISCELLANEOUS POINTS OF THE LOWER LIMB

M-LE-1 *(Lineiting)* 里内庭 "Within Inner Court"

Location: In depression anterior to the metatarsophalangeal joints of the 2nd and 3rd toes, plantar aspect. (Dia. 2-91)
Indications: Pain in toes, infantile convulsions, seizures.
Method: Straight insertion, 0.3-0.5 unit.

M-LE-2 *(Muzhilihengwen)* 踇趾里横纹 "Transverse Crease of Big Toe"

Location: At the middle of the transverse crease of the metatarsophalangeal joint of the big toe, plantar aspect. (Dia. 2-91)
Indications: Orchitis.
Method: Straight insertion, 0.3-0.5 unit.

M-LE-3 *(Qianhouyinzhu)* 前后隐珠 "Hidden Pearls in Front and Back"

Location: 2 points, 0.5 unit posterior and anterior to K-1 *(Yongquan)*. (Dia. 2-91)
Indications: Hypertension, pain in the sole of foot, infantile convulsions.
Method: Straight insertion, 0.3-0.5 unit.

M-LE-4 *(Zuxin)*　足心　　"Sole of Foot"

Location: 1 unit posterior to K-1 *(Yongquan)*. (Dia. 2-91)
Indications: Headache, pain in the sole of the foot, abnormal uterine bleeding.
Method: Straight insertion, 0.5-1 unit.

M-LE-5 *(Shimian)*　失眠　　"Insomnia"

Location: At the center of the heel in the bottom of foot. (Dia. 2-91)
Indications: Insomnia, pain in the sole of the foot.
Method: Straight insertion, 0.3-0.5 unit.

M-LE-6 *(Qiduan)*　气端　　"Qi's Extremity"

Location: At the tip of each toe. (Dia. 2-90)
Indications: Apoplectic coma, beriberi, paralysis of toes, red swollen dorsum of the foot.
Method: Prick the point; or insert straight, 0.1-0.2 unit.

M-LE-9 *(Nuxi)*　女膝　　"Woman's Knee"

Location: On the back of the heel, at the center of the calcaneous bone. (Dia. 2-92)
Indications: Gingivitis, mental illness.
Method: Straight insertion, 0.2-0. unit.

M-LE-10 *(Quanshengzu)*　泉生足　"Spring at the Foot"

Location: On the back of the heel at the middle of the superior margin of the calcaneous bone, in the tendon. (Dia. 2-92)
Indications: Spasm of the esophagus, brain disease, low back pain.
Method: Straight insertion, 0.2-0.3 unit.

M-LE-11 *(Taiyinqiao)*　太阴跷　"Greater Yin Heel"

Location: In the depression at the inferior margin of the medial malleolus. (Dia. 2-93)
Indications: Irregular menstruation, abnormal uterine bleeding, prolapsed uterus, infertility (in women).
Method: Straight insertion, 0.3-0.5 unit.

M-LE-12 *(Xiakunlun)*　下昆仑　"Lower Kunlun (Mountains)"

Location: 1 unit below B-60 *(Kunlun)*. (Dia. 2-92)
Indications: Arthritic pain, paraplegia, low back pain.
Method: Straight insertion, 0.3-0.5 unit.

M-LE-14 *(Zuzhongping)*　足中平　"Level with Mid-Leg"

Location: 1 unit below S-36 *(Zusanli)*. (Dia. 2-90)

Indications: Mental illness, paralysis of lower limb.
Method: Straight insertion, 2-3 units.

M-LE-15 *(Xixia)* 膝下 "Below Knee"

Location: In the patellar ligament, at the middle of the inferior margin of the patella. (Dia. 2-90)
Indications: Diseases of knee joint and surrounding soft tissues.
Method: Straight insertion, 1-1.5 units; or use moxibustion.

M-LE-17 *(Neihuaijian)* 外踝尖 "Tip of Medial Malleolus"

Location: At the prominence of the medial malleolus. (Dia. 2-93)
Indications: Toothache, tonsillitis, muscle spasm on medial aspect of calf.
Method: Use moxibustion.

M-LE-18 *(Zhizhuanjin)* 治转筋 "Heal Turned Muscle"

Location: At the middle of the superior margin of the medial malleolus. (Dia. 2-93)
Indications: Spasm of gastrocnemius muscle, low back pain, pain of the ankle joint.
Method: Use moxibustion.

M-LE-19 *(Shaoyangwei)* 少陽维 "Lesser Yang Link"

Location: 1 unit above the posterior margin of the medial malleolus, between K-3 *(Taixi)* and K-7 *(Fuliu)*. (Dia. 2-93)
Indications: Beriberi, chronic eczema of lower limbs, lupus, paralysis of lower limb.
Method: Slanted insertion, 0.5-1 unit.

M-LE-20 *(Chengming)* 承命 "Support Life"

Location: 3 units above K-3 *(Taixi)*. (Dia. 2-93)
Indications: Seizures, mental illness, edema of lower limb.
Method: Straight insertion, 1-1.5 units.

M-LE-21 *(Jiaoyi)* 交仪 "Exchange Ceremony"

Location: 0.5 unit above medial malleolus. (Dia. 2-93)
Indications: Irregular menstruation, leukorrhea, beriberi.
Method: Straight insertion, 1.5-2 units.

M-LE-22 *(Waihuaijian)* 内踝尖 "Tip of Lateral Malleolus"

Location: At the prominence of the lateral malleolus. (Dia. 2-92)
Indications: Toothache, beriberi, paraplegia, severe headache.
Method: Prick the point.

M-LE-25 *(Linghouxia)*   陵后下   "Below Behind the Tomb"

Location: 0.5 unit below M-LE-24 *(Linghou)*. (Dia. 2-92)
Indications: Sciatica, arthritis of knee, neuralgia of the peroneal nerve, paralysis of lower limb.
Method: Straight insertion, 2-3 units.

M-LE-26 *(Xiwai)*   膝外   "Outside the Knee"

Location: At the lateral end of the transverse crease of the knee, slightly anterior to B-53 *(Weiyang)*. (Dia. 2-92)
Indications: Arthritis of the knee, ulcerations on the lower limb.
Method: Straight insertion, 1-1.5 units.

M-LE-27 *(Heding)*   鹤顶   "Crane's Top"

Location: In the depression at the middle of the superior margin of the patella. (Dia. 2-90)
Indications: Diseases of knee joint and surrounding soft tissues.
Method: Straight or slanted insertion, 0.5-1 unit.

M-LE-28 *(Kuangu)*   髋骨   "Patella"

Location: 2 points, about 1.5 units to the left and right of S-34 *(Liangqiu)* on the thigh. (Dia. 2-90)
Indications: Arthritis of the knee, paralysis of the lower limb.
Method: Straight insertion, 1.5-2 units.

M-LE-29 *(Shenxi)*   肾系   "Kidney's Connection"

Location: 1 unit below S-32 *(Futu)*. (Dia. 2-90)
Indications: Diabetes, paralysis of the lower limb.
Method: Straight insertion, 1.5-2 units.

M-LE-30 *(Guantu)*   关兔   "Hinge and Rabbit"

Location: Midway between S-31 *(Biguan)* and S-32 *(Futu)*. (Dia. 2-90)
Indications: Stomach-ache, enteritis, sequelae of infantile paralysis.
Method: Straight insertion, 1.5-2 units.

M-LE-31 *(Liaoliao)*   髎髎   "Seam of the Seam"

Location: The prominence at the medial condyle of the femur. (Dia. 2-90)
Indications: Irregular menstruation, abnormal uterine bleeding.
Method: Slanted insertion, 1-1.5 units.

M-LE-32 *(Dalun)*   大轮   "Big Wheel"

Location: At the superior margin of the medial condyle of the femur. (Dia. 2-90)
Indications: Arthritis of the knee, puerperal fever.
Method: Straight insertion, 2-3 units.

M-LE-33 *(Zuming)* 足明 "Leg's Brightness"

Location: 2 finger widths above M-LE-32 *(Dalun)*. (Dia. 2-90)
Indications: Same as M-LE-32 *(Dalun)* above.
Method: Straight insertion, 2-3 units.

M-LE-34 *(Baichongwo)* 百虫窝 "Hundred Insects' Nest"

Location: 1 unit above Sp-10 *(Xuehai)*. (Dia. 2-93)
Indications: Urticaria, eczema.
Method: Straight insertion, 2-3 units.

M-LE-35 *(Zuluo)* 足罗 "Leg's Snare"

Location: 3 units above M-LE-32 *(Dalun)*. (Dia. 2-90)
Indications: Irregular menstruation, puerperal fever, pain of thigh and knee.
Method: Straight insertion, 2-3 units.

M-LE-36 *(Chenggu)* 成骨 "Complete Bone"

Location: At the prominence of the lateral condyle of the femur. (Dia. 2-92)
Indications: Low back pain, arthritis of the knee.
Method: Prick the point.

M-LE-37(a) *(Yinwei #1)* 阴委₁ "Yin's Commission #1"

Location: 1 unit above the lateral end of the transverse crease of the knee. (Dia. 2-92)
Indications: Mental illness, hysterical paralysis.
Method: Straight insertion, 2-3 units.

M-LE-37(b) *(Yinwei #2)* 阴委₂

Location: 2 units above the lateral end of the transverse crease of the knee. (Dia. 2-92)
Indications: Same as M-LE-37(a) *(Yinwei #1)* above.
Method: Straight insertion, 2-3 units.

M-LE-37(c) *(Yinwei #3)* 阴委₃

Location: 3 units above the lateral end of the transverse crease of the knee. (Dia. 2-92)
Indications: Same as M-LE-37(a) *(Yinwei #1)* above.
Method: Straight insertion, 2-3 units.

M-LE-38 *(Silian)* 四连 "Four Connection"

Location: 4 units above the lateral end of the transverse crease of the knee. (Dia. 2-92)
Indications: Same as M-LE-37(a) *(Yinwei #1)* above.
Method: Straight insertion, 2-3 units.

M-LE-39 *(Wuling)* 五灵 "Five Spirit"

Location: 5 units above the lateral end of the transverse crease of the knee. (Dia. 2-92)
Indications: Same as M-LE-37(a) *(Yinwei #1)* above.
Method: Straight insertion, 2-3 units.

M-LE-40 *(Lingbao)* 灵宝 "Spirit's Treasure"

Location: 6 units above the lateral end of the transverse crease of the knee. (Dia. 2-92)
Indications: Same as M-LE-37(a) *(Yinwei #1)* above.
Method: Straight insertion, 2-3 units.

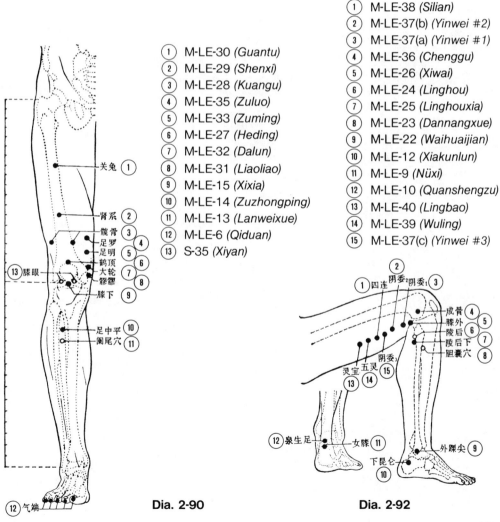

① M-LE-30 *(Guantu)*
② M-LE-29 *(Shenxi)*
③ M-LE-28 *(Kuangu)*
④ M-LE-35 *(Zuluo)*
⑤ M-LE-33 *(Zuming)*
⑥ M-LE-27 *(Heding)*
⑦ M-LE-32 *(Dalun)*
⑧ M-LE-31 *(Liaoliao)*
⑨ M-LE-15 *(Xixia)*
⑩ M-LE-14 *(Zuzhongping)*
⑪ M-LE-13 *(Lanweixue)*
⑫ M-LE-6 *(Qiduan)*
⑬ S-35 *(Xiyan)*

① M-LE-38 *(Silian)*
② M-LE-37(b) *(Yinwei #2)*
③ M-LE-37(a) *(Yinwei #1)*
④ M-LE-36 *(Chenggu)*
⑤ M-LE-26 *(Xiwai)*
⑥ M-LE-24 *(Linghou)*
⑦ M-LE-25 *(Linghouxia)*
⑧ M-LE-23 *(Dannangxue)*
⑨ M-LE-22 *(Waihuaijian)*
⑩ M-LE-12 *(Xiakunlun)*
⑪ M-LE-9 *(Nüxi)*
⑫ M-LE-10 *(Quanshengzu)*
⑬ M-LE-40 *(Lingbao)*
⑭ M-LE-39 *(Wuling)*
⑮ M-LE-37(c) *(Yinwei #3)*

Dia. 2-90

Dia. 2-92

1. M-LE-1 *(Lineiting)*
2. M-LE-4 *(Zuxin)*
3. M-LE-2 *(Muzhilihengwen)*
4. M-LE-3 *(Qianhouyinzhu)*
5. M-LE-5 *(Shimian)*

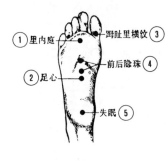

Dia. 2-91

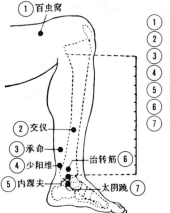

1. M-LE-34 *(Baichongwo)*
2. M-LE-21 *(Jiaoyi)*
3. M-LE-20 *(Chengming)*
4. M-LE-19 *(Shaoyangwei)*
5. M-LE-17 *(Neihuaijian)*
6. M-LE-18 *(Zhizhuanjin)*
7. M-LE-11 *(Taiyinqiao)*

Dia. 2-93

392

Section III

Techniques

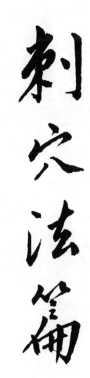

Introductory Comment

Acupuncture and moxibustion are methods of treating disease by stimulating certain points or loci on the body.* As such, they have been known since at least the time of the *Inner Classic* as "outer methods." Acupuncture involves the use of needles, ordinarily inserted beneath the superficial layers of skin, to provide mechanical stimulation of the underlying points. Moxibustion, on the other hand, utilizes the dried, powdered leaves of the moxa plant (mugwort, or *Artemisia vulgaris),* with or without other herbs, which are burned on or above the surface of the skin to provide thermal stimulation. In chapter 7 of *Spiritual Axis* is written: "When needles are unsuccessful, moxa is appropriate."

Since 1949 there have been great advances in the techniques and materials of acupuncture therapy based upon the traditional foundation of the channels and points as well as the principles of modern medicine. Among the discoveries are new forms of stimulation (electrical, pharmacological, surgical), the most important of which will be discussed in separate chapters of this Section.

*The roots of the English word acupuncture refer only to the use of needles to puncture, whereas the common Chinese appellation for what we call acupuncture, *zhenjiu,* literally means to needle and cauterize.—*Editors*

Chapter 1

An Overview of Acupuncture and Moxibustion

ORIGIN AND DEVELOPMENT

It is probable that acupuncture had its beginning in China among Stone Age tribes. In this primitive society, people lived in damp caves and often fought wild animals. It is likely that these early peoples experienced pain from arthritis and injury, and instinctively rubbed or massaged the affected area to relieve the pain. As stone tools were developed, a crude pointed instrument called *bian* was fashioned to tap and pierce the skin. Several of these were found in archaeological diggings at Anyang dating from about 1700 B.C. Their purpose was spelled out in a dictionary of the Han Dynasty:"*Bian* means using stone to treat disease."[1] The *bian* were thus the earliest acupuncture needles.

Cauterization, from which moxibustion is derived, was a development which followed the controlled use of fire. It is speculated that the warmth and sense of well-being which fire afforded from the cold and dampness of cave life, as well as the fortuitous cures which occasionally followed upon touching a live coal or burning stick, were the primitive beginnings of this art.

Cupping was originally known as the horn method. The horns of animals were heated and a partial vacuum was created when they were placed on the skin. The purpose of this was to treat diseases and draw out the pus. By the end of the Neolithic era animal husbandry had become widespread, which facilitated the development of the horn (cupping) method.

What distinguishes these early skills in China from those elsewhere is the extent to which they were subsequently developed within the framework of traditional physiology and pathology, outlined in the Introduction and the first Section of this book.

As for the tools themselves, there followed from the original stone needle a succession of instruments which mirrored the evolution of society and technology. Relatively finer needles were fashioned from bone with the aid of stone tools. These were utilized both in sewing and acupuncture. There were also bamboo needles. One of the ancient forms of the character *zhen* (needle) includes the bamboo radical, suggesting the material from which it was made. With the appearance of ceramics in the Yang Shao or Painted Pottery culture of the late Neolithic period somewhat prior to 2,000 B.C., ceramic needles were introduced.

The use of metal needles began in the Bronze Age (Shang Dynasty, c. 1600 B.C.) and grew with the subsequent introduction of iron. By the Warring States period (5th century B.C.), advances in metallurgy made it possible to manufacture steel needles of a fine, thin quality. The so-called Nine Needles (see below) described in the *Inner Classic* and used by physicians in the early centuries B.C., can thus be considered a development which started in the Bronze Age and was only finished in the Iron Age.[2] Later, gold, silver and alloyed metal needles appeared. During the recent Cultural Revolution in China, a number of needles were discovered while excavating a tomb in Hebei province dating from the Western Han Dynasty (c. 200 B.C.-8 A.D.). Among the needles were several gold and silver specimens, similar in shape to certain of the Nine Needles. This discovery is proof that these

398

metals were used in the manufacture of needles as early as 2,000 years ago. Presently, most acupuncture needles are made of stainless steel, whose strength and relatively low cost make it preferable to other metals.

Since ancient times there have been different needles for different purposes. Both the shapes and uses have changed over the years. For example, there were three types of stone needles: one was thin like a needle, the second looked like a knife, and the third was shaped like an arrowhead. By the time of the *Yellow Emperor's Inner Classic* (2nd century B.C.) there was even more variety.

The classic Nine Needles (Dia. 3-1) were designed to perform different functions. In chapter 7 of the *Spiritual Axis* is written:"Each of the Nine Needles has its appropriate function. Long, short, big, and small, each has a purpose." Many of these needles are still in use, although their design and purpose may have changed somewhat. As described in the *Inner Classic*, the Nine Needles are as follows:

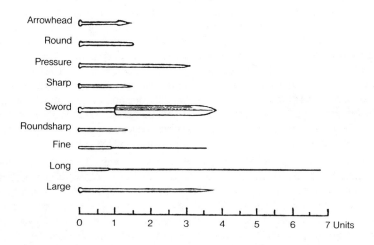

Dia. 3-1 The Nine Needles

1. **Arrowhead needle**
   Shape: 1.6 units* long with a tapered point.
   Function: Superficial puncture for bleeding. Treats Hot conditions.
2. **Round needle**
   Shape: 1.6 units long with a rounded tip
   Function: Rub against the external skin. Treats superficial stagnant Qi.
3. **Pressure needle**
   Shape: 3.5 units long with the tip shaped like a grain of millet
   Function: Press against the channels without deep insertion.
4. **Sharp needle**
   Shape: 1.6 units long with a round body and a sharp, pyramid-shaped tip
   Function: Bleed and drain abscesses.
5. **Sword needle**
   Shape: 4 units long, .25 units wide, shaped like a sword
   Function: Drain superficial abscesses.
6. **Round-sharp needle**
   Shape: 1.6 units long with a thin round body and a slightly large head
   Function: Drain abscesses or eliminate obstruction with deep insertion.

*Unit here refers to a Chinese inch.

7. Fine (or Filiform) needle
   Shape: 3.6 units with a thin shaft
   Function: Eliminate Cold, Heat, pain, and obstruction.
8. Long needle
   Shape: 7 units long
   Function: Deep insertion.
9. Large needle
   Shape: 4 units long with a thick body
   Function: Alleviate arthritis or drain fluids.

The Round and Pressure needles are used for rubbing or pressing against the surface of the skin. The Arrowhead needle was utilized for superficial pricking of the skin and later evolved into the Cutaneous or Plum Blossom needle. It has also been used to introduce herbal preparations beneath the superficial layers of skin, and is therefore called the Painting needle. The Sharp needle is the ancestor of the Pyramid needle, used for letting blood. The Sword needle was used to make surgical incisions and is the forerunner of certain modern surgical instruments. The Fine needle (sometimes called Filiform) was by far the most common of acupuncture needles, and remains so to this day. The Long needle is simply a fine needle of great length used for very deep or extended insertions. Today it is called the Beard of Wheat needle. The Large needle has the shape of a Fine needle but with a much larger diameter. This needle was altered somewhat during the Cultural Revolution to become the Barefoot Doctor needle. A synthesis of the features of the Long and Large needles produced what we know today as the Great needle. It can generally be said, therefore, that the needles presently used in acupuncture, and many of the methods as well, are direct descendants of the ancient Nine Needles. Several of these are discussed in greater detail later in this Section.

Cauterization as a method of curing disease originally utilized twigs and other common, combustible materials. The use of the moxa plant as the principal substance of combustion dates from the late Chou period. This plant is referred to in the book *Mencius* (290 B.C.): "For a disease of seven years, seek three year old moxa." This would suggest that its use was already widespread by that time.

In ancient times, the direct method of cauterization was generally followed, applying the combustible material directly on the skin. Instructions are found in the *Tradition of Zuo* (581 B.C.): "Above or below the Vitals, direct cauterization cannot be used . . ." In the *Book of Bian Que's Secrets,* mention is made of giving moxa to sleeping people. The medical classic of the Eastern Han Dynasty, *Discussion of Cold-Induced Disorders,* also refers to diseases for which direct cauterization is either permitted or prohibited. At that time, the size of the moxa wick or cone was large, and a great number were used for each treatment. Later, in the Tang and Song Dynasties, as many as 100 cones were prescribed. More recently, the number and size of the cones in direct moxibustion has declined. The new criterion distinguishes only whether or not the cauterization leaves a scar.

During the Jin and Tang periods, an indirect method of cauterization was developed. In the Tang classic, *Thousand Ducat Prescriptions,* various methods are discussed including placement of the moxa on top of a wafer of another material such as garlic, soybean, beeswax, salt, or ginger, and then igniting it. In the same book a method is described for treating ear diseases by which a hollow bamboo tube is placed in the ear and moxa burned at the other end. This was called tube or cylinder cauterization and was a forerunner of the modern 'warming cylinder' technique. Another method, devised in the Ming Dynasty (c. 1368-1662), utilized a branch from a mulberry or peach tree which was dipped in sesame oil, lit and blown out. The heated stick was then wrapped with soft paper and used like an iron over the designated area of the skin. In a later development, the powder of dried, crushed moxa and other herbs was rolled together into a cigar-shaped 'stick' to be held by one end in the hand and burned at the other a short distance from the skin. This method is widely practiced today. Also developed during the Ming epoch was a method whereby the stalk of the *Juncus effusus* plant *(dengxincao)* was soaked, ignited and then placed on the skin. Still another method made use of a copper mirror to focus the light rays of the sun for cauterization. In the Song Dynasty (c. 960-1279), references are made in medical books to natural or spontaneous cauterization, by which certain herbs known for their irritant properties (e.g., *Rhus toxicodendron,* mustard plaster, etc.) were rubbed on the skin, producing a blister.

Other methods which are still prevalent today will be described later in this Section.

In early times, cupping was performed with animal horns. Later, better methods of suction were developed as cups were made of bamboo, ceramics, metal or glass. Suction is now obtained by either putting a burning substance into the cup before placing the cup on the skin, by heating the cups in water, or by pumping out the air after a cup has been emplaced. There are many different ways in which cups can be used. Those methods in common use today are described in chapter 5 below.

THE FUNCTIONS OF ACUPUNCTURE AND MOXIBUSTION

The therapeutic functions of both acupuncture and moxibustion result from the stimulation of points and channels. Qi and Blood, the bases of life and movement, circulate through the channels. The combination of Qi and Blood in the channels is called Channel Qi. In addition to coursing through the body to nourish the Organs and tissues, Channel Qi may also reflect disease and transmit stimulation. Spirit is also involved here. In chapter 8 of *Spiritual Axis* is written: "The pulse houses the Spirit." Spirit and Qi have a very close relationship and are sometimes referred to in the singular as Spirit Qi. The importance of the relationship between Spirit Qi and the channels is emphasized in chapter 1 of *Spiritual Axis,* where it is said that the points are "where the Spirit Qi roams in and out."

The functions of both acupuncture and moxibustion are frequently described in the *Yellow Emperor's Inner Classic.* "The use of techniques like acupuncture is to regulate the Qi" *(Spiritual Axis,* chapter 75). "All proper needling first treats the Spirit" *(Simple Questions,* chapter 25). Regulating the Qi includes treatment of both Deficient and Excessive conditions, as well as regulation of the Nourishing and Protective Qi. Treatment of the Spirit is also an important aspect of acupuncture. "Controlling the Spirit facilitates the movement of Qi" *(Simple Questions,* chapter 54). This passage reflects the mutuality between Spirit and Qi. Similarly, chapter 1 of *Spiritual Axis* provides: "Those who use needles must not forget the Spirit."

Clinically, Blood must also be taken into consideration. Bleeding regulates the Qi and heals the Spirit. Congealed Blood often leads to stagnant Qi; treating one thereby treats the other. Essence and Spirit depend on Blood for nourishment, and are adversely affected by diseases of the Blood. In chapter 32 of *Spiritual Axis* is written: "Only when the pulse and Blood are harmonious are the Essence and Spirit secure."

The ancients taught that acupuncture could "localize pain and move pain" *(Ode of the Standard of Mystery).* In chapter 1 of *Simple Questions* it is said: "Injured Qi is pain." In Chinese medicine all pain is said to arise from problems with the flow of Qi and Blood through the channels, Organs and tissues. This is ordinarily caused by external Excesses invading the body, or discordant emotions. The principle that 'if there is no circulation there is pain' is illustrated by the following passage from chapter 39 of *Simple Questions:* "The circulation in the channels and vessels is unceasing; it slows without rest. When Cold Qi enters the channels movement is slowed; when it forms a stagnant obstruction the flow is stayed. When [Cold Qi] resides outside the vessels there is less Blood; when it resides in the vessels the Qi cannot pass and there is sudden pain."

Under different conditions, pain may be caused by constriction of tissues. This type of pain is discussed in chapter 39 of *Simple Questions:* "When Cold Qi lodges outside the vessels, they become cold; when the vessels are cold they contract; when they contract there is constriction; when there is constriction the surrounding small Connecting channels are affected and there is sudden pain." In trauma, local injury interferes with the flow of Qi, and the resulting stagnation of Qi or coagulation of Blood causes pain. The perception of pain is through the Spirit. In Chinese medicine, Spirit is said to be stored in the Heart. In chapter 74 of *Simple Questions* it is said: "All pain, itching, and skin disorders pertain to the Heart."

The analgesic function of acupuncture assumes two principal forms. On the one hand, acupuncture "regulates the Qi and Blood" *(Simple Questions,* chapter 1). This means it removes blockages or obstructions to the flow of Qi. At the same time, acupuncture is said to "restore the Qi" *(Classic of Categories)* and to release constriction of the tissues. But there is another aspect to the capacity of acupuncture for treating pain, which is to change the perception of pain by treating the Spirit. This aspect is reflected in a passage from chapter 74 of *Simple Questions:* "When the Heart is serene [any] pain seems negligible."

Acupuncture is capable of treating diseases of obstruction, which includes atrophy and blockage. In Chinese medicine, atrophy is considered to result from an insufficient flow of Qi and Blood in the channels manifested by wasting of a limb, lack of sensation, and loss of function. "When the Nourishing Qi is Deficient there is a loss of function" *(Simple Questions,* chapter 34). Acupuncture treats these disorders by regulating the Qi so as to facilitate its smooth and harmonious flow. "When the [Nourishing Qi and] Blood are in harmony they flow smoothly through the channels, circulating to nourish the Yin and Yang. Thus the sinews and bones are strong and sturdy and the joints move quickly and easily. When the Protective Qi is harmonious the flesh is supple, the skin soft, and the pores are closed" *(Spiritual Axis,* chapter 47). Blockage disorders are characterized by soreness and pain in the muscles and bones. This pain also arises from improper circulation of Blood and Qi in the channels. The rationale underlying the use of acupuncture for the treatment of atrophy and blockage is similar to that for the treatment of pain.

Acupuncture can regulate the functions of the Organs (i.e., by strengthening Deficiency and draining Excess). As with pain, this is also based upon acupuncture's ability to regulate Qi and treat the Spirit. The Ming Dynasty physician Zhang Jiebing, in his annotation of the phrase 'direct (lead) the Qi' from chapter 34 of *Spiritual Axis,* explained: "Direct the Qi to restore the Source Qi . . . to strengthen, direct the Normal Qi . . . to drain, direct the Abnormal Qi." When the body is Deficient, a strengthening method of acupuncture is used to strengthen the functions of the Organs. When there is Excess, a draining method is used to drain the Excess and increase the body's powers of resistance. By appropriately draining or strengthening, the Abnormal is expelled and the Normal is restored, the Spirit "returns to its abode" *(Spiritual Axis,* chapter 35), the Organs resume functioning and the disease is cured.

Moxibustion is similar to acupuncture in that it works by stimulating the points to strengthen the flow of Qi and Blood and the movement of Spirit. The primary difference is that moxibustion stimulates with heat. In chapter 75 of *Spiritual Axis* is written: "When the Blood in the vessels has become stagnant or has stopped it can only be treated by Fire." Chapter 48 provides: "When the pulse is collapsed, the Blood in the vessels is knotted up inside . . . and the Blood is Cold. Under these conditions, moxibustion is appropriate." These passages illustrate the functions of moxibustion: warming the channels, dispersing Cold, and moving the Blood. The belief that heat helps the Blood move was succinctly expressed in *Secrets of the Cinnabar Creek Master:* "If the Blood encounters Heat it moves, if it encounters Cold it stagnates." However, it should be remembered that 'Qi is the leader of Blood', and that Cold and Heat primarily effect the Qi, and only secondarily the Blood. "For stagnation and rough movement [of the Blood], direct the (Yang) Qi to warm it. In this way the Blood will be in harmony and [the pain] will cease" *(Spiritual Axis,* chapter 64).

Other classic works further detail the use of moxibustion. Here are two examples from the 3rd century, *Discussion of Cold-Induced Disorders:* "In diseases of the Lesser Yin [channels] there is vomiting and diarrhea and the hands and feet are cold . . . If the pulse cannot be felt, burn seven cones of moxa on the Lesser Yin [channels]. After six or seven days of Cold-induced disease when the pulse is faint, the hands and feet cold, and the patient dry and irritable, apply moxa on the Absolute Yin [channels]." These examples illustrate the use of moxibustion in the treatment of exhausted Yang, in the course of febrile diseases. In the Song Dynasty work, *Book of Bian Que's Secrets,* appears the following passage: "If you are able to use moxibustion early [in the course of a disease], the Yang Qi will naturally not become exhausted." The importance of Yang Qi (which includes Source Qi, Ancestral Qi, Protective Qi, etc.) is emphasized repeatedly in classical texts. It is called the "root of Essence and Spirit" in the 15th century collection, *Ten Works of Dongyuan.* In chapter 30 of *Spiritual Axis,* the Yang Qi is said to "spread the essence of food, warm the flesh, fill out the body, and moisten the body hair." In chapter 3 of *Simple Questions* it is written: "The Yang protects against external [Excesses] and stabilizes [the body]." The effectiveness of moxibustion in treating conditions of depleted Yang, cold limbs, 'hidden' pulse, exhausted Yang and Yin, and delirium is thus derived from its ability to regulate Qi and Spirit in such a way as to warm and stabilize the Yang.

The function of warming the Yang also gives moxibustion an important role in health maintenance. This was first noted in the Tang Dynasty work, *Thousand Ducat Prescriptions:* "Whoever has two or three places always being cauterized, so that the scars never heal completely even for a short time, is protected from plagues, epidemics, miasma, and poisonous Qi." That is to say, when the Yang Qi is strong the body's ability to protect itself from harmful influences is greatly enhanced.

In summary, both acupuncture and moxibustion affect the closely allied Qi and Spirit. Both methods are used to restore to normalcy that which is dysfunctioning, i.e., to restore harmony. And even though both stimulate the Qi (a Yang aspect) from the outside, they also beneficially influence the Yin and fluid aspects of the body. This is because when the inner workings of the body are well regulated, those functions which produce the fluids will perform more effectively. In *Simple Questions,* chapter 5 is written: "When the Qi transforms, Essence is produced." The various techniques of acupuncture and moxibustion described in the following pages all regulate and harmonize the functions of the Organs and other aspects of the body, with the object of achieving health and preventing disease.

FOOTNOTES

1. *Analytical Dictionary of Characters (Shuowen jiezi).*

2. This is contrary to the popular belief that the legendary ruler Fu Xi made the Nine Needles, and the Yellow Emperor later taught his method. Fu Xi is thought possibly to have lived in the late Paleolithic, and the Yellow Emperor in the late Neolithic eras, both before the development of metalurgy.

Chapter 2

Needling Technique

THE FILIFORM OR FINE NEEDLE

The most popular acupuncture needle is the fine or filiform needle. In this chapter, basic information concerning the preparation, care and method of manipulating this needle will be discussed. Much of this information, however, is of general relevance to other types of needles treated separately in chapter 3 below.

A typical filiform needle (Dia. 3-2) is made of stainless steel with either a copper or stainless steel wire webbing on the handle for easy gripping. Stainless steel is used because of its superior strength and resiliency, as well as its resistance to rust. While gold and silver also resist rust, they are expensive and soft, and so are seldom used.

The filiform needle varies in length from 0.5 to 6 inches, and the diameter of the body from .23 to .45 mm. The most commonly used needles are 1.5-3.5 inches in length, and #26-#30 gauge. The needles should be needlelike—that is neither too soft (causing unnecessary discomfort to the patient) nor too sharp (cutting through blood vessels and tissues too easily).

Prior to use, needles should be inspected to see that no burrs or tiny cracks appear on the tip which might tear skin tissue or result in breakage of the needle during manipulation. (One method of checking for burrs is to pull the needle by the handle through a ball of cotton. If the tip catches on the cotton fibers, there is often a burr.) Burrs may be filed smooth with extra fine sand paper or grinding stone. Cracked needles should be discarded.

Older needles are usually bent somewhat from use, yet it is important that the needle be straight when inserted. If small, such irregularities may be corrected by hand or with a special frame, but in doing so the elasticity of the needle progressively weakens, making it harder to manipulate. Eventually the needle must be thrown away.

Needles should be stored in such a way that the needle tips are cushioned to avoid blunting or cracking. When sterilized (in boiling water), it is suggested that they be wrapped in cloth so that they do not bump against the sides of the container. Similarly, care must be taken during treatment to avoid striking bones and blunting the tip.

PREPARATIONS

• Needles should be sterilized in an autoclave at 15 lbs. of pressure and temperature of 120°C for at least 15 minutes. Other utensils with which the needles come in contact should also be sterilized.

• Alternatively, if an autoclave is not available, needles may be boiled for 15 minutes after wrapping in cloth to protect the tips. Although this method requires no special equipment, with time it can dull the tips of the needles. However, if boiled in a 2% solution of sodium bicarbonate (baking

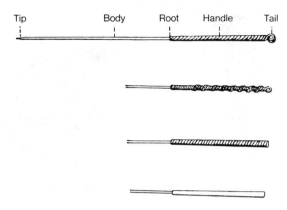

Dia. 3-2 The Filiform Needle

soda) the boiling point is raised to 120°C and the corrosive potential of the water is reduced.*
 • Glass containers or utensils which cannot withstand high temperatures may be placed in a 2% lysol solution for 1 to 2 hours.
 • Another method of sterilization, normally used in addition to boiling or pressure sterilization and just prior to treatment, is to soak the needles for half an hour in alcohol.
 • The physician's hands should be scrubbed with soap, dried, and rubbed with alcohol prior to needling.
 • The areas of skin around points selected on the patient should be cleaned with alcohol, both before and after needling.

POSITIONING THE PATIENT

Whether or not a patient is suitably positioned has a definite effect on the success of treatment. This is particularly true for patients who are very weak or nervous, and who are therefore more subject to fainting from 'needle shock'. It is also more likely, if a patient's position is uncomfortable, that he or she will move while a needle is in place, causing it to bend. The following items should be considered:
 • A position should be chosen for the patient which allows the physician accessibility to the necessary points for needling, and is comfortable enough that the patient can remain without moving for a period equal to the length of treatment.
 • Needling certain points requires a particular posture based upon considerations apart from merely exposing the area. For instance, the head may need to be lowered or an arm held 'akimbo'. (These special instructions are found together with the descriptions of individual points in Section II).
 • Generally, it is preferred that the patient lie down. This is especially true of those who are weak, nervous or hypersensitive, or who are receiving acupuncture for the first time. This is the best defense against fainting.
 • The patient should be encouraged to assume a comfortable position within the limitations of treatment. He or she should be impressed with the necessity of holding still once the needles are in place.
 • Before treatment begins, the procedure should be explained to the patient, who should also be told the feeling that can be expected from the needle. This is important not only to relax the patient, but also to encourage cooperation with the physician in interpreting the patient's response.

The most commonly used positions are shown in Diagram 3-3. Note that in the supine position, a pillow may be placed under the knees for needling points on the legs.

*In North America the general standard of practice is to autoclave the needles at 120°C for at least 30 minutes.—*Editors.*

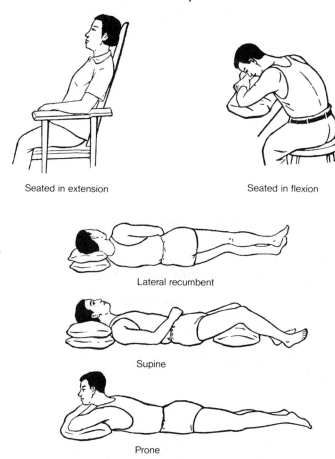

Seated in extension

Seated in flexion

Lateral recumbent

Supine

Prone

Dia. 3-3 Patient's Positions for Acupuncture

PRACTICE

It is important that the physician's skill in inserting and manipulating the needle be proficient before attempting to treat patients. This can only be accomplished with practice. A skilled practitioner inserts the needle quickly, penetrating the epidermis with little or no pain, and manipulates the needle with flexibility as the condition requires. A novice, on the other hand, often has difficulty controlling the needle, inserts it slowly causing discomfort to the patient, and is unable to adjust the method to the needs of the condition being treated, adversely affecting the result.

For practice, a pad of soft, porous paper (toilet paper will do) bound tightly with string, or a ball of cotton, loose on the inside but stretched tightly along the surface, can be used. A pin cushion is ideal. A 1.5 inch needle is recommended.

The handle of the needle is held firmly between the thumb, index and middle fingers and the needle tip placed on the practice pad at right angles to its surface. The needle is then rotated, clock-wise and counter-clockwise, between the fingers, and pressure is applied by the fingers downward so as to penetrate the surface. Attention should be directed toward keeping the needle erect and gradually increasing the downward pressure of the fingers. Then withdraw the needle and select another spot on the pad for practice. (As a method of insertion, this is only one among several. Others are described below. However, the general principles of needle control are the same.)

When a degree of confidence has been reached, students can pratice on themselves and on other students. Sterile technique, as outlined above, should be closely followed. Points on the arm and leg are safest for practice. Those on the head and trunk should be attempted only when familiar with precautions associated with these areas. Ultimately, however, only after a student has needled a point on him or herself, and then on other students, and has in turn been needled by other students, will he or she be able to treat a patient and correctly interpret the patient's response. The skill of an acupuncturist is proportionate to the amount of practice undertaken.

INSERTING THE NEEDLE

Different methods of inserting the needle are suggested, partly on the basis of the region of the body to be treated, and partly according to the preference of the physician (Dia. 3-4). It should always be kept in mind that the majority of pain occurs in the most superficial layers of skin. When these are penetrated, the sensation of pain largely disappears.

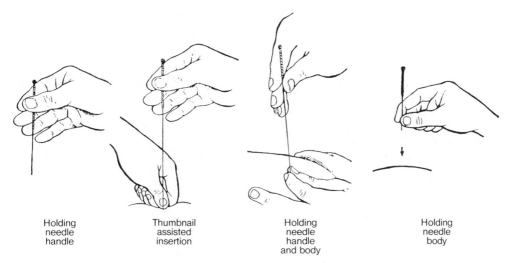

Holding
needle
handle

Thumbnail
assisted
insertion

Holding
needle
handle
and body

Holding
needle
body

Dia. 3-4   Insertion Methods

There are several ways of minimizing the pain of insertion. Most important is that the needles be inserted quickly, with a sudden thrust of the fingers. To assist this action, it is helpful if the skin surface is pulled taut so that it won't 'give' when the needle is thrust into it. Another method is to put pressure on the area adjacent to the point, usually with the thumb or thumbnail. In this way it is possible to insert the needle while distracting the attention of the patient with the pressure of the thumb.

The importance of a quick, painless insertion has been recognized since ancient times. In chapter 78 of the *Spiritual Axis* is written: "The right [hand] is responsible for pushing [the needle] while the left [hand] supports and controls it." The *Ode to the Standard of Mystery* describes the process in more detail: "The left hand is heavy and presses hard. This causes the Qi to disperse. The right hand is light for entry and exit [of the needle]. In this way there is no pain."

The needle may be held at the handle or at the body, 0.2-0.3 inch from the tip. Holding at the body of the needle is particularly recommended for loose, flabby skin (e.g., on the abdomen), or with longer or thinner gauge needles whose bodies tend to bend when pressure is exerted from the handle. Generally, a needle held by the handle can more easily be thrust deeply, whereas one held close to the tip, while penetrating rapidly, does so superficially. If the fingers are then moved to the handle, the needle can be inserted deeper into the flesh. Or, the needle can be held by the handle while the fingers of the other hand spread the skin taut below (Dia. 3-5).

Another method, useful on the face where the tissues overlying the bone are thin, is to pinch the skin

407

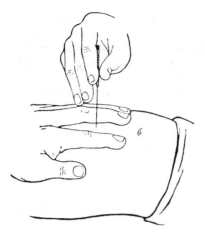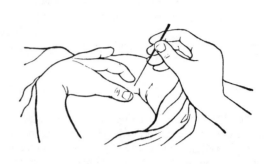

**Dia. 3-5 Pulling Skin Taut for
Needle Insertion**

together with the thumb and index finger of the left hand, while inserting the needle with the opposite hand (Dia. 3-6).

Finally, some acupuncturists prefer to use a needle tube, a device which holds the needle steady over the point while the physician taps it in place from above. The physician then removes the tube and manipulates the needle by hand* (Dia. 3-7).

A versatile physician utilizes more than one technique. With experience, the student will understand the advantages of each.

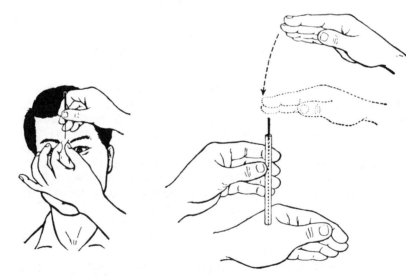

**Dia. 3-6 Pinching Skin for
Needle Insertion**

**Dia. 3-7 Using a Tube for
Needle Insertion**

*This device is especially useful for inserting very thin needles.—*Editors*.

408

ANGLE AND DEPTH OF INSERTION

In the clinic, it is not only important that the needle be inserted painlessly and in the proper position, but equally important to the result is the correct angle and depth. There are certain standards that should be learned, in addition to considering the patient's individual constitution and physique.

Angle

This is largely determined by the position of the point *vis a vis* underlying tissue. There are three general angles of the needle relative to the surface of the skin (Dia. 3-8).

Straight (perpendicular) insertion
This angle is often used when there is plentiful muscle in the area of the point.
Slanted insertion
This angle of insertion has wide applicability for thinner areas of the body, or when 'moving the Qi' in a specific direction.
Transverse insertion
This angle is used most commonly in areas with very little underlying muscle (e.g., the head) and for joining points with one needle.

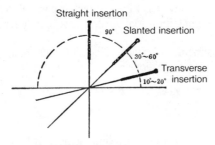

Dia. 3-8   Insertion Angles

Depth

Appropriate depth of insertion varies according to the area of the body, the physique of patient, and the nature of the disease. In chapter 50 of *Simple Questions* it is said: "[The level of] disease is either floating or sunken and [the depth of] insertion is either superficial or deep. Each assumes its appropriate place without overstepping the right path." It is common for the depth of insertion at a single point to vary according to the disease under treatment. For example, when S-7 *(Xiaguan)* is used to treat facial palsy, the needle is inserted just under the skin (transverse insertion) for 2-2.5 units to join with S-6 *(Jiache)*. When used to treat problems with the mandibular joint, a slanted insertion, first anteriorly and then posteriorly 0.5-0.7 units is recommended. And for treating trigeminal neuralgia, a straight insertion 1.5-2 units in depth is employed.

Furthermore, it is usually the case that the deeper the insertion, the stronger the needle sensation. Therefore, deep insertion is not recommended for weak patients or those susceptible to fainting. It is also necessary to be extremely cautious when inserting needles over important organs. Detailed descriptions of needle depths for individual points are set forth in Section II. For further discussion of traditional views with respect to the depth of insertion, see chapter 9 of this Section.

NEEDLING METHODS

Raising and thrusting

This refers to an up-down, push-pull movement of the needle once it is inserted beneath the skin.

When the depth at which the sensation of the point is reached (or the 'Qi is obtained') the needle is pushed and pulled, generally not exceeding about one half inch in vertical movement. The more active this motion, the stronger the stimulation. However, when raising the needle it should not be completely withdrawn from the skin.

Twirling or rotating

Again, after the needle has found its depth use the fingers on the handle to twirl or rotate the needle, first in one direction then the other. Do not exceed a 360° arc as this may cause the needle to bind in fibrous muscle tissue and produce pain. The wider the arc and the more rapid the twirling, the stronger the stimulation. Often, this method and the raising and thrusting method are combined.

Retaining the needle

After the needle has been inserted and manipulated in the manner described above, it is often retained in place anywhere from a few minutes up to an hour or two, depending on the condition. From time to time (usually every five minutes or so) it is manipulated to maintain the needle sensation. Recently in China, the technique of 'rapid' acupuncture has become widely used, whereby a needle is inserted and manipulated with considerable intensity for a few minutes or less, and then withdrawn. The needle is not retained at all. However, when the pain is particularly stubborn, or in conjunction with methods requiring repeated manipulation, the needle is usually retained in place for a period of time.

The length of a single treatment varies according to the condition, the method used and the preference of the physician. Some suggestions are made with respect to specific diseases in Section IV.

Supplementary stimulation methods

The number of special or supplementary needling methods is legion. Chapter 9 of this Section contains a discussion of many traditional techniques. Below are some of those which are still widely used.

'Following'
This is suggested for cases when, after insertion and manipulation of the needle, the patient does not feel the characteristic sensation of 'obtaining Qi'. It was first mentioned in the Ming Dynasty classic, *Great Compendium of Acupuncture and Moxibustion.* After making exploratory probings beneath the skin surface whereby the needle is only partially withdrawn and then thrust again at a slightly different angle, the physician must be satisfied that the location of the needle is not in error. Then, using his or her fingers, the physician lightly presses the skin, 'following' along the course of the channel on which the point is located, both above and below. The purpose is to encourage the movement of Qi through the channel and facilitate its sensation at the point.

'Plucking'
This method is suggested when the Qi sensation is retarded. With the needle in place, the physician uses the index finger to lightly pluck the handle of the needle, causing it to waver back and forth and strengthen the stimulation below.

'Scraping'
With the needle in place, the thumb and index finger of the left hand support the body of the needle where it enters the skin, while the thumb of the right hand is placed on the tail end to hold the needle steady. Then, using either the index or middle fingernail of the right hand, the handle is 'scraped' up and down, creating vibrations throughout the needle. A variation on this method is to use the thumb and index finger of the right hand to circularly rub the handle from bottom to top in a rapid, screwing motion. 'Scraping' strengthens the expansion or dispersal of the Qi sensation.

410

'Shaking'

This is an aid to 'moving the Qi' (see below). If the needle is shaken back and forth when it is erect, the sensation of Qi is strengthened. If the body of the needle is pulled in one direction and shaken (without bending the needle out of shape!), the conduction of the Qi sensation in the direction toward which the needle points is facilitated.

'Flying'

This is a combination of two movements. The first is the basic twirling method using thumb and index finger, with a relatively large amplitude. The second is a release which, like the 'scraping' method above, creates vibration. The needle is twirled 2 or 3 times in rapid succession and then released, then twirled again and released again. This can be repeated several times until the Qi sensation is strengthened.

'Trembling'

The needle is rapidly raised and thrust, but with only the slightest vertical movement, as if the physician's hand (and the needle between his fingers) was 'trembling.' This method strengthens the Qi sensation.

THE NEEDLE SENSATION: OBTAINING AND MOVING THE QI

One of the fundamentals of acupuncture therapy is that the sensation produced by the needle at specific points, variously described as sore, aching, numb, heavy and distended or swollen, is necessary for effective treatment. When this sensation is perceived by the patient, Qi is said to be 'obtained.' The importance of obtaining Qi has been stressed since earliest times. In chapter 1 of *Spiritual Axis* is written: "If after insertion the Qi does not arrive, use as many methods of manipulation as is necessary [to obtain it]. If after insertion the Qi arrives, remove the needle." Although uncomfortable, it is not to be confused with the pain that a needle might produce when it pricks the skin, or that which often accompanies injections. The sensation differs from individual to individual and is affected by the condition of the patient or the anatomical location of the point. A very weak patient may respond less than a strong one. A point needled in shallow tissue, such as on the face, may feel more distended, while another in deep muscle tissue may be predominantly sore.

There are signs which are useful to the physician in determining whether Qi has been "obtained." These objective manifestations may be more reliable than the subjective response of a patient who may be hypersensitive to needles generally, and only too eager to shout, "I feel it!" as soon as the needle is introduced. Frequently, the muscle fibers will respond to effective needle stimulation by tightening around the body of the needle and constricting its movement. The *Ode to the Standard of Mystery* compares this feeling to the sensation of getting a bite on a fishing line. Conversely, when there is no resistance to the needle, as if it were in a hollow, or pushing through butter, it is unlikely that the point has been 'found'. This is of less significance on the face where the muscle tissue is shallow. A reddish discoloration of the skin similar to that around a fresh mosquito bite is another positive indication, although this sign generally appears only after the needle has been retained in place for a period of time.

If there is no response, i.e., no needle sensation, it is doubtful if the treatment will be effective. (In treating conditions such as hemiplegia, or when the patient is extremely weak following a prolonged illness, this rule may not be applicable.) On the other hand, when the patient responds immediately upon insertion of the needle, the likelihood of a favorable result is increased. "When the Qi arrives, the treatment is effective. This is the essential of needling." *(Spiritual Axis,* chapter 1.) Failing to elicit such response in the beginning, the physician should reconsider the location, depth and angle of the needle, or turn to one of the supplementary methods described above.

'Moving the Qi' refers to the conduction of the needle sensation from the local point of stimulation toward a distant site on the body. In the *Great Compendiuim of Acupuncture and Moxibustion,* it is said that when using distant points in acupuncture, it is necessary that the Qi sensation reach the diseased area. The course along which the needle sensation is conducted is the channel system, described in Section I of this book. 'Moving the Qi' is more than a hypothetical description. The patient may actually feel the conduction of local stimulation toward a distant part of the body. The needle sensation can also be controlled somewhat by controlling the angle and direction of insertion, by slanting the needle along the channel in the direction of the disease, or by simultaneously pressing with the thumb on the side of the point away from the disease (thereby closing off conduction in the opposite direction). After the sensation of Qi is felt to be 'moving', it can be boosted by increasing needle stimulation.

THE INTENSITY OF STIMULATION

Several factors which affect the intensity of stimulation from the needle have already been discussed in this Section. These are summarized in Table 3-1 below.

It is very important to determine how much stimulation is required. According to traditional Chinese medicine, the problem is expressed in terms of Deficient (or hypofunction) and Excessive (hyperfunction) conditions, discussed in the Introduction. Deficient conditions should be strengthened or supplemented, while Excessive conditions are drained or reduced. As Table 3-1 reflects, symptoms or conditions which would be characterized as Deficient, indicating that a method of strengthening be used, usually call for mild needle stimulation (or moxibustion in its place). Conversely, Excessive conditions are treated by draining the Excess by means of strong stimulation. Many conditions, neither predominantly Deficient nor Excessive, are treated with moderate stimulation. Other traditional strengthening and draining techniques are described in chapter 9 at the end of this Section.

It should be remembered that the length of time a needle is retained and the frequency of needle manipulation both contribute to the result. With respect to the frequency of needle manipulation once it has been inserted, there are two principal methods: intermittent and continuous.

Intermittent

When the needle is in place, it is alternately manipulated anywhere from 20-30 seconds to a couple of minutes, then 'rested' for a few minutes, then manipulated again. This procedure is repeated for the duration of the treatment. The effect is said to be cumulative. This is probably the most common method and is particularly recommended for its analgesic, anti-inflammatory and sedative effects.

Continuous

When the needle is in place, it is continuously manipulated until the symptoms have been relieved. This may be several minutes (for analgesia, relieving cramps, or reviving from shock) or even an hour or more (during acupuncture anesthesia).

JOINING POINTS

Joining two or more points with a single needle is a means of increasing stimulation, simplifying the physician's procedure and reducing the patient's fear of many needles.

In superficial tissue, such as the face, two points may be joined with a transverse insertion of one needle just beneath the skin surface. When the tissues are deeper, a slanted insertion can be used. On the limbs, one needle can be inserted vertically to join a point on the anterior (medial) with another on the posterior (lateral) side of a limb, in some instances penetrating the interosseous membrane.

Usually only two points are joined. In certain cases, e.g. the shoulder, a needle can be used to join a point on one side first; then, after withdrawing it partially, the direction of the needle can be changed to join with a point on another side, stimulating a wide area with a single needle.

Table 3-1
NEEDLE STIMULATION METHODS

Needle Stimulation	Method	Response	Indicated For
Strong	Needle is twirled, raised and thrust rapidly, with wide amplitude and vertical movement. Supplementary stimulation may be used.	Needle sensation is strong with wide dispersal or conduction some distance along channel.	Patients with strong constitution and high needle tolerance; acute pain, cramps; usually for points on the limbs; 'Excessive' conditions.
Mild	Needle is twirled, raised and thrust slowly, with little amplitude or vertical movement. Sometimes limited to obtaining Qi sensation.	Needle sensation is slight	Weak patients with little needle tolerance or who are particularly nervous, have history of fainting, or taking acupuncture for first time. Use at points above important organs and for 'Deficient' conditions.
Moderate	Between strong and mild methods.	Needle sensation moderate, sometimes extending along channel.	Used in majority of cases, for most diseases.

413

WITHDRAWING THE NEEDLE

If inserted deeply, the needle should be slowly withdrawn with a slight twirling motion to avoid pulling on subcutaneous tissues or tearing capillaries. If superficially inserted, a quick withdrawal is recommended.

During removal of the needle, a sterile cotton ball can be pressed against the skin and around the body of the needle at the level of the skin to prevent binding.

Afterward, clean the area with alcohol.

MANAGING ACCIDENTS DURING ACUPUNCTURE TREATMENT

A careful physician will encounter few accidents with acupuncture. Familiarity with those that might occur should help the physician in taking appropriate precautions.

Stuck or bent needle

The needle may become stuck in place, difficult to manipulate or withdraw. Often this is caused by the application of excessive force when inserting the needle, uneven manipulation, or twirling the needle in one direction only or with too great an amplitude, causing muscle fibers to bind around the needle. Sometimes the muscles of a tense or extremely nervous patient (or one in great pain) will cramp and bind the needle. When the muscles cramp, or if the patient should suddenly move while the needle is in place, it may cause the needle to bend as well.

A stuck needle often loosens itself spontaneously if left alone for a few minutes. This result can be hastened by lightly stroking or massaging the skin near the point, applying a warm, moistened rag, or (if this fails) by inserting another needle an inch or so from the first. (This will scatter the concentration of Qi and Blood according to tradition). If the needle is stuck due to excessive rotation in one direction, it will usually release when the needle is twirled in the opposite direction, although the amplitude should remain small. Never try to force a stubborn needle.

When a needle bends beneath the skin it is unwise to twirl or rotate it as it is withdrawn. Instead, it should be lightly shaken from side to side and pulled directly out. The angle of the needle's handle often reflects the manner in which the needle has bent subcutaneously. When pulled in accordance with this angle, withdrawal is facilitated. Forcing the needle may cause it to break.

Broken needle

This may arise from imperfections in the body of the needle which were neglected by the physician; from sudden movement of the patient when the needle is in place, or strong muscle contractions; from excessive force used during needle manipulation, or when withdrawing a needle that has stuck.

When a break is discovered, it is important that the physician remain calm and that the patient be kept still. If part of the broken needle protrudes from the skin, forceps or tweezers may be used to extract it. If it has broken at or just below the surface of the skin, apply pressure with the thumb and index finger against the skin surrounding the needle. This may cause it to protrude, where it can be removed with tweezers. If it has broken in deep tissue, the needle fragment must be removed surgically.

Fainting

This is often due to excessive nervousness, fatigue, weakness or even hunger. When the needle is inserted, or during manipulation, the patient may become pale, feel dizzy, nauseous, cold in the extremities, or experience palpitations. In severe cases there may be loss of consciousness, cyanosis, or incontinence.

When these symptoms first appear, needling should immediately stop and those needles already in place should be withdrawn. Ask the patient to lie down. Loosen tight clothing. Offer a warm beverage.

If the patient has passed out, needle (or press hard with the finger nail) at Gv-26 *(Renzhong)*, LI-4 *(Hegu)* or K-1 *(Yongquan)*, or use smelling salts to revive, then allow the patient to rest. Do not attempt acupuncture again that day.

The precautionary measures for fainting are suggested by its causes. Patients who are very weak or tired should be encouraged to rest for a time preceding treatment. Hungry patients should eat first. Those who are excessively nervous or taking acupuncture for the first time should have the procedure clearly explained to them beforehand so that they are reassured. It is usually a good idea to have such patients lie down for treatment. Proper ventilation is also important.

Accidental injury to organs

Lung

The danger of puncturing a lung by inserting a needle too deeply into the chest or upper back cannot be overemphasized. Traumatic pneumothorax could result. Symptoms include pain or a sensation of fullness in the chest, difficult breathing, cyanosis, sweating, lowered blood pressure or other symptoms associated with shock. Percussion of the chest, x-ray, and marked changes in the sound of breathing may provide other indications. In serious cases, a movement of the trachea toward the unpunctured side may be observed. In some instances the patient will show no signs of trouble until hours later when chest pain and breathing difficulties begin to appear.

In superficial cases, a patient should be told to lie on his side. If there is coughing, a cough suppressant should be taken. The patient should be closely watched. If there is breathing difficulty, cyanosis, shock, etc., the condition is serious and the patient should be hospitalized immediately, where air may be removed by thoracentesis.

Puncturing the lung is entirely avoidable if the physician adheres strictly to the proper depth and angle of needle insertion recommended under each point (see Section II). Generally speaking, slanted or transverse (rather than straight) insertions are recommended for areas over the lungs. Compensation must be made for thin patients or children.

Brain and spinal cord

When needling points between or beside the upper cervical vertebrae too deeply or at the wrong angle there is danger that the medulla oblongata may be punctured. Between other vertebrae above the 1st lumbar, there is a danger that the spinal cord could be damaged. Puncturing the medulla oblongata may cause convulsions, paralysis or coma. There may also be severe bleeding. Post-treatment symptoms of headache, nausea, vomiting or disorientation may be the first indications of trouble. Pricking the spinal cord causes an electric, 'flash' pain that can be felt in the extremities. If stimulation is prolonged, continued pain may result after treatment.

As in the case of the lung, accidents associated with the brain and spinal cord can be avoided if the proper depth and angle of insertion is observed. Particular caution must be exercised with regard to the points Gv-15 *(Yamen)*, Gv-16 *(Fengfu)* and GB-20 *(Fengchi)*.

Heart, liver, spleen, kidney

Familiarity with anatomy will help the physician exercise care when needling points in the vicinity of these organs. A physical examination will signal changes in the size of these organs which can then be compensated for by shortening the depth, or altering the angle of needle insertion. This is especially significant in cases of cardiac disease or enlargement or either the liver or spleen.

When the liver or spleen is punctured and bleeding ensues, pain will be felt locally, often extending toward the back, and the abdominal muscles will constrict. Puncturing the kidney will result in pain about the waist, and possibly blood in the urine. If the bleeding is serious, blood pressure will decline and shock may follow.

If the damage is only minor, it will usually heal itself with sufficient rest. If there is bleeding, careful observation of the patient (blood pressure, etc.) is required; a cold compress may be applied to stop the bleeding. If serious, the patient should be hospitalized.

The propinquity of other organs to acupuncture loci when specific diseases are present in the body (e.g., enlargement of gall bladder, retention of urine, intestinal adhesion, etc.) must also be taken into consideration.

Nerve trunk

If a nerve trunk is directly stimulated, a 'flash' pain extendng to the extremities will result. This should not be confused with the needle sensation characteristic of acupuncture ('obtaining Qi'). If stimulation is repeated, damage could be done to the nervous tissue and there may be peripheral neuritis, whose symptoms are continued pain and numbness, or functional impairment along the path of the nerve.

In superficial cases massage will help. In more serious instances, vitamin B complex can be injected in the points.

Local hematoma

When capillaries are punctured by the needle there may be a small amount of bleeding or slight discoloration of the skin. Normally, these signs will disappear by themselves and no exceptional measures need be taken. If a larger area is affected, accompanied by pain, impaired movement, etc., a cold compress should be applied to stop the bleeding, after which the area may be lightly massaged or a hot compress substituted so as to help disperse the hematoma.

Sometimes bleeding is caused by a burr or other irregularity on the tip of the needle. Needles must always be inspected prior to use. The skin should also be examined for the location of superficial capillaries and blood vessels before needling. Particular care must be taken when treating old people whose blood vessel walls are less elastic and therefore more likely to puncture.

Chapter 3

Other Needling Techniques

CUTANEOUS ACUPUNCTURE

Cutaneous needles are used to stimulate the skin superficially, without puncturing deeper tissues subcutaneously. The most common varieties are the 'plum blossom' and 'seven star' needles, so called because of the configuration of individual needles in the cluster that forms the head. (Dia. 3-9) Since the Cultural Revolution, another cutaneous instrument called a 'rolling drum' has gained popularity. (Dia. 3-10)

Several needles striking the skin simultaneously cause less pain and stimulate a wider surface area than does a single needle. They are thus more suitable for use on small children than are regular needles whose stimulation (and discomfort) is more concentrated. In fact, the cutaneous needle is nicknamed the 'infant needle', although it is widely recommended for adults as well.

Unlike individual acupuncture needles, the cutaneous needle is rarely used above a single point. Instead it is applied over a broad area, tapping (or rolling) across the skin, more in the manner of pecking than puncturing. Where an area has been stimulated (commonly from 5-10 minutes), the skin is typically reddened and moist. Bleeding is generally to be avoided.

As might be expected the cutaneous needle is described in the ancient medical texts, and its therapeutic properties defined, in terms of traditional theory: "To each of the twelve [Primary] channels belongs a cutaneous region. Thus, the hundred diseases arise first in the skin and pores." *(Simple Questions,* chapter 56) Since each of the channels has its corresponding domain on the skin and is linked to one of the Organ systems, 'tapping' the skin stimulates not only the tissues in the immediate vicinity, but the channel (or channels) which traverse it as well, whose Qi circulates throughout the course of the channel and its associated Organ system.

Sites for cutaneous stimulation (Table 3-2)

Because of the involvement of the channels in the cutaneous regions, an internal disease associated with a certain channel can be treated by tapping along that channel. In practice, points along the

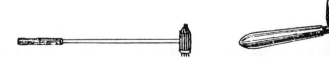

Dia. 3-9 Cutaneous Needle   **Dia. 3-10 Rolling Drum**

Governing channel (which 'governs' all the Yang channels) and particularly along the course of the Bladder channel parallel to the spine are commonly selected. Diseases affecting the Organs are treated by choosing segments along those channels on the same horizontal plane as the affected Organ, with particular emphasis on the Organ's Associated point.

The local area of pain may be tapped (e.g., in the neck region for stiff neck, in the lumbo-sacral region for low back pain) with particular emphasis on principal acupuncture points. Similarly, cutaneous regions above sites of internal diseases (e.g., above the intercostal spaces for diseases of the thoracic cavity, or in the occipital region for occipital headaches) are also stimulated in this manner.

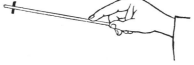

**Dia. 3-11 Holding Cutaneous
Needle**

Method

The area must first be cleaned with alcohol.

The plum blossom or seven star needles are held as shown in Diagram 3-11. The head of the instrument should strike the skin at right angles to the surface, rather than obliquely. This will distribute the force equally among the needles and prevent a single needle from puncturing the skin.

The needle is held 1-2 inches above the surface of the skin and rapidly tapped along the chosen area with a wrist motion only. Holding the needle too high or using the arm in tapping may be too forceful and cause bleeding.

When treating areas on the head and face, for chronic or Deficient disease, or when treating patients who are very weak, old, or of tender years, a relatively mild method of stimulation is indicated. When the skin becomes red, needling should stop. Conversely, patients with strong constitutions and whose diseases are acute (or Excessive) may be treated more vigorously. The skin should become red and moist and occasionally there is slight bleeding. The physician's judgment is necessary in determining the proper amount of stimulation.

Treatments are given daily or on alternating days. Ten to fifteen treatments over a period of 2-3 weeks may be considered an average course of treatment for most chronic diseases.

The same principles apply to the rolling drum except, obviously, that it is rolled over the skin rather than tapped.

Indications

A wide variety of illnesses are amenable to this mode of treatment. Particularly good results have been obtained in cases of hypertension, headache, myopia, dysmenorrhea, intercostal neuralgia, neurasthenia, gastrointestinal disorders and local skin diseases like neurodermatitis. Instructions for specific diseases are provided in Section IV.

Other considerations

• When tapping the needle over an area, the usual sequence is from above to below, medial to lateral.

• This method should not be used where there are ulcerations, or over areas of traumatic injury. Further, it is counter-indicated for acute infectious diseases or acute abdominal disorders.

Table 3-2
COMMON SITES FOR CUTANEOUS ACUPUNCTURE

Area	Location	Indications	Remarks
Back	3 paraspinal lines	1st line: 1 cm. from midline; 2nd line: 2 cm. from midline; 3rd line: 3–4 cm. from midline	Extensive, see entry for M-BW-35 (Jiajixue) in Section II	All serve as principal points
	Supraspinatus area	2 lines running parallel to the supraspinatus muscle	Shoulder and scapula pain, paralysis of upper extremity, diseases of the respiratory organs	Combine with appropriate paraspinal points
	Scapular area	2 lines over the scapula	Same as above	Same as above
	Lumbar area	2-3 lines, 2-3 cm. lateral to the paraspinal lines in the area between the inferior angle of the scapula and the ilium	Low back pain, paralysis of the lower extremities, diseases of the stomach, pancreas, liver, and gall bladder	Same as above
	Sacral area	2-3 curved lines over the sacrum and gluteal region	Lower back pain, urogenital disorders, intestinal diseases and paralysis of the lower extremities	Same as above
Head	Vertex area	5-7 lines from the anterior hairline to a line connecting the tips of the ears	Headache, neurasthenia	Combine with appropriate points according to disease
	Frontal area	3 horizontal lines across the forehead	Same as above	Same as above

Area	Location	Indications	Remarks
Occipital area	3 horizontal lines across the occiput	Headache, neurasthenia	Combine with appropriate points according to disease
Temporal area	1-5 lines spreading over the temples from the ears	Same as above	
Face			
Eye area	1-3 horizontal lines over the orbits	Eye diseases, facial paralysis	
Mouth area	1-2 lines around the mouth	Facial paralysis	Same as above
Mandibular area	1-3 lines across the mandible	Same as above	Same as above
Cheek area	1-3 lines across the zygoma	Same as above	Same as above
Chest and Abdomen			
Intercostal area	1-2 lines across each intercostal space	Disorders of the thorax (including heart and lungs)	Same as above
Sternocostal area	1-2 lines across the sternum and clavicle	Same as above	Same as above
Upper abdomen area	3-7 horizontal lines from the costal angle to a line parallel with the navel	Disorders of the liver, gall bladder, stomach, and spleen	Same as above
Lower abdomen area	3-9 horizontal lines from a line parallel to the pubic symphysis	Urogenital and intestinal disorders	Same as above
Inguinal area	1-2 lines in the inguinal area	Genital disorders	Same as above

Area	Location	Indications	Remarks
Neck	1-3 horizontal lines across muscle bellies	Neck and digestive disorders	Combine with appropriate points according to disease
	Lateral cervical area 1-3 lines across the sternocleido-mastoid muscle	Same as above	Same as above
	Lower cervical area 1-2 lines across suprasternal area	Same as above	Same as above
Extremities	1-2 lines along each channel	See pathology of the channels (Section I)	

421

PRESSURE ACUPUNCTURE

The pressure needle, also called the 'pushing needle', is one of the Nine Needles mentioned in the *Inner Classic.* It is used to press against the external skin above acupuncture points and may therefore be considered a form of cutaneous needle, like the plum blossom. However, unlike other cutaneous needles, the pressure needle is blunt-tipped and does not prick the skin at all. Its stimulation is derived from highly focused pressure similar to, but more specific than, finger-tip massage ('acupressure').

Most needles are made of thick steel wire, though bone or hard wood may be substituted. The average needle length is 3-4 inches.

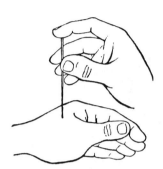

Dia. 3-12   Holding Pressure Needle

Method

The needle is held against the skin and pressed downward as shown in Diagram 3-12, the amount of stimulation being controlled by the pressure of the index finger.

The use of the pressure needle, described in chapter 1 of *Spiritual Axis,* is to "press the vessels and obtain the Qi."

Mild stimulation is provided when the skin in the vicinity of the needle tip becomes red or the symptoms are relieved, after which the pressure on the needle should be slowly diminished and the needle removed. The area may then be lightly massaged. When stronger stimulation is desired, the needle is pressed more rapidly and with greater force, causing a sensation of soreness and distension or pain which may extend beyond the point. The needle is then quickly removed.

Note that there is no twirling or manipulation other than the vertical pressure from the index finger.

Indications

The traditional source for this method is a passage in chapter 7 of *Spiritual Axis:* "When the disease is in the vessels and the Qi is diminished it should be supplemented. For this purpose, apply the pressure needle at the Well and Gushing points." Pressure acupuncture is indicated for Deficient diseases with pain, and weakened Qi in the channels. This would include conditions like stomach-ache, abdominal pain, indigestion, nervous vomiting, morning sickness, and nervous dysfunction. The relative simplicity of this method recommends its use; it may easily be taught to patients who can then treat themselves.

Points for pressing are selected along the channel associated with the disease, or from among those points used in regular acupuncture for the same condition. Points of pain may also be used.

The average course of treatment is about ten visits, on consecutive days, though superficial conditions can be treated in only one or two visits. If after ten treatments the symptoms persist, another method should be considered.

INTRADERMAL ACUPUNCTURE

Intradermal embedding of needles is a modern development of the ancient method of retaining needles in place. Two varieties of needles have been designed for this purpose. (Dia. 3-13) The first, the 'grain of wheat' or straight intradermal needle, is inserted at an angle almost horizontal to the surface of the skin, about 0.8 to 1.3 cm. The handle of the needle, lying flat on the skin surface, is held in place by a piece of adhesive tape. This type of needle is generally used on the back and limbs. The second variety, the intradermal tack, is inserted at an angle perpendicular to the skin surface to a depth flush with the head of the needle. Because the intradermal tack is only a few tenths of a centimeter in length, it is used for only the most superficial punctures, specifically on the ear. Once in place, the tack is secured by adhesive tape.

Because of their size, the needles may be difficult to hold with the fingers. Tweezers are helpful. Another method, particularly useful when inserting tacks on the ear, is to apply the strip of adhesive tape to the back of the needle before insertion.

Points are selected from among the regular acupuncture loci, however consideration should be given to those points that will not interfere with normal body movement. Intradermal needles are commonly retained from one to three days, or as long as a week. To avoid infection, needles should be retained for shorter periods in hot weather.

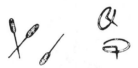

Dia. 3-13   Intradermal Needles

Indications

Intradermal acupuncture is most often used in chronic or stubborn, painful diseases such as tension headache, migraine headache, stomach-ache, bilious colic, neurasthenia, hypertension, asthma, irregular menstruation.

Other considerations

- Usually only 1-2 points are selected unilaterally, or points on both sides may be used in rotation.
- If the needles cause pain or inhibit movement they should be withdrawn and re-inserted. (However, on the ear a hot, numb sensation locally is considered a good sign, whereas no sensation after needle insertion is regarded as useless. See chapter 7 of this Section.)
- It is essential, particularly in hot weather or if the patient is involved in strenuous work, to keep the area around the needle clean so as to prevent infection. The physician may choose to remove the needle daily for sterilization of both the skin and the needle.

THE 'BEARD OF WHEAT' OR LONG NEEDLE ACUPUNCTURE

The 'beard of wheat' needle, so-called because of its shape (Dia. 3-14), is related to the 'long' needle, which is one of the ancient Nine Needles. Its length, varying from 5 inches to 2 feet, makes it possible to join several points along a channel with a single needle. The stimulation it provides is correspondingly large. Because of its size, manipulation is somewhat different from other needles and a physician must practice for a time before attempting to needle a patient.

The needle is generally made of stainless steel wire, 28-32 gauge (.38-.28 mm).

Method

The length of this needle requires the use of both hands. The right hand holds the handle and is used principally in twirling or rotating, while the fingers of the left hand guide the tip and exert vertical pressure near the skin. Thus the hand closer to the tip controls the direction and force of the needle. The same is true when the needle is withdrawn.

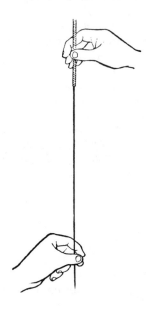

**Dia. 3-14 'Beard of Wheat'
Needle Method**

Direction and depth

These elements are determined by local anatomy and the weight of the patient. Straight, vertical insertions can be made on parts of the abdomen, whereas slanted or transverse insertions are indicated for lower back, buttocks and above or below the knee. On the head, or above vital organs a transverse insertion almost parallel to the skin is required. *All movements of the needle should be performed slowly,* and the patient continually consulted to determine needle sensation. If the patient reports an abnormal sensation, the needle is withdrawn.

For example, a needle inserted along the mid-line of the abdomen, joining points on the Conception channel, should cause the patient to feel a sore, distended sensation extending upward to the throat and ribs and downward to the lower abdomen and waist. If instead there is a sharp pain, the angle of the needle should be changed somewhat toward the horizontal, or the direction altered. The standard is always the obtaining of the Qi sensation, typical of all acupuncture. Patients with Deficient conditions usually show only a mild response, while those with Excessive conditions respond more strongly.

Indications

Because of the difficulty of this method, it is generally reserved for the treatment of chronic diseases, and then only after shorter needles have proved ineffective. Certain mental diseases, gastro-intenstinal disorders, irregular menstruation and rheumatism are among the conditions for which this needle is recommended.

Other considerations

- Particular caution must be exercised when treating very weak or thin patients.
- A thorough knowledge of anatomy is essential so that vital organs and blood vessels are avoided.
- The longer the needle, the greater the patient's apprehension. This should be borne in mind when selecting a needle.

BAREFOOT DOCTOR ACUPUNCTURE

During the Cultural Revolution, a technique that was previously known only in the tradition of the people of Northeastern China, utilizing a variation of the ancient big needle, was further developed by local medical personnel so as to become a part of general acupuncture practice. It is called barefoot doctor acupuncture in recognition of China's paramedical workers who have been encouraged to adopt the traditional folk medicine of their native regions.

In this method, a relatively thick needle is inserted superficially at points along the Governing channel between the vertebrae, and at a few points elsewhere on the body. This method has been proven to have an analgesic, anti-allergic, and anti-inflammatory effect, helping to regulate the nervous and endocrine systems. It is sometimes used in acupuncture anesthesia.

It will be remembered from Section I that the range of diseases within the domain of the Governing channel is large, and that through its connecting channels it is joined to the Bladder channel whose Associated points are linked with many important organs. These connections provide the theoretical explanation for the numerous diseases treated by stimulation of points along the Governing channel.

Needles

Two varieties of needles are commonly used. The first, called a steel needle (Dia. 3-15), ranges from about 2-4.5 inches in length and has a diameter of between 0.6 and 1.2 mm, the thicker needle used on intervertebral points. The tip of the needle is only slightly tapered, allowing shallow insertion, but with maximum stimulation.

The second, a tubular needle (Dia. 3-16), is made of stainless steel tubing and features 2-4 small holes in the body through which medicine can be injected. It is for this purpose that the tubular needle, instead of the steel needle, is used.

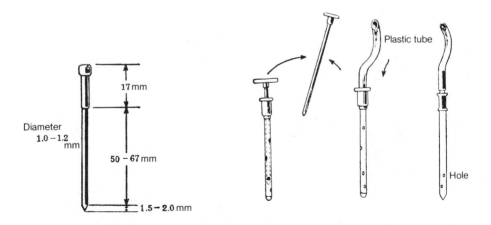

Dia. 3-15 Steel Needle   **Dia. 3-16 Tubular Needle**

425

Selecting points

One of the advantages of using this method is that rather few points are used to treat a broad spectrum of diseases. For simplicity's sake, each of the intervertebral points is given the name of the vertebra above whose spinous process it is located. For example, the point located above the spinous process of the second thoracic vertebra is called Thoracic #2.

There are 10 intervertebral points. (Dia. 3-17) The most important one, used in every treatment, is located above the spinous process of the 6th thoracic vertebra and has been given the special name, 'Barefoot Doctor point.' (This is identical to the regularly listed acupuncture point Gv-11 *(Shendao).)* There are only 7 points in addition to those between the vertebrae: Tip of Tragus (see Ear Points), Posterior *Hegu* (at the base between the 1st and 2nd metacarpal bones), Ankle point (at the inferior margin of the lateral malleolus), N-LE-47 *(Xinhuantiao),* and the Three Needles at the Shoulder points (a group including LI-15 *(Jianyu)* and two points located one unit above the axillary crease, front and back).

Listed below are many diseases and the points which are used in treating them according to the barefoot doctor method.

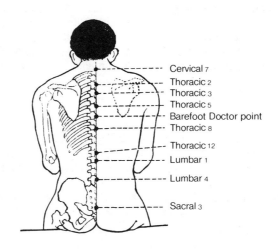

**Dia. 3-17 Barefoot
Doctor Points**

TREATMENT OF DISEASE WITH BAREFOOT DOCTOR ACUPUNCTURE

Points	Disease
Barefoot Doctor point, Thoracic #5	Erysipelas, acute skin infections, lymphangitis, boils, carbuncle, acute mastitis, parotitis, urticaria, neurodermatitis, chronic ulceration of lower limb, pruritus
Barefoot Doctor point. Thoracic #2, #5	Psoriasis, eczema and other skin diseases
Barefoot Doctor point, Thoracic #5, #8, Posterior *Hegu*	Tension headache, nervous dysfunction, trigeminal neuralgia, psychosis, hypertension
Barefoot Doctor point, Cervical #7, Thoracic #5	Acute tonsilitis, pharyngitis, T.B. of lymph gland
Barefoot Doctor point, Thoracic #5, Lumbar #4, N-LE-47 *(Xinhuantiao)*	Acute arthritic pain, low back pain, sciatica
Barefoot Doctor point, Thoracic #3, #5	Asthma, bronchitis
Barefoot Doctor point, Thoracic #12	Nephritis, stomach spasm, gastric ulcer
Barefoot Doctor point, Thoracic #3	Rheumatic heart disease
Barefoot Doctor point, Thoracic #8, #12	Hepatitis, pancreatitis, roundworm in the bile duct
Barefoot Doctor point, Thoracic #5	Arteriole spasm, Buerger's disease, peripheral neuritis, multiple neuritis
Barefoot Doctor point, Lumbar #1, #4	Diabetes, polyuria, incontinence, spermatorrhea, impotence, amenorrhea, prostatitis
Barefoot Doctor point, Lumbar #1, Thoracic #5	Nephritis, leukoderma of external genitals
Barefoot Doctor point, Thoracic #5, #8, Tip of Tragus	Keratitis, traumatic cataract, arteriosclerosis of arteries at base of eye, squint (stabismus)
Barefoot Doctor point, Thoracic #5, Lumbar #4, Sacral #3	Hemiplegia, paraplegia, sequelae of infantile paralysis
Posterior *Hegu,* Three Needles at the Shoulder points	Paralysis of upper limb
Ankle point, N-LE-47 *(Xinhuantiao)*	Paralysis of lower limb

427

Method

For most of the above conditions, acute diseases can be treated once daily for the first three days, then on alternating days, 10 visits to one course of treatment. Chronic diseases should be treated on alternating days, 10-15 visits constituting one course of treatment.

A sitting position is recommended for needling points on the back. (Dia. 3-18) The arms should be crossed on the chest, the head held forward and bowed, and the shoulders pulled forward and down so as to stretch the skin tight on the back. The needle should be inserted with its tip pointed downward at about a 30-40° angle to the surface of the skin. After initial insertion, the needle is further inserted 1.5-2 units almost horizontal to the skin surface along the spine. The needle must not be inserted at an angle vertical to the skin, where it might penetrate the spinal cord or an internal organ. However, caution must also be exercised so as not to allow the needle tip, in the course of a transverse insertion, to break the skin surface in a second location, as the skin above the spine is very shallow.

The Three Needles at the Shoulder points and N-LE-47 *(Xinhuantiao)* should be needled according to the methods provided for each point in Section II.

The Ankle point may be needled with the patient lying on his side, ankle turned inward, needle pointed in a superior, medial direction 1-1.5 units. Ideally, the needle sensation should extend up the leg.

The Tip of Tragus point should be punctured with a fine needle, 0.5 unit in length.

The Posterior *Hegu* point should likewise be punctured with a fine needle, 3 units in length. After the needle sensation (Qi) is obtained with a straight insertion, the needle may be partially withdrawn and the needle pointed between the joint of the 1st and 2nd metacarpal bones.

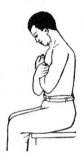

**Dia. 3-18   Patient's
Position for Barefoot
Doctor Acupuncture**

Other considerations

- Because of the diameter of the needles used, the stimulation is quite strong. The likelihood of weaker or more nervous patients fainting is correspondingly greater.
- This method should not be used on pregnant women, or those with hemorrhagic diseases.

GREAT NEEDLE ACUPUNCTURE

This may be considered a hybrid needle, developed from crossing two of the ancient Nine Needles, the long and the big. The length varies from 3 inches to 1 foot, similar to the long needle, however its diameter usually matches that of the big or the barefoot doctor needles. With other lengthy needles it shares the advantage of requiring only one insertion to join many points.

428

The great needle is manipulated in the same manner as the beard of wheat needle, and the same precautions apply. Because of its great diameter, however, the stimulation is stronger. For this reason the great needle is used today primarily in the treatment of paralysis.

This needle is believed to work best in muscular or tendinous tissue. If inserted over a long distance too superficially it causes the skin to buckle around the needle and the needle tip to break the surface in a second location; if inserted too deeply it may strike a bone.

BLOODLETTING

There are numerous references in early medical texts to the technique of pricking superficial blood vessels so as to 'drain Heat' from the body. In practice, this method is also used to 'activate' the Blood and reduce swelling.

Any type of acupuncture needle may be used for this purpose, although a thick filiform (fine) and the pyramid needles are probably the most common, the latter being specifically intended for letting blood. The cutaneous needle, rolling drum, hypodermic needle or scalpel may be preferred for certain kinds of incisions.

Method

Pricking method
Pressure is ordinarily applied to the area first so as to cause slight venous pooling. This makes the blood vessels easier to see. A point or a blood vessel is then chosen and pricked with a quick, deft motion, about 0.1 inch deep. The needle is then immediately withdrawn allowing a few drops of blood to escape. To prevent a deep insertion of the needle, a ball of cotton may be wrapped around the lower part of the needle body exposing only as much of the needle as the physician intends to insert. After pricking, the puncture is pressed with a cotton ball until the bleeding stops. This is the most widely practiced method of bloodletting, commonly used for hematoma, low back pain, fever, tonsillitis, acute gastrointestinal inflammation, heat stroke, apoplexy, etc.

A variation of this method, called 'stirring', is to make a slight incision (rather than merely a needle prick) on a capillary, and squeeze out a few drops of blood. This method is used on the back of the ear, chest and back.

Clumping method
Pyramid needle, scalpel, or cutaneous needle is applied over a small area (rather than a particular vessel), making many tiny pin-prick like punctures, or heavier tapping which causes irritation and slight bleeding. This method is generally used around tender areas of injured soft tissue, abscesses, or the reddened, swollen skin tissue associated with skin diseases like neurodermatitis, allergic dermatitis, and erysipelas.

Dispersing method
Using a cutaneous needle, a wide area of the skin surface is stimulated to induce superficial bleeding. This method is most appropriate for skin diseases like neurodermatitis, allergic dermatitis, and erysipelas.

Indications

Acute and chronic tonsillitis, neurodermatitis, allergic dermatitis, acute sprain, heatstroke, abscesses, febrile diseases, headache, rhinitis, acute conjunctivitis or keratitis, numbness of the fingers or toes, erysipelas, eczema, lymphangitis, phlebitis, hemorrhoids and coma.

Letting blood is counter-indicated for patients with hemorrhagic diseases or vascular tumors, and should be used only with the utmost caution on pregnant or recently-delivered women, or weak, anemic or hypotensive patients.

Frequency

Depending upon the disease, treat once daily or on alternating days, 1-3 visits constituting a course of treatment. For patients who tend to bleed more, treat only once or twice a week.

Other considerations

- Pricking should be performed as gently as possible and the size of the puncture or incision kept small.
- It is important to thoroughly clean the skin with alcohol around the puncture both prior to and following the blood-letting to avoid infection.

WARM NEEDLE ACUPUNCTURE

First mentioned in the Han Dynasty classic, *Discussion of Cold Induced Disorders,* warm needle acupuncture is a mixture of acupuncture and moxibustion. A filiform needle is inserted at a point and then 'warmed' by burning a clump of moxa attached to the other end of the needle. (Dia. 3-19) In this manner, the movement of Qi and Blood through the channels is facilitated. According to traditional pathology, this method is indicated for conditions wherein the channels are Cold or stagnant, or when the circulation of Qi and Blood is obstructed.

Needles made of silver are considered most ideal because of their excellent heat conducting properties. However, regular stainless steel needles may also be utilized. It is important that the moxa be secured on the 'tail' of the needle so that it doesn't fall and burn the skin. A thin slice about 2 cm. in length may be cut from a moxa stick and attached over the tail or inserted in the ring of the needle. (A towel may be placed around the base of the needle to catch falling ashes.) Burning 1-3 slices is generally sufficient to cause the desired warmth below the skin.

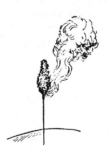

**Dia. 3-19   Warm
Needle Acupuncture**

Indications

Wind Dampness and Cold diseases such as arthritis, generalized weakness or cold, numb limbs, diarrhea, abdominal distension. This method should not be used for conditions in which the needle cannot be retained in place (cramps, spasms), for febrile diseases or for hypertension.

Other considerations

- Once the needle is in place and the Qi sensation obtained, no further manipulation of the needle should be made.

430

● The moxa should be ignited from below so that the thermal conduction is not impeded by as yet unburned material.

HOT NEEDLE ACUPUNCTURE

Hot needle acupuncture is a method whereby the tip of a relatively thick needle is heated with an alcohol lamp, inserted beneath the skin, and then quickly withdrawn. The *Inner Classic* refers to this as a 'tempered needle'. The Ming Dynasty physician, Wu Hegao, recommended this technique for Cold obstruction which has penetrated to the bones. It is currently used in the treatment of abscesses and hardening of the lymph glands, for certain skin diseases and severe arthritis.

Instruments

Needles are generally 3-4 inches in length with a diameter of 0.5-1 mm., the longer and thicker needles being used for deeper insertions. Because the needle must be held by the physician when heated, the handle is usually made of wood or bamboo. For superficial stimulation over a wide area, a cutaneous needle with several tips clustered together may be used.

Method

Deep insertion
Appropriate for surgical diseases like abscesses or hardening of the lymph glands. When lancing an abscess, a relatively thick needle is used, whereas a finer needle should be selected for treating hardening of the lymph glands. After the needle has been heated over an alcohol lamp, it is quickly inserted in the affected tissue and then immediately withdrawn. A cotton ball may then be secured over the puncture.

Superficial insertion
Generally used for arthritic pain or stubborn skin diseases. Instead of lancing the affected area, the needle is used to tap or lightly prick the skin superficially. For arthritic pain or cold and numbness in the skin and muscle tissue, a single needle is sufficient. When treating skin diseases, however, the multi-tipped cutaneous needle is preferred.

Other considerations

● For deep insertions, care must be taken to control the depth of the needle puncture and to avoid local blood vessels.
● Superficial tapping must be even and light to prevent skin lesions.

ELECTRO-ACUPUNCTURE*

After a needle has been inserted at a point and the Qi sensation obtained, an electric current is passed through the needle both to strengthen and alter the nature of stimulation. This is electro-

---

*Our main text, **Acupuncture and Moxibustion,** describes the construction and characteristics of several electro-acupuncture devices. We have omitted this. Several such devices are available on the market in this country with instructions concerning their use.—*Editors*

acupuncture. It was first used in China during the 1930's and is now widely employed throughout the country and abroad.

Electro-acupuncture has certain advantages over ordinary acupuncture. First, it can substitute for the time-consuming hand manipulation, thereby freeing the doctor to treat other patients. Second, the amount of stimulation can be more objectively measured and regulated by adjusting the current, amplitude and frequency. Third, it can, if desired, produce a higher and more continuous level of stimulation than manual manipulation (an important factor in acupuncture anesthesia). And finally, it is possible to apply the current through an electrode on the skin surface without the aid of a needle inserted subcutaneously, i.e., it can supplement or, to some degree, substitute for needle puncture.

Method

The characteristics peculiar to different kinds of electro-acupuncture apparati make it difficult to describe operation in detail. Some general observations can be made.

Because electro-acupuncture involves both needle and electric stimulation, it is best to use this method only when the patient has demonstrated a tolerance for regular acupuncture.

The machine should not be turned on until the needles are in place and the conducting wires have been attached to the needles. At the beginning, the electric potential should be zero and the current only gradually increased so as to monitor the patient's reaction.

The amount of electric stimulation depends entirely on the tolerance of the patient and the nature of the disease. A condition like sequelae of infantile paralysis usually calls for stronger stimulation.

After the treatment has progressed for a minute or two the patient may become accustomed to the electric current such that effective stimulation gradually declines. This often happens when a regular pulse is used. When this occurs, the current should be increased accordingly. On the other hand, when the pulses come at irregular intervals or randomly, this phenomenon does not occur.

Most electro-acupuncture treatments last from 10-20 minutes, although in certain caes they may continue for as long as 4-5 hours.

Selecting points

Point selection for electro-acupuncture is identical to regular acupuncture except that usually only the principal points in a prescription are chosen. If only one point is selected, the other electrode (since there must be two to complete the circuit) can be held in the hand or taped to the skin. For better results, attach the second conducting wire to a lead bar which is wrapped in cloth, moistened with water and placed on the skin. Because of the great difference in surface area between the needle and the plate, the sensation at the point should be quite strong while that at the area of the plate relatively weak.

Commonly observed phenomena during electro-acupuncture

When the needles are placed in areas where there is much muscle tissue, the muscles will contract at the same frequency as the output. When the pulse passes a certain frequency the muscles will go into a weak tetanus accompanied by a numb, swollen and heavy sensation.

Remarks

Electro-acupuncture provides stronger stimulation than regular acupuncture. It is therefore necessary to guard against fainting. Because electro-acupuncture also induces muscle contraction, care should be taken that the needles do not bend or break.

In most acupuncture machines, the potentiometers are nonlinear, i.e., the higher they are turned the larger the increment of power. It is therefore necessary to adjust them very slowly, to avoid giving the patient a sudden burst of stimulation.

When opposing points differ markedly in sensation, switch the outputs. If the one that originally had a strong sensation has a weak one or vice versa, then the problem is in the machine or wires. If there is no change, the difference is due to insertion of the needles in anatomically different structures.

Points below the elbow and knee or on the face are more sensitive to electric stimulation than are other locations.

Indications

Electro-acupuncture is generally indicated for the same diseases as regular acupuncture. However, because its stimulation is usually stronger, it is seldom used when only mild needle stimulation is required. Electro-acupuncture is especially recommended for neuralgia and nervous paralysis.*

Other considerations

• If a needle has been used for burning moxa (see Warm Needle Acupuncture), there is usually some oxidation on the surface of the needle, preventing proper conduction of the electric current. The same is true of needles whose handles are wound with aluminum wire which has since assumed a gold coloration. If this is the case, the clip from the conducting wire should be attached to the body of the needle, rather than to the handle.

• This method is usually counter-indicated for patients with a history of heart disease. It is particularly important in such cases that the electrical path does not cross the heart.

INJECTION THERAPY

This is a relatively new method in which medicine is injected at regular acupuncture points, points of pain (tenderness), or points of 'positive response'.**

Instruments

#20-27 gauge hypodermic needle and 2, 5, 10 and 20 milliliter capacity syringe.

Depending on the disease, various medicines may be chosen to inject in the muscle. Among those commonly used are a 5-10% glucose solution, normal saline, distilled water, 25% magnesium sulphate, vitamin B1 or B12, 0.25-2% procaine hydrochloride, and certain tissue fluids, as well as liquid extracts from herbs such as *Angelica sinesis (danggui), Carthamus tinctoris (honghua)* or *Lingusticum wallichii (chuangxiong)*.

Selection of points

Depending on the disease, the following items should be considered:

On the back and chest, the Associated or Alarm points are palpated for tenderness or 'positive response', in which case they may be injected.

---

*Many acupuncturists believe that continuous, regular frequencies are best for treating pain and spasms, whereas pulses which alternate quick and slow periods are preferrable in treating paralysis and numbness. Others, using traditional terminology, say that regular frequencies drain Excess while irregular frequencies strengthen Deficiency.—*Editors*

**Positive response points are any irregularities that can be palpated on the skin surface whether they be flat, round, strand-like or nodular in shape. Discoloration or local changes of skin temperature are also included; scars are not.—*Editors*

'Positive response points' palpated along the course of the related channel, or acupuncture points of special significance such as the pulmonary tuberculosis point (N-BW-6 *(Jiehexue))*, blood pressure point (N-BW-2 *(Xueyadian))*, or the ulcer point (N-BW-13 *(Kuiyangxue))* may be injected.

In cases of traumatic injury to soft tissues, the point of greatest tenderness can be chosen. Or, inject the origin or insertion of related major muscles or tendons. In cases of 'slipped disc', the injection can be made near the spinal nerve root.

When treating a particular disease, points for injection can be selected from among regular acupuncture points most efficacious in treating that disease. Those points in areas of the body where muscle tissue is thin should be used as little as possible.

Method

After a point has been selected and the skin cleansed with alcohol, the needle is slowly inserted to a depth where the Qi sensation is felt. The syringe should then be drawn to check for evidence of bleeding. If there is none, the medicine may be injected at a moderate rate, or more slowly for patients who are particularly weak or have chronic diseases. If a relatively large amount of medicine is being injected, the needle may be progressively withdrawn to more superficial muscle layers, or the direction of the needle varied.

On the face or ear, 0.3-0.5 milliliters of medicine per injection is the norm; on the limbs and thick muscles of the lower back, from 2-15 ml. The amount will vary according to the concentration of the medicine and the particular condition of each patient. Depending on the location of the point, when determining the depth of insertion, the physician must also take into account the depth of the tender tissue. If a point is tender to superficial pressure, the injection should be correspondingly superficial, whereas a point that is painful only when pressed with some force requires a deeper injection.

Generally speaking, injections may be given daily or on alternating days, 7-12 treatments in a single course. Between two courses of treatment, the patient should be allowed to rest from 3-5 days.

Indications

Certain kinds of low back and leg pain, shoulder pain, pain of joints and surrounding tissues, sprains, sciatica, perifocal inflammation of shoulder joint, arthritis, etc.

Many other diseases for which regular acupuncture is indicated, particularly bronchitis, pulmonary tuberculosis, hypertension, peptic ulcer, hepatitis, neurasthenia, and sequelae of brain concussion.

Other considerations

• There are certain uncomfortable side effects which may accompany injections of medicine. These should be clearly explained to the patient so that he or she is not unduly alarmed. There may be local soreness and distension around the point of injection, and perhaps even temporary exacerbation of symptoms. There may also be a low fever. These side effects should disappear after a few hours or within a day.

• If more than one medicine is used, the physician should take care to see that they are compatible.

• When using medicines for which there is a possible allergic reaction (e.g., procaine), an allergy test should first be given to the patient.

• When first treating weak or older patients, the amount of medicine should be reduced accordingly. Injections should not be given to pregnant women in the lumbo-sacral region.

• Medicine should not be injected into the joint capsule as this may cause severe pain and fever. Glucose should not be injected in superficial tissue, but only in deep muscle tissue.

APPENDIX 1: PALPATING FOR 'POSITIVE RESPONSE POINTS'

Areas on the back, chest, abdomen and limbs can be lightly palpated to examine for 'positive response points'. Certain points or lines are particularly useful for this purpose, as they are often the first to respond to pathological changes in the body.

There are three vertical lines on the back. The first joins the M-BW-35 *(Jiaji)* vertebral points, situated approximately 0.5 unit along both sides of the spine. The second corresponds to the medial course of the Bladder channel, situated 1.5 units lateral to the spine. The Associated points on this channel are of particular importance. The third line coincides with the lateral course of the Bladder channel, 3 units from the spine. Irregularities along this line often indicate disease in an internal organ within the horizontal plane corresponding to that of the point.

On the chest and abdomen, the Alarm points are palpated.

On the limbs, the Accumulating, Source, Uniting and Lower Uniting points are examined. (See chapter 1, Section II)

APPENDIX 2: AIR INJECTION THERAPY

This method is akin to the injection of medicine, except that sterile, filtered air is injected instead of medicine. Slowly injected in the principal acupuncture points nearest sprained or strained soft tissues, the combination of needle stimulation and the irritation caused by the gradual absorption of the air is said to help regulate the functioning of the channels, and thereby to assist the healing of the tissues.

Instruments

#20-27 gauge hypodermic needle, 5-10 ml. capacity syringe.

Method

Similar to medicine injecting method. Usually 3-5 ml. of air is injected once every 2-3 days.

Selection of points

Select major acupuncture points near the site of injury. E.g., for sprained wrist, P-6 *(Neiguan)* or TB-5 *(Waiguan)* may be injected; for sprained ankle, use S-36 *(Zusanli)* or GB-39 *(Xuanzhong)*, etc.

Other considerations

- It is essential that after the needle is inserted, the syringe be drawn first to see if it has punctured a blood vessel. Air injection in a vessel may cause an air embolism.
- The rate of injection must be kept very slow.

INFRARED AND ULTRAVIOLET THERAPY

The primary effect of infrared radiation is heat, while ultraviolet light precipitates certain chemical reactions in cells. Both types of light can be used to stimulate acupuncture points and other areas on the skin. When used to stimulate points, the surrounding area is protected by white cloth. When the therapy is designed to treat a broader surface, the light is centered at the point and the surrounding area

435

(about 60-80 square centimeters, depending on the type of light and technique) is also exposed. For example, in the treatment of asthma, the light may be centered at Gv-12 *(Shenzhu)* and the area as far up as Gv-14 *(Dazhui),* as far down as Gv-9 *(Zhiyang),* and as far to the side as B-38 *(Gaohuangshu)* may be exposed.

Infrared therapy

Method

Usually a 250W infrared bulb is used and placed 20-60 cm. from the skin. Dosage is based upon the amount of exposure necessary to make the patient feel warm, but not hot, for 15-20 minutes. Treat daily or on alternating days, with 15-20 treatments constituting one course. During treatment, it is important to pay close attention to the patient's local skin reaction and to adjust the lamp accordingly.

Indications

Low back pain, joint pain, tendinitis, neuralgia, sprain of soft tissue, asthma, chronic bronchitis, frostbite, acute eczema, chronic pharyngitis.

Other considerations

If, during the course of treatment, the patient experiences lassitude, vertigo, insomnia, etc., treatment should be suspended.

This therapy is counter-indicated for patients suffering from acute tuberculosis, malignancies, cardiovascular insufficiency, hemorrhage, sensory impairment, or bleeding problems.

Ultraviolet therapy

Method

Because patient tolerance to ultraviolet light varies, it is necessary to determine the physiologic dosage for each patient at the first session. (See below.) It is important that both the operator and the patient wear protective goggles while the ultraviolet light is on.

The light is warmed up prior to the beginning of treatment. Usually the dosage begins at 2 physiologic dosages and is gradually increased to 5-6 physiologic dosages. Because the physiologic dosage for children is difficult to determine, the lamp's average physiologic dosage is used as the starting point for them. If this method is used on elderly, weak, or dry-skinned patients, or those with a sensitivity to ultraviolet light, there is a tendency for undesirable reactions to occur. For such cases the initial exposure should be less.

Usually, treatments are given 2-4 days apart, with 5-10 treatments constituting a course. Once an area has been treated, it is not re-exposed until the redness has disappeared.

Indications

Pelvic inflammatory disease, carbuncles, erysipelas, eczema, rickets, insufficient lactation, mastitis, frostbite, burns, asthma, joint pain, functional uterine hemorrhage, neuralgia, autonomic nervous system dysfunction, pruritis.

Other considerations

This form of therapy is counter-indicated in active tuberculosis, arteriosclerosis, severe hepatic or renal dysfunction, hyperthyroidism, malignancies, lupus erythematosus and other conditions.

Determination of physiologic dosage of ultraviolet light

A piece of paper in which six holes have been cut is placed on an area of the body not ordinarily exposed to sunlight (usually the abdomen). A piece of white cloth is then placed over each hole. The ultraviolet lamp is placed a specified distance away (usually 50 cm.) and turned on. At fixed intervals—from 15 seconds to 1 minute—one of the pieces of cloth is removed until one interval elapses after the last piece has been removed. Twenty-four hours later the skin is checked and the exposure which produced the least redness is one physiologic dosage for that patient. If, for example, the interval was one minute and the skin under the 5th piece of cloth was slightly red, two minutes would be the physiologic dosage. The average physiologic dosage of a particular ultraviolet lamp is determined by taking the average of the physiologic dosages of 10-15 healthy young adults.

Chapter 4

Moxibustion

Moxibustion is a method whereby moxa punk (or other herbs) is burned on or above the skin at acupuncture points. The heat warms the Qi and Blood in the channels and is therefore useful in the treatment of disease and maintenance of health. Sometimes moxibustion is more effective than acupuncture, whereas at other times the two have a synergistic effect.

The origin and development of moxibustion was outlined in the first part of this Section. Here we will describe the characteristics of dried moxa *(Artemisia vulgaris)* and the most common methods of moxibustion in current use.

CHARACTERISTICS

In *A New Edition of the Pharmacopoeia* appears the following description: "The moxa leaf is bitter and acrid, producing warmth when used in small amounts and strong heat when used in large amounts. Its nature is pure Yang and can thus restore weakened Yang. It opens the twelve Primary channels, courses through the three Yin, regulates the Qi and Blood, expels Cold and Dampness, warms the Uterus . . . When burned, it penetrates all the channels eliminating the hundred diseases." Hence, moxibustion is used for chronic weakened conditions (exhausted Yang) where the channels have been obstructed by Cold or Dampness, or more generally for stimulation of the circulating Qi and Blood. In *Spiritual Axis* it is written: "When acupuncture is useless, moxibustion is appropriate." This refers to the use of moxibustion in the treatment of Cold patterns (Yin disorders) for which acupuncture alone is relatively ineffectual. Asthma, diarrhea, arthritis, rheumatic pain, vomiting or abdominal pain, and certain gynecological disorders are among the most common diseases for which moxibustion is indicated.

The use of the moxa plant, dried and ground into a powder or moxa 'wool', is considered especially beneficial for this purpose. Moxa is easy to shape into cones or bind together in 'sticks', it burns well, and has a pleasant odor. Its combustion produces a penetrating heat. The plant flourishes in varied climates and is therefore relatively cheap. For these reasons it has been the most popular material used for cauterization during the last 2,000 years.

The fresh leaves of the plant are picked in the spring and set out in the sun to dry. They are then ground into a fine powder, sifted and filtered to remove sand or coarse stems, then set out in the sun again. This process is repeated until the desired consistency is obtained, usually a fine, soft, white powder. Moxa used for direct cauterization must be extremely fine so that it may be kneaded and shaped into cones that won't fall apart, while moxa used for indirect cauterization need not be quite as fine.

Chinese doctors say that the older the moxa the better it is. It is important that it be kept in a dry container and periodically dried in the sun.

438

Moxibustion

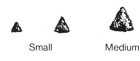

Small   Medium   Large

Used in
indirect moxibustion

Dia. 3-20 Moxa Cones

METHOD

There are two general methods of moxibustion therapy, direct and indirect. The classics generally speak of the direct method, but as time went on indirect methods were developed and are much more popular today.

With either method, the moxa wool is often shaped into little cones that do not crumble if tightly packed (Dia. 3-20). The size and number of cones determine the amount of thermal stimulation. A small cone is perhaps the size of a pea (or smaller), a large one the size of a date cut in half. Generally speaking, for acute diseases or when the patient is relatively strong, more and larger moxa cones are used. Conversely, patients with prolonged diseases, or who are very old or weak usually require fewer and smaller cones. These specifications were recognized as long ago as the Tang Dynasty where they were mentioned in the *Necessities of a Frontier Official*. The direct method more often utilizes small sized cones, the indirect method larger ones.

The location of the site of moxibustion on the body must be considered in determining the amount of stimulation. On the face and chest, fewer and smaller cones are used than on the lower back and abdomen. Where the flesh is rather thin, e.g., on the back and feet and over shallow bones and cartilage, less thermal stimulation is indicated than where the flesh is thick, e.g., the shoulders and thighs. A text of the Qing Dynasty, the *Golden Mirror of Medicine*, explains: "When treating diseases with moxibustion, for there to be any effect the heat must be sufficient to obtain the Qi. Because the skin and flesh on the head and limbs is shallow, repeated moxibustion may render it difficult to sustain [the circulation of] Qi and Blood through and flesh and bones. [In these cases] treatments should be separated by one or two days, the cones should be small, and only a few should be burned during one treatment. If it is necessary to apply moxibustion at Co-14 *(Juque)* or Co-15 *(Jiuwei),* the cones should be the size of grains of wheat and should number no more than three in any single treatment, for it is feared that the Fire Qi might otherwise injure the Heart. The skin and flesh on the back and lumbar region are thick; thus, when moxibustion is given there, the cones should be large in size and many in number so as to obtain the Fire Qi and expel the coagulated Cold."

If a patient is extremely weak, or if a patient is fearful of moxibustion, it is best to use less moxa but compensate with more treatments. When older books speak of using as many as 100 cones of moxa in the treatment of certain diseases, it means over the entire course of treatment and not for a single visit. The physician should be flexible in determining both the amount of stimulation and the frequency of moxibustion treatments.

Direct cauterization

Utilizing the direct method, the moxa cone is placed directly on the skin at selected points and burned. This method is again subdivided into pustulating (or blister forming) and non-pulsating techniques.

The pustulating method is more intense inasmuch as the cone is completely burned and causes considerable pain. Only small cones about a centimeter in diameter are used. As with other methods of moxibustion, it is important that the cone be placed on a level surface so that it doesn't fall off or cause inadvertent burns elsewhere on the body.

The moxa powder can be mixed with powdered cloves or cinnamon to increase thermal penetration. Garlic oil can be smeared around the moxa site, both to hold the cone in place and further stimulate the skin.

As the cone burns and the patient begins to feel pain, the physician should lightly tap the skin around the point which will lessen the pain somewhat. When the cone has fully burned, a rag soaked in cold, sterilized water may be used to gently clean the skin. Then another cone can be prepared and the process repeated. Seven to nine cones is considered average.

When the treatment is completed, a salve may be applied over the area which should be changed daily. After a few days a blister will appear. If there is much fluid in the blister, the ointment must be conscientiously changed to prevent infection. At the same time, the nutritional intake of the patient can be increased to accelerate the healing process and increase the efficacy of the treatment. After about one month to forty days, the blister should disappear and be replaced by a small scar.

The therapeutic effect of this treatment is due to an improvement in the body's general health and resistance to disease. In ancient times the raising of a pustule and scarring was regarded as the key to effective treatment. At present this method is used in the treatment of asthma, chronic gastrointestinal problems, general weakness of the body, and developmental disorders. However, the pain and danger of infection, as well as the formation of a scar tissue, has made this method unpopular.

The non-pustulating method of direct moxibustion provides the concentrated, scorching stimulation of the previous technique, without actually burning the skin and causing a blister. When the burning cone begins to cause the patient pain, it is quickly removed with tweezers, leaving the skin reddened but unburned. Three to seven cones are generally applied in succession. This method is used for relatively mild Deficient Cold conditions.

A third method, somewhat intermediate to the others, is to burn tiny cones the size of a grain of wheat, hence the name 'grain of wheat moxibustion'. The cones (usually 3-7 in number) are placed on skin which has been smeared with petroleum jelly, then burned completely. Because they burn quickly, the likelihood of a blister or a noticeable scar is diminished. Still, an ointment is applied after treatment. This method is used for Deficient Blood, dizziness, and warts.

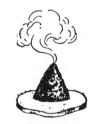

**Dia. 3-21   Indirect
Moxibustion**

Indirect cauterization

For indirect cauterization, a medium is placed between the burning moxa and the skin. It is less painful than direct methods, and creates little risk of infection. Several mediums are used. Among the most common:

Ginger
A flat slice of ginger about 0.3 inch thick is cut and perforated in several places with a needle. (Dia. 3-21) This is placed above the point to be cauterized. Then a moxa cone is set securely on the ginger wafer and ignited. When the patient feels that the heat is too painful, the whole wafer is lifted from the skin, either with the fingers or tweezers. After a moment's respite, it is replaced on the skin. This procedure is repeated until the skin beneath the wafer is red and moist. If the first moxa cone was insufficient to cause this response, additional cones may be used.

This method is relatively simple and should not burn the skin. It is recommended for conditions such as abdominal pain, diarrhea, pain or soreness in the joints and Deficient Cold conditions in general.

Garlic

Prepared like the ginger wafer (above), garlic may be placed either on an acupuncture point or directly over cutaneous swellings (e.g., non-ulcerated carbuncle). After 4-5 moxa cones have been burned, the garlic wafer must be replaced. Burning 5-7 cones above a single point is average. Because of the irritant property of garlic, the formation of blisters is common. In *Thousand Ducat Prescriptions,* this method is recommended for the treatment of scrofula. It is presently used in treating pulmonary tuberculosis, abdominal masses, and non-ulcerated carbuncles.

Salt

This technique is only used in the umbilicus. The umbilicus is filled with salt until level with the surface of the abdomen. A ginger wafer is then placed on the salt and a moxa cone on the wafer. The moxa is ignited. (If the moxa is placed directly on the salt it will probably burn the skin.) This technique is indicated for acute abdominal pain accompanied by vomiting or diarrhea, dysentery, 'abandoned' stroke, etc.

Aconite

A slice of aconite (root of *Aconitum carmichaeli)* or a paste one centimeter thick made of ground aconite and yellow wine is placed on the point and moxa burned on top of it. Aconite is an acrid and very hot herb that warms the Kidneys and strengthens the Yang; thus, this method is used in the treatment of various Deficient Yang conditions, including skin ulcerations that resist healing or Yin abscesses and carbuncles where the pus will not disperse. Recently, aconite and similar hot, aromatic drying herbs have been ground up and made into dry cakes which are separated from the skin by layers of gauze, to prevent scorching when the herbs are burned. This method is used in the treatment of conditions for which indirect moxibustion is suitable.

Pepper

A paste is made of white pepper powder mixed with flour and spread over a point in a layer about 0.1 inch thick. A slight hollow may be left in the center, into which another powdered herb (like cinnamon or cloves) can be placed if desired. A moxa cone is then set upon the paste medium and burned. This method is indicated for arthritic pain, local numbness and stiffness.

Mud plasters

Mud plasters may also be used as a medium for treating localized eczema and other skin diseases.

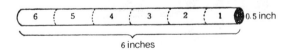

Dia. 3-22   Moxa Stick

Moxa sticks

The use of the moxa stick or roll was first developed in the Ming Dynasty as a convenient, less time consuming and more easily controlled method than other forms of moxibustion. Moxa sticks are commercially manufactured today, and this method has come to enjoy widespread popularity. (Dia. 3-22)

As one of the indirect methods of moxibustion, the dried moxa is not placed on the skin surface; neither is it shaped into cones. Instead, the powder (usually together with stems) is rolled tightly in a paper wrapper about six inches in length, looking very much like a giant cigarette. The powder of certain other medicinal herbs may be mixed with the moxa. The most commonly used moxa sticks contain 24 grams of moxa punk and 6 grams of a powder made from equal amounts of the following ground herbs: cinnamon, dried ginger, cloves, Sichuan pepper, realgar *(xionghua)*, *Saussurea lappa (muxiang)*, *Angelica sp. (duhuo)*, *Asarum sieboldi (xixin)*, *Angelica dahurica (baizhi)*, *Atractylodes iancea (cangshu)*, myrrh and frankincense. The moxa stick is lit at one end and held about half an inch from the surface of the skin, the distance varying with the tolerance of the patient and the amount of thermal stimulation desired. Normally, the moxa stick is burned from 5-10 minutes, or until the skin becomes red in the vicinity of the point. This method is used for the pain associated with blockage or obstruction disorders (analogous to arthritic pain). The burning end of the stick may then be snipped off and the unburned portion saved for later treatments.

A circular motion of the stick around the point is a variant technique used to spread the focus of thermal stimulation in the treatment of blockage pain over large surface areas, soft tissue injuries, skin disorder, etc. (Dia. 3-23) Another method is called 'sparrow pecking', whereby the moxa stick is rapidly 'pecked' at the point (without touching the skin). (Dia. 3-24) It is said that this method facilitates heat penetration and is therefore used when strong stimulation is desired.

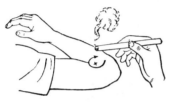

**Dia. 3-23   Circular
Method of
Moxibustion**

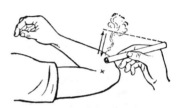

**Dia. 3-24   'Sparrow
Pecking' Moxibustion**

Warming cylinders

A metal container may be used for burning moxa. This method is most often used when treating children or those who are afraid of other cauterization methods. After the moxa has been ignited inside the container, it is placed briefly on the selected point, then removed, then replaced until the skin becomes red. A flat bottomed container is used for large, flat body surfaces, a pointed container for more angular locations.*

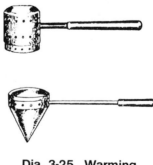

**Dia. 3-25   Warming
Cylinders**

*Many plastic warming cylinders are currently available.—*Editors*

442

Electric warming method

A rather recent invention, this method simply substitutes a specially designed electric heating device for the moxa to produce warmth at specific points. The device is available on certain electro-acupuncture machines.

'Heavenly' cauterization

This method involves the application of various plasters that irritate the skin. The plasters are placed on acupuncture points until the area becomes congested and red; in some cases blisters arise. Garlic is commonly used for this purpose. For example, in the treatment of throat blockage (swollen, painful throat), garlic paste may be applied on the skin at L-10 *(Yuji)* until a blister is raised. *Brassica alba (baijiezi)* is an herb that is pungent and warm and contains volatile oils that irritate the skin. When ground and mixed with water, it possesses excellent blister-forming properties and is often used in the treatment of arthritis. If mixed with other herbs and applied on back points, it can be used to treat asthma. Another method is recorded in the Yuan Dynasty work, *Extensive Treasures to Protect Life:* "To treat Cold asthma, the following are ground into powders and combined: One *liang* [approximately 37g] of *Brassica alba (baijiezi)* and *Corydalis bulbosa (yenhusuo),* 5 *qian* [about 19g] of both *Euphorbia kansui (gansui)* and *Asarum sieboldi (xixin),* and 1g of musk. The resulting mixture is placed on B-13 *(Feishu),* B-38 *(Gaohuang),* and M-HN-30 *(Bailao).* [The patient] will experience sensations of numbness and pain after application. The herbs must not be removed until the time it takes two cones of incense to burn. Ten days later the process is repeated. After two treatments the disease will be cured."

Other considerations

- Precautions must be taken to avoid inadvertent burns and to properly treat those which do occur.
- Moxibustion is counter-indicated for patients with febrile diseases, and must not be used on the lower back or abdomen of pregnant women.
- Moxibustion is generally not used in the vicinity of the sensory organs or mucous membranes. The direct method should not be used on the face, the region of the breast, over large blood vessels, prominent tendons, or major creases in the skin.
- When giving moxibustion to unconscious patients or over areas that are numb, care must be taken to avoid giving too much stimulation.

Chapter 5

Cupping

Cupping is a method of treating disease by causing local congestion. A partial vacuum is created in jars, usually by means of heat, which are then applied to the skin, drawing up the underlying tissues and forming blood stasis. In ancient times, animal horns were used, principally in draining pustulated sores. Later this method was utilized in treating consumptive and rheumatic diseases. For example, in the Tang Dynasty work, *Necessities of a Frontier Official,* cupping is prescribed for the treatment of a condition similar to pulmonary tuberculosis. Bamboo, ceramic, iron and brass 'cups' were developed. Today, cups made of glass or bamboo are by far the most common. (Dia. 3-26) They are available in many sizes, and selected according to the skin surface and method of treatment. Both the range of indications and the variety of instruments have grown since the beginning of the Cultural Revolution.

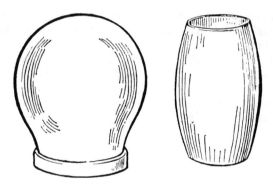

Dia. 3-26   Cups

CUPPING METHODS

Attach a cotton ball to a stick and dip it in alcohol. Ignite the cotton, and insert the burning cotton into the mouth of the cup. This will evacuate some of the air, causing a partial vacuum within the cup. Withdraw the cotton stick and quickly place the mouth of the cup firmly against the skin at the desired location. Suction should hold it in place. This is the most popular method of cupping. (Dia. 3-27)

Though less convenient, a strip of paper may be used in place of the stick and cotton. Or, a small, thin piece of cotton can be dipped in alcohol and attached to the top of the cup on the inside surface. After the cotton is ignited the cup is placed on the skin. If this method is used, it is important that only a very small piece of cotton be utilized, otherwise a fragment of burning cotton may fall on the skin. (Dia. 3-28)

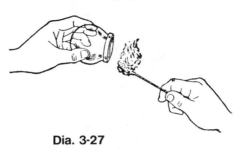

Dia. 3-27

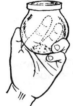

Dia. 3-28

A third method is to first place a thin wafer of some non-combustible, non-heat conducting material on the skin. A small ball of cotton soaked in alcohol is set atop a wafer and ignited. The cup is then placed over both. This produces a relatively strong suction. (Dia. 3-29)

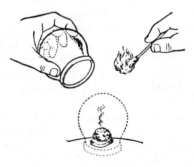

Dia. 3-29

Finally, by cutting off the bottom of a medicine ampul and smoothing the edges, a special 'cup' can be fashioned from which the air is evacuated with a hypodermic syringe. This is called 'suction method'. (Dia. 3-30) Cups need only be retained in place from 5-15 minutes, depending on the strength of suction. Especially in hot weather, or when cupping over shallow flesh, the duration of treatment should not be too long.

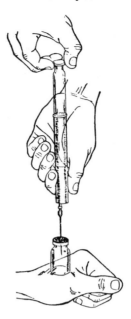

**Dia. 3-30 Suction
Method**

Point selection and use of the cups

• Single cups may be applied on smaller areas or specific points of tenderness, e.g., at Co-12 *(Zhongwan)* for certain stomach diseases, or at LI-15 *(Jianyu)* for supraspinatus tendinitis.

• Several cups may be indicated for disorders over a wider area, e.g., along a strained muscle, or arranged horizontally and vertically in rows on the skin above a diseased internal organ. The cups should not be placed too close together.*

• A cup can be alternately placed, lifted, and replaced in rapid succession, producing many small suctions, until the underlying skin is reddened. This method is most commonly used over local areas of numbness or declining function, associated with Deficient conditions.

• Moving the cups is a technique that is utilized over large, flat body surfaces like the back or thigh. Only glass cups with relatively wide mouths are used. First, a lubricant is smeared around the mouth of the cup. Then, after the cup has been applied to the skin, the physician moves it back and forth by holding the cup at its base and slightly raising the front edge in the direction of movement (without breaking the suction 'seal') while applying force along the back edge. This movement continues until the skin has reddened. (Dia. 3-31)

• Herbal medicine preparations such as ginger juice, hot pepper water, etc., can be placed in either a regular cupping instrument (1/3 to 1/2 full of the medicinal fluid) or a vial. If a cup is used, suction is first created with the heat from a burning cotton ball as described above. Turning the cup over and onto the skin must be performed with dexterity, but some of the medicine is bound to escape anyway. If an ampul is used, suction is created by drawing out the air once the bottle and medicine are in place on the skin. These methods are often used for arthritic pain, coughing, asthma, common cold, ulcers, chronic gastritis, indigestion, psoriasis.

• Cupping can be combined with regular acupuncture. (Dia. 3-32) First the needle is inserted until the Qi sensation is obtained, then retained in place. A cup is prepared and placed over the needle on the surrounding skin. This method may be further combined with the application of herbal medicines

*The rims should ordinarily be at least 5 cm. apart.—*Editors*

(see above). Cupping with acupuncture is often used for rheumatism and is considered more effective than cupping alone in the treatment of this disease.

- Cupping may also be combined with the blood letting technique, first letting blood, then cupping. This method is used in cases of injury to soft tissues, neurodermatitis, pruritis, neurasthenia, and gastrointestinal nervous dysfunction.

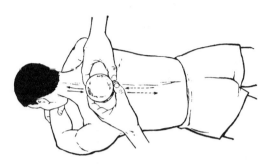

Dia. 3-31 Moving the
Cups

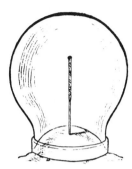

Dia. 3-32 Cupping
and Acupuncture

General indications

Arthritic pain, abdominal pain, stomach-ache, indigestion, headache, hypertension, common cold, cough, low back pain, painful menstruation, eyes red, swollen, and painful, poisonous snake bite, non-ulcerated furuncle.

Cupping is counter-indicated for high fever, convulsions or cramps, allergic skin conditions or ulcerated sores; over areas where the muscle is thin or the skin is not level because of bony angles and depressions; on the abdomen or lower back of pregnant women.

Other considerations

- Where the skin is not smooth, it is difficult to maintain suction under the cups which may then fall off. Around joints, because of the rounded or angular surface, smaller cups are therefore preferred.
- When using many cups, avoid placing them too close together. This will pull the surrounding skin too tightly and cause pain.
- When 'moving the cups', bony prominences should be avoided.
- To remove cups, first press with a finger against the flesh at the base of the cup so as to break the 'seal'. Don't try to pull the cup off from the top.
- Cupping often leaves a purplish mark where the rim of the cup has pressed against the skin. This is normal and will disappear without special treatment. If very pronounced, cups should not be applied at this site a second time.
- Cups should be left in place only until there is local congestion (usually 5-15 minutes). If retained too long a blister may form. If a large blister does form, it should be punctured to drain the fluid and then dressed to avoid infection.

Chapter 6

Surgical Techniques

There are several methods which combine traditional acupuncture channel theory with modern surgical technique, among them piercing, burying thread or threading points, incisions, stimulation of the nerve trunks, and piercing the lymph nodes.

PIERCING ('STIRRING') METHOD

Also called 'cutting the root method', this is regarded as a form of the traditional 'piercing the vessels,' a blood letting technique first mentioned in *Spiritual Axis*. Either a needle or surgical instrument is used to pierce or sever the fibrous tissue at specific locations beneath the skin. Sites are chosen at skin eruptions, papules, stasis in small blood vessels, related acupuncture points or locations which experience has shown are associated with a particular disease.

Instruments

Suture needle, forceps, sterile coarse silk thread or surgical gut, scalpel.

Selecting the point

Eruptions on the skin, often associated with a particular disease, are frequently chosen for piercing. This is particularly true on the back. A typical eruption (for this purpose) is described as a papule, slightly elevated from the skin surface, about the size of a pin-head. It can be grey, dark or light red in color which does not change when pressed by the finger. Some involve hair follicles. The location of the eruption often differs with the disease. For example, eruptions indicating hemorrhoids are frequently found in the lumbo-sacral region and on the lip; those indicating a stye, between the shoulder blades. Scrofula is often reflected in eruptions above the inferior angle of the scapula, at both sides of the spine or at the site of the disease itself.

If eruptions cannot be found, a second choice is to pierce acupuncture points associated with the disease. For example, in the case of hemorrhoids, B-25 *(Dachangshu)*, B-27 *(Xiaochangshu)*, Gv-1 *(Changqiang)* or B-31 - 34 *(Shangliao, Ciliao, Zhongliao)* may be pierced; for prostatitis, pierce B-28 *(Pangguangshu)*; for conjunctivitis, pierce Gv-14 *(Dazhui)*.

Finally, certain regions of the body have been associated, in traditional experience, with particular diseases. Points in these regions can be pierced. A survey of such areas together with indications and piercing methods is set forth in Table 3-4.

Method

1) First, clean the area with alcohol.

2) Insert the needle almost horizontally to the skin. Once the needle tip is beneath the surface, the physician can use the left hand to carefully press the skin against the tip, while continuing to push the needle with the right hand until it reemerges from the skin at a second site. Thus in place, the needle should be moved back and forth or rotated several times, slowly causing the underlying fibrous tissue to wind around the needle's 'tail'. Finally, the needle is pulled through the skin and removed, as if one were sewing. A thread may be attached to the needle and pulled back and forth through the two needle holes, pulling fibrous tissue with it.

3) A local anesthetic may be used, e.g., 1-2 milliliters of 0.5% procaine, and the chosen point incised with a scalpel to a depth of less than 0.1 inch. The tip of a needle can then be manipulated so as to pull up and sever underlying fibrous tissue.

4) When the operation is completed, the incision should be properly dressed with a sterile bandage.

5) Usually, therapeutic results will appear within several days of the operation (30-40 days for lymphogenous tuberculosis). If after 7-10 days there is no result, another point should be selected for treatment. If the same point is selected, at least 2-3 weeks should be allowed between operations.

Other considerations

- It is best to have the patient lie down during treatment to prevent fainting.
- Rigorous sterile technique is essential.
- It is recommended that the patient not participate in strenuous activity, nor eat spicy foods on the day of the operation.
- This method is counter-indicated for pregnant women, or patients with serious heart disese or hemorrhagic conditions.

449

Table 3-4   Sites for Piercing Therapy

Name	Location	Indications	Method
Frontal branch of the superficial temporal artery	At the temple, along the frontal branch of superficial temporal artery.	Migraine, vertigo, common cold, neurasthenia, conjunctivitis, febrile diseases.	Using medium or large suture needle, points along the branch may be selected for piercing. Needle inserted downward. Once inserted, the needle can be jiggled back and forth several times. Each point can be pierced 3-6 times as desired.
Parietal branch of the superficial temporal artery	Along parietal branch of superficial temporal artery, anterior and superior to the ear, approximately at hairline on the temple.	Migraine, vertigo, febrile diseases.	Same as above.
Supratrochlear artery	Along supratrochlear artery, from above the eyebrow to the hairline.	Migraine, neuralgia of frontal nerve, common cold, eye diseases, febrile diseases.	Same as above.
Supraorbital artery	Along supratrochlear artery, from above the center of eyebrow to the hairline.	Same as above.	Same as above.
Glabella	Between the eyebrows.	Headache, vertigo, eye diseases, febrile diseases, infantile convulsions.	Using a large gauge suture needle, pierce skin from below, upward. Jiggle needle in all directions to enlarge opening and let a few drops of blood.

Name	Location	Indications	Method
Occipital artery	Along occipital artery, from the inferior margin of the occipital bone upward.	Neurasthenia, headache, vertigo.	Hair should be shaved at site of piercing. Method same as for superficial temporal artery above.
Upper eyelid #1	In middle of upper eyelid, opposite pupil, on the medial palpebral artery. With the patient's eye closed, the thumb and index finger can be used to carefully stretch the eyelid taut. This will reveal the capillaries on the eyelid to be pierced.	Acute or chronic conjunctivitis, trachoma, stye, ulcer of cornea, nebula, myopia, astigmatism, diseases of optic nerve.	Using a thin, long suture needle, the eyelid is pulled taut with left hand and needle tip placed on lid surface. The lid is then released, causing force to be exerted against tip of needle and effecting a shallow insertion.
Upper eyelid #2	About 0.3 inch medial to #1.	Same as above.	Same as above.
Upper eyelid #3	About 0.3 inch lateral to #1.	Same as above.	Same as above.
Upper eyelid #4	Above and between #1 and #2, at apex of equilateral triangle formed by 3 points.	Same as above.	Same as above.
Upper eyelid #5	Above and between #1 and #3, at apex of equilateral triangle formed by 3 points.	Same as above.	Same as above.
Laryngeal region #1	In the depression above the laryngeal prominence.	Acute or chronic laryngitis, pharyngitis, tonsillitis, inflammation of upper respiratory tract.	The patient's head should be held back. Use a relatively thin suture needle. Method is same as above. Important that needle manipulation be performed slowly.

451

Name	Location	Indications	Method
Laryngeal region #2	In the depression at the anterior, middle part of the border between thyroid and cricoid cartilage.	Same as above.	Same as above.
Laryngeal region #3	At Co-22 (*Tiantu*) in the suprasternal notch.	Same as above.	Same as above.
Laryngeal region #4	In the depression formed by the thyroid cartilage and the anterior margin of sternocleidomastoid muscle at S-9 (*Renying*).	Same as above.	Same as above.
Laryngeal region #5	In the depression formed by the sternocleidomastoid muscle and the side of the intersection of thyroid and cricoid cartilage.	Same as above.	Same as above.
Below the ear #1	Below and posterior to the earlobe. Approximately at TB-17 (*Yifeng*).	Eye disease, headache with fever.	Same as above. Let blood for the best result
Below the ear # 2	About a finger width below #1.	Same as above.	Same as above.
Below the ear #3	About a finger width below #2, in front of the sternocleido-mastoid muscle.	Same as above.	Same as above.
Behind the ear	Posterior to the upper half of the root of the auricle.	Acute conjunctivitis, bleeding beneath the eye or around optic nerve.	Use common sewing needle to pierce prominent capillaries posterior to the root of the auricle.

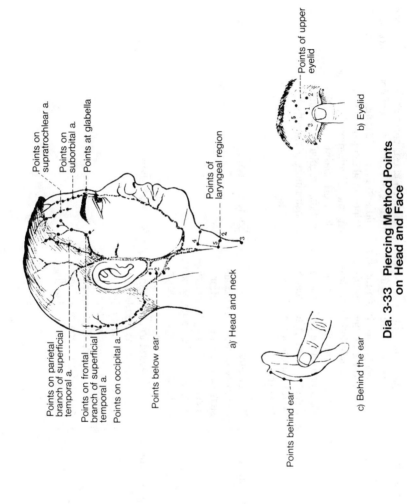

Points on
supratrochlear a.

Points on
suborbital a.

Points at glabella

Points on parietal
branch of superficial
temporal a.

Points on frontal
branch of superficial
temporal a.

Points on occipital a.

Points below ear

Points of
laryngeal region

a) Head and neck

Points of upper
eyelid

b) Eyelid

Points behind ear

c) Behind the ear

**Dia. 3-33 Piercing Method Points
on Head and Face**

453

Name	Location	Indications	Method
Abdominal-thoracic median line	Along a straight line from above the manubrium sterni to the pubic symphysis. From manubrium to navel there are six points equidistant from each other (the navel being #6). Below navel are 2 more, an equal distance apart. Altogether 8 points (navel is not pierced, however).	Points on chest: chest pains, intercostal neuralgia, common cold and Hot conditions. Points on abdomen: acute or chronic GI inflammation, peptic ulcer, GI spasm or neuralgia, cystitis, irregular or painful menstruation, peritonitis.	Use common sewing needle and normal surgical method.
1st lateral abdominal-thoracic line	2 units lateral to median line (midway between nipple and sternum), from the inferior margin of clavicle to superior margin of pubic bone, 9 points equidistant from each other.	Same as above.	Same as above.
2nd lateral abdominal-thoracic line	2 units lateral to above line, beginning at the middle of the clavicle, intersecting the nipple, and continuing toward the inguinal canal. 8 points equidistant from each other, level with 8 points on median line.	Same as above.	Same as above.

454

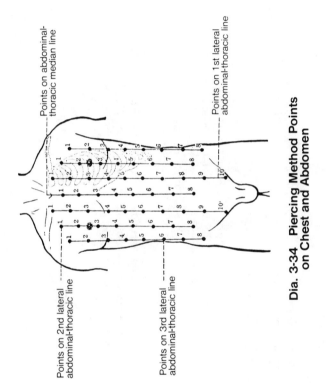

Points on abdominal-thoracic median line

Points on 1st lateral abdominal-thoracic line

Points on 2nd lateral abdominal-thoracic line

Points on 3rd lateral abdominal-thoracic line

Dia. 3-34. Piercing Method Points on Chest and Abdomen

455

Name	Location	Indications	Method
3rd lateral abdominal-thoracic line	2 units lateral to above line, from the shoulder joint to anterior, superior iliac spine. Eight equi-distant points.	Same as above.	Same as above.
Median line of back	Along the spine, below each spinous process from the 1st cervical to the 4th sacral vertebra. Altogether 27 points.	For all lines on back: rheumatic pain, back pain, stomach-ache.	Normal piercing method.
1st lateral line of the back	Above each transverse process from the 1st thoracic to the 3rd sacral vertebra. Altogether 20 points.	From the 1st to the 7th point on the 1st lateral line: acute, chronic stye and eye diseases generally; from the 7th to the 10th point: scrofula.	Normal piercing method.
2nd lateral line of the back	From the superior margin of the 1st rib to about 2 units below the posterior, inferior iliac spine. Altogether 19 points.	For 2nd and 3rd points on median line: infantile convul-sions and high fever, antitoxic function.	Same as above.
3rd lateral line of the back	From the supraspinous fossa to the iliac crest. Altogether 16 points.	Same as above.	Same as above.
Posterior axillary line	With the arm held at the side, from below the shoulder joint to the posterior axillary crease. Altogether 3 points.	Same as above.	Same as above.

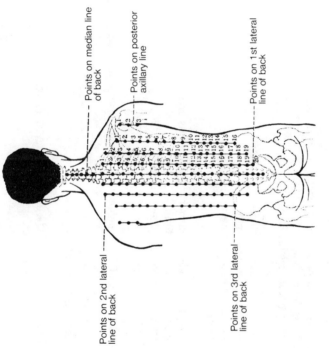

Points on median line of back

Points on posterior axillary line

Points on 1st lateral line of back

Points on 2nd lateral line of back

Points on 3rd lateral line of back

Dia. 3-35   Piercing Method Points on Back

457

Name	Location	Indications	Method
Anterior midline of upper limb	Along middle of anterior aspect of upper limb, from shoulder joint to the wrist. Altogether 13 points.	Neuralgia, rheumatic pain, muscular paralysis, arthritis.	Same as above.
Posterior midline of upper limb	Along middle of posterior aspect of upper limb, from shoulder joint to the wrist. Altogether 13 points.	Same as above.	Same as above.
Ulnar line of upper limb	Along ulnar side of anterior aspect of upper limb, from shoulder joint to wrist joint. Altogether 13 points.	Same as above.	Same as above.
Radial line of upper limb	Along radial side of anterior aspect of upper limb, from shoulder joint to wrist joint. Altogether 13 points.	Same as above.	Same as above.
Thenar point	At the middle of thenar eminence above 1st metacarpal bone, at the border of light and dark flesh. (Same as L-10 (*Yuji*))	Infantile malnutrition syndrome.	Normal piercing method. (If a little serous fluid is drawn, results are best.)
Infantile malnutrition syndrome points	On the palm, in the middle of the metacarpophalangeal crease of 2nd-5th fingers.	Same as above.	Same as above. (Let blood for best result.)
Finger seam points	In the middle of the proximal phalangeal crease on the palmar surface of 2nd-5th fingers.	Infantile indigestion, chronic peritonitis, infantile malnutrition syndrome.	Same as above.

Name	Location	Indications	Method
Fingernail seam points	On dorsum of hand, just proximal to fingernails of all fingers.	Same as above.	Same as above.

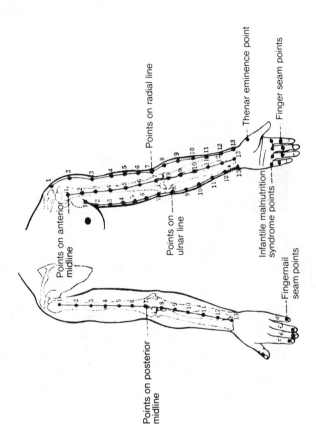

Dia. 3-36 Piercing Method Points on Upper Limb

Labels on figure: Points on radial line; Points on anterior midline; Points on ulnar line; Thenar eminence point; Finger seam points; Infantile malnutrition syndrome points; Points on posterior midline; Fingernail seam points

459

Name	Location	Indications	Method
Anterior line of lower limb	Along middle of anterior aspect of lower limb, from inguinal canal to transverse crease at ankle. Altogether 19 points equidistant from each other.	Neuralgia, rheumatic pain.	Same as above.
Posterior line of lower limb	Along middle of posterior aspect of lower limb, from transverse crease below the buttock to base of Achilles tendon. Altogether 19 points equidistant from each other.	Muscular palsy, etc.	Same as above.
Medial line of lower limb	Along medial aspect of lower limb, from the medial end of inguinal canal to the medial malleolus. Altogether 18 points equidistant from each other.	Same as above.	Same as above.
Lateral line of lower limb	Along lateral aspect of lower limb, from anterior, superior iliac spine to anterior part of lateral malleolus. Altogether 12 points equidistant from each other.	Same as above.	Same as above.

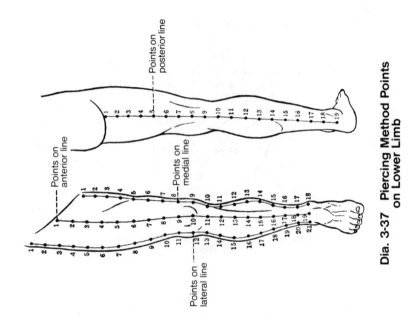

Points on posterior line

Points on anterior line

Points on medial line

Points on lateral line

Dia. 3-37 Piercing Method Points on Lower Limb

INCISION METHOD

Also called 'cutting the fat', this method involves making surgical incisions at points on the skin, removing a small amount of fatty tissue, and then manually massaging the open wound so as to strengthen the body's capacity to resist disease and improve its functioning.

Instruments

Surgical knife, vascular forceps, sterile gauze, bandages.

Sites for incision

The seven sites listed below, all on the palmar surface of the hand, are the most common sites for incision. (Dia. 3-38)

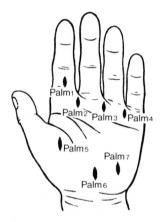

Dia. 3-38   Incision Method Points on Palm

Name	Location	Indications
Palm 1	In the center of the crease of the metacarpo-phalangeal joint of the index finger	Bronchial athma
Palm 2	About 0.5 cm. proximal to the webbing between index and middle fingers	Chronic bronchitis, bronchial asthma
Palm 3	About 0.5 cm. proximal to the webbing between middle and fourth fingers	Bronchitis, bronchial asthma
Palm 4	About 0.5 cm. proximal to the webbing between fourth and little fingers	Neurasthenia, headache, GI disease
Palm 5	On the ulnar margin of the thenar muscle	Bronchial asthma, infantile malnutrition syndrome

Palm 6	About 1.5 cm. from P-7 *(Daling)* toward the center of the palm (Do not cut too deeply)	Chronic gastritis, nervous stomach, gastric ulcer, round worm in the bile duct, indigestion, segmental enteritis
Palm 7	About 1.5 cm. from H-7 *(Shenmen)* toward the palm between the 4th and little fingers	Nervous stomach, gastric ulcer

Acupuncture points may also be incised in the treatment of certain illnesses. Among the most common are Co-17 *(Shanzhong)* and Gv-14 *(Dazhui)* for bronchial asthma or chronic bronchitis; Co-15 *(Jiuwei)* and K-1 *(Yongquan)* for scrofula; B-18 *(Ganshu)*, B-20 *(Pishu)*, Co-13 *(Shangwan),* and Co-12 *(Zhongwan)* for peptic ulcers; S-25 *(Tianshu)* and S-36 *(Zusanli)* for tuberculosis of mesenteric lymph nodes; Sp-4 *(Gongsun)* and K-2 *(Rangu)* for tumors.

Method

1) First, sterilize the area, then inject local anesthetic. Use the thumb of the left hand to press firmly against the skin below the site of incision, then open the skin with a surgical knife (not too deeply), making the incision about 0.5-1 cm. in length (smaller for children).

2) Use vascular forceps to open the wound and expose underlying fatty tissue. Remove a small portion, about the size of a soy bean or pea.

3) Use the forceps to further stretch the incision and massage all sides of the opening, causing a numb, sore and distended sensation extending outwards from the incision. Alternatively, the forceps may be utilized to pinch the underlying or neighboring tissue several times, or the handle of the surgical knife can be used to stroke the underlying periosteum (e.g., when incising Co-17 *(Shanzhong))*, producing very strong stimulation.

4) When the operation has been completed, dress the wound with sterile gauze.

5) If a second incision is necessary, 7-10 days should be allowed between treatments.

Further considerations

• It is important that this method not be used on patients with histories of heart disease or hemorrhagic conditions. It is also not advised for patients in critical condition or with prolonged high fever, or at site of local infection or edema.

• Incisions must not be too deep, to avoid severing blood vessels, nerves, or tendons.

• It is not uncommon for patients to show a reaction to this operation, generally within 3 days, but perhaps as long as a month afterward. Symptoms usually include general discomfort, soreness in the joints and reduced appetite. There may also be specific changes due to the original illness of the patient. These side effects usually disappear after a few days. If not, further measures should be taken.

• Patients should be advised to rest for a few days after the operation. They should also watch what they eat and keep warm.

THREADING THE POINTS, EMBEDDING SUTURES, AND LOOP-TYING THE POINTS

By means of these three methods, surgical gut is introduced at subcutaneous locations corresponding to acupuncture loci to provide prolonged therapeutic stimulation. Experimental studies have found that the stimulation caused by the thread at these sites led to an increase in muscle anabolism and a decrease in catabolism, to higher levels of muscle protein and carbohydrate synthesis, and lower levels of lactic acid and creatine; in short, to an improvement in muscle nutrition and metabolism. Studies of the loop-tying method showed increases in local blood vessel supply and blood flow, and an improvement of circulation leading to conditions of better nourishment in the limbs. At the same time there was an increase in the number of muscle fibers and improved adhesion, which served to improve the tone of previously flaccid muscles. Within the muscle, newly generated nerve fibers were found.

These methods are used primarily in the treatment of peptic ulcer, bronchial asthma and sequelae of infantile paralysis, all with generally good results.

Methods

Threading the points

A site is selected within 1.5-2.5 cm. from an acupuncture point associated with the disease under treatment, and an infiltration anesthetic of procaine is injected so as to cause a wheal about 0.3-0.5 cm. in diameter. Then a threaded triangular needle is inserted at one side of the wheal, penetrating the underlying muscle tissue in the vicinity of the acupuncture locus and emerging from the skin on the other side of the wheal. (Dia. 3-39) The thread is then snipped at the skin level and left in place below. (Dia. 3-40) The area should be bound with sterile bandages for 5-7 days.

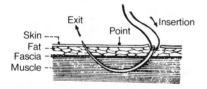

Dia. 3-39 Threading Point Method

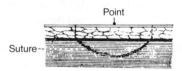

Dia. 3-40 Threaded Point

Embedding sutures

An infiltration anesthetic of procaine is injected at an acupuncture point and a surgical knife used to make an incision about 0.5-1 cm. in length at this site. Vascular forceps are then inserted through superficial tissues to the point of tenderness in the muscle tissue associated with the acupuncture point. The area is massaged with the forceps for a few seconds, then rested. This is repeated about 3 times. Small strands of surgical gut, less than a centimeter in length and perhaps 4-5 in number, are then buried or embedded in the muscle. The sutures should not be embedded in fatty tissue nor inserted too deeply in the muscle, where they may either be difficult to absorb or cause infection. The incision is then stitched and the area covered with a sterile dressing. After a week the stitches may be removed. (Dia. 3-41)

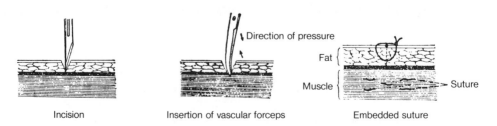

Dia. 3-41 Embedding Point Method

Loop-tying

This method is similar to the threading method, except that a small incision is made on the wheal to the side of the acupuncture point, and the anesthetic wheal itself must be somewhat larger. The incision should be about 0.3-0.5 cm. in length. Curved forceps are inserted to the deep position of the acupuncture point in the muscle, where they are vibrated 40-50 times to stimulate the point and then removed. Thereafter, a threaded suture needle is inserted along the same path, emerging on the other side of the acupuncture point. It is then reinserted, this time penetrating the superficial tissues just below the fatty layer, and withdrawn through the original incision. (Dia. 3-42) The two ends are then pulled taut and tied with a surgical knot which is itself embedded. Finally, the incision is stitched and the area bandaged. (Dia. 3-42)

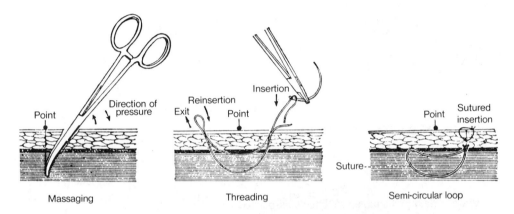

Massaging   Threading   Semi-circular loop

Dia. 3-42 Loop-tying Point Method

There are several variations in the shape of the threading pattern, which are chosen on the basis of the site of the operation. Among them:

Figure '8' loop (Dia. 3-43) used at Gv-14 *(Dazhui)* and Gv-3 *(Yaoyangguan)*.

Letter 'K' figure '8' loop (Dia. 3-44) used at GB-30 *(Huantiao)*, with one loop toward N-BW-37 *(Huanyue)* and the other toward B-34 *(Xialiao)*.

Letter 'K' with double figure '8' loops (Dia. 3-45) also used at GB-30 *(Huantiao)*.

Circular loop (Dia. 3-46) used in the deltoid muscle from SI-10 *(Naoshu)* through LI-15 *(Jianyu)*.

Generally, these methods are performed once every three weeks to a month. Depending on the progress of treatment and the general strength of the patient, this period may be extended or shortened.

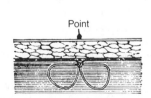

Dia. 3-43 Figure '8' Loop

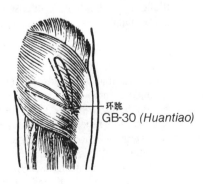

环跳
GB-30 *(Huantiao)*

Dia. 3-44 'K' Figure '8' Loop

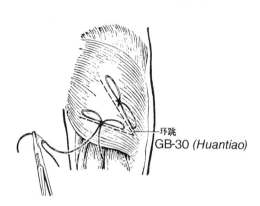

① LI-15 *(Jianyu)*
② SI-10 *(Naoshu)*

Point of tying thread

① 肩髃
② 臑俞

环跳
GB-30 *(Huantiao)*

Dia. 3-45 'K' Double Figure '8' Loops   **Dia. 3-46 Circular Loop**

Patient Reaction

There are certain predictable side effects associated with these methods.

Normal reactions
● Local reactions: During both the surgical operation and later from the irritation caused by the embedded thread, there is commonly a local aseptic inflammation which appears within 1-5 days of the operation, and is accompanied by reddening, swelling, pain and fever. A more serious reaction, arising from irritation of the fatty tissue, could produce a small amount of milky exudate, but this too is a normal reaction requiring no special treatment. If the exudate is enough to cause swelling with external draining, it can be cleaned with alcohol and re-bandaged with another sterile dressing. Such reactions are not only considered normal, but positive signs of stimulation.
● Systemic reaction: A minority of patients will show an increase in temperature within 4-24 hours following the operation, generally about 38°C, in fewer cases as high as 39° or 40°C, which usually subsides within 2-4 days. There is also an increase, to varying degrees, in the leukocyte and neutrophil cell count.

Abnormal reactions
● Pain: If after treatment there is intense pain in the vicinity of the wound, or a numb pain in the limbs, it could be that the loop is too tight. If this is the case the thread must be cut so as to relieve the pressure.
● Bleeding: Usually arises from excessive stimulation or because the suture needle punctured a blood vessel. Treat it as you normally would bleeding.
● Nerve damage: Injury to sensory nerves manifests as impediment to or loss of feeling in associated cutaneous regions. Injury to motor nerves is reflected in paralysis of muscle groups innervated by the damaged nerve. This problem usually arises because of excessive stimulation or severance of a nerve or blood vessel. Caution must be exercised.
● Infection, allergic reaction: Infection is ordinarily caused by poor sterilization procedures during or after the operation. Allergic reaction may result either from the anesthetic or the surgical gut thread. There is local itching, redness and swelling or systemic fever. There may be degeneration of fatty tissues which continues until the thread is extruded. Normal procedures should be taken to treat the infection or allergy.

Other considerations

- The surgical methods are counter-indicated for patients with heart conditions, diabetes, high fever or for women during pregnancy. Caution should also be exercised when using this method on women during menstruation.
- Blood vessels and nerves should be carefully avoided.
- Along the side of the spine, in the sacral region, or in atrophied muscles on the limbs the threading or embedding methods should be used, rather than the loop-tying method.
- When operating in muscle or muscle tendon, it is important to massage the acupuncture loci before proceeding to embed the thread. In flaccid muscle, the loop-tying method should be used, the tightness of the loop depending upon the degree of tension in the muscle. In tight, spastic muscle it is best to massage first, and then imbed. Looping is not recommended in this case.
- Patients with paralysis should be encouraged to exercise in addition to receiving this treatment.

DIRECT STIMULATION OF NERVE TRUNK

With this method, incisions are made over certain acupuncture points that are contiguous to major nerve trunks. The exposed nerve is then massaged with the forceps, providing direct and intense stimulation. This method is used to stimulate and revive nervous tissue that has been injured due to disease. (It does not revive dead cells.) Results have been comparatively good in treating cases of muscle paralysis caused by diseases like infantile paralysis and encephalitis.

Method

An acupuncture site is selected according to the location of the condition under treatment. After sterilization with alcohol, a 0.5-1% procaine anesthetic is injected superficially and an incision 1-3 cm. in length is made, deeply enough to expose the nerve trunk. Vascular forceps are inserted into the wound, massaging the surrounding tissues until a sore, distended sensation characteristic of acupuncture stimulation is felt by the patient. Then the tip of the forceps is used to massage the nerve trunk itself for perhaps a minute, followed by a few moments' rest. This procedure may be repeated 3-5 times. To protect neighboring blood vessels, the nerve can be moved somewhat toward the opening of the incision. When the stimulation has been completed, the incision should be stitched. As soon as possible after the operation the patient should begin functional exercises and physical therapy, if necessary.

Below are several of the most common acupuncture points selected for treatment in this manner, with their associated nerves.

SI-9 *(Jianzhen).* The ulnar and median nerves are massaged. (Dia. 3-47) For patients who have difficulty raising the arm at the shoulder, the axillary nerve at the posterior, medial margin of the deltoid muscle may be stimulated as well.

LI-11 *(Quchi).* Radial nerve. If the response to stimulation of the median nerve at SI-9 *(Jianzhen)* is unsatisfactory, that nerve may also be probed from this site. (Dia. 3-48)

LI-4 *(Hegu).* Radial nerve branch. For patients who cannot extend the fingers or make a fist, the tip of the forceps can be further inserted into deeper muscle membranes in the palm to the neighborhood of P-8 *(Laogong)* where branches of the median and ulnar nerves can be massaged. (Dia. 3-49)

GB-30 *(Huantiao).* Superior gluteal nerve branch; and, between the ischial tuberosity and greater trochanter, the inferior gluteal and posterior, cutaneous nerve of the thigh, as well as the sciatic nerve. (Dia. 3-50)

GB-34 *(Yanglingquan).* Superficial peroneal nerve (anteriorly) and the common peroneal nerve (posteriorly). (Dia. 3-51)

S-36 *(Zusanli).* Deep branch of common peroneal nerve. (Dia. 3-51)

Other points may be selected for specific problems on the basis of associated neural supply (e.g., the tibial nerve below B-57 *(Chengshan)* for drop foot).

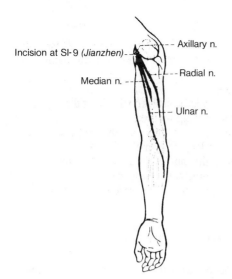

Incision at SI-9 *(Jianzhen)*
Axillary n.
Radial n.
Median n.
Ulnar n.

Dia. 3-47   Incising SI-19 *(Jianzhen)*

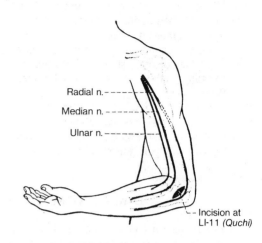

Radial n.
Median n.
Ulnar n.
Incision at LI-11 *(Quchi)*

Dia. 3-48   Incising LI-11 *(Quchi)*

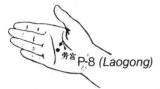

劳宫 P-8 *(Laogong)*

Incision at LI-4 *(Hegu)*

**Dia. 3-49   Incising at LI-4 *(Hegu)* and
Joining to P-8 *(Laogong)***

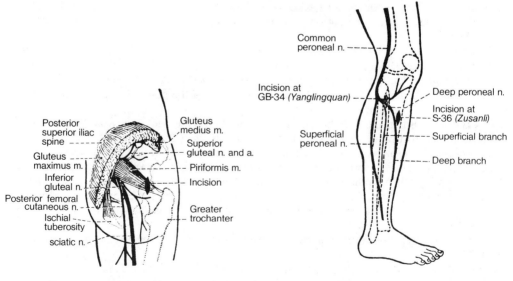

Posterior superior iliac spine
Gluteus maximus m.
Inferior gluteal n.
Posterior femoral cutaneous n.
Ischial tuberosity
sciatic n.
Gluteus medius m.
Superior gluteal n. and a.
Piriformis m.
Incision
Greater trochanter

Dia. 3-50   Incising GB-30 *(Huantiao)*

Common peroneal n.
Incision at GB-34 *(Yanglingquan)*
Superficial peroneal n.
Deep peroneal n.
Incision at S-36 *(Zusanli)*
Superficial branch
Deep branch

**Dia. 3-51   Incising GB-34 *(Yanglingquan)*
and S-36 *(Zusanli)***

Other considerations

• The patient should be warned of the rather intense stimulation he or she should expect from this method.

• There are four sensations which most patients encounter during stimulation of the nerve trunk. These are also described as 'stages' of intensity, from relatively weak to strong: Distended soreness similar to acupuncture point massage), numbness (caused by direct stimulation of nerve trunk), heat (with continuous stimulation, this sensation is perceived throughout the area supplied by the nerve), and burning (repeated stimulation causes this intense reaction, similar to being scalded by water, along the course of the nerve).

• It is recommended that if more than one point is selected, the first be that which is closest to the heart and the others progressively distal. For example, on the lower limb the order might be GB-30 *(Huantiao),* GB-34 *(Yanglingquan),* S-36 *(Zusanli);* on the upper limb, SI-9 *(Jianzhen),* LI-11 *(Quchi),* LI-4 *(Hegu).* In this manner the most important nerves on the limbs are 'activated' and their excitability strengthened.

• When a local anesthetic is used, do not allow the numbness to go too deeply as this will cause a block that will affect the therapy.

• The technique of nerve stimulation is described as 'plucking', as one would a stringed instrument, with small amplitude but high frequency.

• The patient must be carefully observed for any early signs of shock, should the stimulation prove too strong.

• Injections of vitamin B1 and B12 are often given to aid recovery of nerve function.

APPENDIX: ELECTRIC STIMULATION

Instead of opening the skin and probing the nerve trunk manually, two acupuncture points either on, or contiguous to a nerve which innervates a paralyzed muscle may be selected for electric stimulation. Filiform needles are inserted at the points and conducting wires from an electroacupuncture apparatus are attached. The current is then gradually increased and its wave pattern selected to produce a plucking sensation similar to that described above. This is continued for several seconds, then the current is reduced for a moment allowing the patient to rest, after which it is resumed. The procedure is ordinarily performed 3-5 times.

Alternatively, one of the needles can be inserted transversely along the affected muscle, and a second on the nerve trunk.

Precautions for electro-acupuncture apply.

This method is simpler and more convenient than surgical 'plucking', and the results are considered good.

PIERCING THE LYMPH NODES

Piercing the lymph node therapy is a collective term for cold needle, hot needle, injection, medullary scraping, and threading therapies that involve piercing the lymph nodes. These therapies strengthen the body's powers of resistance and have anti-inflammatory and antimicrobic functions. They utilize a combination of Western and Chinese medicine and are based on the traditional hot needle treatment for scrofula. Presently, these therapies are used for the treatment of acute inflammation upon which they have a definite effect.

Sites of operation

Usually the node that drains the affected area is selected. For example, in the treatment of head diseases the cervical nodes are used; for oral and throat conditions the submandibular nodes are used, etc. If the nodes that serve the affected area are relatively inaccessible, the superficial nodes are utilized instead.

469

Methods

Cold needle
Equipment: Same as for ordinary acupuncture.

Technique: After surgical preparation, the left hand holds the node to be pierced in place or raises it from the underlying tissue. A relatively thick needle slowly pierces the node to its center and is lightly raised and thrust several times. The needle then pierces through the other side of the node, and is then twirled every 3-5 minutes. After repeating this procedure 3-4 times, the needle is withdrawn.

Hot needle
Equipment: A special needle made of an amalgam of 15% copper and 85% silver is used. These needles are manufactured in 25 and 26 gauges, and 2-4 inch lengths.

Technique: After preparing the area, the special needle is inserted through the node so that the node is in the middle of the needle. Pads made of rubber or other insulating material are placed between the protruding ends of the needle and the skin to prevent burns. The electro-acupuncture apparatus is attached to the needle (one wire to each end), the apparatus is turned on and warmed up for about one minute, and then the power is turned up until the patient feels that the area is hot or painfully swollen. Usually, the temperature of the needle reaches 55-56°C at a current of 10-15 amps. After 15 minutes turn the machine off, remove the wires, pads, and needle, and lightly massage the area.

Lymph node injection
Ringer's solution is generally used.

Technique: After preparing the area, the head of the hypodermic needle is inserted into the medulla of the node and the solution is injected (0.5-1 ml). This causes the patient to feel distension locally. After the needle is withdrawn the area is gently massaged.

Medulla scraping therapy
Equipment: Scalpel, small scraper, suture needle, surgical gut.

Technique: After the area is prepared, a local anesthetic is given. The skin and subcutaneous tissue are cut through and the node is exposed. An incision 2-3 cm. in length is made in the cortex. The small scraper is used to gently scrape the medulla. Then the surgical gut is used to suture the node. (Usually only one stitch is required; when the node is small it is unnecessary to tie the stitch). The node is replaced, the skin sutured and bandaged. Five to six days later, the skin sutures can be removed.

Threading therapy
Equipment: See threading the points method.

Technique: After preparing the area, one hand is used to hold the node in place. The other hand passes the threaded needle in one side of the node, through the center, and out the other side. The gut is then pulled back and forth a few times and then cut so that both ends are buried beneath the skin. The area is then bandaged.

Duration of treatment

Cold needle, hot needle, and injection therapies are given once a day until the condition stabilizes. Thereafter, treatment is given 2-3 times a week. In acute, serious cases, treatment can be given up to twice a day until there is improvement. A period of treatment is 7-10 days. Periods of treatment are separated by one week.

Medulla scraping therapy is performed once every 20-30 days. Scrape 1-2 nodes each visit.

Threading therapy is performed once every 7-10 days.

Indications

Pneumonia, bronchitis, tonsillitis, multiple boils, bacillary dysentery, acute colitis, appendicitis, prostatitis, cystitis, osteotuberculosis (combined with surgical excision), and to counter infection from surgery or trauma.

Other considerations

- When performing these therapies it is important to note the state of the affected area and organs. If the disease is very severe, these methods are inappropriate. (The immune system is too weak to respond effectively.) Nerves and blood vessels must not be damaged during the operation. In the performance of the medulla scraping method, one must be careful to avoid damaging the hilus.
- Lymph node injection therapy is the most commonly used technique. It should be performed only after the patient has eaten.
- Supportive therapy is necessary before these techniques can be performed on patients who are weak or whose resistance to disease is low.
- Except where noted it is best not to use anesthetics, hormones, analgesics, or drugs which inhibit the autonomic nervous system before or after treatment.
- Lymph nodes should be selected in rotation.

Chapter 7

Ear Acupuncture

A large number of sites have been identified on the ear which become spontaneously tender or otherwise react to the presence of disease or injury elsewhere in the body. Stimulation of these ear points in turn exerts certain therapeutic effects on those parts of the body with which they are associated.

The range of indications in ear acupuncture is broad, the method is relatively simple and economical, and there are few side effects. For these reasons, ear acupuncture has become increasingly popular both in China and abroad.

DEVELOPMENT

The theoretical origins of auriculotherapy derive in the first instance from classical descriptions of the pathways of the channels (see Section I). Of the twelve Primary channels, the six Yang channels traverse or skirt portions of the ear, either directly or through a branch channel; the six Yin channels, having no direct connections, are nevertheless indirectly linked through their Inner/Outer relationships with the Yang channels. See, e.g., the passage from chapter 4 of *Spiritual Axis*, quoted on p. 82 above.

Among the Miscellaneous channels, the Yin and Yang Heel channels as well as the Yang Linking channel have connections with the ear. Thus, in chapter 28 of *Spiritual Axis*, it is written: "All the vessels congregate in the ear."

Similarly, traditional medical literature abounds with references to the close relationship between the ear and specific Organs. E.g., *Spiritual Axis*, chapter 17: "The Kidney Qi communicates with the ear." *Simple Questions*, chapter 4: "The Heart opens at the ear." *Simple Questions*, chapter 22: "As for diseases of the Liver . . . when there is Deficiency, the ears cannot hear . . . when the Qi is rebellious, there are headaches and the ears are deaf."

There are traditional references to treating certain diseases by direct manipulation of the auricle. The famous Tang Dynasty physician, Sun Simo, in his *Thousand Ducat Prescriptions*, recommended that a site corresponding to the modern Lower Abdomen point above the opening of the external auditory meatus be needled or warmed with moxa to treat jaundice and Cold contagious diseases most common in the summer. The Ming Dynasty classic, *Great Compendium of Acupuncture and Moxibustion*, prescribed that moxa be burned at the apex of the ear to treat membranes on the eye. In addition, there are prescriptions in traditional folk medicine for treating redness of the eye by pricking the ear lobes or by letting blood from the posterior auricular vein in the treatment of pain and redness in the eye. The ear lobes were pulled upward as one means of coping with headache, or massaged in the treatment of infantile convulsions.*

As a comprehensive system of diagnosis and treatment, however, ear acupuncture is of recent origin. A French physician by the name of Nogier, writing in a German acupuncture periodical in 1957, first drew serious attention to the correspondences between specific sites on the auricle and other parts of the body. After years of careful observation relating points of tenderness, reduced electrical resistance, morphological and coloration changes on the ear to disease elsewhere in the body, more than 200 sites were charted on the auricle by Chinese medical workers. Ear acupuncture is not only effective in the treatment of a wide range of common diseases, it can also be used with good results in the treatment of difficult diseases or as an analgesic during surgery.

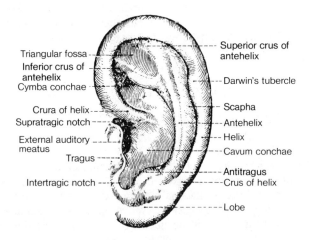

Dia. 3-52   Surface Anatomy of Auricle

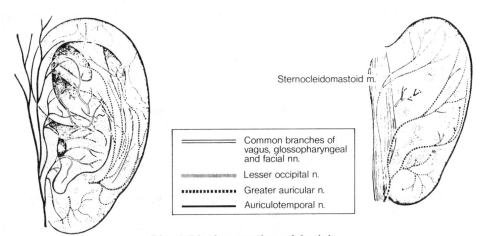

Dia. 3-53   Innervation of Auricle

---

*Although it is true that many of the channels cross the ear and there are several important acupuncture points around its perimeter, ancient practitioners did not place even one of the 365 traditional points on the auricle itself. Furthermore, although traditional Chinese doctors, like their Western counterparts, noted the relationship between diseases of the Organs and manifestations at the ear, these were by and large symptoms of the middle and inner ear such as tinnitus, deafness and vertigo rather than alterations on the auricle itself. —*Editors*

LOCATION AND FUNCTION OF THE EAR POINTS

Unlike most traditional acupuncture points on the body, the ear points have been named according to their associated anatomical position or pathologic indications, e.g., the Lung point or the Hepatitis point. Because their arrangement on the ear often parallels the anatomy of a fetus, the location of many of the principal points is relatively easy to learn. About 180 auricular points together with their primary indications are shown in Table 3-5 below. It is important to remember that because of the differences among ears on different individuals, the locations of the points vary somewhat from person to person.

Most significant when exploring for the point are sites which are unusually sensitive or appear abnormal (see Appendix to this chapter). 'Point' is perhaps a poor choice of words to describe a site which more often has a spatial dimension much larger than the head of a pin. Nevertheless, if a physician is unable to find an alteration in the region of the ear associated with the disease, he may still needle the 'point' he has learned here.

SELECTION OF POINTS

The following methods should be considered when selecting points for a specific disease.
  • According to the associated anatomical location of the disease. E.g., selecting the Stomach point for stomach ache, or the Elbow point for pain in the elbow.
  • According to Western physiological and pathological relationships. E.g., selecting the Endocrine point for irregular menstruation, or the Sympathetic and Cerebrum points for ulcers.
  • According to concepts of Chinese traditional medicine (discussed in Introduction). E.g., because the Liver is said to 'open' at the eyes, diseases of the eyes can be treated by stimulating the Liver point; or, because the Lungs control the skin, cutaneous diseases are often treated by means of the Lung point.
  • According to points of clinically proven effectiveness, i.e., points whose functions are varied or whose name bears little if any relation to the disease. E.g., selecting the Parotid Gland point for neurodermatitis, or pricking the Ear Apex point to treat fever.

The examples cited above are illustrative of the principles which should be considered when selecting a point. Usually, more than one point is chosen. Specific prescriptions are listed under individual diseases in Section IV.

METHODS

Methods previously introduced for regular acupuncture points on the body such as simple needling, embedding or warming the needle, electro- and injection acupuncture, as well as moxibustion and blood letting can all be used on the ear. Below are some special considerations for auriculotherapy.

Needling

1) Once the point has been located, apply the head of the needle at the point, leaving a mark that can be found for inserting the needle. Then clean the area with alcohol.

2) Usually a #28 gauge needle, half an inch in length is used on the ear (larger and thinner needles tend to fall out). The needle is inserted with a quick motion to a depth of approximately 0.1 inch, reaching but not penetrating the ear cartilage. The needle is then twirled a few times to elicit the Qi sensation characteristic of acupuncture. The needle is usually retained, depending on the disease, from 30-60 minutes. For certain acute, inflammatory or painful diseases as well as those characterized by seizures, the needle may be retained for longer periods (up to 2 hours). While the needle is in place it should be manipulated once every 5-10 minutes.

3) Treatments are given once a day or on alternating days. Ten treatments is considered an average course, although most chronic diseases may require from 10-20 treatments (acute cases, 5-10). If

another course or cycle of treatments is necessary, 5-15 days should be allowed to elapse in between.

4) Unlike acupuncture on the body, needling the auricle often causes pain in addition to the characteristic sensations of soreness, distension, warmth, heaviness and perhaps numbness.

5) It is preferable to use only a few (3-5) points at a single session. Usually only points on one ear corresponding to the side of the disease are selected, although in a minority of cases the opposite ear or both ears are used.

6) If the needle is inserted transversely, it is possible to join two or more neighboring points.

Embedding the needle

Special intradermal ear needles or tacks (see Dia. 3-13) can be embedded in ear points and held in place with adhesive tape, usually from one day to a week or more. While in place, the patient should be instructed to press them several times each day so as to stimulate underlying tissues. The ear will otherwise adapt itself to the needle's pressure. Care must be exercised to see that the ear is kept clean during this period so as to avoid infection. During hot weather or if the patient is engaged in strenuous physical activity, it is best not to use this method.

Embedding is utilized for certain chronic diseases, or diseases with repeated seizures. However, it is not considered as effective as regular needling.

Moxibustion

Moxibustion (usually above the inserted needle) may be used in cases of chronic rheumatic or Cold diseases, if the physician so desires. Usually 3-5 minutes of moxa warmth is sufficient.

Pricking

Pricking auricular points with the tip of a surgical knife or pyramid needle to let blood is a common technique in the treatment of certain acute inflammatory diseases. Usually 3-5 drops of blood is sufficient, once a day, with 3-5 visits constituting a course of treatment.

Electro-acupuncture

When electrical stimulation is used for ear acupuncture, usually only two needles are utilized. The level of stimulation is raised to the patient's tolerance and continued for 15-30 minutes.

Injection therapy

Various substances are injected in amounts ranging from 0.1-0.3 ml., daily or on alternating days. Indicated for pulmonary tuberculosis, bronchial asthma, and anesthesia.

OTHER CONSIDERATIONS

When the ear needles are in place there is usually a sensation similar to that of an insect bite (local soreness, warmth and distension). If this sensation is absent, it is generally believed that the effects of the treatment will be negligible. For this reason, once the needle is in place, it should be manipulated from time to time so as to restore the needle sensation.

If, while the needle is retained, there is suddenly pain at a location unrelated to the disease, the angle or position of the needle can be changed slightly and the reaction should disappear.

As with all medicine, proper diagnosis is essential in identifying the fundamental source of a disease. If points are selected which only affect superficial symptoms, the physician may find that the patient shows some relief at first but no further improvement despite continued treatment.

Similarly, although a patient may respond well to initial treatment and his condition appear to have been cured, he should be encouraged to continue treatments through the duration of the recommended course.

A physician should not be discouraged if, after apparent success, the condition returns. Studies have shown that the condition is rarely as severe the second time, indicating that some progress has been made.

Strict measures must be taken to assure that the ear is properly cleaned both before and after treatment. Auricular infections are quite serious and stubborn to cure.

APPENDIX: FINDING POINTS ON THE AURICLE

Examination of the ear can serve either as an aid in diagnosis, or, having already diagnosed a disease and selected appropriate points, examination can help to pinpoint the most sensitive or tender site within the selected area. There are three general methods of finding the points:

Direct examination

The physician looks for alterations in the color or morphological changes on the surface of the skin. The ear should not be cleaned or otherwise disturbed prior to the examination.

Alterations which may be caused by disease should be distinguished from scars, marks, or diseases (boils, ulcers, etc.) which are purely local in nature. Often, the latter do not respond painfully to pressure and show no reduction in electrical resistance.

The site of an alteration may directly correspond to a pathologic change in the organ with which it is associated, or it may be related indirectly to a disease in a body system or through traditional Inner/Outer connections between important Organs.

Both ears should be examined, and features compared. The thumb and index finger can be used to palpate for differences in thickness, ridges, etc., on the surface of the ear. The age, environment, and occupation of the patient must be taken into consideration before drawing any conclusions from the ears.

In examining the ear the following are said to be signs of 'positive response':

Color changes: The area has a different color than the surrounding region—either more pale, redder, or darker. If the color does not change upon pressure, then it is not a 'positive response' point (i.e., the color is an intrinsic property of the area).

Shape changes: The area may have a nodule, strand, protuberance or depression.

Rashes: Often there is a white or red macular rash, or a small blister in the area.

Accumulations: Normal wax or dirt accumulations in the ear are easily wiped away and have no significance. When the accretions are not easily wiped away, they may be signs of a 'positive response' point.

Probing

Use a blunt-tipped probe or head of a pin to lightly press against a site which the physician has determined through diagnosis to be related to a certain disease. The most tender spot, often quite painful, is the point used for therapy. Care must be taken to see that all points are probed with uniform pressure and for a similar length of time, long enough for the patient to make a comparative judgment.

If points of tenderness cannot be found, the physician may still needle those sites on the ear associated with the illness.

Measuring electrical resistance

A special electrical probing device, often included as an accessory on electro-acupuncture machines, may be used to measure changes in the electrical resistance of the skin at various sites on the ear. Points at which the electrical resistance is significantly lower than other points are selected for therapy since this often indicates disease in the related Organ or region of the body. The probe is simple to use and the method is by and large painless.

The ear should be cleaned with alcohol and allowed to dry before beginning. The examination should take place in a quiet room. Electric current is adjusted to the individual patient by placing the probe on the Spinal Cord point at the back of the auricle and increasing the current until there is a slight stinging sensation.

There are several factors which have a considerable influence on the electrical resistance of the ear, including changes in the weather (resistance greater in cold weather), age (younger people whose ears are more moist and soft have a lower electrical resistance), and location (the Uterus, Bladder, Large Intestine, Esophagus, Triple Burner, and Endocrine points usually have low resistance; likewise, areas where overlying skin is relatively soft usually have a somewhat lower electrical resistance than more 'exposed' and less soft areas, e.g., the helix and tragus.) These factors must be kept in mind and compensated for in practice. Areas with typically lower electrical resistance are pressed with less force than those which are predictably higher.

Finally, if one point is probed repeatedly, or pressed too long, it will become tender and the electrical resistance will decline, causing it to be misinterpreted as a point for therapy.

It should be remembered that the physician is measuring a relative difference so as to discover those points which react most to a disease and whose manipulation might in turn be expected to affect that disease most significantly. It is not an absolute measurement, and other methods of observation should not be neglected.

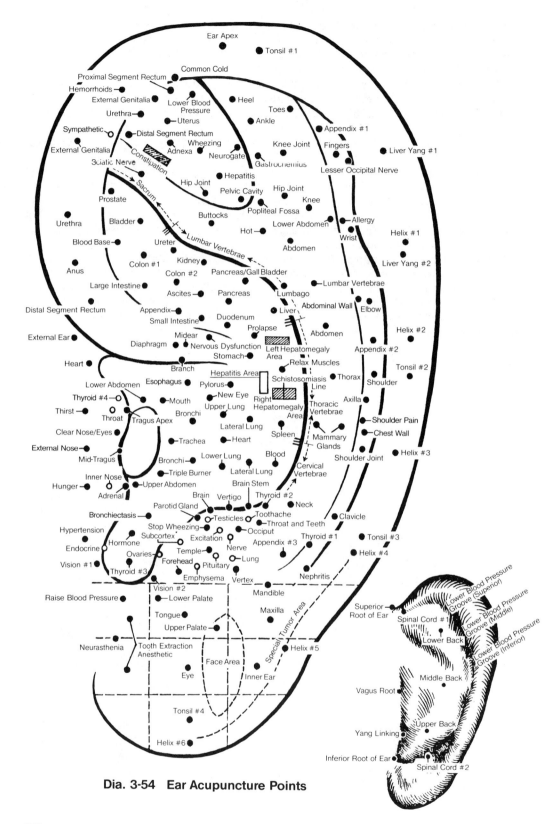

Dia. 3-54 Ear Acupuncture Points

478

TABLE 3-5 EAR POINTS

Points on helix and crus of helix

Name	Location	Indications
Diaphragm	On crus of the helix	Spasms of diaphragm, hemorrhage, pruritis, hemorrhagic skin disorders, hemotological diseases
Branch	On crus of helix, midway between Bladder and Brain points	Usually used for incontinence
Midear	Center of crus of helix	Indications not listed
Nervous Dysfunction	Superior aspect of crus of helix	Indications not listed
Distal Segment Rectum	On helix, almost level with Large Intestine point on the cymba conchae	Dysentery, enteritis, prolapsed anus, fissure of anus, hemorrhoids, constipation
Urethra	On helix, level with Bladder point on the cymba conchae	Urinary tract infection, incontinence
Anus	On helix, midway between Distal Segment Rectum and Urethra points	Itching around anus, anal fissure, hemorrhoids, prolapsed anus
External Genitalia	On helix, level with inferior crus of antehelix	Sexual dysfunction, inflammation of scrotum or penis, cervicitis, low back pain, sciatica
Common Cold	On the margin of helix, slightly anterior to superior margin of superior crus of antehelix	Common cold (prick point)
Hemorrhoids	On helix bordering lateral margin of triangular fossa	Hemorrhoids, fissure of anus
Ear Apex	When ear is bent toward tragus, this point can be found at tip of fold on superior aspect of helix	Prick point for fever, inflammation, hypertension, revival from hepatic coma, or for analgesic or sedative effect. Use moxibustion for keratitis.
Tonsil #1	On helix, posterior to Ear Apex point	Tonsillitis, pharyngitis
Liver Yang #1	Superior border of Darwin's tubercle	Chronic hepatitis
Liver Yang #2	Inferior border of Darwin's tubercle	Same as Liver Yang #1 above

479

Name	Location	Indications
Helix #1-6	Six points evenly spaced along helix from inferior margin of Darwin's tubercle to inferior margin of earlobe	Tonsillitis, pharyngitis
Tonsil #2	On helix, level with the Shoulder point on the scapula	Same as Helix #1-6 above
Tonsil #3	On the 'tail' of the helix	Same as Helix #1-6 above

Points on scapha

Name	Location	Indications
Appendix #1	On scapha, midway between the Toe and Finger points	Appendicitis
Fingers	On scapha, above Darwin's tubercle	Pain or hindered movement of finger joints
Wrist	On scapha, level with prominence on Darwin's tubercle	Pain or hindered movement of the wrist
Allergy	On scapha, medial to Wrist point	Allergic diseases
Shoulder	On scapha, level with supratragic notch	Pain or hindered movement of shoulder
Elbow	On scapha, midway between Shoulder and Wrist points	Pain of elbow joint
Appendix #2	On scapha, midway between Shoulder and Elbow points	Appendicitis
Shoulder Joint	On scapha, midway between Shoulder and Clavicle points	Pain or hindered movement of shoulder
Clavicle	On scapha, level with Neck point on antehelix	Diseases of clavicle
Shoulder Pain	On scapha, superior and medial to Shoulder Joint point	Shoulder pain
Axilla	On scapha, above Shoulder Pain point	Swelling of subaxillary lymph glands and other diseases of this region
Chest Wall	On scapha, above Shoulder Joint point	Pain of chest and ribs, gallstones
Abdominal Wall	On scapha, above Shoulder point on border of antehelix and scapha	Abdominal pain, pain in hypochondriac region, renal colic

480

Name	Location	Indications
Nephritis	Lateral and inferior to the Clavicle point, in the depression on lower margin of scapha	Nephritis, pyelonephritis
Thyroid #1	On border of scapha, lateral to Neck point on antehelix	Regulates function of thyroid gland; may also be used in shock to raise blood pressure.
Appendix #3	On scapha, medial and inferior to Clavicle point	Appendicitis

Superior crus and inferior crus of antehelix

Name	Location	Indications
Toes	On the lateral, superior angle of superior crus of antehelix	Pain or functional hinderance of the toes
Ankle	On the medial, superior angle of superior crus of antehelix	Pain or functional hinderance of the ankle
Heel	On the medial, superior angle of superior crus of antehelix	Pain or functional hinderance of the heel
Knee	On the superior crus of antehelix, level with superior border of inferior crus of antehelix	Pain or functional hinderance of the knee
Knee Joint	On the superior crus of antehelix, 1/3 the distance from the Ankle to the Knee point	Pain or functional hinderance of the knee
Hip Joint	On the superior crus of antehelix, 1/3 the distance from the Knee to the Ankle point	Pain or functional hinderance of the hip
Gastrocnemius	On the superior crus of antehelix, medial and inferior to the Knee Joint point	Pain or functional hinderance along the gastrocnemius muscles
Popliteal Fossa	On the superior crus of antehelix, medial to the Knee point	Pain or functional hinderance in the popliteal fossa
Sympathetic	At the intersection of the superior border of the inferior crus of antehelix and the medial border of the helix	Used for numerous diseases related to disruption in autonomic (both sympathetic and parasympathetic) nervous system. Strong analgesic and relaxant effect upon internal organs. Specifically, for relieving pain associated with ulcers, stomach spasm, round worm in bile duct, gall and urethral stones. Dilates blood vessels. Useful in treating circulatory and ophthalmological diseases, and excessive sweating. Important point of anesthesia.

481

Name	Location	Indications
Sciatic Nerve	Slightly medial to mid-point on superior margin of inferior crus of antehelix	Sciatica
Buttocks	Slightly lateral to mid-point on superior margin of inferior crus of antehelix	Pain of hip and sacroiliac joints, atrophy of gluteal muscles
Hot	On antehelix directly below Popliteal Fossa point	Low-grade fever
Lower Abdomen	On antehelix, lateral and inferior to Knee point	Pain of lower abdomen

Points on antehelix

Name	Location	Indications
Lumbar Vertebrae	On the prominence of the antehelix, level with Distal Segment of Rectum point	Low back pain
Abdomen	On the antehelix, level with the inferior border of the inferior crus of antehelix	Pain of mid- or lower abdomen
Lumbago	Near medial border of antehelix, level with Lumbar Vertebrae point	Acute low back sprain, chronic low back pain
Chest	On antehelix, level with supratragic notch	Intercostal neuralgia, soreness or depressed sensation in chest
Abdomen [same name, different point than above]	On antehelix, between Lumbar Vertebrae and Chest points	Pain of upper abdomen
Mammary Glands	Two points on antehelix, both below Chest point, one medial, the other lateral	Acute mastitis, lumps in the breast
Neck	In notch at the intersection of the antehelix and antitragus	Pain or dysfunction of the neck
Thyroid #2	On medial margin of antehelix, medial to Neck point	Same as Thyroid #1 above
Sacral, Lumbar, Thoracic and Cervical Vertebrae	These vertebral points are found along the curved, medial margin of the antehelix from a point level with the Urethra point (above) to Shoulder Joint point (below). The curved line	Each segment corresponds to pain or dysfunction along that part of the spine

Name	Location	Indications
	can be divided into four segments each corresponding to one of the vertebral groupings, from the Sacral (above) to the Cervical (below)	

Points on tragus and antitragus

Name	Location	Indications
External Ear	In depression slightly anterior to supratragic notch	Tinnitus, deafness
Heart	On tragus, posterior and inferior to External Ear point	Tachycardia, arrhythmias, and other heart disorders
Tragus Apex	The prominence on superior part of tragus	Inflammation, fever, hypertension, pain (in general). Prick point.
Adrenal	At the prominence on inferior part of tragus (if the ear has only one such prominence, the point is on the inferior border)	Functions to stimulate adrenalin and adrenocortical hormones. Used for inflammation, allergies, shock, rheumatism and serious poisoning symptoms resulting from bacterial infection. Affects the dilation and constriction of blood vessels, hyper- and hypotension, capillary hemorrhage. Regulates excitation or inhibition of respiratory function. Used for fever, certain skin diseases, and chronic illnesses.
External Nose	At the middle of the anterior aspect of the tragus	Brandy-nose
Thirst	Above External Nose point on tragus	Relieves thirst, diabetes, polyuria
Hunger	Below External Nose point on tragus	Relieves hunger, diabetes, compulsive eating
Clear Nose/Eyes	On tragus, behind Thirst point	Acute and chronic rhinitis, eye inflammation
Hypertension	On tragus, below Hunger point	Hypertension
Throat	On upper half of medial aspect of tragus	Acute and chronic laryngitis, hoarseness, tonsillitis, edema of the uvula
Inner Nose	On lower half of medial aspect of tragus	Rhinitis, nosebleed
Thyroid #4	On tragus, lateral and superior to Throat point	Same as Thyroid #1 above
Forehead	On anterior, inferior part of antitragus	Frontal headache, rhinitis

Name	Location	Indications
Occiput	On posterior, superior part of antitragus	Used for neuropsychiatric disorders and symptoms due to meningeal irritation: convulsions, locked jaw, stiffness along nape of neck, psychosis, etc. Also useful in preventing motion or sea sickness. Used for various skin and eye diseases, inflammation, pain, shock.
Temple	On antitragus, between Forehead and Occiput points	Headache at the temple, migraine headache, vertigo, lassitude
Vertex	On antitragus, between and below Temple and Occiput points	Headache at the vertex, vertigo
Stop Wheezing	At apex of angle of antitragus (if angle unclear, mid-point on medial border of antitragus)	Regulates excitation or inhibition of respiratory center. Used for coughing, panting, and/or itching.
Parotid Gland	On antitragus, medial to Stop Wheezing point	Parotitis, obstruction of parotid ducts. Effective in relieving itching symptoms of many skin diseases.
Brain	On antitragus, between Stop Wheezing and Brain Stem points	Regulates excitation or inhibition of the cerebral cortex. Used for disease of nervous, digestive, endocrine, and urogenital systems; hemorrhage.
Brain Stem	On the border of the lower segment of the antitragus, near Neck point	Disorders of the cerebral blood vessels and meninges, e.g., apoplexy, hemiplegia, convulsions, stiffness along nape of neck, etc. Also used for sequelae of cerebral shock, incomplete development of the brain.
Vertigo	On antitragus, between Brain point and Brain Stem point	Aural vertigo, prevents motion sickness
Throat and Teeth	On antitragus, superior and posterior to Occiput point	Toothache, swelling of gums, pharyngitis, tonsillitis
Vision #1	Inferior and anterior to the intertragic notch	Glaucoma, atrophy of optic nerve, diseases below the eyes
Vision #2	Inferior and posterior to the intertragic notch	Astigmatism and other ophthalmological diseases
Endocrine	At the extreme anterior portion in the bottom of the intertragic notch	Regulates disturbance of endocrine function, aids in metabolic function of absorption and excretion. Has antiallergic and antirheumatic function. Used for gynecological and urogenital diseases, for dysfunction of the digestive system, blood and skin diseases, malaria.

Name	Location	Indications
Ovaries	On anterior, inferior part of the inner wall of the antitragus	Irregular menstruation, painful menstruation, infertility, developmental gynecological disorders
Subcortex	On anterior side of the inner wall of the antitragus	Regulates excitation and inhibition of cerebral cortex. Often used for insomnia, lassitude and other neuropsychiatric disorders. Also for inflammation, excessive sweating, and pain.
Hormone	On medial side in the bottom of the intertragic notch	Inflammation, allergies, shock, rheumatism
Testicles	On superior part of inner wall of antitragus	Sexual dysfunction, orchitis, eczema of scrotum
Excitation	On inner wall of antitragus below Testicles point	Narcolepsy, depression, emotional withdrawal
Nerve	On inner wall of antitragus, below and posterior to Excitation point	Facial nerve paralysis, severe muscle weakness, oculomotor nerve paralysis
Toothache	On inner wall of antitragus, below and posterior to Nerve point	Toothache
Pituitary	At the bottom of inner wall of antitragus	Regulates function of pituitary. Used for dwarfism, acromegalic gigantism, polyuria. Also used for shock, improper contraction of uterus after childbirth, sexual dysfunction, and disease resulting from disturbances of endocrine function.

Points on triangular fossa

Name	Location	Indications
Uterus	Slightly above the parting of the two crura of the antehelix, in the triangular fossa	Obstetrical and gynecological diseases, sexual dysfunction in the male
Pelvic Cavity	In the lateral angle of the triangular fossa near the intersection of the superior and inferior crura of the antehelix	Pelvic cavity inflammation, painful menstruation
Neurogate	In the triangular fossa, medial and superior to the Pelvic Cavity point	Regulates excitation and inhibition of the cerebral cortex. Sedative, analgesic, anti-allergy effects. Used for neuropsychiatric disorders (hysteria, psychosis, etc.), hypertension, coughing, allergic asthma, itching symptoms, and pain. Important point for anesthesia.

Name	Location	Indications
Wheezing	In the triangular fossa, between the Uterus and Pelvic Cavity points	Anti-allergy, suppresses wheezing, bronchial asthma
Hepatitis	In the triangular fossa, between the Wheezing and Pelvic Cavity points	Acute and chronic hepatitis
Hip Joint	In the triangular fossa, below the Hepatitis point	Often used for pain of lower limb joints or buttocks
Adnexa	In the triangular fossa, lateral and inferior to the Uterus point	Inflammation of the adnexa, painful menstruation
Constipation	In the triangular fossa, below the Adnexa point	Constipation, bleeding from hemmorhoids
Lower Blood Pressure	In the superior angle of the triangular fossa where the superior crus meets the helix	Hypertension, headache (due to hypertension)
(New) Distal Segment Rectum	At the inferior angle of triangular fossa where the inferior crus of the antehelix meets the helix	Enteritis, constipation, hemmorhoids, prolapsed anus
(New) Urethra	In the triangular fossa, medial to Uterus point and near the border of helix	Frequent and urgent urination, painful urination, incontinence, retention of urine
(New) External Genitalia	In the triangular fossa, anterior and superior to Uterus point	Sexual dysfunction, leukorrhea, excessive menstruation
(New) Proximal Segment Rectum	In the triangular fossa, above the (new) Urethra point	Functional disturbance of the colon

Points on cavum and cymba conchae

Name	Location	Indications
Mouth	On superior, posterior wall of the opening of the external meatus	Ulcers in the mouth, stiffness in the tempero-mandibular joint
Esophagus	In the cavum of conchae, below midpoint of the crus of helix	Functional constriction of larynx, difficulty in swallowing due to hysteria, belching
Pylorus	In the cavum of conchae, below the crus of helix and posterior to the Esophagus point	Pyloric spasm, belching, constriction of diaphragm causing regurgitation

Name	Location	Indications
Stomach	In the cavum of conchae, where the crus of helix 'disappears'	Diseases of stomach including indigestion, acute and chronic gastritis, peptic ulcer, distension of stomach, belching, insomnia, etc.
Prolapse	In the cymba of conchae, above the Stomach point and posterior to the Duodenum point	Prolapse of the viscera
Duodenum	In the cymba of conchae, between Prolapse and Small Intestine points	Duodenal ulcer, pyloric spasm, hypoacidic stomach
Small Intestine	In the cymba of conchae, above midpoint of crus of helix	Indigestion, enteritis, distension of intestine by gas, heart disease
Large Intestine	In the cymba of conchae, above crus of helix, anterior to Small Intestine point	Enteritis, dysentery, diarrhea, constipation, hemmorrhoids, diseases of respiratory system
Appendix	In the cymba of conchae, between Large and Small Intestine points	Acute and chronic appendicitis
Colon #1	In the cymba of conchae, between Large Intestine and Bladder points	These 3 points treat allergic colitis, ulcer of the colon, intestinal polyps, bleeding in lower digestive tract, diarrhea due to schistosomiasis
Colon #2	In the cymba of conchae, between Appendix and Ureter points	Same
Blood Base	In the cymba of conchae, between the Prostate and Large Intestine points	Same
Prostate	In the cymba of conchae, medial to the Bladder point	Prostatitis, urinary tract infection, blood in the urine, painful urination, spermatorrhea, premature ejaculation
Bladder	In the cymba of conchae, above the Large Intestine point	Cystitis, frequent and urgent urination, incontinence, retention of urine, enuresis, low back pain, neck pain
Kidney	In cymba of conchae, above the Small Intestine point	Strengthening point, beneficial to the cerebrum, Kidneys, and hematopoietic system. Used for incomplete development of brain, amnesia, neurasthenia, vertigo, headache, lassitude, nerve deafness, tinnitus, advancing deafness, loss of hair, diseases of the eyes, gynecological and urogenital system diseases, assists in bone mending, loose teeth, aplastic anemia, leukemia, edema, chronic pharyngitis, electrolyte imbalance, etc.

Name	Location	Indications
Ureter	In cymba of conchae, between Bladder and Kidney points	Kidney stones, renal colic
Ascites	In cymba of conchae, above Small Intestine point	Electrolyte imbalance, ascites, cirrhosis of liver, intestinal adhesions
Pancreas	In cymba of conchae, above Duodenum point	Acute and chronic pancreatitis, diabetes, indigestion, pancreatic diarrhea
Relax Muscles	In cymba of conchae, posterior to Stomach point	Used for relaxing muscles, and is important point in anesthesia; also for hepatitis and cirrhosis of liver
Left Hepatomegaly Area	Above Relax Muscles point and lateral to Prolapse point (approximately 5 mm. long and 2 mm. wide)	Hepatitis, enlargement of liver (hepatomegaly)
Liver	In cymba of conchae, above Left Hepatomegaly Area	Acute and chronic hepatitis, eye diseases, iron deficient anemia and other blood diseases, arthritic pain, neuralgia, headache, vertigo, stomach gas and pain, gas in the GI tract, hemiplegia, seizures, muscle spasms
Pancreas/Gall Bladder	In cymba of conchae, between Liver point and Kidney point	Indigestion, pancreatitis, diabetes, cholecystitis, gall stones, round worm in bile duct, chest and rib pain
Right Hepatomegaly Area	In the cavum of conchae, between Relax Muscles and Spleen points (approximately 5 mm. long and 2 mm. wide)	Hepatitis, enlargement of liver (hepatomegaly)
Schistosomiasis Line	A straight line from Relax Muscles point to the Right Hepatomegaly Area in the cavum of conchae	Cirrhosis of liver due to schistosomiasis, as well as enlargement of spleen, diarrhea, indigestion
Hepatitis Area	Between Stomach point and Right Hepatomegaly Area, in the cavum of conchae	Acute and chronic hepatitis
Spleen	Between Blood point and Right Hepatomegaly Area, in the cavum of conchae	Indigestion, muscle atrophy (in general), blood diseases, abnormal uterine bleeding, prolapsed anus, weakness following a disease, prolapse of viscera, muscle weakness
Blood	In the cavum of conchae, below the Spleen point and level with the Neck point	Hemorrhagic diseases
Heart	In depression at the center of	Strengthens heart, anti-shock, regulates blood

Name	Location	Indications
	the cavum of conchae	pressure. Used for various mental diseases, heart disease, glossitis, Buerger's disease, anemia
Upper Lung, Lower Lung	Two points, one above and one below the Heart point, near the center of cavum of conchae	Various respiratory system and skin diseases, rhinitis, mutism, night sweats, spontaneous sweating. Also used as analgesic points in acupuncture anesthesia.
Lateral Lung	Posterior to and between the Lung points, near the cavum of conchae	Same
Bronchi	Two points anterior to and between the Lung points, near the center of cavum of conchae	Acute and chronic bronchitis, asthma
New Eye	Between and below the Esophagus and Pylorus points, above the Lung point	Ametropia, diseases below the eye
Trachea	Between and medial to the two Bronchi points	Diseases of trachea
Triple Burner	Below Trachea point, above Bronchiectasis point, in the cavum of conchae	Hepatitis, tracheal disorders, diseases affecting mesentery or peritoneum; diuretic function
Bronchiectasis	Above Hormone point in the cavum of conchae	Bronchiectasis
Emphysema	Anterior and inferior to Pituitary point in the cavum of conchae	Emphysema, wheezing
Lung	Posterior to the Pituitary point	Same as other Lung point

Points on ear lobe

Name	Location	Indications
Eye	If the earlobe from below the intertragic notch is divided by three parallel, horizontal lines, then sub-divided by two parallel vertical lines, the lobe will be comprised of 9 sections (numbered left to right, top to bottom). The Eye point is in section 5.	Eye diseases
Tooth Extraction Anesthetic	Using the system outlined above under Eye point, one Tooth Extraction Anesthetic	Toothache, anesthesia for tooth extraction

Name	Location	Indications
	point is in section 1, and the other Tooth Extraction Anesthetic point in Section 4.	
Neurasthenia	Using system outlined above under Eye point, this point is between sections 1 and 4.	Neurasthenia
Tongue	Using system outlined above under Eye point, this point is in the center of section 2.	Glossitis, nervous aphasia
Upper and Lower Palate	Using system outlined above under Eye point, the Lower Palate point is in the anterior, superior part of section 2, and the Upper Palate point in the posterior, inferior part of section 2.	These points are used for toothache, swelling of gums, stiffness in temporomandibular joint, ulcers in the mouth, swelling of submaxillary lymph glands. Also anesthesia points for tooth extraction.
Maxilla and Mandible	Using system outlined above under Eye point, the Mandible point is at the top of section 3, the Maxilla point in the lower part of section 3.	Same
Inner Ear	Using system outlined above under Eye point, this point is in section 6.	Aural vertigo, tinnitus, deafness
Tonsil #4	Using system outlined above under Eye point, this point is in section 8.	Tonsillitis, pharyngitis
Face Area	An elongated region stretching between the Eye and the Inner Ear points on the earlobe	Facial paralysis, spasms of facial muscles, trigeminal neuralgia, parotitis
Special Tumor Area	A line extending from Helix #4 to Helix #6 on the earlobe	Definite analgesic effect for pain from tumors

Points on back of ear

Name	Location	Indications
Lower Blood Pressure Groove	In trough along the backside of antehelix on the back of ear. This groove is divided into upper, middle and lower segments.	Hypertension (prick point)
Upper Back	On back of ear, on lower cartilaginous prominence	Acute sprain of lower back, back pain; pruritis

490

Name	Location	Indications
Lower Back	On back of ear, on upper cartilaginous prominence	
Middle Back	On back of ear, between Upper and Lower Back points	
Vagus Root	At midpoint on back of ear where the auricle intersects the mastoid process	Diseases of internal organs
Superior Root of Auricle	At intersection of superior border of auricle with the skin of face	Hemiplegia, hardening of funiculus lateralis spinalis
Inferior Root of Auricle	At intersection of inferior border with the skin of face	
Spinal Cord #1	Posterior border of superior annicular root	Muscle atrophy, paralysis
Spinal Cord #2	Superior border of inferior annicular root	
Yang Linking	Lateral and inferior to Vagus Root point, on back of ear	Tinnitus

Chapter 8

Face, Nose, Head, Hand and Foot Acupuncture

FACE AND NOSE ACUPUNCTURE

One of the features of traditional diagnosis is the identification of color changes on the skin with pathology in a particular Organ or Organ system.* Although not always apparent, these color changes are most often reflected in the face. Channel theory ascribes to those areas traversed by the various channels (many cross the face or connect with others that do) the characteristics of their associated Organs. The distribution of channels and color characteristics formed the theoretical basis of face acupuncture.

The nose is situated in the center of the face. The ancients called it the "Bright Hall." In chapter 49 of *Spiritual Axis* is written: "It is in the Bright Hall that the five colors are resolved." It is believed that the nose reflects the health of the body in general, and the Heart and Lungs in particular: "The five Qi's enter the nose and are stored in the Heart and Lungs." *(Simple Questions,* chapter 11) In recent times, ancient theory has been coupled with clinical experience in the development of face and nose acupuncture, which can be used to treat disease anywhere in the body. This is an example of using observation to develop a method of treatment.

Location of face and nose points

The seven midline and seventeen pair of bilateral face and nose acpuncture points are described in Tables 3-6 and 3-7, and are illustrated in Diagrams 3-55 and 3-56.

Principles of point selection

A point on the face or nose may be selected because its name corresponds to the location of a disease in the body, e.g., selecting the Stomach point for problems of the stomach. Or a point can be chosen because it relates indirectly to a disease according to a principle of traditional physiology. This is particularly important in acupuncture anesthesia, e.g., needling the Lung point as a cutaneous analgesic because the Lungs control the skin and pores; or the Kidney point in orthopedic surgery because the Kidneys control the bones according to traditional medicine. Finally, a point may be selected because it becomes spontaneously tender or sensitive to the presence of disease in a certain

---

*Green is associated with the Liver and its related Yang Organ, the Gall Bladder; red with the Heart and Small Intestine; white with the Lung and Large Intestine; black with the Kidneys and Bladder. For a more detailed description of the Five Phases system of correspondences, see Introduction.—*Editors*

part of the body. Such points of tenderness (or 'positive response') are found in the same manner as those on the ear. (See chapter 7)

Method

Because of the shallow depth of flesh over much of the face, the needle is usually inserted at a transverse or slanted angle to the surface. A #28-32 gauge needle, 0.5-1.5 inches in length is ordinarily used.

After the needle sensation (Qi) has been obtained, the needle is retained for 10-30 minutes. The physician should manipulate the needle a few times every 5-10 minutes so as to maintain stimulation. Generally, ten treatments constitute one course, on consecutive or alternating days. If it is necessary to begin a second course, a week's rest should be allowed during the interim.

Other considerations

- Acupuncture sites must be rigorously cleaned. Scars and sores should be avoided.
- As on the ear, areas on the nose which are typically moist or oily are expected to show lower electrical resistance than surrounding areas. These areas in particular must be thoroughly cleaned and dried if the physician intends to use the electric probing device for diagnosis.
- The face—and particularly the nose—is very sensitive to needle stimulation. Many sites are simply painful to needle. The physician can help somewhat by avoiding deep insertion on the nose, and minimizing the manipulation of the needle once in place.

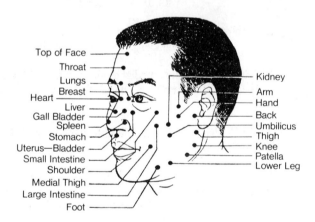

Dia. 3-55   Facial Acupuncture Points

Table 3-6   FACE ACUPUNCTURE POINTS

Area	Point	Location
Midline from Forehead to Upper Lip	Top of Face	On midline of forehead, 1/3 the distance from the natural hairline to a point midway between the eyebrows
	Throat	On midline of forehead, 2/3 the distance from the natural hairline to a point midway between eyebrows

493

Area	Point	Location
Midline from Forehead to Upper Lip	Lung (same as M-HN-3 *(Yintang)*	At midpoint between eyebrows
	Heart (same as M-HN-4 *(Shangen)*)	At lowest point on bridge of nose (the nasion), midway between inner canthi of eyes
	Liver	Just below highest point on nasal bone, midway between the Heart and Spleen points of the nose
	Spleen	Just above the knob at the tip of the nose, on the midline
	Uterus and Bladder (same as Gv-26 *(Renzhong)*)	One third the distance from the base of the nose to the top of the upper lip, in the philtrum
Nose, Eye, Mouth and Cheek	Gall Bladder	At the side of the nose, directly below the inner canthus at the inferior margin of the nasal bone, level with the Liver point
	Stomach	Slightly above middle of ala nasi directly below Gall Bladder point, level with Spleen point
	Breast (same as B-1 *(Jingming)*)	Just medial to inner canthus, in depression on lateral margin of nasal bone
	Medial Thigh (same as S-4 *(Dicang)*)	0.5 unit lateral to the corner of mouth
	Small Intestine	At the medial margin of the zygomatic bone, level with the Liver and Gall Bladder points
	Large Intestine	At the inferior margin of the zygomatic bone, directly below the outer canthus of the eye
	Shoulder	At the superior margin of the zygomatic arch, directly below the outer canthus, midway between the outer canthus and Large Intestine point
	Arm	On superior margin of zygomatic arch, at posterior, superior margin of zygomatic bone, posterior to the Shoulder point
	Hand	On inferior margin of zygomatic arch, at posterior, inferior border of zygomatic bone, directly below the Arm point

Area	Point	Location
Cheek	Kidney	Level with the ala nasi, directly below M-HN-9 *(Taiyang)*
	Umbilicus	About 0.7 unit directly below the Kidney point, approximately level with Gv-26 *(Renzhong)*
	Back (same as SI-19 *(Tinggong)*)	In front of the tragus of the ear, between the anterior aspect of tragus and the temporomandibular joint
	Thigh	1/3 the distance from the ear lobe to the angle of the mandible
	Knee	1/3 the distance from the angle of the mandible to the ear lobe
	Patella (same as S-6 *(Jiache)*)	In depression above angle of mandible
	Lower Leg	On superior margin of mandible, anterior to the angle of mandible
	Foot	On superior margin of mandible, directly below the outer canthus and anterior to the Lower Leg

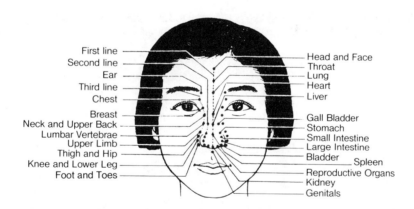

Dia. 3-56   Nose Acupuncture Points

Table 3-7   NOSE ACUPUNCTURE POINTS

Line	Point	Location
1st Line: From mid-line of forehead, down bridge of nose to philtrum (9 points)	Head and Face	In the middle of forehead, 1/3 the distance from the natural hairline to a point between eyebrows

495

Line	Point	Location
1st line, cont.	Throat	On midline of forehead, 2/3 the distance from the natural hairline to a point between eyebrows
	Lung (same as M-HN-3 *(Yintang)*)	Between eyebrows
	Heart (same as M-HN-4 *(Shangen)*)	On bridge of nose, at midpoint between inner canthi of eyes
	Liver	Just below highest point on nasal bone, midway between the Heart and Spleen points
	Spleen	Just above the knob on the tip of the nose
	Kidney (same as Gv-25 *(Suliao)*)	On the tip of the nose
	Genitals	Just below the nasal septum, above Gv-26 *(Renzhong)*
	Reproductive Organs	On either side of Kidney point at the tip of nose
2nd Line: From medial angle of orbit, along the sides of bridge of nose to bottom of ala nasi (5 points)	Gall Bladder	Lateral to Liver point, directly below medial angle of orbit
	Stomach	Lateral to Spleen point, directly below Gall Bladder point
	Small Intestine	At the upper third of ala nasi, directly below the Stomach point
	Large Intestine	In the middle of ala nasi, directly below Small Intestine point
	Bladder	Directly below Large Intestine point, on the inferior wall of ala nasi
3rd Line: From medial tip of eyebrow, along ala nasi lateral to the 2nd line (9 points)	Ear (Same as B-2 *(Zanzhu)*)	At medial end of eyebrow
	Chest	Below Ear point, on the margin of the orbit

Line	Point	Location
3rd line, cont.	Breast	Above B-1 *(Jingming)*, near the inner canthus of eye
	Neck and Upper Back	Below B-1 *(Jingming)*, near the inner canthus of eye
	Lumbar Vertebrae	Lateral to Gall Bladder point, lateral and inferior to Neck point
	Upper Limb	Lateral to Stomach point, lateral and inferior to Lumbar Vertebrae point
	Thigh and Hip	Lateral to and level with the superior margin of the ala nasi
	Knee and Lower Leg	Lateral to middle of ala nasi, below Thigh and Hip point
	Foot and Toes	Lateral to and level with the inferior part of ala nasi, below Knee and Lower Leg point

HEAD ACUPUNCTURE

The importance of the head has been recognized since earliest times. In chapter 70 of *Simple Questions* is written, "The head is the seat of the Essential Brightness." The famous Ming dynasty physician Zhang Jiebin wrote, "All the Essential Qi of the Yin and Yang Organs rises to the head."

Recently, combining traditional acupuncture techniques with modern knowledge about the representative areas of the cerebral cortex gave rise to head acupuncture. Much of the pioneering work in this field was conducted during the Cultural Revolution at the Jishan County Peoples' Hospital of Shanxi province where excellent results were obtained in treating certain diseases of the central nervous system. The following presentation is based upon their work.

Location of areas for needling

See Table 3-8 and Diagram 3-57 below for location of head acupuncture areas and indications for their use. For purposes of head acupuncture, the midline of the head is defined as a line from the glabella to the occipital protuberance. The other major line runs between the upper border of the midline of each eyebrow to the occipital protuberance. The intersection of this second line with the hairline is the end of the Motor area. If the hairline is not present in the area, the point is directly above the midline of the zygomatic arch. In head acupuncture measurements are based upon the metric system.

Principles of site selection

For diseases affecting only one limb, a site is selected on the contralateral side of the head. Diseases affecting the limbs bilaterally are treated by stimulating sites on both sides of the head. Diseases of the internal organs or those which are systemic in nature (e.g., hypertension, arteriosclerosis accompanied by numbness in the limbs, urticaria, etc.), or those illnesses which are difficult to distinguish as being on one side or the other (e.g., vertigo, incomplete maturation of the brain) are treated by stimulating sites on both sides of the head.

Generally, a principal site is selected which corresponds directly to the representative area on the cerebral cortex for a certain disease, and a supplementary site may be added which is less directly related. For instance, when treating paralysis of the lower limb, the principal site is the Lower limb and trunk area in the Motor area; a supplementary site would be the Leg motor and sensory area.

Method

1) The area to be stimulated must be carefully delineated, the scalp exposed and the area cleaned with alcohol.

2) #26-28 gauge filiform needles between 2.5-3 inches in length are recommended. The needle is inserted almost horizontally to the scalp (not touching the bone) and slowly rotated until the requisite portion of the needle has been inserted. Once in place, the needle should *not* be further raised or thrust. Instead, it should be rapidly twirled (200 times per minute is ideal) with a wide amplitude (2-3 rotations forward, 2-3 rotations backward) until the characteristic needle sensation (Qi) is obtained. Twirling may then be continued for 3-4 minutes after which the needle is left in place for 5-10 minutes, then twirled again. After repeating this procedure 2-3 times, the needle is withdrawn. A cotton ball may be pressed against the puncture to prevent bleeding.

3) The most common response to needling is a hot sensation, usually on the limbs opposite the needling site. Less frequently, this sensation will be perceived over the entire body, or only at a single joint or muscle. Other responses include numbness and a tightening sensation (a minority of cases report cold and pain, however these sensations usually disappear as needling continues). Generally, if these responses accompany the needling, the result will be good, although in some cases treatment is effective despite their absence.

Other considerations

• Precisely locating the stimulation areas on the scalp bears directly on the result.

• Needle stimulation must generally be strong and the response somewhat intense to obtain a satisfactory result.

• It is best to have the patient lie down for treatment to prevent fainting.

Table 3-8
HEAD ACUPUNCTURE POINTS

Name	Location	Indications
Motor Area	A line starting from a point 0.5 cm. posterior to midpoint of midline and stretching diagonally across the head to a point at the intersection of the zygomatic arch (superior margin) with the hairline at the temple.	
Lower limb and trunk area	Upper fifth of Motor area line.	Paralysis of lower limb (opposite side)
Upper limb area	Second and third fifths of Motor area line.	Paralysis of upper limb (opposite side)
Facial area (includes Speech #1)	Lower two fifths of Motor area line.	Upper motor neuron paralysis of face (opposite side), motor aphasia, dribbling saliva, impaired speech

498

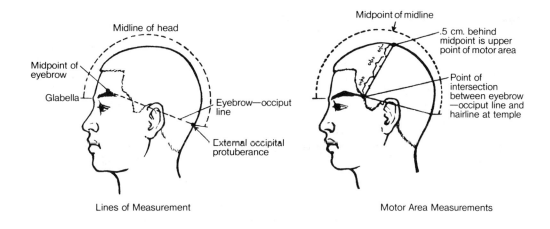

Lines of Measurement

Motor Area Measurements

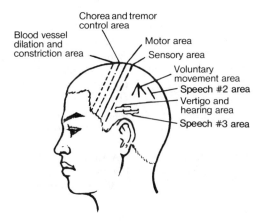

Stimulation Areas—Side View

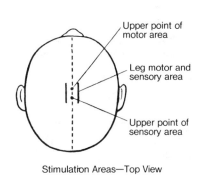

Stimulation Areas—Top View

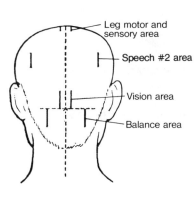

Stimulation Areas—Back View

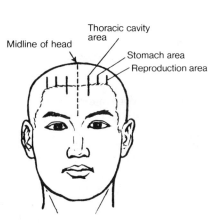

Stimulation Areas—Front View

Dia. 3-57   Head Acupuncture Areas

Name	Location	Indications
Sensory Area	A line parallel and 1.5 cm. posterior to the Motor line.	
Lower limb, head and trunk area	Upper fifth of Sensory area line.	Low back pain (opposite side), numbness or paresthesia in that area, occipital headache, stiff neck, vertigo
Upper limb area	Second and third fifths of Sensory area line.	Pain,numbness or other paresthesia of upper limb (opposite side)
Facial area	Lower two fifths of Sensory area line.	Migraine headache, trigeminal neuralgia, toothache (opposite side),arthritis of the temporomandibular joint
Leg motor and sensory area	Parallel with midline of head, 1 cm. beside midpoint (bilaterally), about 3 cm. long.	Paralysis, pain, or numbness of lower limb, acute lower back sprain, nocturnal urination, prolapsed uterus
Chorea and tremor control area	Parallel with and 1.5 cm. anterior to Motor area line.	Syndenham's chorea, tremors, palsy and related syndromes
Blood vessel dilations and constriction area	Parallel with and 1.5 cm. to Chorea and tremor control area.	Superficial edema, hypertension
Vertigo and hearing area	Horizontal line 1.5 cm. above and centered on the apex of ear, 4 cm. in length.	Tinnitus, vertigo, diminished hearing, Menier's syndrome
Speech #2	Vertical line 2 cm. beside tuber parietale on back of head, 3 cm. in length.	Nominal aphasia
Speech #3	Overlaps Vertigo and hearing area at midpoint and continues 3 cm. posteriorly.	Receptive aphasia
Voluntary movement area	With the tuber parietale origin, three needles can be inserted inferiorly, anteriorly and posteriorly to a length of 3 cm. Between them, the 3 lines will form a 40° angle.	Apraxia
Vision area	One cm. lateral to external occipital protuberance, parallel to midline of head, 4 cm. in length extending upward.	Cortical blindness

500

Name	Location	Indications
Balance area	Three cm. lateral to the external occipital protuberance, parallel to midline of head, 4 cm. in length, extending downward.	Loss of balance due to cerebellar disorders
Stomach area	Beginning at the hairline directly above pupil of eye, parallel with midline of head, 2 cm. in length extending posteriorally.	Discomfort in upper abdomen
Liver and gall bladder area	A line 2 cm. in length extending anteriorally from the Stomach area.	Pain in upper right quadrant of the abdomen and/or right rib cage; chronic hepatitis
Thoracic cavity area	Midway between and parallel with Stomach area and midline of head, bilaterally, 2 cm. in length.	Asthma, chest pain, intermittent supra-ventricular tachycardia
Reproduction area	Parallel and lateral to the Stomach area at a distance equal to that between Stomach area and the Thoracic cavity area, 2 cm. in length	Abnormal uterine bleeding, combined with Leg motor area for prolapsed uterus

HAND AND FOOT ACUPUNCTURE

The concentration of the channels in the hands and feet reflects the importance of these areas in acupuncture therapy. According to traditional theory, the relationship of the hand and foot to diseases of the trunk and head is that of Root or Origin to the Branch or End (see Section I, chapter 4). The Qi which circulates through the channels of the body is said to arise in the hands and feet. Thus, stimulation of points on the hands and feet affects, through the channels, diseases in distant parts of the body.

Location of hand and foot points

See Tables 3-9 and 3-10 and Diagrams 3-58 and 3-59.

Selection of points

Hand points
As far back as the *Inner Classic* it was suggested that certain diseases could be treated by stimulating points on the side of the body opposite that of the disease. (See *Simple Questions,* chapter 63) This principle is generally applied to hand acupuncture. A disease affecting the left side of the body is treated by inserting needles in the right hand, and vice versa.

Hand acupuncture points are named according to either a part of the body which they affect, e.g., the Sciatic Nerve point is named for its effect upon the sciatic nerve, or according to a disease for which they are indicated, e.g., the Malaria point for malaria. Points should be selected on the same

501

basis. A point selected for the primary condition or symptom can be matched with a point indicated for a secondary symptom.

Foot points

Foot points are usually selected in pairs, by matching points with similar or related indications. For example, #1 and #2 are both indicated for neurasthenia and are therefore a natural pair in the treatment of that condition. Another pair might include one of these points and a second indicated for a symptom associated with neurasthenia, e.g., headache (point #46 or #47). One to three pair of points is the norm.

Method

1) A #28-30 gauge needle, 1-2 inches in length is recommended. After cleaning the site with alcohol, the needle is usually inserted to a depth of 0.3-0.5 inch. Moderate to strong stimulation is applied. The needle is ordinarily retained for only 3-5 minutes.

2) When needling the Lumbar and Leg point on the hand, the needle should be inserted at a 15°-30° angle to the surface of the skin, between the tendon of the extensor digitorum and the metacarpal bone, to a depth of 0.5-0.8 inch.

3) When treating lower back sprain or sprain of the soft tissues at other joints, needling should be accompanied by massage or exercise of the affected part.

4) When treating painful diseases, after the pain has stopped, manipulation of the needle should continue for 2-3 minutes. If necessary, the needle can be retained for longer periods, or an intradermal needle embedded in the skin.

5) Electro-acupuncture may also be used in cases where extended periods of stimulation are required.

Other considerations

• The stimulation from hand and foot acupuncture is usually quite intense, causing the patient some pain. This should be explained to the patient in advance, and precautions taken to prevent fainting.

• When inserting a needle along the surface of a bone, the physician must be careful to avoid damaging the periosteum.

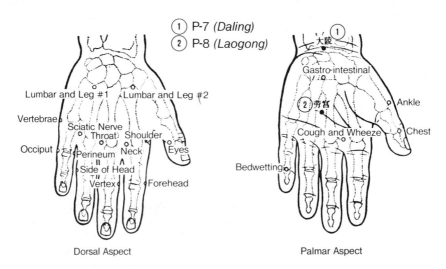

Dia. 3-58 Selected Hand Acupuncture Points

502

Table 3-9   HAND ACUPUNCTURE POINTS

Name	Location	Indications
Raise Pressure	At mid-point of transverse crease on dorsum of wrist	Low blood pressure
Lumbar and Leg	1.5 units anterior to transverse crease on dorsum of wrist, at radial side of the tendon of the 2nd extensor digitorum manus (1st point), and the ulnar side of 4th (2nd point)	Pain of lower back and leg, lower back sprain
Ankle	At the border of the light and dark skin on radial side of thumb at the metacarpophalangeal joint	Pain of ankle joint
Chest	At the border of the light and dark skin on radial side of thumb at the interphalangeal joint	Chest pain, vomiting and diarrhea, seizures
Eye	At the border of the light and dark skin on ulnar side of thumb at the interphalangeal joint	Eye pain, eye diseases
Shoulder	At the border of the light and dark skin on radial side of index finger at the metacarpophalangeal joint	Shoulder pain
Forehead	At the border of the light and dark skin on the radial side of index finger and the first interphalangeal joint	Frontal headache, stomach spasms, acute gastroenteritis, acute, uncomplicated appendicitis, pain of knee joint
Vertex	At the border of the light and dark flesh on medial side of middle finger at the first interphalangeal joint	Nervous headache, headache at vertex
Side of Head	At the border of the light and dark flesh on ulnar side of fourth finger at the first interphalangeal joint	Migraine headache, pain of chest and ribs, pain in region of spleen and liver, colic of the gall bladder
Hiccough	At the mid-point of transverse crease on dorsum of middle finger at the second interphalangeal joint	Hiccoughs
Reduce Fever	In the web at radial side of middle finger on dorsum of hand	Fever, impaired vision
Perineum	At the border of the light and dark skin on radial side of small finger at the first interphalangeal joint	Pain in perineal region
Occiput	At the border of the light and dark skin on ulnar side of little finger at the first interphalangeal joint	Occipital headache, acute tonsillitis, arm pain, jaw pain, hiccoughs
Vertebrae	At the border of the light and dark skin on ulnar side of little finger at metacarpophalangeal joint	Acute sprain of inter-spinous ligaments,

503

Name	Location	Indications
Vertebrae (cont.)		'slipped' disc, post-operative low back pain, coccygeal pain, tinnitus, occluded nose
Sciatic Nerve	At the ulnar margin of 4th metacarpophalangeal joint on dorsum of hand	Sciatica, pain of hip joint and buttocks
Throat	At the ulnar margin of 3rd metacarpophalangeal joint on dorsum of hand	Acute tonsillitis, pharyngitis, trigeminal neuralgia, toothache
Neck	At the ulnar margin of 2nd metacarpophalangeal joint on dorsum of hand	Stiff or sprained neck
Diarrhea	1 unit proximal to the mid-point of a line between the 3rd and 4th metacarpophalangeal joints on the dorsum of hand	Diarrhea
Palm of Hand		
Malaria	At the articulation of the 1st metacarpal bone with the wrist (trapezium), on the radial margin of the thenar eminence	Malaria
Tonsil (same as L-10 *(Yuji)*)	At the mid-point on ulnar side of 1st metacarpal bone on the palm	Tonsillitis, pharyngitis
Cough and Wheeze	On the ulnar side of index finger at metacarpophalangeal joint on the palm	Bronchitis, bronchial asthma, tension headache
Infantile Indigestion	At the middle of transverse crease on the 1st interphalangeal joint of the middle finger, palmar surface	Infantile indigestion
Revive	At the tip of middle finger, about 0.2 unit from fingernail	Revive from coma
Toothache	Between the 3rd and 4th metacarpal bones, about 1 unit proximal to transverse crease of metacarpophalangeal joint, palmar surface	Toothache
Bedwetting	At the mid-point of transverse crease on the 2nd interphalangeal joint of the little finger, palmar surface	Bedwetting, frequent urination
Stop Convulsions	At the mid-point of the intersection of the thenar and the hypothenar, palmar surface	Convulsions due to high fever
Gastro-intestinal	Midway between P-8 *(Laogong)* and P-7 *(Daling)*, on the palm	Chronic gastritis, ulcers, indigestion, round worm in bile duct

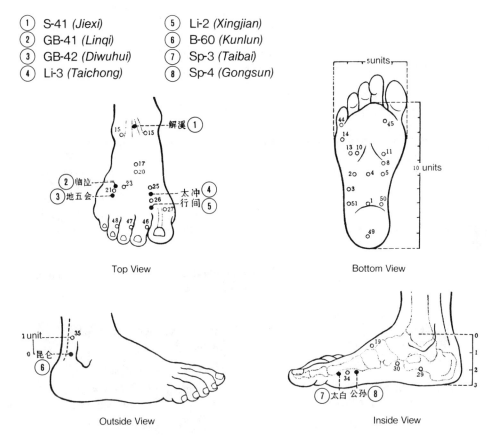

① S-41 *(Jiexi)*   ⑤ Li-2 *(Xingjian)*
② GB-41 *(Linqi)*   ⑥ B-60 *(Kunlun)*
③ GB-42 *(Diwuhui)*   ⑦ Sp-3 *(Taibai)*
④ Li-3 *(Taichong)*   ⑧ Sp-4 *(Gongsun)*

Top View

Bottom View

Outside View

Inside View

Dia. 3-59 Selected Foot Acupuncture Points

Table 3-10   FOOT ACUPUNCTURE POINTS

Point	Location	Needling Method	Indications
1	Bottom of foot at mid-point between medial and lateral malleoli	Straight insertion or slanted distally, 0.5-1 unit	Neurasthenia, hysteria, insomnia, low blood pressure
2	Bottom of foot, 5 units distal from heel, 1 unit lateral to midline	Straight insertion or slanted medially, 0.5-1 unit	Insomnia, hysteria, neurasthenia
3	Bottom of foot, 4 units distal from heel, 1.5 units lateral to midline	Straight insertion or slanted distally, 1-1.5 units	Sciatica, pain of lower back and leg
4	Bottom of foot, 5 units distal from heel on midline	Straight or slanted insertion, 0.5-1 unit	Insomnia, hepatitis with jaundice, asthma, incomplete maturation of brain

505

Point	Location	Needling Method	Indications
5	Bottom of foot, 5 units distal from heel, 1 unit medial to midline	Straight insertion or slanted distally, 1-1.5 units	Dysentery, diarrhea
8	1 unit distal to #5	Same as #5 above	Same as #5 above
10	3 units proximal to mid-point of line, between 3rd and 4th toes, plantar surface	Straight insertion or slanted medially, 1.5 units	Abdominal pain, acute, chronic GI inflammation, painful menstruation
11	3 units proximal to mid-point of line between 1st and 2nd toes, plantar surface	Straight insertion, 1 unit	Acute, chronic GI inflammation, stomach spasms
13	3 units proximal to head of 4th metatarsal bone, plantar surface	Straight insertion or slanted distally, 0.5-1 unit	Sciatica, urticaria, shoulder pain
14	1 unit proximal to head of 5th metatarsal bone, plantar surface	Straight insertion or slanted distally, 0.5-1 unit	Toothache
15	0.5 unit inferior to S-41 *(Jiexi)*, in depression on either side	Join points or slanted insertion inferiorly or superiorly, 0.5-1 unit	Low back pain, spasm of gastrocnemius muscle
17	2.5 units inferior to S-41 *(Jiexi)*	Straight insertion, 0.1-0.5 unit, or prick point	Angina pectoris, asthma, common cold
19	In depression above the tubercle of the navicular on medial aspect of foot	Straight insertion, 0.5 unit	Hypertension, parotitis, acute tonsillitis
20	3 units proximal to mid-point of line between the 2nd and 3rd metatarsal bones on dorsum of foot	Straight insertion or slanted superiorly, 2 units	Acute, chronic GI inflammation, gastric, duodenal ulcer
21	At mid-point between GB-41 *(Zulingqi)* and GB-42 *(Diwuhui)* on dorsum of foot	Straight insertion or slanted, 0.5-1 unit	Sciatica, parotitis, tonsillitis
23	2 units proximal to mid-point of line between 3rd and 4th metatarsal bones on dorsum of foot	Straight insertion or slanted, 1.5 units	Stiff neck
25	In the depression medial and anterior to the base of the 1st metatarsal bone on dorsum of foot	Straight insertion or slanted, 1-2 units	Acute sprain of lower back

Point	Location	Needling Method	Indications
26	At mid-point between Li-2 (*Xingjian*) and Li-3 (*Taichong*) on dorsum of foot	Straight insertion or slanted proximally, 1-2 units	Acute tonsillitis, parotitis
27	On medial aspect of extensor hallucis longus tendon at metatarsophalangeal joint on dorsum of foot	Prick or shallow insertion, 0.1-0.5 unit	Same as #26. Also eczema, urticaria
29	2 units directly below middle of medial malleolus	Straight insertion or transverse, 1-2 units	Functional uterine bleeding
30	In depression posterior and inferior to the tubercle of navicular on medial aspect of foot	Straight insertion, 1 unit	Painful menstruation, abnormal uterine bleeding, pelvic inflammatory disease
34	Mid-point between Sp-3 (*Taibai*) and Sp-4 (*Gongsun*)	Transverse insertion, 1-2 units	Hysteria, seizures, neurasthenia
35	1 unit directly above B-60 (*Kunlun*) on lateral aspect of ankle		Sciatica, headache, abdominal pain
44	Mid-point of transverse crease of each metatarsophalangeal joint, plantar surface	Straight insertion or slanted proximally, 0.5 unit	Incontinence, frequent urination
45	1 unit posterior to mid-point of line between base of big toe and 2nd phalanx, plantar surface	Straight insertion, 0.5-1 unit	Toothache
46	At border of light and dark skin on medial aspect of 2nd interphalangeal joint of 2nd toe	Prick 0.1-0.3 unit	Headache
47	At border of light and dark skin on medial aspect of 2nd interphalangeal joint of 3rd toe	Prick 0.1-0.3 unit	Headache
48	At border of light and dark skin on medial aspect of 2nd interphalangeal joint of 4th toe	Prick 0.1-0.3 unit	Headache
49	1 unit above mid-point at base of heel, posterior aspect	Straight insertion, 0.5 unit	Common cold, headache, sinusitis, rhinitis
50	1 unit medial to #1, on plantar surface	Straight insertion, 0.5 unit	Trigeminal neuralgia
51	1 unit directly posterior to #3, on plantar surface	Straight insertion, 0.5 unit	Intercostal neuralgia, chest pain, fullness in chest

Chapter 9

Description and Analysis of Ancient Acupuncture Techniques

The needling methods devised in ancient times were based on the long and varied experience of practitioners of acupuncture in China. These methods are described in the *Yellow Emperor's Inner Classic* and later works. They have provided a foundation for the continuing development of acupuncture therapy in the modern epoch. However, due to historical limitations, certain idealistic and metaphysical elements are reflected in the ancient techniques which must be critically analyzed if they are to serve the purpose of improving the practice of acupuncture.

STANDARDS OF NEEDLING

The standards governing acupuncture practice refer generally to how and when needling can be used and when it is prohibited. That acupuncture is to be used only under certain conditions was stated as early as the 2nd century B.C. in the *Spiritual Axis*. The clinical application of acupuncture depends on such factors as the status of the disease and the constitution of the patient. Some of the more important standards and prohibitions found in the *Inner Classic* with respect to the use of acupuncture are discussed below.

Depth of needle insertion and amount of stimulation

In the first chapter of *Spiritual Axis* it is written: "If you needle and the Qi is not obtained, do not ask the number [of insertions]. If you needle and the Qi is obtained, then remove the needle and do not needle again." This passage reflects the belief that 'obtaining Qi' is the goal of needling, to which the rules governing the depth and duration of needle insertion are subordinate. The methods outlined below must therefore be used flexibly. The importance of the needing site, the location and nature of the disease, and the physiological characteristics of the patient must all be considered.

Points are situated in shallow and fleshy (deep) tissue. Chapter 40 of *Spiritual Axis* sets out the general rule: "Into that which is Yin, insert deeply and retain the needle. Into that which is Yang, insert superficially and quickly remove the needle." Yin and Yang refer here to parts of the body. The abdomen, flanks and medial aspect of the limbs correspond to Yin (fleshy tissue), while the head, chest, back, and lateral aspect of the limbs are Yang (shallow tissue). Generally, these guidelines are followed in practice, although one should not be inflexible with regard to the distinction between the medial and lateral aspect of the limbs.

Concerning the location of a disease, chapter 50 of *Simple Questions* provides: "The location of a disease is either superficial or deep; needle insertions are [likewise] superficial or deep. Each [insertion should] reach to its proper [depth] without exceeding its proper path . . . . If the depth of insertion is

508

wrong, great harm will result." Similarly, a passage in chapter 62 of *Simple Questions* instructs that diseases in the Blood vessels should be treated by letting blood, those of the Blood and Qi by superficial needle insertions, and those of the flesh by deep insertions. Pain is regarded as a deep (Yin) symptom and requires a deep insertion of the needle, while itching is considered to be a shallow (Yang) symptom for which a superficial insertion is indicated. This standard does not apply to diseases of the internal organs, about which more is said below.

The general physical characteristics of a patient and the nature of the disease being treated have a direct bearing on the depth of needling and the length of time a needle is retained. The following guidelines have been drawn from chapters 4, 5, 9, 10 and 38 of *Spiritual Axis:* The needle should be inserted deeply and retained for a relatively long time, and the number of needles as well as the frequency of treatment should be greater when treating patients who are heavy, big or of robust health, or for whom the needling sensation is not strong. On the other hand, children or patients who are thin, weak and very sensitive to needle stimulation should be needled superficially, quickly, less frequently and with fewer needles. Furthermore, Cold or Excessive conditions require strong needling, whereas mild needle stimulation is indicated for Deficient or Hot conditions.

These directions retain a certain degree of usefulness in the modern clinic.

Prohibitions in the use of acupuncture and moxibustion

The ancients proscribed needling in areas near the important organs or large blood vessels. Such prohibitions abound in both *Simple Questions* and *Spiritual Axis.* For example, from chapter 16 of *Simple Questions:* "When needling the chest or abdomen it is imperative to avoid the Five Organs." Elsewhere, there are injunctions against injuring the joints, eyes, and ears by improper needling technique.

Of course, we must realize that many of the prohibitions regarding acupuncture in ancient texts are related to such factors as the use of needles much thicker than those available today, as well as a very limited knowledge of anatomy, and the absence of sterilization techniques. Because modern clinical conditions far surpass those of previous ages, we should not, except for certain points, feel overly constrained by these ancient prohibitions.

Nevertheless, under certain conditions acupuncture is not to be used. In chapter 52 of *Simple Questions* is written: "Don't needle those who are very drunk as this leads to disordered Qi. Don't needle those who are very angry as this leads to rebellious Qi. Don't needle those exhausted by work; don't needle those who have just eaten; don't needle those who are very hungry; don't needle those who are very thirsty; don't needle those who are very upset." This chapter also instructs that before needling begins, the physician should ask the patients who were transported to the clinic to wait for the period of time it takes to eat a meal, and for those who came on foot to rest for the time it takes to walk three miles. Precautions such as these are exceedingly important in preventing fainting and other abnormal reactions to acupuncture therapy.

For certain particularly severe diseases, or those in which the pulse did not correspond with the symptoms, the ancients thought it improper to perform acupuncture or use strong stimulation. The following illustrations are taken from chapter 61 of *Spiritual Axis* (entitled "Five Prohibitions"). There are Five Removals [of substances from the body]—emaciation, severe hemorrhage, excessive sweating, severe diarrhea and childbirth—where the Normal Qi is injured and during which a strong needling method should not be used. There are Five Rebellions, serious conditions in which the pulse is opposite that which would ordinarily accompany the other symptoms. The ancients regarded these as inappropriate for acupuncture treatment:

1) Febrile disease accompanied by a calm pulse, or where perspiration has broken out but the pulse is very hasty. The first shows that the Excess is growing and the Normal diminishing, while the second is a sign that the body's fluids have been depleted.

2) Diarrhea with a huge pulse. The Yin has drained downward and the Yang has ascended. This signifies a separation of Yin and Yang and is very serious.

509

3) Dampness obstructing Qi (pain in joints), with muscular atrophy and fever accompanied by an extremely fine pulse. A tiny pulse with these symptoms reflects depleted Qi.

4) Emaciation due to excessive sexual intercourse, with fever and pallid complexion followed by blood in the stool. These symptoms indicate severe deficiency of Blood, Qi and Essence which represents a perilous condition.

5) Alternating fever and chills with a tight pulse. This condition shows that the Excess is very strong while the Normal Qi is weak.

Elsewhere in the *Inner Classic* other critical conditions are described wherein the body is so weak that acupuncture is counterindicated. Later generations of acupuncturists often extended these restrictions until they became wary of treating almost any serious condition. It is again important to remember, however, that in modern clinical practice we must not be overly constrained by such proscriptions. Especially since the development of combined Chinese-Western medical techniques, many effective treatments have been devised for diseases previously regarded as 'extremely grave' or 'incurable'. For example, rheumatic heart disease, shock and delirium are now considered amenable to acupuncture therapy.

CLASSIFICATION OF NEEDLING METHODS IN THE *INNER CLASSIC*

Descriptions of different needling methods abound in the *Inner Classic*. For example, in chapter 7 of *Spiritual Axis* various classifications of needling methods are set forth including the five, nine, and twelve needling methods. Essentially, these methods provide a rationale for combining points in a prescription, the depth of insertion, the direction of needling and the number of needles used. Additionally, the techniques of letting blood, expelling pus and hot needle acupuncture are described. All of these modalities arose from the ancients' recognition of the diverse location and nature of disease. Most of these methods are suitable for clinical use and have in recent times undergone further development.

Methods of matching or combining points

Needling the Transport points (one of the nine needling methods)
  The Transport points of the Inner (Yin) Organs located below the knee and elbow, particularly the Gushing and Transporting points in this group (see Section II, chapter 1), are needled in conjunction with the Associated points of the affected Organs. This method is described, among other places, in chapter 6 of *Spiritual Axis* and chapter 39 of *Simple Questions*. In modern clinical practice, this method typifies the way that points are selected for treating diseases of the Inner (Yin) Organs. For example, in the treatment of Lung diseases, L-9 *(Taiyuan)*, the Transporting point of the Lung channel, and B-13 *(Feishu)*, the Lung Associated point, are used together. For Kidney diseases, K-3 *(Taixi)*, the Kidney Transporting point, and B-23 *(Shenshu)*, the Associated point of the Kidney, are combined.

Needling distant points (one of the nine needling methods)
  Originally, this designation referred to needling points on the lower limbs, specifically the Lower Uniting points [see Section II, chapter 1], to treat diseases of the trunk or head which were related with the Outer (Yang) Organs. It is also described in chapter 4 of *Spiritual Axis* and chapter 39 of *Simple Questions*. This method is commonly used today. For example, to treat diseases of the Stomach, needle S-36 *(Zusanli)*, the Lower Uniting point of the Stomach; GB-34 *(Yanglingquan)* is used in its capacity as the Lower Uniting point of the Gall Bladder for diseases affecting that Organ; diseases of the Small and Large Intestine can be treated via their Lower Uniting points, S-39 *(Xiajuxu)* and S-37 *(Shangjuxu)* respectively. Since the Jin and Yuan dynasties (c. 12th and 13th centuries), the

510

treatment of any disorder of the trunk or head by means of points below the elbow or knee has been referred to as an application of the distant point method. For example, needling Li-3 *(Taichong)* for headache at the vertex, or S-44 *(Neiting)* for toothache can be called using the distant point method even though neither of these points is a Lower Uniting point.

Needling coupled points (one of the twelve needling methods)

This method involves palpation of the chest and back to locate points of tenderness on both sides which are then needled, care being taken to avoid the internal organs. Originally, this method was used to treat severe congestion of Qi in the Heart (analagous to angina pectoris). It is also known as the Yin/Yang needling method. Since its early conception, it has evolved into the Alarm point—Associated point combination method and has proven to be effective in the treatment of a wide range of diseases.

Great needle method (one of the nine needling methods)

Select points on one side (right or left) of the body to treat a disease on the other. Two such methods are described in the *Inner Classic*. One, the great needle method, is used when the Excess is in the Primary channels, and although there is only pain on one side, there is a disturbance in the pulse on both sides. In this case, channel points on the side opposite the pain are needled. The other method is called the precautionary needling method. It is used when the Excess is in the Connecting channels and there is pain, but the pulse is normal. Under these conditions, the Well points on the extremities where the channels connect, and areas where hematomas are visible along the paths of the Connecting channels are needled.

Utilizing different needling methods for diseases in different tissues

Cutaneous needling: local, superficial insertion

1) Hairline insertion method (one of the nine needling methods). Very slight insertions are made in only the most superficial layers of the skin. This method is indicated for treating numbness of the skin. In ancient times, the arrowhead needle was used to perform this technique, but more recently the cutaneous needle and 'rolling drum' have been used.

2) Half-insertion method (one of the five needling methods). The needle is rapidly inserted and withdrawn, somewhat deeper than the hairline method, but still not penetrating into deep muscle tissue.

Subcutaneous needling: local, superficial insertion

Direct method (one of the twelve needling methods). The needle is inserted superficially, at an angle almost parallel to the skin, by first using the fingers of one hand to pinch the skin so that it can be more easily needled. Originally used for treating pain caused by superficial attack of the Cold Excess, it is now used at any point for which a transverse insertion is required.

Muscle needling: local, relatively deep insertion

1) Shallow method (one of the twelve needling methods). The needle is inserted at an angle across the grain of the muscle. It is shallow only in relation to the other muscle needling methods. In the *Inner Classic*, this method is recommended for the treatment of constricted muscles and sensitivity to cold. Today, it is used to treat spasms of the superficial muscles.

2) Deep muscle insertion method (one of the nine needling methods). The needle is inserted straight into deep muscle tissue. This method is used for muscle soreness and pain.

3) 'Joining valleys' method (one of five needling methods). The needle is inserted at a slant in one direction, then partially withdrawn and inserted in another direction. This procedure may be repeated several times. The technique is utilized for pain, numbness and debility of the muscle. Its name is derived from what ancient physicians described as confluences of valleys in the muscle tissue. This

511

method is still widely used and may be combined with the shallow or deep-muscle insertion techniques described above.

Tendon needling: local, relatively deep, or deep insertion

1) Joint method (one of the five needling methods). Straight insertion of the needle near the tendon. Bleeding is to be avoided. This method is used for pain and numbness of the connective tissue.

2) Large method (one of the twelve needling methods). Needle is inserted from the side across the tendon. Indicated for spasms, pain, and/or debility of the joints. Often used in conjunction with the joint needling method. Great needle acupuncture is a modern development of this technique and is used to treat muscle spasm and contraction.

Bone needling: local, deep insertion

1) Reaching method (one of the five needling methods). The needle is inserted and withdrawn perpendicularly to the skin, with no lateral movement, until it 'reaches' the surface of the bone. This technique is used to treat pain in the bone accompanied by paralysis and/or a feeling of heaviness. The technique prevalent today of inserting a needle deep within the tissues surrounding a joint, such as through the shoulder from LI-15 *(Jianyu)* to H-1 *(Jiquan),* may be said to belong to this category of technique.

2) Hurried method (one of the twelve needling methods). Similar to the preceeding method except that the needle is agitated from side to side as well as up and down, creating a stronger needle sensation. In the *Inner Classic,* this method is prescribed for treating the same bone problems as the reaching method above, and may be considered supplementary to it. (The agitation must be performed carefully so as to prevent the needle from striking the bone too hard, chipping or bending the needle and injuring the bone.)

Primary channel needling: deep insertion along the channels

Channel method (one of the nine needling methods). Needles are inserted at points along the channels at which alterations such as hardening of the underlying tissues, hematoma, or local tenderness occur. This method has been of considerable interest recently and has been used as a method of diagnosis (palpation of the skin) and treatment.

Connecting channel needling: superficial insertion, letting blood

1) Connecting channel method (one of the nine needling methods). This is a method of needling a hematoma at the Minute Connecting channels on the body's surface. Presently, the use of any kind of needle (triangular, cutaneous, etc.) to let blood is said to belong to this method. Sometimes it is combined with cupping.

2) Assisting method (one of the twelve needling methods). At several points in the same area, the needle is inserted superficially and then rapidly withdrawn to induce bleeding. In the *Inner Classic,* this method is recommended for the treatment of abcesses, ulcers, boils, etc. The use of the triangular needle to treat erysipelas is an example of the contemporary application of this method.

3) Leopard-pattern method (one of the five needling methods). Insertions are made on all four sides of a hematoma along a channel and allowed to bleed. The method is named after the pattern so formed. This and the preceding technique may be considered supplementary to the Connecting channel needling method above.

Other specific needling methods

Multiple needle insertions

1) Aligned insertion method (one of the twelve needling methods). After the first needle is inserted, one needle is placed on each side thereof, forming a line. This technique is used for treating pain where the area affected is not large but deep. Today this method is regarded as effective when used at points of local tenderness.

2) Spread insertion method (one of the twelve needling methods). One needle is inserted in the center, perpendicularly, and four needles are slanted toward it by insertion from four sides. This method has been used for treating superficial pain over relatively large surfaces. Today, the method is used in the treatment of subcutaneous lumps and nodules. The plum blossom (cutaneous) needle, with its cluster of needle points, serves a similar purpose.

3) Bordering needle insertion method (one of the twelve needling methods). After a needle is inserted perpendicularly, another is placed beside it at a slant so as to increase local stimulation. Recommended in the *Spiritual Axis* for treatment of stubborn pain, this method is very similar to the aligned insertion method above. The modern practice of inserting needles along a muscle or on both sides of a blood vessel is derived from this ancient technique.

Intermittent needling (one of the twelve needling methods)

In the *Spiritual Axis,* this method is suggested for the treatment of pain which is not fixed in one place but moves around. When the pain migrates up and down, the needle is inserted at one point and the areas above and below are massaged. The needle is then removed and the procedure repeated elsewhere along the path of pain. The contemporary method is similar to the traditional technique, the major difference being that the first needle is not removed before successive ones are inserted.

Hot needle method (one of the twelve needling methods)

A needle is heated until very hot, then inserted as quickly as possible into the body. This method is used for rheumatic type conditions caused by Cold (painful and/or swollen joints, feeling of heaviness, sometimes accompanied by soreness in the muscles) and is counter-indicated for those caused by Heat (skin in the affected area is hot, patient is feverish, or the muscles are flaccid). In contemporary practice, this method is still used to treat such conditions as scrofula and breast abcess.

Lancing

Great draining method (one of the twelve needling methods)

The *pi* or sword needle was traditionally used to lance an abscess or boil for the purpose of draining pus and Blood. It is no longer performed as this type of operation is now left to surgeons.

Yin insertion method (one of the twelve needling methods)

Here, the same point is needled on both sides of the body. In the *Spiritual Axis,* certain points were specified on the Yin channels to be punctured so as to treat Cold (Yin) disorders. An example is the use of K-3 *(Taixi)* to treat a condition of cold hands and feet accompanied by a faint pulse. Presently, the method is used in conjunction with the techniques of retaining the needle and intermittent manipulation so as to strengthen the sedating and analgesic functions of acupuncture.

Passage method (one of the twelve needling methods)

The needle is inserted deeply and then withdrawn slowly so as to drain the Heat Excess. This technique provides a 'passage' for the drainage of Heat from the body. It is similar in function to the strong stimulation methods used today.

Three distinct 'passage' methods are described in chapter 7 of *Spiritual Axis.* The first, one of the nine needling methods, is utilized in the treatment of diseases of the five Yang Organs. One or more of the Transport points (typically the Gushing and Transporting points) on the affected channel below the elbow or knee is selected for treatment.

The second 'passage' method, one of the twelve needling methods, is used in the treatment of febrile diseases. The needle is inserted perpendicularly to a deep position, then slowly withdrawn.

The third 'passage' method, one of the five needling methods, was applied in the treatment of bone blockage. The needle is inserted perpendicularly until it touches the underlying bone.

NEEDLING METHODS IN THE *CLASSIC OF DIFFICULTIES* AND LATER WORKS

In addition to those methods in the *Inner Classic* introduced above, there are many other needling techniques developed by later practitioners of acupuncture. Beginning with the *Classic of Difficulties* (c.3rd century) and continuing through the Tang, Song, Yuan and Ming periods (i.e., through the 17th century), a variety of both new and combined techniques and theories was developed. As might be expected, owing to differences in experience, learning and outlook among the formulators of the new methods, only some of the ideas are clinically useful while others, divorced from reality, are not.

Here, we introduce needling methods found in representative works of these periods.

Needling methods in the *Classic of Difficulties*

The *Classic of Difficulties* was probably written during the later Han Dynasty and has been attributed to the earlier, semi-legendary doctor, Bian Que. This book is primarily an amplification of some of the problems initially posed in the *Inner Classic*.

Chapters 69-81 of the *Classic of Difficulties* are concerned exclusively with needling methods. Chapter 78 emphasizes the importance of using both hands in the needling process: "One who is knowledgeable about acupuncture relies on the left; one who is not knowledgeable about acupuncture relies on the right. When needling, it is first necessary to use the left hand to press the area of the point, pinch and grab [the skin], press it down . . . and needle it." This passage expands upon the instructions in chapter 3 of the *Spiritual Axis* regarding the use of the hands, and has been stressed as an important aspect of needling technique by practitioners of the Jin and Yuan periods.

Chapter 70 of the *Classic of Difficulties* amplifies the teaching in the *Inner Classic* that there is a relationship between the seasons and Qi and Blood: "In spring and summer, the Yang Qi [in nature] is above. The Qi in man is also above and should therefore be sought superficially [when needling]. In autumn and winter, the Yang Qi is below. The Qi in man is also below and should therefore be sought deeply." That is to say, because the movement of Qi and Blood is related to the heat or cold of the seasons, the depth of needle insertion should vary accordingly. However, Hua Shouyi, a physician of the 13th century, wrote that practitioners should not be bound by this concept, indicating that it is not a reliable clinical standard.

Needling methods in *Ode of the Subtleties of Flow*

The *Ode of the Subtleties of Flow* is a condensation of the *Discussion of the Subtleties of Flow* by He Ruoyu (c. 12th century). Although the latter work is now lost, parts of the former are found excerpted in later medical texts.

One reference to needling methods in the *Ode of the Subtleties of Flow* provides: "Insert the needle with noble speed then proceed (to the point) slowly; withdraw the needle with noble slowness as haste will cause injury." In other words, the needle should penetrate the skin quickly, minimizing pain, then advance slowly to the proper depth, increasing needle stimulation. Slowly withdrawing the needle helps prevent bleeding. This method is consistent with modern clinical practice.

Needling methods in the *Guide to the Classics of Acupuncture*

Another famous doctor of the Jin-Yuan period, Dou Hanqing, wrote a book entitled *Guide to the Classics of Acupuncture*. Although not widely disseminated in his own time, parts of this book are found in later Yuan and Ming medical texts. One part, entitled *Ode to the Standard of Mystery,* discourses upon all the different theories of acupuncture up to its time and has been commented upon by many medical writers since. Below, we shall briefly discuss those principles in the *Guide to the Classics of Acupuncture* concerned with needling methodology.

1) Emphasis on preliminary massage and slow insertion. The left hand should be used to apply pressure above the point so that Qi and Blood in the area are dispersed. Insertion should be performed slowly with a light touch of the needle. This is regarded as the basis of painless insertion and is, of course, different from the method described in the *Ode of the Subtleties of Flow* of quickly piercing through the skin. Both methods, however, may be useful in the clinic.

2) Joining points. Another distinctive technique found in this work is that of joining points, whereby one needle is inserted over a long enough distance, either transversely or perpendicularly, to 'join' one point to others using the same needle. An example mentined in the *Guide to the Classics of Acupuncture* is inserting a needle from TB-23 *(Sizhukong)* to GB-8 *(Shuaigu)* in the treatment of migraine headache. This method simplifies the performance of acupuncture. The modern practice of joining points is based on this technique.

3) The 14 methods of insertion. These methods were derived from the experience of acupuncturists up to the time of the *Guide to the Classics of Acupuncture.* Most of them have a practical clinical application. Drawing from commentaries in the Ming works, *Questions and Answers about Acupuncture and Moxibustion* and the *Great Compendium of Acupuncture and Moxibustion,* the content of these methods is summarized in the table below.

Name	Method	Clinical Value	Traditional Function
Moving	After the needle is inserted, if the Qi does not move, agitate the needle by shaking, raising and moving it from side to side.	Later called 'wagging the green dragon's tail'; useful in controlling needle sensation.	Moves the Qi
Withdrawing	When the needle is to be removed, first withdraw it to a position just beneath the skin, then remove it using either a strengthening or draining technique.	Usually reduces bleeding.	Clears the Qi
Twisting	Once the needle is inserted, it is twisted like yarn, but not too tightly. The needle is twisted to the right for Cold, and to the left for Hot conditions.	The concept of right for Cold, left for Hot has no clinical value. However, the wide amplitude with which the needle is twisted is effective in strengthening stimulation.	Hot and Cold conditions
Entering	If, after inserting the needle, Qi is not obtained, rotate the needle to the left for a man and to the right for a woman while pressing the needle more deeply.	The distinction between left and right for men and women is baseless. However, the method does help stimulate the Qi.	Benefits Qi
Bowling	Once a needle has been inserted in the soft flesh of the abdomen, it is rotated as if inscribing an imaginary bowl in the air for 5 rotations. The needle is inserted more deeply and rotated to the left to strengthen; it is raised and rotated to the right to drain.	The distinction between left and right has no basis in reality, but the method does strengthen needle stimulation.	Strengthens a Deficient condition; drains an Excessive condition.

515

Name	Method	Clinical Value	Traditional Function
Shaking	The needle is shaken as it is withdrawn so as to drain an Excessive condition.	Augments stimulation.	Drains Qi
Plucking	The thumbnail lightly plucks the tail of the needle causing the Qi to move quickly. A strengthening method.	Corresponds to mild or moderate stimulation techniques.	Strengthens Qi
Turning	Turning the needle to the left strengthens and treats diseases above a point; turning the needle to the right drains and treats diseases below a point.	No practical value.	Strengthens, drains and moves Qi.
Following	Use the fingers to rub up and down the channel below the point needled.	A supplemental method to obtain Qi.	Regulates Qi and Blood
Covering	After the needle is withdrawn, a finger is placed over the point as a strengthening method.	No effect except to help stop bleeding.	Strengthening method
Assisting	If, after the needle is inserted, the muscle tissue contracts around it, press with the fingernail along the affected channel.	Can be used when needle is stuck.	Spreads Qi
Pressing	To tighten up the rotation of an emplaced needle without either advancing or withdrawing it, the finger can be used to press against the body of the needle as if loading a crossbow.	Strong stimulation method.	Augments Qi
Scratching	At the point where the needle is to be inserted, press the skin with the fingernail to mark the spot.	Currently used to mark the point of insertion.	Finding the point
Cutting	Before needling, press the thumbnail [of the opposite hand] hard against the skin beside the point; then insert the needle.	Commonly used method. Reduces pain and possibility of bleeding.	Spreads Qi and Blood

Needling Methods in the *Classic of Divine Resonance*

The *Classic of Divine Resonance* was written by Chen Hui, a physician of the Ming Dynasty. It is a work which contains many acupuncture prescriptions. Here, the special needling methods described in the book will be introduced.

Urging the Qi

A combination of basic techniques including agitating, lifting, thrusting and rotating. The thumb and index finger of the right hand hold the needle and delicately agitate, rotate and move it up and down. This movement resembles that of trembling hands, and is intended to help obtain the Qi.

Equally strengthening and draining

The *Classic of Divine Resonance* instructs: "Whenever there is disease, the Excesses invade. Although the person is thin and weak, one must not solely use the strengthening method . . . only equally strengthening and draining is suitable. It is necessary first to drain and then to strengthen, i.e., first to drain the Excess and then strengthen the Normal Qi." This technique is different from the contemporary moderate stimulation method, wherein a balance is struck between strengthening and draining techniques. (Strengthening and draining are discussed below.)

Needling methods in the *Ode of the Golden Needle*

The *Ode of The Golden Needle,* a part of the Ming work by Xu Feng entitled *Complete Collection of Acupuncture and Moxibustion,* is devoted entirely to needling methods. A few of its more important ideas are introduced below.

Lifting the needle to regulate (and move) the Qi

The *Ode of the Golden Needle* provides: "To regulate the Qi, after inserting the needle to the earth [i.e., the deep position], raise it to the human [i.e., middle] position. If it is desired that the Qi move upward, rotate the needle to the right [i.e., clockwise]; if downward, rotate to the left [i.e., counter-clockwise]. If the area in front of the point of insertion is pressed, the Qi will move behind the point; if the area behind the point is pressed, the Qi will move in front." This method is presently used in the clinic for controlling the needle sensation. Although no apparent purpose can be discerned from the difference between left and right rotation, massage as described in this passage has a definite influence on the conduction of the needle sensation.

Waiting for relaxation before withdrawing the needle

The *Ode of the Golden Needle* provides: "Method of removing the needle: When the strength of the diseae has subsided, the needle Qi [i.e., its manner of movement] will be loose; if the disease has not yet subsided, the needle Qi will be as if rooted—pushing will not move it, twisting will not turn it. This is because the Excess holds the needle and the Normal Qi has not arrived. At this time, the needle should not be withdrawn; if it is, the disease will return. Moreover, when strengthening or draining, one must wait until there is some loosening before the needle can be removed." This passage indicates that when the needle is stuck or the needle sensation is still strong, hasty removal of the needle will adversely affect the result. This observation is consistent with modern clinical experience.

Fourteen consolidated needling methods

The *Ode of the Golden Needle* collected a number of the fundamental strengthening, draining, and moving the Qi techniques from prior ages and combined them into 14 needling methods which are discussed later in this chapter.

Needling methods in the *Gatherings from Outstanding Acupuncturists*

Gatherings from Outstanding Acupuncturists, by the Ming author Gao Wu, is a critique of many of the needling methods practiced by his contemporaries. Among the criticisms are the following:

517

Practices such as selecting points on the basis of the circulation of the Heavenly Stems and Earthly Branches

Gao wrote: "People nowadays . . . absurdly maintain that today being a certain day, at a certain hour a certain point will open, and at that time all diseases can be treated by acupuncture and moxibustion at that point. Tomorrow being a certain day, at a certain time a certain point will open and all diseases will be able to be treated by acupuncture and moxibustion at that point. [This doctrine] deceives many people!" He also condemned many idealistic and feudal superstitions and practices which had crept into acupuncture, although not mentioned in the classics.

The relationship between needling and breathing

Gao Wu took exception to the prevailing interpretation during his era of certain passages in *Simple Questions* which provide: "Wait until inhalation to insert the needle," and "Wait until exhalation to withdraw the needle." Some writers of the Jin-Yuan period interpreted this to mean that the patient had to be told when to inhale and exhale. Inhalation upon insertion and exhalation upon withdrawal of the needle was thought of as a draining method, while the opposite was regarded as a strengthening method. Gao believed this to be unrealistic and interpreted the passages to mean simply that the doctor should await the inhalation or exhalation of the patient before using the needle.

Strengthening and draining methods of the "Rhyme of the Golden Needle"

Gao Wu thought these techniques were nothing but clever names. However, he did not proceed to differentiate those parts of the methods which are useful from those which are merely fanciful.

Needling methods in *Questions and Answers about Acupuncture and Moxibustion*

A Ming physician, Wang Ji, discussed needling methods, moxibustion, channels and points in his book, *Questions and Answers about Acupuncture and Moxibustion.* Basing his views on the early classics, he criticized certain contemporary practices. Many of his ideas are similar to those of Gao Wu.

Flexibility concerning the depth and duration of needling and the number of cones of moxa to be burned

Wang Ji believed it was unnecessary to strictly adhere to the rules in certain texts stipulating how many tenths of a unit a needle was to be inserted at a certain point, or for how many breaths of the patient the needle was to be retained, or how many moxa cones were to be burned at a certain point. Wang contended that these factors had to be determined from the particular circumstances of each case: the depth of insertion according to the depth of the disease; the duration of needling according to the time it takes to obtain Qi; and the number of moxa cones according to the severity of the disease and the thickness of the flesh at the point being needled. These views are consistent with modern clinical practice.

Simplification of the confusion surrounding needling methods

Wang Ji criticized the mushrooming in the number of needling methods (such as the 14 methods of the *Ode of the Golden Needle)* as unnecessary obfuscation and window dressing. He maintained that the methods described in the *Classic of Difficulties* were sufficient both for purposes of strengthening and draining. His practical attitude and skepticism toward useless accretion was admirable.

Needling methods in the *Great Compendium of Acupuncture and Moxibustion*

Two of the principal aspects in the area of needling methodology are discussed in the *Great Compendium of Acupuncture and Moxibustion,* written by the Ming Dynasty acupuncturist, Yang Jizhou.

Degrees of strengthening and draining

Yang Jizhou differentiated not only between strenthening and draining techniques but also between the degrees of each. Moderate strengthening and draining methods require relatively little stimulation; strong strengthening and draining methods necessitate greater stimulation. The basic idea of matching the degree of Deficiency or Excess present in a disease to the intensity of stimulation is correct. However, Yang's methods of strengthening and draining included instructions with respect to the direction of needle rotation, the manner of raising and thrusting the needle, the number of times the needle is to be rotated, etc. Thus, the results from these methods were difficult to predict.

The twelve methods and eight methods of inserting the needle

Yang consolidated the fourteen methods in the *Guide to the Classics of Acupuncture* with the popular methods of his day. The result was the twelve methods, of which all but the four described below have been previously discussed. Later, this grouping was further simplified, and in some ways supplemented, to emerge as the eight needling methods: scratching, twisting, plucking, shaking, covering, following, turning, and probing. All but probing were described earlier.

Name	Purpose	Method	Clinical Value
Grasping	Quick insertion	Hold the needle with the right hand, thrust and rotate it into the body with force.	Rapid insertion is still used today.
Warming	To prevent a struggle between Heat and Cold	Warm the needle in the mouth before inserting.	Not suitable when infection is widespread.
Entering	To concentrate the minds of patient and doctor	Before needling, the patient and physician should breathe evenly a few times to calm the Spirit. The point is then located accurately, the physician makes an indentation with his thumbnail, and the needle is inserted in either a strengthening or draining manner.	Pressing the nail into the skin at the point prevents pain upon needle insertion, but one should not be bound by the strengthening and draining methods.
Pulling	To prevent soreness after withdrawing the needle	When withdrawing the needle, be sure that it is not stuck tightly, but is a little loose. Then use the fingers to lift the needle out as if "pulling a tiger's tail"—very carefully.	In agreement with the *Ode of the Golden Needle*

From the brief discussion above, we can see that since the time of the *Classic of Difficulties,* there has been a proliferation of needling techniques. However, due to the limitations of social conditions of the times, certain superstitious and idealistic elements influenced the reasoning of these writers. For example, in the *Classic of Divine Resonance* and the *Ode of the Golden Needle* there are elaborate rules with respect to strengthening and draining techniques based upon perceived differences in the flow of Qi and Blood in the morning and afternoon, between men and women, between the right and left sides of the body, the Leg channels and the Arm channels, the front and back of the trunk, etc. Such factors must be further investigated in some detail in order to determine their possible significance in the clinic. However, such investigation is beyond the scope of this book.

519

TECHNIQUES OF MOVING THE QI,
STRENGTHENING AND DRAINING

Techniques of moving the Qi, strengthening, and draining are important constituents of needling methodology. Ancient physicians sought to move and regulate the Qi and Blood, strengthening what was Deficient, and draining what was Excessive, by utilizing a variety of needling methods. This rationale is a simple, dialectical one. However, because the ancients were influenced by the mysticism prevalent in their times, it was inevitable that certain subjective elements and mechanistic extrapolations from the Yin/Yang and Five Phases doctrines became incorporated in the methodology. The result is that these methods do not completely coincide with clinical experience.

An analysis of the techniques of moving the Qi

These are also referred to as methods of regulating the Qi. Their purpose is to regulate the flow of Qi and Blood in the channels and control the needle sensation. The ancients believed that the phenomenon of needle sensation was one manifestation of the movement of Qi and Blood, and that in the course of treatment the Qi should be made to flow toward a particular area. The statement in the *Great Compendium of Acupuncture and Moxibustion*—"When using the distant point method it is first necessary to cause the Qi to reach straight to the diseased area"—is what 'moving the Qi' is all about. Some specific techniques are described below.

Directing the needle
In the *Great Compendium of Acupuncture and Moxibustion* it is observed: "Turn the needle [tip] upward and the Qi will move upward. Turn the needle downward and the Qi will move downward." This method of controlling the needle sensation was previously discussed in chapter 2 of this Section. It has a definite, practical use.

Massage
The *Ode of the Golden Needle* provides: "Pressing in front causes the Qi to be behind; pressing behind causes the Qi to be in front." This means that massaging the area above the point will cause the needle sensation to be directed downward from the point, while if the area below the needle is massaged the opposite effect will occur. This method has definite clinical value in controlling needle sensation.

Twisting
This refers to the twisting method, one of the fourteen needling methods discussed above. It is based on a theory which correlates right and left with Yin and Yang. In our experience, the differentiation between right and left rotation as a means of controlling needle response has no real significance. Rotation does have the function of tightening the needle sensation and strengthening its conduction when used in tandem with the directing the needle method.

Raising and thrusting
This method is described in a passage from the *Great Compendium of Acupuncture and Moxibustion:* "Slowly pushing the needle, the Qi will depart; slightly drawing the needle up, the Qi will come." The word "depart" here means to move against the flow, while "come" means to move with the flow. The ancients believed that needling an acupuncture point was like closing a sluice on a waterway. Needling was supposed to temporarily prevent the flow of Qi and Blood, keeping that which was behind the point behind, and preventing the Qi and Blood in front of the point from reversing its flow. By this means, one can direct the needle sensation so that it is transmitted in the opposite direction from the flow of Qi and Blood in the channels (as in the 'white tiger shaking its head' method below), or one can cause the needle sensation to reach a certain distance beyond a point and then shut it off (as in the 'receiving Qi' method below). Drawing the needle up is like opening the sluice and letting the Qi and Bloood flow unimpeded. It is therefore used when it is desirable for the needle

sensation to travel along the channel (also found in the 'white tiger shaking its head' method).

This 'sluice' theory of conductivity is merely an extension of the theory of Qi and the channels (see Section I), and is not really helpful. The process can better be understood by realizing that the needle sensation relies for its conduction upon certain distinct structures at the site of a point. When the needle is pushed into the area of the point, the needle sensation is strengthened and spread; when the needle is withdrawn, it leaves the area of the point and the needle sensation correspondingly weakens or disappears.

Breathing

The ancients believed that inhalation and exhalation moved the Qi and Blood, and that the needle sensation could be controlled by causing the needling to coincide with the appropriate stage of breathing. The *Ode of the Golden Needle* provides: "If the disease is above (the point), withdraw the needle when the patient inhales. If the disease is below (the point), advance the needle when the patient exhales." In our clinical experience, we have yet to observe any appreciable effect from the utilization of this method.

An analysis of the basic strengthening and draining techniques

The strengthening and draining methods used by the ancients can be distinguished according to certain characteristics: the speed of needle insertion and withdrawal, the manner of raising and thrusting the needle, the direction of rotation, the direction of the needle point, the number of needles used, the duration of needling, and the selection of points. From the *Inner Classic* through the works of successive generations of physicians, the techniques of strengthening and draining have became more numerous and complex.

To begin with, let us look at the fundamental characteristics of strengthening and draining techniques.

Method	Distinction	Strengthening Technique	Draining Technique
Slow or Quick	The needle is inserted and/or withdrawn quickly or slowly	Slow, gradual insertion; quick withdrawal	Quick insertion; slow, gradual withdrawal
Raising and Thrusting	After insertion the needle is raised or thrust either gently or with force	Thrust forcefully; raised gently	Thrust gently; raised forcefully
Rotation	The needle is rotated to the left or right	Left rotation (counter-clockwise)	Right rotation (clockwise)
Direction	The needle is pointed either with or against the flow of Qi and Blood in the channels	Point needle with the flow	Point needle against the flow
Breathing	Conforming insertion, withdrawal and rotation of the needle to the patient's breathing	Insert needle during exhalation, rotate and withdraw during inhalation	Insert during inhalation, rotate and withdraw during exhalation

Techinques

Method	Instruction	Strengthening Technique	Draining Technique
Opening and Covering	The puncture is either pressed or not pressed with the finger after withdrawal of the needle	The needle is quickly withdrawn and the point is pressed	The needle is slowly withdrawn with shaking (to enlarge hole), and the point is not pressed
9 and 6	Rotation and/or thrusting of needle performed either 9 (Yang) or 6 (Yin) times	Perform procedure 9 times	Perform procedure 6 times
Mother and Son points	'Mother' or 'Son' points Select 'Mother' or 'Son' points from among the 5 Transport points according to progression of the Five Phases	Select the 'Mother' point	Select 'Son' point
12 time periods	'Mother' or 'Son' points selected according to the times of day associated with each of the 12 Primary channels	When the time associated with a particular channel is past, select the 'Mother' point	During the time associated with a particular channel, select the 'Son' point

Differences of opinion regarding the nine basic strengthening and draining techniques described above still exist in acupuncture circles. Clinical and experimental data is still insufficient to justify any definitive conclusions. The analyses below are only preliminary views based upon investigation of the theories themselves, their historical evolution and the manner in which they have been utilized in the clinic. The analyses may well be incorrect and must await further verification.

Strengthening and draining with respect to slow or quick, raising or thrusting techniques

These methods are derived from the association of the superficial and deep positions of needling with Yang and Yin respectively. It was thought that a slow insertion and quick withdrawal of the needle, or a forceful thrusting and gentle raising of the needle would strengthen the body by leading the Yang Qi in the superficial layers of the body into deeper tissue. In the *Great Compendium of Acupuncture and Moxibustion,* it is observed: "Lowering the Yang constitutes strengthening." Conversely, a quick insertion and slow withdrawal, and a gentle thrusting with forceful raising of the needle are draining methods because they are said to bring the deep Yin Qi to the surface. Thus, the *Great Compendium of Acupuncture and Moxibustion* notes: "Raising the Yin constitutes draining." The ancients felt that using this method would result in the regulation of Qi at the points and thereby relieve any problem of Deficiency or Excess caused by an imbalance in the Organs. The actual value of these methods with respect to Yin and Yang correlatives has yet to be determined.

Furthermore, there are differences of opinion in the ancient literature with respect to which methods strengthen and which drain. The earliest reference to the slow and quick method (chapter 1 of *Spiritual Axis)* instructs: "Slow then quick [for] Excess; quick then slow [for] Deficiency." Although this does not clarify the actual technique, chapter 3 explains that a slow insertion and quick withdrawal strengthens, while the opposite procedure drains. However, in chapter 54 of *Simple Questions* these instructions are reversed. It would seem that on this point, *Spiritual Axis* and *Simple Questions* are inconsistent.

The texts are similarly confused regarding the raising and thrusting techniques in relation to strengthening and draining. In chapter 73 of *Spiritual Axis* it is said that a strengthening method consists of slightly twisting the needle while thrusting it, whereas raising and 'meeting' it is a draining technique. The *Classic of Difficulties,* chapter 78, supplements this instruction by providing that the action of thrusting and entering strengthens, while shaking and raising drains. Subsequent generations of physicians reduced this to the formulae: 'tightly thrust and slowly raise' to strengthen, and 'tightly raise and slowly thrust' to drain. However, there is a passage in *Song of the Eight Methods* which contradicts this: "Quickly thrusting and slowly raising, the Yin Qi ascends (draining); quickly raising and slowly thrusting, the Yang Qi descends (strengthening)." The *Ode of the Golden Needle* provides: "For men . . . raising the needle is Hot (strengthening), thrusting the needle is Cold (draining). For women . . . thrusting is Hot, raising is Cold." And the *Introduction to Medicine* states: "For men, in the morning raising the needle is Hot, thrusting is cold; in the afternoon raising the needle is cold, thrusting is Hot. For women, the opposite is true."

The mutual contradictions in these accounts clearly show that these techniques are mere extensions of Yin/Yang theories. However, it is true that slowly inserting and thrusting the needle results in a relatively mild stimulus, while quickly inserting and thrusting the needle produces a relatively strong stimulus. These differences have a definite reference value in the clinic.

Strengthening and draining with respect to rotation techniques

The division of rotation techniques into strengthening and draining characteristics is found as early as the writings of Dou Hanqing (Jin/Yuan period). In *Ode to the Standard of Mystery,* it is written that rotation to the right (clockwise) drains, while rotation to the left (counter-clockwise) strengthens. The *Great Compendium of Acupuncture and Moxibustion* provides: "Leftward rotation after midnight [the period of Yang ascendancy] can move all the Yang [Qi] outward; rightward rotation after noon can move all the Yin [Qi] inward." This passage is clearly an extension of the idea that right is Yin and left is Yang. Because of this, the relationship between needle rotation and strengthening or draining became even more confused. For example, the *Ode of the Golden Needle* instructed: "For men, leftward rotation with the thumb advancing during exhalation strengthens; rightward rotation during inhalation drains." The opposite is said to be true of women, for whom everything is reversed in the afternoon. The *Introduction to Medicine* gathered a variety of factors which it related to strengthening and draining including distinctions between left and right, Arm and Leg, Yin and Yang, male and female, before and after noon, inhalation and exhalation, etc. The *Questions and Answers about Acupuncture and Moxibustion* teaches that in the ascending channels (the 3 Arm Yang, 3 Leg Yin and Conception channels), leftward rotation of the needle strengthens and rightward rotation drains. The opposite is said to occur in the descending channels (3 Arm Yin, 3 Leg Yang and Governing channels).

It should therefore be apparent that there are many contradictions among the various sources describing different techniques of draining and strengthening by differentiating between directions of needle rotation. Further clinical investigation is warranted.

Strengthening and draining with respect to techniques based upon the direction of the needle

First mentioned in *Selected Materials Beneficial to Life* (Yuan Dynasty), this method differentiates strengthening and draining by the opposition or conformity of the direction of needling to the flow of Qi and Blood in the channels. When the direction in which the needle is inserted coincides with that of the flow of Qi and Blood in the channels, the flow is aided and there is a strengthening effect; when it is inserted against the flow, the movement of Qi and Blood is hindered and draining occurs. This method is obviously removed from clinical reality and is the product of baseless speculation. There have been attempts to link this type of strengthening and draining technique with the *Inner Classic* by pointing to certain passages therein, e.g.,"welcome and guide it" and "follow to benefit." However, these are but general guidelines to strengthening and draining and do not specifically refer to the direction of needling.

Strengthening and draining with respect to the breathing technique

This technique was first mentioned in chapter 27 of *Simple Questions*. Inserting the needle as the patient exhales and withdrawing it as she inhales is a strengthening method; the opposite procedures induce draining. The first action is intended to retain the Qi from the air in the body, while the latter is supposed to release it. If there is, in fact, a relationship between breathing and insertion and withdrawal of the needle, it has yet to be proven.

Strengthening and draining with respect to techniques which open and cover the needle puncture

This distinction was first mentioned in chapter 73 of *Spiritual Axis*. To drain, the needle is rotated and agitated vigorously so as to enlarge the hole before the needle is withdrawn. This allows more of the (Excess) Qi to escape. To strengthen, the hole made by the needle is pressed with a finger immediately upon withdrawal of the needle, thereby preventing the Normal Qi from escaping. In chapter 53 of *Simple Questions*, it is said that when needling Excessive conditions the hole is to be left uncovered, whereas when needling Deficient conditions the hole should be covered. Based on this instruction, later generations of physicians determined that quickly withdrawing the needle and immediately covering the hole strengthens, while slowly withdrawing the needle and leaving the hole uncovered drains.

The idea of retention or expulsion of Qi from the body is clearly a deduction based upon a theory without empirical support. However, the two methods do produce different amounts of stimulation and conform with clinical experience in this sense: that in most circumstances, a relatively mild degree of stimulation has a strengthening effect, while a strong amount of stimulation drains. Because of this difference, these techniques possess a definite clinical value.

Strengthening and draining with respect to techniques based upon counting the times the needle is manipulated

During the Jin-Yuan period, physicians believed that six rotations, raisings, thrustings or other manipulations of the needle constituted a technique of draining, while nine manipulations constituted a strenthening technique. Even numbers were associated with Yin and considered appropriate for draining; odd numbers were associated with Yang and deemed best for strengthening. (This type of numerology can be traced to the *Book of Change*.) The number six was called a 'young Yin', nine an 'old Yang'. Seven was a 'young Yang', eight and 'old Yin'. In practice, these numbers were squared. A variant of this technique discussed in the *Introduction to Medicine* (Ming Dynasty) claimed: "After midnight, nine manipulations will strengthen the Yang; from afternoon on, six manipulations will strengthen the Yin. On Yin [even-numbered] days, perform six manipulations when needling a Yang channel. On Yang [odd numbered] days, perform nine manipulations when needling a Yin channel." This passage clearly reflects the influence of Neo-Confucian thought on medicine. In addition to causing confusion regarding needling techniques, such correspondences have no clinical value whatever.

Strengthening and draining with respect to techniques utilizing the 'Mother' and 'Son' points in conjunction with the 12 time phases

This is a system of matching points based upon correlations between the 12 time phases (named after the 12 Earthly Branches) of two hours each into which the day was divided, and the circulation of Qi in the 12 Primary channels. Accordingly, the time-phase *yin* (from 3-5 a.m.) corresponds to the Lung channel, while the eleventh time phase after that, *chou*, corresponds to the Liver channel. To strengthen, the 'Mother' point* is needled during the time-phase immediately following that corresponding to the channel. This is when the Qi in the channel is said to be exhausted. For example, to strengthen the Lungs, L-9 *(Taiyuan),* the Earth point on the Lung channel, would be needled between 5-7 a.m. To drain, the 'Son' point is needled during the time-phase which corresponds to the channel. This is when the Qi in the channel is said to be ascendant. To drain the Lungs, L-5 *(Chize),* the Water point on the Lung channel, would be needled between 3-5 a.m.

This description stands in opposition to that of the *Inner Classic* which states that the Qi and Blood circulate through the 14 channels 50 times a day. It reflects the influence of the Tang and Song school of phase energetics. A method of strengthening and draining based on these theories is difficult to reconcile with clinical practice.

An analysis of combined needling methods

The combined needling methods represent a synthesis of the techniques of moving the Qi, strengthening and draining described above. They are primarily the creation of physicians from the Jin, Yuan and later dynasties. The earliest examples are found in the *Ode of the Golden Needle,* wherein 14 types are described. Later physicians supplemented this number with 6 additional methods, bringing the total to 20. Of these, some are strengthening techniques, some are draining, others are both draining and strengthening, some hasten the Qi, others move the Qi, and still others combine elements of all of these techniques. Below, they are introduced with a preliminary critique.

Strengthening and draining by needling in stages ('mountain-burning fire' and 'penetrating-heaven coolness')

The most important aspect of these methods is the insertion or withdrawal of the needle in stages, either quickly or slowly. Variations in speed as well as the force with which the needle is raised or thrust determine whether the technique strengthens or drains. In the strengthening method ('mountain-burning fire'), the needle is inserted slowly in three stages and then quickly withdrawn. While in place, it is thrust with force and raised gently. The needle is inserted during exhalation, withdrawn during inhalation, and manipulated a total of nine or nine-squared times. After the needle is withdrawn, the hole is covered.

In the draining method ('penetrating-heaven coolness'), the needle is inserted quickly with one motion and withdrawn slowly in three stages. While in place, it is raised with force but thrust gently. The needle is inserted during inhalation, withdrawn during exhalation, and manipulated six or six-squared times. After the needle is withdrawn, the hole is left uncovered.

It is thought that by these methods, the Yang Qi can be made to penetrate (strengthen), or the Yin Qi to ascend (drain). Because 'Yang produces Heat,' when utilizing the 'burning-mountain fire' method the patient may feel a warm sensation. And because 'Yin produces Cold,' the 'penetrating-heaven coolness' method may induce a feeling of coolness. It is therefore used in treating Hot conditions. At present, there is no unanimity of opinion regarding the clinical value of these methods.

Combined strengthening and draining methods ('Yin hidden in Yang' and 'Yang hidden in Yin').

Each of these methods has both strengthening (Yang) and draining (Yin) characteristics. The first ('Yin hidden in Yang') is primarily a strengthening method, wherein a strengthening technique is followed by a draining one. The needle is inserted slowly, 0.5 unit, and at that position thrust with force, then raised gently nine times. This is the strengthening phase. The needle is then inserted further to a depth of 1 unit, thrust gently and raised forcefully six times, then withdrawn quickly. This is the draining phase. This method is used for Hot conditions which contain Excessive aspects.

---

*That point belonging to the phase immediately preceding the phase of the affected channel in the 'production cycle' of the Five Phases. See Introduction and Section II, chapter 1.—Editors

The second method ('Yang hidden in Yin') is primarily a draining method, whereby a draining technique is followed by a strengthening one. The needle is inserted quickly to a depth of 1 unit, gently thrust and forcefully raised six times, then withdrawn to a depth of 0.5 unit. At this position, the needle is forcefully thrust and gently raised nine times, then slowly withdrawn. This method is used for Cold conditions preceded by Hot conditions, or for Excessive conditions with Deficient aspects.

Strengthening and draining by rotation ('dragon and tiger joined in battle')

Strengthening and draining are combined through repeated rotation of the needle, first nine times to the left, then six times to the right. If necessary, this may be done at each of the three depths of insertion. This technique is intended to facilitate the circulation of Qi and to alleviate pain. Although the effect of this particular number and manner of rotation has yet to be verified, the method itself increases the needle sensation and has definite clinical value.

Strengthening and draining by rotation, thrusting and draining ('midnight-midday threshing')

This method is similar to 'dragon and tiger joined in battle,' except that the vertical motion of raising and thrusting ('threshing') is emphasized. This increases the amount of stimulation. After the needle is inserted, it is first thrust forcefully, raised gently, and rotated to the left (counterclockwise) nine times. Then it is raised forcefully, thrust gently and turned to the right six times. This procedure is repeated several times. The purpose is to harmonize the Yin and Yang and facilitate the passage of Qi through the channels. It is considered effective for conditions requiring strong stimulation. However, one need not be bound by the rules of precedence in thrusting and raising, the direction of rotation, or the number of revolutions.

Rotating above and below to move the Qi ('dragon and tiger ascending and descending')

A number of techniques are employed at varying depths. First, at the 'heaven' (most superficial) position, the needle is rotated once to the left, then thrust firmly to the middle or 'human' position, and gently raised back to the position of 'heaven.' The needle is rotated one revolution to the right, then thrust and raised as before. This procedure is repeated nine times. Its purpose is to cause the Yang Qi to descend. In the second stage, the needle is inserted to the 'earth' (deep) position, rotated one revolution to the right, raised forcefully and thrust gently, then rotated once to the left and raised and thrust as before. This second stage is repeated six times so as to induce the Yin Qi to ascend. Finally, the middle finger is pressed against the body of the emplaced needle, bending it back like a crossbow. Bending the needle forward causes the Qi to move behind; bending the needle behind causes the Qi to move forward. The net effect of all these operations is to harmonize an imbalance of Yin and Yang and facilitate the movement of Qi through the channels. In practice, this method has definite value as a means of strong stimulation. However, the direction of rotation, order and strength of raisings and thrustings, and number of procedures need not be rigidly adhered to.

Four methods of moving the Qi

1) 'Wagging the tail.' (Originally called 'green dragon wags its tail.') After obtaining Qi, the needle is slanted in the direction of the disorder. The needle is neither thrust, raised nor rotated. Instead, the 'tail' of the needle is 'wagged' back and forth, either nine or twenty-seven times. This is a Yang method and therefore specifically moves Yang Qi. Although the association of nine with Yang is specious, the method does control and strengthen the conduction of the needle sensation.

2) 'Shaking the head.' (Originally called 'white tiger shakes its head.') The needle is thrust with a leftward rotation, and 'shaken' when the patient exhales. When the needle is raised, it is rotated to the right and 'shaken' upon inhalation. These operations are repeated six or eighteen times. This is a Yin method and therefore is intended to move the Blood, which is Yin. Shaking the needle certainly strengthens needle sensation; however, the references to breathing and numerology are without value.

3) Searching for the point. (Originally called 'green turtle searches for the point.') The needle is inserted slowly (in 3 stages) and withdrawn quickly. This procedure is repeatedly performed, each time altering the direction and angle of insertion. This is an easy method of obtaining Qi. The stages of insertion and withdrawal, however, are unimportant.

4) Meeting the source. (Originally called 'scarlet phoenix meeting the source.') The needle is repeatedly thrust, first to the deep ('earth') position, then raised to the superficial ('heaven') position and finally thrust to the middle ('human') position. While this is being done, the needle should be shaken back and forth and rapidly twirled to hasten the Qi. If the disease is above the point, the needle is rotated to the right and raised as the patient inhales. If the disease is below the point, the needle is rotated to the left and thrust as the patient exhales. This technique is definitely useful in obtaining Qi.

The animals mentioned in the original names for the techniques above are representative of the Five Phases. Each one belongs to a direction. According to the Five Phase theory of correspondences, the techniques fancifully named after the animals of the east and south (dragon and phoenix) are meant to strengthen, while those named after the animals of the west and north (tiger and turtle) are prescribed for draining.

Four methods of benefitting the Qi.

1) Flowing Qi. The needle is inserted to a depth of 0.7 unit and is raised and thrust in accordance with strengthening techniques nine times. Then, when Qi has been obtained, the needle is further inserted to a depth of 1 unit, and raised and thrust in accordance with draining techniques six times. Performed repeatedly, this is a treatment for 'masses (lumps) of Qi' which are migratory areas of painful nodules that are soft to the touch, or not even palpable. In actual clinical practice, the instructions concerning the depth of insertion and the enumeration of thrust are irrelevant.

2) Raising Qi. The needle is raised forcefully and thrust slowly six times so as to drain an Excess. The needle is left in place until the muscle tightens and the needle is 'settled.' This indicates that Qi has been obtained. The needle is then rotated slightly, and gently raised. It is believed that this technique is effective in the treatment of numbness, cold limbs, and persistent pain accompanied by difficulty in movement. It is thought to facilitate the circulation of Protective and Nourishing Qi. It is definitely effective in strengthening local needle sensation.

3) Circulating Qi. Raise the needle forcefully and thrust it slowly six times to drain. When Qi has been obtained, slant the needle in the direction of the disorder, and ask the patient to inhale five times to cause the Qi to flow towards the problem area. Although the inhalation itself does not control the needle sensation, deep breathing during acupuncture treatment does relax the patient and reduce pain. This method can be used for any type of pain.

4) Receiving Qi. This method utilizes the technique of 'circulating Qi' as its basis. After performing the 'circulating Qi' procedure (see above) and Qi has been obtained at the site of the disease, the needle is held perpendicular to the skin, pressed straight down, and the area on the side of the needle away from the affected part of the body is pressed. It is believed that this procedure prevents the Qi from flowing back toward the point. This method is clinically useful in directing the conduction of needle sensation.

Of the needling methods described above—those to move the Qi, strengthen, drain, and the combined methods—some are based upon the actual clinical experience of our predecessors, while others are only based upon theoretical speculation. The latter group inevitably includes methods which are inconsistent with clinical practice. Still, even some of these techniques have certain limited value, as we have pointed out. We must continue to pursue a concrete analysis of ancient methodologies based upon clinical experience.

We feel that the true meaning of 'strengthening that which is Deficient and draining that which is Excessive' must be found in actual clinical practice. The needle sensation, and the strength and duration of that sensation, will depend in each case upon such diverse factors as the particular patient and disease, the channels and points thereon chosen for therapy, as well as the specific type of needle and method of treatment used. When these factors are properly taken into account, the needle sensation, mediated through the channel system, will result in a strengthening effect when the Normal Qi is weak, or a draining effect when Excess prevails.

This strengthening or draining function is primarily dependent upon the ability of the organism to regulate itself. However, the method of needle stimulation is an important condition for the promotion of the organism's regulatory capacity. In chapter 75 of *Spiritual Axis* is written: "The use of methods like acupuncture is in regulating the Qi." As we have seen, the various techniques of strengthening and draining recorded in medical texts through the ages include elements which have no empirical basis (direction of rotation, number of operations, time of needling, sex of patient, etc.) as well as elements based upon actual clinical experience (depth and direction of needle insertion, strength of stimulation, duration of needling, and the extent of conduction of the needle sensation). It is essential that the physician have a good understanding of the appropriate forms of acupuncture stimulation so as to best treat each individual condition. Only then can the body's regulatory capabilities be brought into play, and Deficiencies strengthened or Excesses drained. Any attempt to resolve the complexities of Excessive or Deficient conditions which ignores the particular state of the body or of the disease by mechanically applying a few set methods will surely fail.

Regarding the ancient needling methods, we must continue through observation and experimentation to critically examine our heritage. Only in this way can these methods be used to the greatest advantage in the clinic.

Chapter 10

A Summary of Research Concerning the Effects of Acupuncture

THE EFFECTS OF ACUPUNCTURE ON THE DIGESTIVE SYSTEM

There is considerable material available from both clinical studies and experimental research showing the excellent results obtained from acupuncture treatment on the diseases of the digestive system. For example, after needling S-36 *(Zusanli)* on a normal subject, the amplitude and frequency of peristalsis in the stomach increased, the tension was raised, the stomach emptying time was shortened and the period of contraction of the stomach lengthened. Needling S-36 *(Zusanli)* and related points on patients with gastric ulcers will, in most cases, cause an increase in peristalsis, open the pyloris and accelerate the emptying of the stomach. (1-5) In research carried out by Xian No. 1 Hospital it was found that needling certain points caused a retardation of stomach functions, while needling other points can cause an acceleration of the gastric functions. (6) Most of the researchers believe that the effect produced by needling is dependent upon the original level of gastric function. For example, when needling S-36 *(Zusanli)* and LI-10 *(Shousanli)* on both healthy and sick subjects, it was discovered that when the stomach was previously relaxed the needling caused a strengthening of the waves of contraction in the stomach, whereas if the stomach was tense before needling, the effect was to relax the stomach. Furthermore, this effect was more pronounced among sick subjects than healthy ones. The Shanghai College of Traditional Medicine proved in their experiments on animals that needling S-36 *(Zusanli)* and related points would stimulate gastrointestinal activity in cases originally found to be hypoactive, and inhibit those cases which were originally hyperactive. (7-9) Clinical evidence has shown that needling certain points plays a regulatory role in regard to the secretion of gastric juice and aids in restoring balance to a diseased stomach. For example, needling S-36 *(Zusanli)* and related points on patients suffering from gastric ulcers reduces the secretion of gastric juices or tends to bring the general level of free acids, and the acidity of the gastric contents, to a normal level.

Among patients with indigestion, needling S-36 *(Zusanli)*, LI-4 *(Hegu)*, Sp-6 *(Sanyinjiao)* and related points quickly restores what were previously low levels of stomach acidity, free stomach acids, pepsin, and gastric lipase to normal levels. After needling M-UE-9 *(Sifeng)* the activity of pepsin increases, and if the general acidity of the stomach was previously low, it is raised; if previously high, it is lowered slightly. Needling LI-4 *(Hegu)* on patients with chronic gastritis and cholecystitis can cause an increase in gastric secretions, thereby increasing the level of acidity in patients whose gastric acid level is low. Those patients with depleted levels of gastric juice show the appearance of free acids after needling LI-4 *(Hegu)*. Patients with excessive gastric acid will, in most cases, show the acid level returned to normal.

Acupuncture also has a regulatory effect upon the functions and motility of the small intestine. For instance, in research done by the Shanghai Hospital of Thoracic Medicine, healthy subjects who were needled at Co-12 *(Zhongwan)* showed an increase in intestinal peristaltic noises. It was also observed through the use of x-ray examination, that the activities of the empty intestine increased, and that the movement of a barium meal through the intestine was accelerated. It was also found that peristalsis of the small intestine previously described as "relatively weak" or of "medium strength," was increased after acupuncture. On the other hand, although needling a patient with "relatively strong" peristalsis did not increase the activity still further, neither was any inhibitory effect demonstrated.

The effects of acupuncture on patients with intestinal tract disorders were even more pronounced. (10) For instance, clinical studies in Guangdong province among patients with intestinal obstruction due to roundworm, or with partial intestinal obstruction, showed that after stimulation of M-UE-9 *(Sifeng),* there was expansion of certain segments of the intestinal tract, relief from intestinal cramps and generally an acceleration of peristalsis as well as the speed with which the intestines were emptied. That needling S-36 *(Zusanli)* and related points can strengthen intestinal peristalsis was proven in numerous experiments and clinical studies on animals. As for the route along which this stimulus is transmitted, some believe it is communicated by the sympathetic nerves surrounding the blood vessels, others that it is transmitted by the sciatic and femoral nerves, and still others believe it is a combination of sciatic and femoral nerves together with the nerve plexus in the walls of the femoral artery.

A number of observations were made clinically concerning the effects of acupuncture on the motility of the gall bladder, bile juice and secretions of pancreatic juice. It was found that stimulation of GB-34 *(Yanglingquan),* S-36 *(Zusanli),* B-15 *(Xinshu),* B-19 *(Danshu),* Li-14 *(Qimen),* GB-24 *(Riyue)* and related points caused a strengthening of the contraction of the gall bladder and speeded up the emptying of that organ. Needling GB-40 *(Qiuxu),* GB-34 *(Yanglingquan),* GB-24 *(Riyue)* and related points caused a strengthening of peristalsis in the common bile duct of the gall bladder. After needling Li-14 *(Qimen)* and GB-24 *(Riyue),* the sphincter of Oddi (gall bladder) was observed to tightly contract. When the needling was stopped, however, the sphincter relaxed. (11-12) It was also reported that needling Li-3 *(Taichong),* S-36 *(Zusanli)* and GB-34 *(Yanglingquan)* can relieve morphine-induced spasms of the sphincter of Oddi. (13)

It has been observed that needling the lower limb points on patients who have undergone a cholecystectomy but have developed biliary fistulas, causes a clear increase in the flow of bile, while needling points on the upper limbs or upper back causes the flow of bile to either decrease or stop altogether. Needling GB-40 *(Qiuxu),* GB-34 *(Yanglingquan),* GB-24 *(Riyue)* and related points on a patient with gall stones also causes a distinct increase in the flow of bile. In other research, it was found that after needling M-UE-9 *(Sifeng)* on patients with roundworm, the level of trypsin, pancreatic amylase, and pancreatic lipase in the intestines was increased. (14) Experiments with animals brought similar results.

A considerable amount of research was done both clinically and experimentally on animals to determine the effect of acupuncture in treating appendicitis. In Shanghai, using both healthy subjects and others with appendicitis, examinations were made both with x-ray and through direct surgical observation, to study the effects of needling S-36 *(Zusanli),* M-LE-13 *(Lanwei),* LI-11 *(Quchi),* Co-6 *(Qihai),* K-7 *(Fuliu)* and related points. It was found that the movements of the diseased appendix were strengthened, the tension increased, or the radius of the appendix itself was altered. It was also noted that there were earlier movements, or segmental bubbles, and that the fecaliths or other contents of the appendix were passed out of the appendix. However, in cases of adhesive appendix these effects were not significant. (15)

Acupuncture has also proved effective in increasing the transportive function of the large intestine. For example, the frequency and amplitude of peristalsis in the colon is increased. (16) Among constipated patients acupuncture can cause increases, sometimes very strong, in the peristalsis of the colon.

THE EFFECTS OF ACUPUNCTURE ON THE CIRCULATORY SYSTEM

Acupuncture has a definite effect upon the functioning of the circulatory system. Most of the clinical and experimental research has been concerned with the changes which occur in the activities of the blood, heart and blood vessels after acupuncture stimulation. (17-18)

The effect of acupuncture on the leukocytes differed widely according to the acupuncture points selected for needling, the method of needling and the functional condition of the organism. In reports of experiments on animals, it was found that after needling S-36 *(Zusanli)* on a rabbit (i.e., the anatomical equivalent of this point on the rabbit) the leukocyte count increased, reaching its highest level three hours after needling. However, needling points on the rabbits' bodies which do not correspond to known acupuncture points produced no visible change in the leukocyte count. According to some reports, using an 'inhibitory method' of needling first caused a slight decrease in leukocytes, followed later by an increase. The peak level was maintained from one to three hours. In the clinic, it was shown that needling certain points that are commonly used in various inflammatory diseases (like appendicitis or pancreatitis) would shortly thereafter produce a gradual decrease in the high white blood cell count induced by the inflammation, as well as bring about a corresponding decline in the percentage of neutrophils. Furthermore, in certain cases of leukopenia caused by radiation or chemical therapy, it was discovered that needling common points such as S-36 *(Zusanli)*, LI-4 *(Hegu)*, and Gv-14 *(Dazhui)* would quickly produce an increase in leukocytes. The percentage of neutrophils would also correspondingly increase. In different diseases, when the leukocyte level was either increased or decreased after acupuncture, there was an improvement in the clinical presentation. If there was no change in the leukocyte count, there was likewise no improvement in the symptoms.

As for the effects of acupuncture on red blood cells, definite results were recorded in treating cases of anemia and weakness. According to reports, daily needling of S-36 *(Zusanli)* and B-38 *(Gaohuang)* on patients with pernicious anemia raised the red blood cell count after five days from 1 mil./cu. mm. to 3.37 mil./cu. mm., and the hemoglobin in the blood registered an increase of anywhere from 30% to 70.9%. In illnesses involving an excess of red blood cells, there was both a reduction in the red blood cell count and in the amount of hemoglobin after acupuncture. The time required to release the poisonous carbon monoxide from a hemoglobin cell with which it has combined is hastened by acupuncture, leading to an earlier revival of consciousness in patients suffering from carbon monoxide poisoning.

The effect of acupuncture on blood platelets and coagulation was used clinically to treat thrombocytopenic purpura, hypersplenic anemia, and related diseases. According to clinical reports, the symptoms accompanying these illnesses improved, while there was a simultaneous increase in the platelet count. In cases of thrombocytopenia following the removal of the spleen, there was a similar increase in platelets after acupuncture therapy. It was also reported that tapping with a Plum Blossom (cutaneous) needle on the neck in the region of the carotid artery for the treatment of coughing blood in tuberculosis can cause an increase in the number of blood platelets, thus having an important effect in stopping the bleeding.

According to reports made by the Electro-acupuncture Research Department of the Xian School of Hygiene on the effects of electro-acupuncture stimulation upon the chemical components of normal blood, it was found that components which were normally in abundance declined, whereas normally low amounts increased. However, the increase and decrease were still within limits. In another report it was stated that the globulin, albumin, thrombin and amylase levels in the serum, as well as the potassium, sodium, calcium and phosphorus in the blood of sick subjects showed little or no change after electro-acupuncture stimulation. The cholesterol level was generally reduced, and the period of coagulation was generally extended. At the same time, the blood ammonia and sugar levels were raised.

The effect of acupuncture on the rate of the heart beat is regulative: a fast heart beat is decreased, a slow one increased. However, the general tendency is to slow down the heart beat. When using acupuncture for the treatment of heart diseases, it was found beneficial in reducing the excessive burden on the heart as well as raising the cardiac output, thus leading to an improvement of the patient's condition.

The influence of acupuncture on the rate of heart beat is often related to the selection of points for stimulation. For instance, needling P-6 *(Neiguan)*, P-5 *(Jianshi)*, B-15 *(Xinshu)*, S-9 *(Renying)*, B-1 *(Jingming)*, B-2 *(Zanshu)*, S-1 *(Chengqi)* and similar points usually caused a reduction in the heart rate. On the other hand, needling H-5 *(Tongli)*, Gv-25 *(Suliao)* and related points usually caused an increase. Needling such points as TB-17 *(Yifeng)*, SI-19 *(Tinggong)* and GB-2 *(Tinghui)* showed no significant effect at all. (19) Most researchers believe that the regulatory stimulation was principally relayed through the nerves of the autonomous nervous system.

The effects of acupuncture as shown on electrocardiograms is more pronounced on patients with irregular heart activities than on normal subjects. Furthermore, from an analysis of the altered features on the electrocardiograms, it was found that the primary effect of acupuncture is a beneficially regulative one. For example, after needling B-15 *(Xinshu)* and Co-5 *(Shimen)* on subjects with heart disease, the electrocardiograms showed an extension in the P—P interval, the QRS complex became narrower, the Q—T interval was shortened, and the T waves became higher and increased in width. (20) These changes all reflect the improvement in the functioning and nourishment of the heart. Other tests measured the effects of needling H-7 *(Shenmen)*, P-7 *(Daling)* and similar points on the cardiac activities of heart patients. These tests were conducted with the use of vectorcardiography and other cardiac measuring methods. In most cases, systole increased in strength. Furthermore, whereas before acupuncture the peaks at the left ventricle and aortic waves were low and of varying shape, and the swelling of the diastolic curve as well as the rise of the systolic curve were weak, after acupuncture the peak of the left ventricle wave was raised, the slope of the systolic curve remained weak, but the swelling of the diastolic curve increased. All of these changes indicate that acupuncture is capable of causing an increase in the strength of heart contraction and an improvement in the functioning of the heart itself.

Concerning the influence of acupuncture on vasoconstriction and vasodilation and the rules by which this is governed, reports differ. Most of the evidence suggests that acupuncture lowers the degree of tension and relaxes the walls of blood vessels in patients with high levels of vasoconstriction. When the tension is too low, acupuncture induces an increase in tension and vasoconstriction. Of all the points chosen for stimulation, those on the extremities of the upper limbs proved most effective. Measurements taken on the fingers and ears showed that needling LI-4 *(Hegu)* and TB-5 *(Waiguan)* caused vasodilation, while needling P-6 *(Neiguan)* caused vasoconstriction. It was also discovered that needling at different depths and with varying intensities of stimulation brought different results.

The researchers believe that acupuncture has a distinct regulative effect on the permeability of the capillaries, i.e., when the permeability of the capillaries is high, acupuncture lowers it. The opposite response is found when a subject with low capillary permeability is needled.

After examining the effects of acupuncture on the lymph circulation in dogs, it was reported that acupuncture could relieve spasms in the lymph vessels, improve the circulation of the lymph, and lessen the effusion and formation of swelling that accompanies inflammation.

Acupuncture also clearly demonstrates a regulative effect upon blood pressure. It has been used clinically to treat both high and low blood pressure. (21-22) Not only can acupuncture regulate diastolic, systolic and mean arterial pressure, it also has a regulatory effect on pulse pressure. However, its greatest and most rapid effect is upon systolic pressure. After treating various kinds of shock, or conditions of low blood pressure, the blood pressure usually begins to increase from five to thirty minutes after needling, and its rise is rather steady. (23) At the same time that the blood pressure is raised, the functioning of the heart and other organs also generally improves. Acupuncture has proven most effective in cases of mild shock. In treating high blood pressure most researchers believe that from seven to ten treatments will reduce the blood pressure to its lowest level. After that, continued needling will bring only marginal gain. However, if treatment is resumed after a rest period of two or three weeks there will be a further reduction in blood pressure.

THE EFFECTS OF ACUPUNCTURE
ON THE RESPIRATORY AND URINARY SYSTEMS

The metabolic and excretory functions of the respiratory and urinary systems are affected in varying degrees by acupuncture.

At the Dalian Medical School and elsewhere, it was discovered that needling S-36 *(Zusanli)* on a healthy subject increased the ventilation capacity by 6.6%. The maximal breathing capacity increased 20%, with a 22% increase in expiratory volume. Needling S-42 *(Chongyang)*, S-45

(Lidui), Co-12 *(Zhongwan)* and related points also showed an increase in respiration and metabolism; however, the results were generally not as pronounced as when S-36 *(Zusanli)* was needled. Needling S-25 *(Tianshu),* S-21 *(Liangmen)* and related points, on the other hand, caused an inhibition of respiration. (24)

Zhongqing Medical School and others found the following evidence from experiments on animals: needling Gv-25 *(Suliao),* Gv-26 *(Renzhong)* and Co-1 *(Huiyin)* on laboratory animals (rabbits, cats, dogs) uniformly caused an immediate strengthening in breathing; if breathing is temporarily halted acupuncture can induce its resumption. Of these three points, Gv-25 *(Suliao)* and Gv-26 *(Renzhong)* showed a considerably higher rate of response than Co-1 *(Huiyin).* (92% of the cases responded to Gv-25, and 85% to Gv-26, compared with only a 43% response rate from Co-1. Furthermore, the degree of response after needling the former two points was more pronounced.) In the experiments it was also observed that the response to needling during inhalation was a strengthening of inhalation because the respiration center in the brain that controls inhalation is already in a state of excitation. Also, if the needling is performed during exhalation, the already excited state of the exhalation controlling center is further excited, and exhalation is correspondingly strengthened. (25)

With respect to the course along which the stimulus from the needle is transmitted to stimulate breathing, most researchers believe it is generally an immediate reflex action of the nerves. Stimulation of B-11 *(Dazhu),* B-12 *(Fengmen),* B-13 *(Feishu)* and similar points in which the effects were more delayed, are believed not to be reflexive in nature, however. The acupuncture stimulation which is used to treat bronchial asthma by relieving breathing difficulties and increasing the flow as well as the maximal breathing capacity, is believed to be primarily a nervous reflex. Acupuncture can reduce the activity of the parasympathetic nervous system while raising the level of excitation of the sympathetic nerves. This causes the bronchioles to expand and the mucous membranes to contract, thereby reducing effusion and leading ultimately to an improvement in the flow of air. Furthermore, in bronchial asthma, where the increase in the amounts of histamine and acetylcholine in the blood and the decrease in the amounts of substances such as adrenaline are interrelated, some people have suggested that acupuncture lowers the first two factors while causing an increase in the latter, jointly curing the condition.

At the Dalian Medical School and elsewhere, observations were made of the effects of acupuncture on the micturation of a healthy subject after drinking water. It was found that after needling K-6 *(Zhaohai)* the micturating function of the kidneys was strengthened. Using as a standard the average amount of urine passed during a 3 hour period after drinking water on an empty stomach, the acupuncture group showed a 19% increase over the control group. After S-36 *(Zusanli),* B-21 *(Weishu)* and related points were needled, however, there was no significant change. Needling B-23 *(Shenshu),* K-7 *(Fuliu)* and related points showed an inhibitory effect on micturation from the kidneys. (26) Based on clinical observations, some have found that needling B-23 *(Shenshu)* and related points on patients with nephritis caused a clear increase in the micturating function of the kidneys and in the amount of phenolsulfonphthalein excreted. This response can be maintained from two to three hours and, in exceptional cases, for several days. The degree of effectiveness of acupuncture in such cases is related to the condition of the kidneys themselves. Harbin Medical College's experiments on animals concluded that needling B-23 *(Shenshu)* to inhibit micturation caused a clear reduction in the filtration rate of the Bowman's capsules in the kidneys; using a novacaine block around B-23 *(Shenshu)* resulted in the disappearance of this response. It is believed that the needle stimulation possibly passes by means of a nervous reflex, altering the amount of blood flow through the Bowman's capsules and regulating their filtration rate. In addition, according to a report from the Shenxi Province Traditional Medicine Research Institute, using electro-acupuncture on animals can cause an increase in ADH. For this reason it is believed that acupuncture stimulation affects the tubular reabsorption of water via the function of ADH.

The principal influence of acupuncture on the bladder is related to its effect on bladder pressure. According to a report from the Second Shanghai Medical School, needling Co-4 *(Guanyuan),* K-15 *(Zhongzhu)* and related points on patients suffering from incontinence, causes various levels of reduction in the pressure of the bladder. On those patients with urine retention, acupuncture caused an increase of pressure. (27) Experiments on animals made at the Shanghai College of Traditional Medicine revealed that needling B-54 *(Weizhong)* on rabbits with high levels of bladder tension induced relaxation of this organ. Conversely, where bladder tension was low, acupuncture caused a contraction of the bladder. (28) Experiments have shown that this kind of regulatory effect occurs through a nervous reflex. (29)

THE EFFECTS OF ACUPUNCTURE ON THE IMMUNE SYSTEM

Acupuncture is effective in treating certain aspects of infectious diseases. Experimental research has clearly shown that acupuncture may reduce fever, increase the production of antibodies, and increase the body's resistance to inflammation.

The Jilin Medical College and others have performed experiments which show that moxibustion has a curative effect on arthritis. They applied acupuncture and moxibustion to S-36 *(Zusanli)* and other points on white rats with inflammatory granuloma on their backs. When they measured the amount of fluid that had effused from the sacs after eight days of treatment, they found that the moxibustion group averaged 3.59 ml., the electro-acupuncture group 3.45 ml., and the control group 7.03 ml. This shows that moxibustion and electro-acupuncture can inhibit effusion. (30) The Shenxi Provincial Research Institute investigated the effects of acupuncture on bacterial peritonitis in rabbits. They discovered that, under acupuncture treatment, the time needed for the inflamed cells to stop effusion, and for a culture made from the tissue to show a negative response to bacterial tests, was much shorter than in the control groups.

They also investigated how acupuncture can relieve spasms in the lymphatic vessels and lower capillary permeability. This can be particularly beneficial in cases of hemorrhagic inflammations. Investigating necrosis in white rats on which granuloma had formed, it was found that acupuncture not only checks and reduces the area of necrosis, but may also delay or prevent its development. It was shown that this was due to the ability of acupuncture to stimulate the phagocytic function of the reticuloendothelial system. (31-32) Acupuncture may also hasten the formation of granular tissue, strengthen the ability of cells to repair themselves and produce scar tissue. It was discovered after needling S-36 *(Zusanli)* and S-41 *(Jiexi)* on cats with ulcers of the cecum, that the alkaline phosphate reactions in the production of new epidermal skin cells occurred stronger and sooner. (33) This is helpful in the regeneration and return of function to the tissues.

When treating infection or inflammation with acupuncture, it was discovered that as the other symptoms improved, the accompanying fever was usually reduced to normal. In experimental investigations on animals, moxa was burned above M-BW-25 *(Shiqizhuixia);* alternatively, Gv-14 *(Dazhui)* and M-BW-25 *(Shiqizhuixia)* were stimulated with electro-acupuncture for three days, and on the fourth a fever inducing agent was injected. The fever responses in the groups treated with moxibustion and electro-acupuncture were much weaker than that of the control group, and the duration of the fever was shorter. Investigation was also pursued into the effects of acupuncture in lowering the temperature of experimentally induced fever. When animals were given electro-acupuncture at Gv-14 *(Dazhui)* for thirty seconds immediately after injection of a fever-inducing agent, the temperature of the animals declined markedly, then rose again slowly. The duration of the fever reaction was shorter and its intensity weaker than in a control group, and was in some cases effectively controlled. Investigating the effect of electro-acupuncture on prolonged fever caused by suppurative wounds, it was discovered that in the beginning, giving electro-acupuncture at S-36 *(Zusanli)* and other points would bring a marked drop in temperature, and that the average temperature of the experimental animals for the whole day was lower than in the animals of the control group. However, if this treatment was continued into the latter stages of the disease, it would cease to have any effect. (34)

The use of acupuncture in preventing infections is derived from its effect upon phagocytosis and the production of antibodies. Studies by the Beijing Medical School have shown that when S-36 *(Zusanli)* and Li-4 *(Zhongfeng)* are needled on a healthy person, phagocytization of Staphylococcus Aureus by leukocytes increased from one to two times (after moxibustion alone, it increaed by one-half). The ability of the cells to phagocytize is also raised. The highest value occurs twenty-four hours after needling. Using acupuncture to cure bacillary dysentery in the clinic, it was discovered that the phagocytic function of the leukocytes began to increase three hours after needling, and reached its highest point after twelve hours. The Shenxi Province Traditional Medicine Research Institute investigated the bacteriocidal capability of leukocytes before and after acupuncture on animals. They found that three to six hours after electro-acupuncture, the bacteriocidal function was at its highest and was above normal even after forty-eight hours. The regular acupuncture group achieved a similar level after three hours, but the duration was shorter, so that after forty-eight hours the level had essentially returned to normal. The moxibustion group showed still less effect. (35) Acupuncture generally increases the phagocytosis by the reticuloendothelial system, as was shown in experiments on animals conducted at the Jilin Medical College and elsewhere using moxibustion or electro-acupuncture at Gv-14 *(Dazhui)*, M-BW-25 *(Shiqizhuixia)*, S-36 *(Zusanli)* and other points. (30) The Shanghai College of Traditional Medicine found that needling S-36 *(Zusanli)*, B-23 *(Shenshu)*, B-18 *(Ganshu)*, or B-19 *(Danshu)* all stimulated phagocytosis. Studying the importance of the strength of stimulation, it was found that a deep penetration at Gv-14 *(Duzhui)* had the desired effect, but that a superficial one did not. (32)

In experiments performed by the Shenxi Province Traditional Medicine Research Institute, it was found that after needling a rabbit's S-36 *(Zusanli)* and Gv14 *(Dazhui)* there was an increase in the opsonin present in the blood, a substantial increase in phagocytosis by the leukocytes, and consequently an increase in the body's resistance to disease. The Jilin Medical College researched the effect of acupuncture combined with preventative injections. They twice injected a combined cholera/typhoid/paratyphoid AB vaccine at S-36 *(Zusanli)* for a total of 0.2 ml. (one-seventh the normal intradermic dosage). Afterwards they needled the point three times weekly and examined the blood three times at fixed intervals. The rate at which the bacteria were lysed by the acupuncture-vaccinated group was considerably higher than that of the control group, and the duration of the effect was longer. The Shenxi Province Traditional Medicine Research Institute investigated the use of acupuncture or electro-acupuncture on rabbits which had received diptheria vaccine, and found that the antibody titer went up, thereby indirectly raising the hemaglutination titer. (36)

THE EFFECTS OF ACUPUNCTURE ON THE ENDOCRINE SYSTEM

The hormones secreted by the endocrine glands play an important role in the body. Experiments have shown that acupuncture exerts varying degrees of influence on the endocrine glands and thereby indirectly influences other organs.

Acupuncture can affect the pituitary-adrenal cortex system. During clinical use of acupuncture in the treatment of appendicitis, it was discovered that within one or two days after acupuncture treatment began, the twenty-four hour urine count of 17-hydroxycorticosterone and 17-ketosteroid generally increased. (37) A blood test taken twenty minutes after needling S-36 *(Zusanli)* and LI-4 *(Hegu)* on healthy subjects showed that the 17-hydroxycorticosterone steroids content in the blood rose significantly, sometimes by as much as a factor of two or three, and was maintained at these levels for a considerable time. Simultaneously, the blood content of the eosinophils showed a corresponding decline. All of these changes show that the secretion of ACTH (adrenocorticotropic hormone) increased. Similar results have been obtained in experiments on animals. After regular acupuncture or electro-acupuncture, the blood content of 17-ketosteroids increased, the adrenal cortex became thicker and heavier, and the content of cholesterol and ascorbic acid in the adrenal cortex declined. (38) The Shenyang Scientific Medical Research Institute, using direct measurement methods, found that the ACTH content of the blood of white rats rose markedly after receiving electro-acupuncture. (39) This demonstrates that acupuncture can strengthen the functioning of the pituitary-adrenal cortex system and thereby raise the power of resistance of the body and hasten its recovery from disease. The effect that acupuncture induces upon the functions of the pituitary-adrenal cortex system has a direct relation to the original state of the system, with acupuncture serving a regulatory function.

Acupuncture can also regulate the thyroid gland. The Shenxi Province Traditional Medicine Research Institute found that when acupuncture was used in the treatment of endemic goiter, not only did the goiter shrink and the symptoms improve or disappear, but also the amount of iodine in the urine markedly decreased and the ability of the thyroid to absorb and use iodine was increased. In cases of hyperthyroidism, acupuncture can shrink the thyroid and reduce the basic metabolism. Experiments conducted on animals by the Jilin Medical College and others also show that acupuncture generally has a regulatory effect on metabolism, raising the tension of individual tissues and cells of the glands, increasing the rate at which the organism uses the body's iodine, and thereby satisfying the body's need for thyroxine under conditions when the supply of iodine is not increased and the thyroid gland is still small.

It has been shown in experiments on animals that electro-acupuncture reflexively releases oxytocin, vasopressin, and norepinephrine. After performing acupuncture on animals in shock at Gv-25 *(Suliao)*, the blood pressure slowly returned to normal and stayed there. Giving electro-acupuncture will raise the blood sugar level if it is low, or lower it if it is too high. In addition to passing through nerve reflexes, this kind of regulatory effect may also involve the participation of insulin and adrenalin regulation.

Acupuncture also has an influence on sex hormones. For example, if one gives acupuncture to women with certain diseases which prevent conception, it will hasten the normalization of the ovulation and menstruation cycles. In experiments on rabbits, after acupuncture the cells around the ovaries became luteinized and the follicle membrane became thicker, which shows that the secretion of the luteinizing hormone increased. (40) The Shanghai Physiological Research Institute has proven that after needling Co-17 *(Shanzhong)*, SI-1 *(Shaoze)*, LI-4 *(Hegu)* and related points on mothers who lacked milk, the prolactin in the blood increased. (41) This shows that perhaps the ability of acupuncture to increase the production of milk is due to its capacity to increase the secretion of prolactin by the anterior pituitary, and the secretion of oxytocin by the posterior pituitary.

THE EFFECTS OF ACUPUNCTURE ON THE NERVOUS SYSTEM

Acupuncture has a curative effect on nervous diseases. It is generally believed that acupuncture, by using a method suitable to the stimulation of the nerve receptors in the area of a point, transmits a signal to a particular level of the central nervous system, which in turn influences the target organ. When the local tissue is stimulated by acupuncture, it gives rise to some of the same biochemical changes that accompany inflammation, thereby prolonging the stimulation around the point which, mediated through the nerves or a combination of nerves and body fluids, prevents and cures disease.

The special characteristic of nerves is excitability. Experiments on animals have shown that using an acupuncture needle to stimulate the outer surface of the nerve trunk from five to thirty times, excited the nerves and made the muscles they controlled contract. When the nerve trunks themselves were needled, half of the time the muscles were stimulated and, in the remaining half, some showed no particular effect while in others the level of muscle contraction diminished. The increase in the nerves' excitability continues for several minutes after needling has ended. If the needling continues before the level of excitability returns to normal, one can raise the excitability of the nerve trunks still higher. This shows that acupuncture has a continuous and cumulative effect. (43)

Clinically, acupuncture is often used to treat nervous disorders. The Chinese Academy of Medical Science and the Shanghai College of Traditional Medicine have demonstrated in experiments on animals that acupuncture can restore the functioning of muscles in which part of the nerves have been injured. In these experiments, the muscles' electrical potential was used as the measure of their health. Twenty days after the nerves were injured, the electrical potential of the muscles in the group which was treated with acupuncture returned to 50% of pre-operative levels. After fifty days it had returned to 103% of pre-operative levels. The control group returned to about 65% of pre-operative levels after fifty days, and there was no further improvement even after four months. (44) This recovery effect may be due to acupuncture causing acceleration in the growth of the wounded nerve fibers' buds, or to its causing the tissue to release a non-specific substance that stimulates the growth of the bud. Experiments performed by the Jilin Medical College have shown that biochemical changes associated with hastening the regeneration of nerves and the recovery of their function occur after acupuncture treatment.

The Shenxi Province Acupuncture and Moxibustion Research Institute used an oscillograph to investigate the influence of differing intensities and durations of electrical stimulation on the action potential of the sciatic nerves of toads. With the frequency of stimulation set at fifty times per minute, the rate of change in the nerves' electrical potential rose with the gradual increase in the strength of the stimulation. When the degree of stimulation passed a certain limit, the action potentials were at their greatest. This shows that the excitability of nerve activity and the strength of stimulation are closely related. After stimulation for a period of time at the point of maximum action potential, with the frequency and strength of stimulation still constant, the action potential will manifest a progressive decline, usually within the first fifteen minutes. In the beginning the rate of change is small, but at thirty minutes the decline becomes rather rapid. (45) This phenomenon shows that a thorough knowledge of the strength, frequency, and duration of stimulation is very important.

Different strengths of needling manifest different effects on the central nervous system. According to a report by the Hebei Medical School, differences in the strength of stimulation regularly result in different changes in the visual cortex. Strong stimulation causes the development of inhibitory processes in the area, whereas weak stimulation is half of the time stimulating and half of the time inhibitory. When the central nervous system is in a significantly inhibitory state, strong stimulation will weaken or remove the state of inhibition, while weak stimulation will produce the opposite effect. When the stimulatory processes are stronger than the inhibitory ones, both weak and strong stimulation have an inhibitory effect, and cause the processes to return to balance. (46) These experimental results are basically consistent with clincial experience. They show that when the active processes of the central nervous system surpass a certain level and are influenced by strong needling, they move toward balance.

It is very common to see stimulation of the same strength produce different results because of the differing functional states of the nervous system. The Shenxi Province Traditional Medicine Research Institute conducted experiments on dogs to investigate the effects of electro-acupuncture on differing states in certain areas of the central nervous system. Before the experiments, medium dosages of caffeine sodium benzoate were injected intradermally. After electro-acupuncture, the excessive secretion of saliva (a reaction to the injection) was reduced or eliminated. Prior to another experiment, dogs were given a small dosage of sodium bromide orally and the secretion of saliva decreased. After electro-acupuncture, the level of secretion continued to decline, but then slowly returned to normal levels. (47)

We can see that the regulatory function of electro-acupuncture encompasses both stimulation and inhibition, and is capable of producing either response, depending on the original state of the cerebral cortex. The state of the cerebral cortex also influences the effect of electro-acupuncture upon the activity of the higher levels of the nervous system. Some experiments have shown that when the central nervous system is under the stimulating effects of caffeine, acupuncture therapy, particularly where a lengthy period of stimulation is used, has an inhibitory effect. Conversely, experiments on subjects under the inhibitory influence of sodium bromide showed that shorter periods of stimulation will cause a decline or disappearance of the inhibitory state more effectively than longer periods of stimulation.

Clinically, acupuncture has demonstrated a broad effect in the treatment of digestive, respiratory and circulatory diseases. It has been proved experimentally that this is due to the influence of acupuncture on the autonomic nervous system. The autonomic nervous system, working within the higher nervous centers, regulates the internal organs. In general, those tissues which are stimulated by sympathetic nerves are inhibited by parasympathetic nerves, and vice versa. As stated above, the effect of acupuncture is usually related to the original state of the body. Some researchers using histamine and adrenalin to conduct experiments with skin tests and ocular pressure reflexes, found that during the period when the autonomic nervous system was over-excited in patients with gastric ulcers, acupuncture caused a decline in the level of excitement. If the autonomic nervous system was functioning abnormally, acupuncture brought it back to normal. In the treatment of gastrointestinal spasms, acupuncture raises the parasympathetic tone, increases the strength of peristalsis, and has a marked regulatory effect on the functions of the autonomic nervous system. In experiments on animals, after raising the blood pressure by an injection of adrenalin, it was found that acupuncture reduces it rather quickly. On the other hand, after injecting acetylcholine (which lowers the blood pressure), acupuncture raises the blood pressure. (48) After strengthening intestinal peristalsis by injections of pilocarpine (a cholinomimetic drug), acupuncture was shown to weaken the peristalsis. (49) Some experiments have been designed to investigate the changes in the body fluids after acupuncture, and have demonstrated that acupuncture has a homeostatic effect. In some circumstances the stimulation of the sympathetic nerves is most important; in others, the release of histamine and acetylcholine is most important. When acupuncture is given to induce labor, the cholinesterase content of the mother's blood will rise. During acute appendicitis, the acetylcholine content of the blood rises; after acupuncture treatment, it falls. These substances all have an important regulatory effect on the body's physiological processes.

Other experiments were used to study the changes in metabolic chemistry of the brain tissue to see what effect acupuncture has on the activities of the higher nervous centers of the cerebrum. The Shenxi Province Traditional Medicine Research Institute measured the changes in the brain amines before and after acupuncture, and discovered that there is a marked increase in the ammonia content of the brain after needling, which disappears within fiften minutes. This shows that acupuncture can temporarily place the brain in an excitory state where the protein metabolism is increased. Five minutes after needling there is a marked increase in the glutamine content, which is related to the restoration of excitory processes. (50) Experiments have also shown that acupuncture has an effect on the metabolism of glucose in the brain tissues. Acupuncture increases the concentration of lactic acid (an intermediary product of glucose metabolism) in the brain of normal animals, with a twenty minute period of stimulation giving the best results. If needling is continued for thirty to forty minutes, the level will fall below normal. Within thirty minutes after stimulation ends, the concentration of lactic acid returns to normal. Acupuncture can raise the low level of lactic acid in the brain during anesthesia, and lower the high level of lactic acid in the brain during convulsions. (51) Again, this demonstrates that the different physiological effects of acupuncture are dependent upon the different organic states of the body.

The processes of nervous stimulation and inhibition share a close relationship with the chemical transmitters in the nervous tissue. When the central nervous system's activities are in an inhibitory state, there is an abundance of acetylcholine in the brain tissue; in a state of excitation, on the other hand, the amount is reduced. The clinical use of acupuncture anesthesia has verified the inhibitory effect of acupuncture. Experiments with animals proved that the acetylcholine content of the brain in the groups given electro-acupuncture was greater than that of control groups. In a state of deep anesthesia, the activity of the brain is reduced and there is a great amount of acetylcholine present. Acupuncture can lower that content and revive the anesthetized animals earlier than usual. (52) Other experiments have investigated the influence of acupuncture on the amount of norepinephrine in animals' brains. It was found that after thirty minutes of electro-acupuncture, the level of norepinephrine significantly decreased. (53) Norepinephrine is most prevalent in the brain stem and hypothalamus; thus there are those who think that acpuncture stimulation has its greatest effect on these locations.

Much research has been done concerning the relationship between acupuncture and the function of the reticular formation in the brainstem, which includes ascending and descending systems. These systems have a close relationship with the sensory, motor and visceral activities and serve an important regulatory function. The ascending system projects to every center in the cerebrum (called non-specific projection) and maintains the state of excitement in the cerebral cortex. The group that descends influences the functioning of the spinal cord and of the autonomic nervous system. The Shanghai College of Traditional Medicine has shown in experiments on animals that giving acupuncture at S-36 *(Zusanli)* and S-37 *(Shangjuxu)* suppresses pain and regulates the function of the stomach and intestines. If the reticular formations are injured or anesthetized, however, this does not occur. (54-55) the Guangxi Medical School showed in experiments on animals that acupuncture has a regulatory effect on blood pressure, but that if the nerve trunks to the points are cut, or if the connection between the medulla and spinal cord is severed, this effect ceases. If neither the nerve trunks nor the brain stem are injured, but only the cerebrum is removed, causing the acupuncture stimulation to be transmitted only to the brain stem, then the effect of regulating blood pressure remains.

The Shanghai Physiological Research Institute has divided nerve fibers into three groups by diameter. Modern research has discovered that the path of every sensory signal is different, and that the pain signal is carried by the thinnest kind of nerve. The thicker nerve fibers have an inhibitory effect on the thinner nerve fibers' activities, and among these fibers, the inhibitory effect of the second group on the thinnest group is most pronounced. Tiny electrodes were planted in single cells of an animal's spinal cord or thalamus, and when the animal received a strong pain stimulation, the electrical response in the cell lessened or disappeared. From this we can see that the ability of acupuncture to suppress pain and anesthetize may be derived from the capacity of the non-pain signal to override the pain signal. (57) According to investigations made by the Shanghai College of Traditional Medicine of electro-acupuncture, the electrical discharge of the pain reactive cells in the reticular formation decreases during electro-acupuncture but slowly returns to normal when the treatment is stopped. This process of slow change strongly suggests that an analgesic chemical may exist. In tests involving the exchange of blood between white rats, it was discovered that the pain threshold of rats which had received acpuncture was raised. Later, the pain threshold of rats which had not been given acupuncture but which had received the blood of those which had, was also raised. This demonstrates that some substances in the body fluids participate in the analgesic function of acupuncture.* (58)

The basis of acupuncture is still being studied from many different aspects. Some preliminary views include:

The analgesic function of acupuncture derives from the clashing of the biochemical lines of acupuncture and those of the pain stimulus in the transmitting processes of the central nervous system, the former overriding the latter.

Acupuncture strengthens the cerebral cortex's inhibiting processes and raises the pain threshold.

Acupuncture has an effect on the reticular structures of the brain stem and the limbic system of the cerebrum.

Acupuncture stimulates the sympathetic nerve centers of the hypothalmus, and its functions are mediated by the sympathetic nerves.

Acupuncture's effect is transmitted through the chemicals in the body's fluids.

However, none of these hypotheses can completely explain the basis on which acupuncture and acupuncture anesthesia operate, or fully answer the question of the existence and nature of the channels.

---

*Recently there has been a considerable amount of research conducted with respect to the physiological effects of acupuncture. The results of this research are published in English. Much of this research deals with the relationship between acupuncture and the endorphins. Endorphins are chemicals produced by the body which perform many functions, most notably as analgesics. (Endorphin means endogenous opiate.) As a supplement to this section, we have included a list of references to research reports available in English, including those on endorphins. This list follows the bibliography to this chapter.—*Editors*

BIBLIOGRAPHY (Chinese Sources)

1. Yangpu District Central Hospital, Shanghai, et al. Investigations by x-ray into acupuncture induced changes in the strength of stomach movements. *Selected Material from the National Traditional Medicine, Channel and Acupuncture Conference,* 1959; X-ray investigations into the influence of stimulating S-36 *(Zusanli)* on peristalsis of the stomach. *The Shanghai Journal of Traditional Medicine,* 7, 1964.

2. The Second Military Medical College. Preliminary discussion on x-ray investigations into the effect of needling a dog's S-36 *(Zusanli)* on the movement of its pylorus. *Selected Materials from the National Traditional Medicine, Channel and Acupuncture Conference,* 1959.

3. Guangzhou Second People's Hospital. Preliminary discussion on barium fluorscopic investigations into the effect of needling S-36 *(Zusanli)* on gastric peristalsis and its clinical application. *Guangdong Traditional Medicine,* 3, 1962.

4. Shanghai College of Traditional Medicine. Preliminary discussion on x-ray investigations into the effect of acupuncture on gastric peristalsis and the selection of points. *Compilation of the Scientific Research of the Shanghai College of Traditional Medicine,* Vol. 2, 1959.

5. The First Teaching Hospital of the Jiangxi Medical School. Preliminary x-ray investigations into the effects on the function of the stomach of needling B-21 *(Weishu)* and S-36 (Zusanli). *Jiangxi Traditional Medicine,* 4, 1959.

6. Xian Number One Hospital. X-ray research into the effects of acupuncture on changes in the function of the stomach and the expelling of liquids from the stomach. *A Selection of Essays on Acupuncture,* 1961.

7. Shanghai College of Traditional Medicine. Analysis of the relationship between needling S-36 *(Zusanli)* of rabbits and the movements of the small intestine. *Materials from the National Conference to Exchange Experiences Related to Combined Traditional Western Medical Work,* 1960.

8. Shanghai Number One Hospital. Preliminary discussion on the ability of acupuncture to cure appendicitis. *Op. cit.* Ref. 7.

9. Shanghai Number Two Hospital. Research into the effect of acupuncture on changes in intestinal peristalsis. *Op cit.* Ref. 7.

10. Shanghai Hospital of Thoracic Medicine. Investigation into the effect of needling Co-12 *(Zhongwan)* on the function of the gastrointestinal tract. *The Shanghai Journal of Traditional Medicine,* 10, 1959.

11. Yangpu District Central Hospital, Shanghai, et al. X-ray investigations into acupuncture and changes in the strength of the gall bladder. *Op. cit.* Ref. 7.

12. Shenxi Province Traditional Medicine Research Institute. Preliminary report concerning the effect of acupuncture on the state of the gall bladder. *The Journal of Traditional Medicine,* 2, 1963.

13. Shanghai Number Two Hospital. The effect of acupuncture on changes in the pressure of the bile duct. *The Chinese Journal of Surgery,* 11-4, 1973.

14. Guangdong College of Traditional Medicine, et al. The effect of needling M-UE-9 *(Sifeng)* on the bile and secretions of the armpits. *Selections from the Guangdong Conference to Exchange Experiences Related to Combined Traditional and Western Medical Work,* 1961.

15. The Shanghai City Coordinating Group to Research the Curing of Appendicitis with Acupuncture. A preliminary discussion on the effectiveness of acupuncture in curing acute appendicitis and its mechanisms. *Op. cit.* Ref. 2.

16. Shanghai College of Traditional Medicine. A preliminary investigation into the effects of different needling techniques on the colon. *Compilation of the Scientific Research of the Shanghai College of Traditional Medicine,* Vol. 3, 1961.

17. The effect of acupuncture on the blood. Abstract from *The Jiangxi Medical Journal,* 11 (4), 1964.

18. Acupuncture Research Institute of the Academy of Traditional Medicine, et al. Research concerning the effects of needling points of different channels on human eletrocardiograms, electroencephalograms, respiration, and on electrical reflexes of the skin. *Tenth Anniversary of the Founding of the People's Republic of China Commemorative Collection of Selections of Scientific Papers of the Academy of Traditional Medicine,* 1959.

19. Shanghai College of Traditional Medicine. A preliminary report on the effect of acupuncture on the action electrical current of the heart. *Op. cit.* Ref. 2.

540

20. Heilungjiang Provincial Research Institute of Our Motherland's Medicine. Experimental report of the effect on the electrocardiogram of needling B-15 *(Xinshu)*. *Harbin Traditional Medicine*, 6, 1961; The effect of giving acupuncture and moxibustion at Co-5 *(Shimen)* on the electrocardiograms of hypertensive patients. *Heilungjiang Research on Traditional Medicine*, 3, 1963.

21. Shanghai Institute of Physiology. A preliminary discussion on the ability of acupuncture to hasten the restoration of blood pressure to a normal level and its mechanisms in the central nervous system. *Op. cit.* Ref. 7.

22. Shanghai College of Traditional Medicine. The influence of moxibustion on the capacitance of the fingers in hypertensive patients. *The Shanghai Journal of Traditional Medicine*, 8, 1964.

23. The Second Shanghai Medical School. Experimental research on and clinical application of moxibustion in the prevention and treatment of shock. *The Chinese Journal of Surgery*, 1, 1963.

24. Dalian Medical School. Discussion of the effect of acupuncture on the activities of the inner organs and the mechanism of its function. *Materials from the National Conference to Exchange Experiences Related to Combined Traditional Western Medical Work*, 1961.

25. Zhongjing Medical School. The reflexive effect of needling sensitive points on the body's surface and the respiratory function. *Op. cit.* Ref. 2.

26. Harbin Medical College. Research into the nature of the channels and the mechanisms of acupuncture. *Op. cit.* Ref. 2.

27. The Second Shanghai Medical School. The effect of acupuncture on the pressure of the bladder. *Op. cit.* Ref. 2.

28. Shanghai College of Traditional Medicine. The effect of acupuncture on tension of the bladder: A preliminary report on the effect of acupuncture on the urinary functions of the kidneys. *Op. cit.* Ref. 7.

29. The Seventh Military Medical School. Research on the mechanisms involved in the effect on the bladder of acupuncture. *The Chinese Journal of Surgery*, 7, 1961.

30. Jilin Medical College. The effects of acupuncture on the main immune and adaptive functions of the body. *Op. cit.* Ref. 24.

31. Guangxi Medical School. Research concerning the effects of acupuncture on the functions of the reticuloendothelial system and its related mechanism. *Op. cit.* Ref. 24.

32. Shanghai College of Traditional Medicine. The effects of acupuncture and moxibustion on the phagocytic function of the reticuloendothelial system in rabbits. *Shanghai Journal of Traditional Medicine*, 4, 1965.

33. Zhongjing Medical School. Some materials on the effects of acupuncture on the organism's immune reactions. *Op. cit.* Ref. 24.

34. Shenxi Province Xian School of Hygiene. The effect of electro-acupuncture on the phagocytic function of leukocytes. *Selected Materials on Electro-acupuncture*, Vol. 1, 1959.

35. Shenxi Province Traditional Medicine Research Institute. The effects of acupuncture on the bacteriocidal ability of the blood in rabbits. *A Collection of Research Materials Concerning Traditional Medicine*, 1964.

36. The occurence of immune responses under the influence of electro- and regular acupuncture. *Chinese Medical Journal*, 12, 1958.

37. A preliminary discussion of the treatment of acute appendicitis using acupuncture in Shanghai City, and its related mechanisms. *Op. cit.* Ref. 2.

38. Hebei Medical School. Organic chemical investigations into the effect of needling S-36 *(Zusanli)* on the function of the adrenal gland in rabbits. *Shanghai Journal of Traditional Medicine*, 12, 1963.

39. Shenyang Medical Science Research Institute. The effects of acupuncture stimulation on the blood content of ACTH in normal rats and in those whose adrenal gland has been removed. *A Selection of Papers on the Study of Acupuncture*, 1964.

40. Department of Obstetrics and Gynecology, Wuhan Medical School. The effect of acupuncture on the functioning and condition of the ovaries. *Chinese Medical Journal*, 11, 1961.

41. Shanghai Institute of Physiology. The effect of acupuncture and moxibustion on the prolactin content of the blood in mothers who lack milk. *Shanghai Journal of Traditional Medicine*, 12, 1958.

42. Shenxi Province Traditional Medicine Research Institute. The influence of regular and electro-acupuncture on the endocrine system. *A Collection of Research Materials Concerning Traditional Medicine,* Vol. 1, 1964.

43. Liaoning Branch of the Chinese Medical Association. Experimental research on acupuncture and the body's senses. *Selection of Papers from the Acupuncture Study Conference,* 1964.

44. Experimental Medical Research Institute of the Chinese Academy of Medical Sciences. The effect of acupuncture on experimentally injured peripheral nerves. *Op. cit.* Ref. 2; Shanghai College of Traditional Medicine. The ability of acupuncture to restore function in muscles whose nerves have been partially removed. *Op. cit.* Ref. 7.

45. Shenxi Province Traditional Medicine Research Institute. The effect of differing strengths and durations of acupuncture stimulation on the action potential of the sciatic nerve in toads. *Materials from the Conference on Study Reports of the Shenxi Province Acupuncture Research Institute,* [no date].

46. Hebei Medical School. On the question of the mechanism of acupuncture treatment and the nature of the channels. *Op. cit.* Ref. 24.

47. Shenxi Province Traditional Medicine Research Institue. *Op. cit.* Ref. 24.

48. Lanzhou Medical School. Some research into the channels and their relation to the mechanism of acupuncture. *Development of Physiological Science,* 2, 1960.

49. Shanghai College of Traditional Medicine. Preliminary discussion on the effect of needling S-36 *(Zusanli)* on the movements of rabbits' stomachs and related mechanisms. *Op. cit.* Ref. 2.

50. Shenxi Province Traditional Medicine Research Institute. Looking at the biochemical basis of the mechanisms of regular and electro-acupuncture through changes in the brain ammonia content. *Journal of Acupuncture,* 2, 1966.

51. Shenxi Province Traditional Medicine Research Institute. The effects of regular and electro-acupuncture on glucose metabolism in animals' brains. *A Collection of Research Materials Concerning Traditional Medicine,* Vol. 2, 1965.

52. Shenxi Province Traditional Medicine Research Institute. The effects of regular and electro-acupuncture on the amount of acetylcholine in the brain under different functional states in animals. *Op. cit.* Ref. 51.

53. Shenxi Province Traditional Medicine Research Institute. The effect of regular and electro-acupuncture on the level of norepinephrine in the brain tissue. *Op. cit.* Ref. 51.

54. Shanghai College of Traditional Medicine. The reason for the saying "Leave the needle in S-36 *(Zusanli)* to benefit the abdomen." *A Collection of Papers Discussing the Basis of Acupuncture Anesthesia,* Vol. 1, 1972.

55. Shanghai College of Traditional Medicine. Discussion of the function of the reticular structures of the midbrain in acupuncture anesthesia. *Op. cit.* Ref. 54.

56. Guangxi Medical School. The activities of the reticular structures of the brain stem and acupuncture anesthesia. *Op. cit.* Ref. 54.

57. Shanghai Institute of Physiology. The struggle between the feeling and non-feeling of pain in acupuncture anesthesia. *Op. cit.* Ref. 54.

58. Shanghai Traditional Medicine Research Institute. Investigations into the fluid factor in acupuncture analgesia. *Op. cit.* Ref. 54.

EDITORS' SELECTED BIBLIOGRAPHY OF CURRENT RESEARCH
CONCERNING THE EFFECTS OF ACUPUNCTURE
(English Sources)

General

Chang H.T. Acupuncture analgesia today. *Chinese Medical Journal* 92:7, 1979.

Chung S. H. and Dickensen, A. Pain, encephalin and acupuncture. *Nature* 283:243, 1980.

Liao S.J. Recent advances in the understanding of acupuncture. *The Yale Journal of Biology and Medicine* 51:55, 1978.

Lu G.D. and Needham, J. *Celestial Lancets: A History and Rationale of Acupuncture and Moxa.* New York: Cambridge University Press, 1980. pp. 184-262.

Wei L.Y. Scientific advances in acupuncture. *American Journal of Chinese Medicine* 7:53, 1978.

Points

Hou Z.L. A study of the histologic structure of acupuncture points and types of fibers conveying needling sensation. *Chinese Medical Journal* 92:223, 1979.

Oleson, T.D. et al. An experimental evaluation of auricular diagnosis: the somatotopic mapping of musculoskeletal pain at ear acupuncture points. *Pain* 8:217, 1980.

Plummer, J.P. Anatomical findings at acupuncture loci. *American Journal of Chinese Medicine* 8:170, 1980.

Central Nervous System

Acupuncture Anesthesia Coordinating Group, Hua Shan Hospital of Shanghai 1st Medical College. Observation on electrical stimulation of the caudate nuclei of human brain and acupuncture in treatment of intractable pain. *Chinese Medical Journal* 3:117, 1977.

Cheng, R. and Pomeranz, B. Electro-acupuncture analgesia could be mediated by at least two pain relieving mechanisms: endorphin and non-endorphin systems. *Life Sciences* 25:1957, 1979.

Chiang Chen-yu, et al. Effects of electrolytic lesions on intracerebral injections of 5,6—dihydroxytryptamine in raphe nuclei on acupuncture analgesia in rats. *Chinese Medical Journal* 92:129, 1979.

Ghia, J.N. et al. Acupuncture and chronic pain mechanisms. *Pain* 2:285, 1976.

Lu, G. et al. Role of peripheral afferent nerve fiber in acupuncture analgesia elicited by needling point zusanli. *Scientia Sinica* 22:680, 1979.

Hans, J.S. et al. Central neurotransmitters in acupuncture analgesia. *American Journal of Chinese Medicine* 8:333, 1980.

Chang H.T. Neurophysiological basis of acupuncture analgesia. *Scientia Sinica* 21:829, 1978.

Mayer, D.J. et al. Antagonism of acupuncture analgesia in man by the narcotic antagonist naloxone. *Brain Research* 121:368, 1977.

Peets, J. and Pomeranz, B. CXBK mice deficient in opiate receptors show poor electro-acupuncture analgesia. *Nature* 273:675, 1978.

Pomeranz, B. Do endorphins mediate acupuncture analgesia? *Advances in Biochemical Psychopharmacology* 18:351, 1978.

Pomeranz, B. et al. Electro-acupuncture is mediated by stereospecific opiate receptors and is reversed by antagonists of Type I receptors. *Life Sciences* 26:631, 1980.

Shen, E. et al. Involvement of descending inhibition in the effect of acupuncture on the splanchnically evoked potential in the orbital cortex of cat. *Scientia Sinica* 21:677, 1978.

Sjolund, B. et al. Increased cerebrospinal fluid levels of endorphins after electro-acupuncture. *Acta Physiologica Scandinavia* 100:382, 1977.

Toda, K. and Iriki, A. Effects of electro-acupuncture on thalamic evoked responses recorded from the ventrobasal complex and posterior nuclear group after tooth pulp stimulation in rat. *Experimental Neurology* 66:419, 1979.

543

Wen H.L. et al. The influence of electro-acupuncture on naloxone-induced morphine withdrawal. *American Journal of Chinese Medicine* 7:237, 1979.

Wen H.L. et al. Immunoassayable beta-endorphin level in the plasma and CSF of heroin addicted and normal subjects before and after electro-acupuncture. *American Journal of Chinese Medicine* 8:154, 1980.

Physiology

Cheng R. et al. Electro-acupuncture elevates blood cortisol levels in naive horses: sham treatment has no effect. *International Journal of Neuroscience* 10:95, 1980.

Chu Y.M. and Affrontic, L.F. Preliminary observations on the effects of acupuncture on immune responses in sensitized rabbits and guinea pigs. *American Journal of Chinese Medicine* 3:151, 1975.

Kline, R.L. et al. Role of somatic nerves in the cardiovascular responses to stimulation of an acupuncture point in anesthetized rabbits. *Experimental Neurology* 61:561, 1978.

Liao Y.Y. et al. Effect of acupuncture on adrenal hormone production: I. variation in the ability for adrenocortical hormone production in relation to the duration of acupuncture stimulation. *American Journal of Chinese Medicine* 7:362, 1979.

Liao Y.Y. et al. Effects of acupuncture on the citrate and glucose metabolism in the liver under various types of stress. *American Journal of Chinese Medicine* 8:354, 1980.

Liao Y.Y. et al. Effect of acupuncture on adrenal hormone production: II. Effect of acupuncture on the response of adrenocortical hormone production to stress. *American Journal of Chinese Medicine* 8:160, 1980.

Sodipo, J.O. and Falaiye, J.M. Acupuncture and gastric acid studies. *American Journal of Chinese Medicine* 7:356, 1979.

Wu C.C. and Hsu C.J. Neurogenic regulation of lipid metabolism in the rabbit: a mechanism for the cholesterol-lowering effect of acupuncture. *Atherosclerosis* 33:153, 1979.

Clinical

Berger, D. and Nolte, D. Acupuncture in bronchial asthma: bodyplethysmographic measurements of acute bronchospasmolytic effects. *Comparative Medicine East-West* 5:265, 1977.

Caesarean Section Acupuncture Anesthesia Unit, Beijing Obstetrics and Gynecology Hospital. Clinical analysis of 1,000 cases of cesarean section under acupuncture anesthesia. *Chinese Medical Journal* 93:221, 1980.

Chiao S.F. Scalp acupuncture in brain diseases. *Chinese Medical Journal* 3:325, 1977.

Coan, R.M. et al. The acupuncture treatment of low back pain: a randomized controlled study. *American Journal of Chinese Medicine* 8:181, 1980.

Hyodo M. and Gega O. Use of acupuncture anesthesia for normal delivery. *American Journal of Chinese Medicine* 5:63, 1977.

Kane, J. and DiScipio, W.J. Acupuncture treatment of schizophrenia: report on three cases. *American Journal of Psychiatry* 136:297, 1979.

Mao W. et al. High versus low intensity acupuncture analgesia for treatment of chronic pain: effects on platelet serotonin. *Pain* 136:297, 1979.

People's Liberation Army 202nd Hospital. Acupuncture point injection in pediatric pneumonia: report of 4,060 cases. *Chinese Medical Journal* 4:51, 1978.

Reuler, J.B. et al. The chronic pain syndrome: misconceptions and management. *Annals of Internal Medicine* 93:588, 1980.

Stern, J.A. et al. A comparison of hypnosis, acupuncture, morphine, valium, aspirin, and placebo in the management of experimentally induced pain. *Annals of New York Academy of Science* 296:175, 1977.

Tashkin, D.P. et al. Comparison of real and simulated acupuncture and isoproterenal in methacholine-induced asthma. *Annals of Allergy* 39:379, 1977.

Tsuei J.J. et al. The influence of acupuncture stimulation during pregnancy: the induction and inhibition of labor. *Obstetrics and Gynecology* 50:479, 1977.

Wong S. and Ching R. The use of acupuncture in ophthalmology. *American Journal of Chinese Medicine* 8:104, 1980.

Yip S.K. et al. Induction of labor by acupuncture electro-stimulation. *American Journal of Chinese Medicine* 4:257, 1976.

Yu D.Y. and Lee S.P. Effect of acupuncture on bronchial asthma. *Clinical Science and Molecular Medicine* 51:503, 1976.

Section IV

Therapy

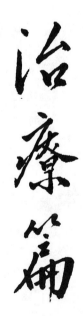

Chapter 1

Principles of Acupuncture Therapy

Treating the Disease and Treating the Person

The curing of disease depends primarily upon the body's internal powers of resistance and only secondarily on treatment. The fundamental view of therapy in Chinese medicine is expressed in the phrase "support what is normal, expel what is abnormal." "Normal" refers to a balance within the organism, the capacity to defend and adapt itself to a changing environment. "Abnormal" refers to harmful elements which upset the normal functioning and development of the body, thereby causing disease. Generally speaking, "supporting what is normal" occupies a more important place than "expelling what is abnormal." This is consistent with Chairman Mao's teaching: "The basic cause in the development of things is not to be found externally, but rather internally, that is, upon internal contradictions." When practicing medicine, doctors must resist the practice of examining the disease but ignoring the patient, or examining the patient but ignoring his attitude. Instead, they should actively encourage the patient to maintain a spirit of optimism and confidence in order that the patient may help himself to the fullest.

This approach has taken on fresh significance in the field of acupuncture anesthesia where the patient receives surgery while fully conscious. For example, when the chest cavity is opened during pneumonectomy, the patient can cooperate by maintaining slow, abdominal breathing, thereby reducing the occurance of mediastinal flutter.

With its high regard for internal factors in the treatment of disease, traditional medicine focuses on the capacity of acupuncture therapy to regulate the Qi. One can thereby balance the Yin and Yang, i.e., the reciprocal relationships among the material and functional activities of the tissues and organs of the body. Disease is manifested by an imbalance in the system, either of Excess or Deficiency. Acupuncture effectively regulates the functioning of the body and strengthens its resistance to disease. Thus: "Because it has been regulated, the Normal Qi is stabilized and the Excessive Qi destroyed." [1]

Local and Systemic

"When a Marxist views a problem, he looks not only at the parts but also at the whole." (Mao Zedong) A symptom appearing at one place in the body is often only a part of a systemic disorder. For example, abdominal pain may not only appear as a local manifestation of disease in an organ of the digestive or urogenital systems, but is often found in diseases of the respiratory, circulatory or nervous systems as well. Therefore, when treating a disease, one must consider the relationship between the parts and the whole.

When stimulating points or channels in the course of acupuncture therapy, not only will there be a local effect upon neighboring tissues and organs, but also a systemic effect upon the organism in general. For instance, the Stomach channel connects the face with the chest, abdomen, and lower limbs on the front of the body. Each of the points on this channel can be used to treat disorders in the area near the point, e.g., points on the face treat disease of the face, those on the abdomen treat abdominal disease, etc. However, a point may also be used to affect conditions quite distant from its location. Thus, for example, the points on the Stomach channel below the knee are commonly selected for treating disease of the chest, abdomen, throat and face. And, owing to the Yang/Yin relationship between the Stomach and Spleen channels, stimulation of points on the Stomach channel has a definite effect on the Spleen. For this reason, only when one understands the relation between the parts and the whole, and can select points and administer treatment based on the integrated view of channel theory, will one be able to avoid the narrow approach of merely treating the head when the head hurts, or the foot when the foot hurts. The following passage aptly expresses this view: "Knowing the left but not the right, or the right but not the left, knowing what is above but not that which is below, or what preceded but not that which follows, the cure will not last." [2]

Treating the Root and Treating the Branch

"When examining any complex process involving more than a single contradiction, one must strive to find the principal contradiction." (Mao Zedong) The contradictions appearing in the course of a disease are complex. To treat the disease properly, one must grasp its main contradiction. For example, when treating deaf-mutism, only by first treating the deafness can the entire condition be successfully cured.

In Chinese medicine, emphasis is placed upon distinguishing the relative importance of the Root and Branch. (See also Section I, chapter 4) In terms of disease, the first to be contracted is considered the Root, and later complications the Branch. Between the Organs and their pertaining channels, the former are considered the Roots and the latter the Branches. Points on the limbs are Roots, those on the trunk and head are Branches.

Sometimes the Root is treated before the Branch, but at other times this sequence is reversed. Occasionally, both may be treated simultaneously, or one treated exclusive of the other. Generally, an acute illness is treated first, a chronic illness second, Exterior disease first, Interior complications second. However, the more general balance between the normal and abnormal forces in the body must also be taken into account. For example, if the Normal Qi is particularly Deficient, i.e., the body is very weak, the most immediate concern is to "support the normal," since the expulsion of the Abnormal Qi from the body depends primarily upon the organism's ability to resist disease.

Strengthening What is Deficient and Draining What is Excessive

Two fundamental principles of traditional therapy are to strengthen or reinforce that which is Deficient, and drain or sedate that which is Excessive. These ancient principles, however, were in the past often abused by inflexible rules and practices which disregarded the actual differences in the nature of diseases, or the points chosen for therapy. (See Section III, chapter 9)

Acupuncture serves to regulate the functioning of the entire organism. By carefully observing internal factors such as the strength of the body and the vigor of the disease, a physician may then select appropriate points along the channels, determine the direction, angle and depth of needle insertion and choose the most appropriate technique with respect to the amount and duration of stimulation desired. All of these factors contribute to the 'strengthening' of a Deficiency, or the 'draining' of an Excess.

For example, relatively mild stimulation is usually indicated for strengthening a Deficiency, and stronger stimulation for draining an Excess. However, because of variations in the physical strength and needle tolerance among patients, the amount of stimulation needed in any particular case differs widely. That is to say, 'strengthening' and 'draining' are not absolute in measure, but are relative to the case at hand. For instance, muscle atrophy due to intrinsic muscle disease, as well as that caused by neural paralysis, are both regarded as Deficient conditions. However, in the first case, a mild degree of needle stimulation is applied to strengthen the Deficiency, while in the second case strong stimulation is used to the same end. Pain caused by inflammation of an internal organ and pain which accompanies external injury, such as sprained back, are both symptoms of Excess. Yet, the first is treated with relatively mild stimulation and the needles are retained for a rather lengthy period of time; in the second, the stimulation should be strong and the needles retained only briefly. Even in surgery where acupuncture is used for the single purpose of suppressing pain, the amount of stimulation varies. In minor operations like tonsillectomy the needles can be retained in place (after Qi is obtained) without further manipulation. But, in major surgery like lobectomy, continuous or intermittent needling is required.

Sometimes, even when the same point is used to treat similar diseases, differences must be considered with respect to the angle, direction and depth of the needle insertion so as to cause the needle sensation to be conducted toward the affected tissue. For example, simple arthritis of the shoulder, inflammation of the shoulder joint, and supraspinatus tendinitis are all conditions of Excess that can be treated at point LI-15 *(Jianyu).* But in each case the angle, direction and depth of needle insertion differs. Other points, however, may require less variation.

There may also be differences in the choice of methods used at different points for treating the same disease. For example, alternative methods like cupping or warming the needle may be used at points near the site of a disease of the shoulder. The same methods would never be used at distant points associated with shoulder disease further down the arm (LI-4 *(Hegu),* LI-11 *(Quchi),* etc.). Yet both the placement of cups on the shoulder and the insertion of needles at points on the lower arm may serve equally well in treating the shoulder condition.

It has also been observed that the same point on opposite sides of the body may react differently to the same stimulus. For example, when needling P-6 *(Neiguan)* bilaterally for a disease of the Stomach, if the response at the two points is different, then at the point of weaker response the physician might compensate with stronger manipulation of the needle, and at the point of greater response with less manipulation. The effect of both methods is equally to drain the Excessive condition.

As these examples illustrate, the principles of strengthening that which is Deficient and draining that which is Excessive must be applied with flexibility. One should not adhere mechanically to the use of only one method for each disease or point.

CHANNEL AND POINT DIAGNOSIS

Before acupuncture treatment can begin, it is necessary to correctly diagnose the disease. Below, a few methods of clinical diagnosis based specifically on the channels and points are briefly introduced.

Palpation

Acupuncture physicians have always given careful attention to examination of the body surfaces, so as to detect abnormalities such as points of tenderness, warmth, skin eruptions and subcutaneous nodules. These phenomena are then linked to the pathology of a neighboring channel. At present, this system of diagnosis is most frequently used in conjunction with cutaneous acupuncture and injection therapy.

Method of examination.

The thumb is rubbed lightly over the skin along the course of a channel, or the thumb and index finger are used together to gently knead the skin in order to detect alterations in the superficial cutaneous layers. Somewhat more pressure may be applied to probe deeper layers of the skin. It is important that the pressure be uniform and that the physician consider differences between the same channel on the left and right sides of the body. Ordinarily, examination begins along the channels of the back and then proceeds to those of the chest, abdomen and limbs. Particular attention should be given to special points such as the Associated points on the back, the Alarm points on the chest and abdomen, the Accumulating and Uniting points on the limbs, etc.

Abnormalities.

These include subcutaneous nodules, areas of tenderness, hard or flaccid muscle tissue, and indentations or changes in the color or temperature of the skin. Once discovered, the physician determines whether the abnormality reflects a symptom of Excess or Deficiency in the related channel.

Clinical application.

This is used in examination of the back. The thumb is pressed along the left and right sides of the spinous processes of the back (the medial course of the Bladder channel), generally beginning beside the 12th thoracic vertebra and working upward to the 1st thoracic vertebra, and then from the sacral to the lumbar vertebrae. When this is completed, skin surfaces in the vicinity of the ilium and shoulder blades may be similarly palpated.

In addition to those abnormalities discussed above, the physician should pay attention to the position of the spinous processes and tissue tension abnormalities of the paraspinal musculature. Such areas may be sensitive to the touch. The physician should also check to see if the vertebrae are evenly spaced or if there is a scolliosis.

Once abnormalities are found, those which indicate a strictly local problem are treated accordingly. The remainder may be regarded as external manifestations of an internal disease. Commonly, abnormalities discovered between the 1st and 3rd thoracic vertebrae suggest an illness related to the Heart; between the 1st and 4th related to the upper limbs; between the 2nd and 5th related to the Lungs and bronchioles; between the 5th and 8th related to the Stomach and duodenum; between the 8th and 10th related to the Liver, Gall Bladder or pancreas; between the 10th and 12th related to Stomach and Intestinal diseases; between the 12th thoracic and the 2nd lumbar related to the Kidneys and urinary system; between the 1st and 4th lumbar vertebrae related to the lower limbs; in the sacral region related to the reproductive organs.

Because the area paralleling the spine corresponds to the course of the Bladder channel, the Associated points along this channel are frequently palpated for diagnostic purposes, as are the Alarm points on the chest and abdomen. These points are identified in Table 4-1 according to the vertebra parallel to which each is located on the back, chest and abdomen.

In practice, these points are considered the primary diagnostic indicators. Neighboring acupuncture points may also be checked for reaction. For example, both the Alarm point L-1 *(Zhongfu)* and the neighboring point K-27 *(Shufu)* may respond to disease of the Lungs or bronchioles; the Alarm points Co-14 *(Juque)* and Co-12 *(Zhongwan)* as well as the neighboring points S-19 *(Burong)* and S-21 *(Liangmen)* may react to diseases of the Heart and Stomach; the Alarm points Co-4 *(Guanyuan)* and Co-3 *(Zhongji)* below react to diseases of the urogenital system.

When palpating points on the limbs, the Accumulating points are considered to be of primary importance, and the Uniting and other neighboring points are secondary. Thus, for example, the Accumulating point S-34 *(Liangqiu)* and the Uniting point S-36 *(Zusanli)* may both react to Stomach disease; the Uniting point Sp-9 *(Yinlingquan)* and the Accumulating point Sp-8 *(Diji)* may both react to diarrhea, a disorder of the Spleen.

Since ancient times, palpation of principal pulses has been used as a means of diagnosis. At first, the radial artery at the wrist was palpated for diseases of the Yin channels, and the carotid artery at the neck for diseases of the Yang channels. In *Simple Questions,* chapter 20, three locations on each of the upper, middle and lower parts of the body were designated for palpation. On the head, the superficial temporal artery at TB-21 *(Ermen),* the frontal branch of the superficial temporal artery at points S-8 *(Touwei)* and GB-4 *(Hanyan),* and the facial artery at S-5 *(Daying)* were used. On the upper limb, the radial artery at the wrist, the dorsal branch of the radial artery of the hand at LI-5 *(Yangxi)* and LI-4 *(Hegu),* and the ulnar artery at H-7 *(Shenmen)* were designated. And on the leg, the dorsalis pedis artery at S-42 *(Chongyang),* the first dorsal metatarsal artery at Li-3 *(Taichong),* and either the posterior tibial artery at K-3 *(Taixi)* or the femoral artery at Li-10 *(Wuli)* and Sp-11 *(Jimen)* were palpated. Later, this was simplified such that palpation at the wrist became the principal

Table 4-1
Point Palpation Diagnosis

Vertebral Level	Associated Point	Related Organ	Alarm Point
3rd thoracic	B-13 *(Feishu)*	Lung	L-1 *(Zhongfu)*
5th thoracic	B-15 *(Xinshu)*	Heart	Co-14 *(Juque)*
9th thoracic	B 18 *(Ganshu)*	Liver	Li-14 *(Qimen)*
10th thoracic	B-19 *(Danshu)*	Gall Bladder	GB-24 *(Riyue)*
11th thoracic	B-20 *(Pishu)*	Spleen	Li-13 *(Zhangmen)*
12th thoracic	B-21 *(Weishu)*	Stomach	Co-12 *(Zhongwan)*
2nd lumbar	B-23 *(Shenshu)*	Kidney	GB-25 *(Jingmen)*
4th lumbar	B-25 *(Dachangshu)*	Large Intestine	S-25 *(Tianshu)*
1st sacral	B-27 *(Xiaochangshu)*	Small Intestine	Co-4 *(Guanyuan)*
2nd sacral	B-28 *(Pangguangshu)*	Bladder	Co-3 *(Zhongji)*

method. (See Introduction) However, other blood vessels are still occasionally examined in connection with channel theory to check the circulation of Qi and Blood. For example, the posterior tibial artery at K-3 *(Taixi)* on the inside of the ankle is palpated to ascertain if the Kidney Qi is Deficient or Excessive, and likewise the dorsalis pedis artery at S-42 *(Chongyang)* for the Stomach Qi.

Measuring Electrical Phenomena of Acupuncture Points

Recent studies of the electrical properties of the skin have shown that the electrical resistance over acupuncture points is generally lower than over other areas of the body. Special electrical detection devices (milliameters) measure the amount of electrical resistance at representative points along each of the channels. The relative Excess or Deficiency of Qi and Blood in each of the channels is believed to be reflected in the high or low levels of electrical resistance in the skin over a channel's representative point. Generally, the Source point of each channel (on the hand or foot) is chosen as representative of that channel's health. The Well, Accumulating, Associated and other special points may also be used.

A number of general rules for measurement of electrical phenomena of the skin are suggested:

1. Before examination, the patient should rest quietly for 20-30 minutes, longer if preceded by strenuous physical activity. If circumstances permit, the best time for examination is shortly after the patient gets out of bed in the morning.

2. The examination room must be quiet and the air temperature comfortable.

3. The patient's skin must be dry.

4. During examination, the physician should avoid touching the metallic portion of the electric probe.

5. The electric current should be set low at the beginning, and increased only gradually to avoid a sudden burst of current.

6. When probing different points on the patient's skin with the electrode, care must be taken to insure that both the amount of time and pressure at each point is uniform. Otherwise, the accuracy of the measurement will be affected.

7. The electrode should be presssed lightly against the skin, not rubbed.

8. After the examination, the electric probe should be covered and stored in a dry place.

The measurements are checked for particularly high or low figures (expressed in ohms) and significant differences between identical points on the left and right sides of the body. Evaluation of the numbers is made according to the following criteria:

High figures.

Generally speaking, a high figure is one which is at least one third greater than most other points. This does not mean that figures somewhat less are without significance, only that those one third higher can be more easily judged. Lower numbers must be subject to further examination. Among the high figures, the greatest may be selected as the most significant. High figures ordinarily indicate a condition of Excess.

Low figures.

Low figures are those which measure at least one third below most other points. Among these, the smallest is the most significant. Low figures ordinarily indicate a condition of Deficiency.

Differences between left and right.

Large differences between the electrical resistance at the same point on the left and right sides of the body often indicate a disease related to the channel on which the point is found. This is particularly true if the difference is greater than 100%. Differences between left and right may be significant even in the absence of other high or low figures.

When analysis has been completed and the suspect channel(s) further examined for symptoms of disease, the physician should verify the results with other diagnostic methods, including both the traditional Four Diagnostic Methods (see Introduction) and Western techniques.

Measuring Heat Sensitivity

This method, developed in Japan by Akabane, involves the application of heat at the Well or Associated points on each of the twelve Primary channels, bilaterally, so as to measure differences in heat sensitivity. By this means, an Excess or Deficiency in a channel, or an imbalance between the left and right sides of the same channel, can be ascertained.

Ordinarily, the heat source is a specially made 'thread incense'. However, a pointed, electric heating element can be used in its place. The important thing is that the temperature of the heat source be stable, without high or low fluctuations.

Most of the Well points are found on the sides of the finger and toenails. The Kidney channel's Well point K-1 *(Yongquan),* is on the sole of the foot, however, and is considered inappropriate for this kind of measurement. Instead, a point on the medial side of the little toenail opposite B-67 *(Zhiyin)* is used for this channel. The Japanese also believe that a point on the ulnar side of the middle fingernail opposite P-9 *(Zhongchong)* corresponds to the Associated point B-17 *(Geshu).* Another point at the lateral corner of the middle toenail, at the same position on the middle toe as S-45 *(Lidui)* on the second toe, corresponds to the Associated point M-BW-12 *(Yishu).*

The heat source is applied by lightly tapping the Well point at uniform intervals of about one half second, tapping the skin, then lifting, then tapping again. This is repeated until the patient experiences a burning sensation, at which time the heat source is removed and the number of 'taps' recorded. This number constitutes the measure of the point's heat sensitivity, which is compared with that of other points.

Another method of measurement is to hold the heating element at a constant height above each of the Well points, without tapping, until the patient feels the burning sensation. The number of seconds which elapse before the burning response is the number assigned to that point.

554

Each of the Well points is measured in this fashion, first on one side of the body and then the other. If for any reason a Well point cannot be used, the channel's Associated point may be substituted.

A difference between the left and right sides of the same channel indicates a condition of relative Excess or Deficiency in that channel. A high number (i.e., greater heat tolerance) is generally a symptom of Deficiency, whereas a low number indicates Excess in the channel. If both sides of the same channel are equally high or low, compared to other channels, both sides are considered Deficient or Excessive. The Associated or other points on the affected channel may then be stimulated with acupuncture or moxibustion to restore balance.

SELECTION OF ACUPUNCTURE POINTS

Acupuncture treatment is administered at specific points or sites on the body. For this reason, the selection and combination of points in an acupuncture prescription is most important. At the same time, the physician must be able to choose flexibly between one or more acupuncture methods, depending upon the characteristics of the disease. Below is a summary of point selection and combination strategies, together with clinical application.

Principles of Point Selection

Point selection may be divided into three broad groupings: local points chosen in the vicinity of the disease, distant points chosen away from the disease, and points chosen for particular symptoms. In practice, each may be used in combination with, or independent of the others.

Local point selection
Local refers to the vicinity of the pain. Thus, pain in the head, neck, forearm, lower abdomen, foot, etc., can be treated via points in the same locality. Diseases of the limbs and superficial diseases of the body are commonly treated by this method. Examples: pain of the elbow can be treated at local points LI-11 *(Quchi)* and TB-10 *(Tianjing)*; pain of the knee at S-35 *(Xiyan)* and GB-34 *(Yanglingquan)*; and pain of the wrist at TB-4 *(Yangchi)* and TB-5 *(Waiguan)*. Many diseases of the head and body may also be treated through local points. Eye diseases can be treated at B-1 *(Jingming)* and GB-20 *(Fengchi)*; ear diseases at TB-21 *(Ermen)* and TB-17 *(Yifeng)*; wheezing at Co-22 *(Tiantu)* and B-13 *(Feishu)*; stomach-ache at Co-12 *(Zhongwan)*, S-21 *(Liangmen)* and B-21 *(Weishu)*; and diseases of the Bladder at Co-3 *(Zhongji)*, Co-4 *(Guanyuan)* and B-32 *(Ciliao)*.
Points over scars, wounds, inflammation or directly above diseased organs should not be used. Neighboring points should be substituted.

The efficacy of needling local points to treat disease can be explained not only on the basis of traditional channel theory, but more recently by neural segment theory as well. For example, in acupuncture anesthesia, the point SI-18 *(Quanliao)* is used for surgery on the cranium, and the point LI-18 *(Futu)* for operations on the thyroid. Similarly, in the clinical treatment of diseases of the Viscera, it is common to select a vertebral point M-BW-35 *(Jiaji)* in the same horizontal plane as the affected Organ. As these examples illustrate, choosing a point in the same or neighboring neural segment as that of the pain or disease is compatible with the rules of traditional local point selection.

Distant point selection
Distant refers to a location far from the site of pain, usually a point below the elbow or knee. This method is commonly used to treat diseases of internal Organs. Examples: needle L-5 *(Chize)* for coughing blood, P-6 *(Neiguan)* for chest pain, and S-36 *(Zusanli)* for abdominal pain. This method may also be used for diseases of the head and trunk: LI-4 *(Hegu)* for toothache, SI-3 *(Houxi)* for stiff neck, and B-54 *(Weizhong)* for lower back pain.

The technique of needling distant points is related to the channel theory of Root and Branch, whereby a disease above is treated by a point below, and vice versa. Because of the bilateral distribution of the Primary channels, and their junctions with the Conception and Governing channels, a disease on the left side of the body can be treated on the right, or a disease on the right by a point on the left. The efficacy of this method has been recognized since at least the 2nd century B.C.

In addition to selecting distant points according to traditional theory, they may also be selected on the basis of nerve distribution. Generally, this is most useful for treatment of disorders on the limbs, whereby a point located on a nerve trunk or root above the disease is selected for needling. For example, diseases of the fingers may be treated via points on related nerves: P-6 *(Neiguan)* on the median nerve near the wrist, and LI-11 *(Quchi)* on the radial nerve near the elbow, as well as points on the more distant brachial plexus. Diseases of the lower leg may be treated at GB-34 *(Yanglingquan)* on the peroneal nerve, at B-54 *(Weizhong)* on the tibial nerve, and, more distantly, at points along the sciatic nerve or sacral plexus.

This method of distant point selection has also been called "selecting points above the site."

Symptomatic point selection

Local and distant point selection are based upon the distance of the points from the site of the disease. However, some diseases are not local but systemic in nature, and can be treated at points long associated with relieving a particular disease. Prominent among such points are the Meeting points first mentioned in the *Classic of Difficulties:* B-17 *(Geshu)* for diseases affecting the Blood, Co-17 *(Shanzhong)* for diseases of the Qi, L-9 *(Taiyuan)* for diseases of the vessels, GB-34 *(Yanglingquan)* for diseases of the muscles and connective tissues, B-11 *(Dazhu)* for diseases of the bones, GB-39 *(Juegu)* for diseases of the marrow, Li-13 *(Zhangmen)* for diseases of the Yin Viscera (Lungs, Spleen, Heart, Kidneys, Liver), and Co-12 *(Zhongwan)* for diseases of the Yang Viscera (Large and Small Intestine, Stomach, Bladder, Triple Burner, Gall Bladder). Stimulation of these points has proven effective in relieving the disorders with which each is associated. The same is true of other special point groups introduced in Section II, chapter 1.

Certain individual points have also traditionally been useful in treating specific symptoms: Gv-14 *(Dazhui)* for reducing fever, Gv-26 *(Renzhong)* for reviving patients from unconsciousness, S-36 *(Zusanli)* for nausea, Co-4 *(Guanyuan)* for 'warming the Yang', etc. Some of the more commonly used 'symptomatic points', as they are called, are listed below.

Table 4-2
Selected Points for Common Symptoms

Symptom	Common Points
Fever	Gv-14 *(Dazhui)*, LI-11 *(Quchi)*, LI-4 *(Hegu)*
Fainting	Gv-26 *(Renzhong)*, M-UE-1 *(Shixuan)*
Shock	Use moxibustion at Gv-20 *(Baihui)*, Co-8 *(Qizhong)*, Co-4 *(Guanyuan)*; needle S-36 *(Zusanli)*
Spontaneous sweating	LI-4 *(Hegu)*, K-7 *(Fuliu)*
Night sweats	SI-3 *(Houxi)*
Insomnia	H-7 *(Shenmen)*, Sp-6 *(Sanyinjaio)*, K-3 *(Taixi)*
Excessive dreaming	B-15 *(Xinshu)*, H-7 *(Shenmen)*, Li-3 *(Taichong)*
Hoarse voice	LI-18 *(Futu)*, LI-4 *(Hegu)*, P-5 *(Jianshi)*
Spasm of the masseter muscle ('lockjaw')	S-7 *(Xiaguan)*, S-6 *(Jiache)*, LI-4 *(Hegu)*

Symptom	Common Points
Paralysis of hyoglossus muscle	Gv-15 *(Yamen)*, Co-23 *(Lianquan)*, LI-4 *(Hegu)*
Congested throat	Co-22 *(Tiantu)*, LI-18 *(Futu)*, LI-4 *(Hegu)*
Salivation	Gv-26 *(Renzhong)*, S-6 *(Jiache)*, LI-4 *(Hegu)*
Palpitations	P-6 *(Neiguan)*, P-4 *(Ximen)*
Chest pain	Co-17 *(Shanzhong)*, P-6 *(Neiguan)*
Cough	Co-22 *(Tiantu)*, L-7 *(Lieque)*
Dysphagia	Co-22 *(Tiantu)*, P-6 *(Neiguan)*
Fullness in chest	Co-12 *(Zhongwan)*, P-6 *(Neiguan)*
Nausea, vomiting	P-6 *(Neiguan)*, S-36 *(Zusanli)*
Hiccough	B-17 *(Geshu)*, P-6 *(Neiguan)*, P-8 *(Laogong)*
Abdominal distension	S-25 *(Tianshu)*, Co-6 *(Qihai)*, P-6 *(Neiguan)*, S-36 *(Zusanli)*
Rib pain	TB-6 *(Zhigou)*
Indigestion	S-36 *(Zusanli)*, Sp-4 *(Gongsun)*
Retention of urine	Sp-6 *(Sanyinjiao)*, Sp-9 *(Yinlingquan)*
Spermatorrhea, impotence, premature ejaculation	Co-4 *(Guanyuan)*, Sp-6 *(Sanyinjiao)*
Enuresis	Co-2 *(Qugu)*, Sp-6 *(Sanyinjiao)*
Constipation	S-25 *(Tianshu)*, TB-6 *(Zhigou)*
Prolapsed anus	Gv-1 *(Changqiang)*, B-57 *(Chengshan)*
Spasm of gastrocnemius muscle	B-57 *(Chengshan)*
Pruritis	LI-11 *(Quchi)*, Sp-10 *(Xuehai)*, Sp-6 *(Sanyinjiao)*
General weakness	Co-4 *(Guanyuan)*, S-36 *(Zusanli)*

Combining Points: The Acupuncture Prescription

In addition to the methods of individual point selection outlined above, there are several traditional methods of combining one point with others in an acupuncture prescription. These techniques are flexible, permitting many variations according to the particular needs of the case.

Combining points on the front with points on the back

The front refers to the chest and abdomen, the back to the back and waist. Points on both the front and back appropriate to a particular disease can be used in combination. For example, in the case of Stomach disease, both Co-12 *(Zhongwan)* on the abdomen and B-21 *(Weishu)* on the back could be needled in tandem.

Among the most commonly used front/back points are two special point groups: the Associated points on the back, and the Alarm points on the chest and abdomen. Because these points are associated with the major Organs of the body and related lesser organs and tissues, the therapeutic domain of each point is correspondingly broad.

For diseases of the Organs, front/back points are selected according to the local point method, and for diseases of the limbs or sensory organs, according to the symptomatic point method. Furthermore, because points contiguous to the Alarm points have similar therapeutic properties, they may be used interchangeably with the Alarm points. For instance, S-21 *(Liangmen)* could be used in place of the Alarm point Co-12 *(Zhongwan),* or S-28 *(Shuidao)* in place of the neighboring Alarm point Co-4 *(Guanyuan).*

Combining Yang channel points with Yin channel points

As we know, the Primary Yang channels are connected with the Primary Yin channels in a Yin/Yang relationship. By combining a point on a Yang channel with another on its paired Yin channel, the cumulative effect is greater than needling either point separately. Examples: combining S-36 *(Zusanli)* on the Stomach channel (Yang) with Sp-4 *(Gongsun)* on the Spleen channel (Yin) for Stomach disease; or combining L-9 *(Taiyuan)* on the Lung channel (Yin) with LI-4 *(Hegu)* on the Large Intestine channel (Yang) for coughing.

The most well known combinations of this kind are between the Source point on the channel primarily affected by a disease, and the Connecting point on the channel paired with the first in the Yin/Yang relationship. In this combination, the Source point is called the 'host', and the Connecting point the 'guest'. For example, a disease affecting the Lung channel may be treated through that channel's Source point, L-9 *(Taiyuan),* in combination with the Connecting point, LI-6 *(Pianli),* of its Yang partner the Large Intestine channel. Conversely, a disease affecting the Large Intestine channel could be treated by that channel's Source point, LI-4 *(Hegu),* together with the Connecting point, L-7 *(Lieque),* of its Yin partner the Lung channel.

This method would also encompass the use of a single point on a Yang channel for disease affecting a Yin channel, or vice versa.

Combining points above with points below

Above refers to points on the arms and above the waist, below to points on the legs or below the waist. This method of point combination is most commonly practiced on the limbs. For example, in the case of Stomach disease, P-6 *(Neiguan)* on the arm may be combined with S-36 *(Zusanli)* on the leg. For sore throat or toothache, LI-4 *(Hegu)* on the hand can be combined with S-44 *(Neiting)* on the foot.

Traditionally, a distinctive use of the above/below combination was made with respect to the Meeting points of the eight Miscellaneous channels. A Meeting point on a Miscellaneous channel affected by a disease above, would be combined in an acupuncture prescription with a Meeting point on a Miscellaneous channel below. For example, diseases of the Heart, chest and abdomen are related to the Yin Linking channel and the Pentrating channel, P-6 *(Neiguan),* the Meeting point of the former on the arm (above), and Sp-4 *(Gongsun),* the Meeting point of the latter on the foot (below), were both selected for needling. Similarly, diseases of the Lungs, throat and diaphragm are related to the Conception and Yin Heel channels. The channels' Meeting points, L-7 *(Lieque)* on the wrist, and K-6 *(Zhaohai)* on the ankle, are often used in combination for treating those diseases. Physicians of the Jin and Yuan periods (12th-14th centuries) particularly favored this method.

Combining points on the left with points on the right

Because channel points are bilateral, it is common to treat diseases of the internal Organs by manipulating the same point on both sides in order to strengthen the effect. For example, B-21

(Weishu) on both left and right sides of the spine, or S-36 *(Zusanli)* on both legs, can be needled to treat diseases of the Stomach. Further, because of the intersection of the channels on the right side with those on the left, a point on the right may be chosen to treat disease or pain on the left side of the body, and vice versa. For instance, in the case of hemiplegia, not only may a point on the side affected by the paralysis be selected, but the same point on the healthy side may be used as well.

Combining local with distant points
This technique combines local points with distant points. For example, when there is Stomach disease, the local points Co-12 *(Zhongwan)* and B-21 *(Weishu),* or the distant points P-6 *(Neiguan),* S-36 *(Zusanli)* and Sp-4 *(Gongsun)* could be used separately. The combination method, however, uses both the local and distant points together.

Another combination takes the Meeting point of the Miscellaneous channel affected by a disease as the principal point, then adds supplementary points according to the symptoms. For example, P-6 *(Neiguan),* the Meeting point of the Yin Linking channel, may be utilized as the principal point for a Stomach complaint. Co-12 *(Zhongwan),* P-7 *(Daling),* S-36 *(Zusanli),* etc., may be added according to the particular symptoms.

A list of the most common distant and local point combinations appears in Table 4-3.

Clinical Application

Acupuncture therapy may be used by itself or in combination with other therapeutic methods, depending on the specific requirements of the case. Acupuncture stimulation is effective only insofar as it produces a functional response in the body. The physician must be able to control both the nature and amount of stimulation in conformance with the particular patient's health. A few pointers:

Alternating the points
Each of the acupuncture points has its own distinctive characteristics, yet those on the same channel or in the same locality can produce certain effects in common. When selecting points for a prescription, it is improper to choose a large number for any single treatment. Instead, after a few initial treatments, points may be added or subtracted as conditions require. In a complex illness, those symptoms which are most acute are treated first.

It is wrong to needle the same points for too many treatments in succession, as the efficacy of these points will diminish. Rather, other points with similar characteristics should be substituted, or a similar prescription made up of different points should be used instead. When treating a patient for the first time, especially a nervous one, the physician should needle fewer points, increasing the number in later treatments when the patient feels more accustomed to acupuncture.

Utilizing different methods
Just as each type of acupuncture needle is recommended for a particular kind of treatment, so each mode of acupuncture therapy has its proper therapeutic domain. Although prescriptions for several different techniques may be found under disease headings later in this Section, the physician should be thoroughly familiar with the advantages and disadvantages of a technique before using it.

Frequency of treatments
A small number of acute diseases require more than one treatment in a single day. Most chronic illnesses are treated once every one to three days. After receiving acupuncture for a period of weeks, treatments should be suspended temporarily to rest the body. Recommmended frequencies of treatment and rest intervals are provided for most of the diseases in this Section.

FOOTNOTES

1. *Simple Questions,* chapter 35
2. *Simple Questions,* chapter 80

Table 4-3

Local and Distant Point Combinations

Site of Disease	Local Points	Distant Points
Frontal region	M-HN-3 (Yintang), GB-14 (Yangbai)	LI-4 (Hegu), S-44 (Neiting)
Temporal region	M-HN-9 (Taiyang), GB-8 (Shuaigu)	TB-3 (Zhongzhu), GB-41 (Zulinqi)
Occipital region	GB-20 (Fengchi), B-10 (Tianzhu)	SI-3 (Houxi), B-65 (Shugu)
Vertex	Gv-20 (Baihui)	Li-3 (Taichong)
Eyes	B-1 (Jingming), S-1 (Chengqi), GB-20 (Fengchi)	LI-4 (Hegu)
Nose	M-HN-3 (Yintang), LI-20 (Yingxiang)	LI-4 (Hegu)
Mouth and gums	S-6 (Jiache), S-7 (Xiaguan), S-4 (Dicang)	LI-4 (Hegu)
Ears	TB-17 (Yifeng), SI-19 (Tinggong), GB-2 (Tinghui)	TB-3 (Zhongzhu), TB-5 (Waiguan)
Tongue	Co-23 (Lianquan)	LI-4 (Hegu)
Throat	SI-17 (Tianrong)	LI-4 (Hegu)
Trachea	Co-22 (Tiantu)	L-7 (Lieque)
Lungs	B-13 (Feishu), Co-17 (Shanzhong), Co-22 (Tiantu)	L-7 (Lieque), L-5 (Chize)
Heart	B-15 (Xinshu), B-14 (Jueyinshu), Co-17 (Shanzhong)	P-6 (Neiguan), H-7 (Shenmen), P-5 (Jianshi), P-4 (Ximen)

Site of Disease	Local Points	Distant Points
Stomach	B-21 (*Weishu*), Co-12 (*Zhongwan*)	P-6 (*Neiguan*), S-36 (*Zusanli*)
Liver	B-18 (*Ganshu*)	Li-3 (*Taichong*)
Gall Bladder	B-19 (*Danshu*)	M-LE-23 (*Dannangxue*), GB-34 (*Yanglingquan*)
Intestines	B-25 (*Dachangshu*), B-27 (*Xiaochangshu*), S-25 (*Tianshu*), Co-4 (*Guanyuan*)	S-37 (*Shangjuxu*), S-36 (*Zusanli*)
Kidneys	B-23 (*Shenshu*), B-47 (*Zhishi*)	K-3 (*Taixi*)
Bladder	B-32 (*Ciliao*), Co-3 (*Zhongji*)	Sp-6 (*Sanyinjiao*)
Reproductive organs	Co-3 (*Zhongji*), Co-4 (*Guanyuan*), M-CA-18 (*Zigong*)	Sp-6 (*Sanyinjiao*)
Anus	Gv-1 (*Changqiang*), B-49 (*Zhibian*)	B-57 (*Chengshan*)
Upper limb	LI-15 (*Jianyu*), LI-11 (*Quchi*), LI-4 (*Hegu*)	M-BW-35 (*Jiaji*) from the 5th cervical to the 1st thoracic, M-HN-41 (*Jingbi*)
Lower limb	GB-30 (*Huantiao*), B-54 (*Weizhong*), GB-34 (*Yanglingquan*), GB-39 (*Xuanzhong*)	M-BW-35 (*Jiaji*) from the 3rd lumbar to the 1st sacral

Chapter 2

Acupuncture Anesthesia

Acupuncture anesthesia was developed by the revolutionary medical workers of China as a distinctive method of anesthesia. Both prior to and during surgery, needles are inserted at various points on the body. This safely and effectively reduces or entirely eliminates the pain accompanying many operations on the head, chest, abdomen and limbs. The most distinctive feature of acupuncture anesthesia is that the patient remains conscious and is therefore able to play an active role throughout the operation. Not only is pain suppressed, but other physiological functions are maintained at normal levels, and the body's power to resist disease is itself strengthened as a result of needle stimulation. The side effects associated with other forms of anesthesia are absent. Thus, the period of post-operative recovery is accelerated. Those patients who, because of abnormal functioning of the liver, kidney or lung, or because of old age, debility, shock, critical illness or allergic reaction to anesthetics are unable to tolerate conventional modes of anesthesia may consider acupuncture anesthesia as an effective substitute.

Prescription

Acupuncture anesthesia is widely practiced throughout China. As a result, there exists a rich reservoir of experience. Prescriptions are numerous, reflecting variations among medical units in different regions. Only those prescriptions for the most common clinical operations which have proven most effective are set forth in this chapter.

Method

After the needles are inserted, they are manipulated for a period of usually 10-20 minutes prior to the beginning of surgery. Electro-acupuncture, adjusted to the tolerance of the patient, may also be used. During surgery and depending on the particular circumstances, the needles are either retained without further manipulation, or continuously manipulated. Similarly, with electro-acupuncture either a continuous or intermittent current is applied. When surgery is completed, the needles are withdrawn.

Items for Consideration

1. At the outset, the patient should be fully informed of the nature of acupuncture anesthesia, both to allay anxiety and gain patient cooperation during surgery.
2. Depending both upon the patient and the operation to be performed, auxilliary drugs may be needed. These are generally given by intramuscular injection in small amounts, 5-30 minutes prior to

surgery. When a nerve is to be severed or there is acute local pain, a .5-1% injection of lidocaine can be given.

3. Surgery under acupuncture anesthesia requires the particular attention of the surgeon toward proceeding "firmly, precisely, deftly and quickly."

4. At present, there remain certain undesirable aspects to acupuncture anesthesia. Analgesia may be incomplete. During abdominal surgery, the abdominal muscles are often insufficiently relaxed. Operating upon certain organs involves an uncomfortable "pulling" reaction which as yet cannot be effectively controlled. However, current research has shown some gradual improvement when the patient's initiative is exercised by cooperating during surgery, as more suitable points and needling methods are used, and as improved surgical techniques are brought to bear.

Selected Acupuncture Anesthesia Prescriptions

Cranial surgery

1) S-43 *(Xiangu)*, GB-41 *(Zulinqi)*, Li-3 *(Taichong)*, SI-18 *(Quanliao)*. Needle points on affected side.

Eye surgery

1) Detached retina: LI-4 *(Hegu)*, TB-6 *(Zhigou)*. Needle points on affected side. A second prescription is, on the ear, Forehead joined to Vision #2 and Vision #1; on the body, join GB-14 *(Yangbai)* to M-HN-6 *(Yuyao)*.

2) Correction of inward turned eyelid and inverted eyelash: LI-4 *(Hegu)*. Needle both sides.

3) Correction of strabismus: The first prescription is LI-4 *(Hegu)*, TB-6 *(Zhigou)*, join GB-14 *(Yangbai)* to M-HN-6 *(Yuyao)*, and S-2 *(Sibai)* to S-1 *(Chengqi)*. Needle points on affected side. Use electro-acupuncture. A second prescription is LI-4 *(Hegu)*, TB-6 *(Zhigou)*, SI-3 *(Houxi)*, GB-25 *(Jingmen)*.

4) Lens extraction in cataract: The first prescription is LI-4 *(Hegu)*, join TB-5 *(Waiguan)* toP-6 *(Neiguan)*. Needle points on affected side. A second prescription is LI-4 *(Hegu)*, TB-6 *(Zhigou)*. Needle points on affected side.

5) Enucleation of eyeball: LI-4 *(Hegu)*, TB-5 *(Waiguan)*, SI-3 *(Houxi)*. Needle points on affected side. If eyeball is particularly sensitive, cotton soaked in 1% decicaine may be applied for surface anesthesia.

6) Iridectomy: LI-4 *(Hegu)*, TB-5 *(Waiguan)*. Continuous needling on both sides. Also insert at S-44 *(Neiting)* on both sides. After Qi is obtained at this point, cease further needle manipulation.

7) Shortening of sclera: The first prescription is LI-4 *(Hegu)*, TB-6 *(Zhigou)*, join GB-14 *(Yangbai)* to M-HN-6 *(Yuyao)*, and S-2 *(Sibai)* to S-1 *(Chengqi)*. Needle points on affected side with electro-acupuncture. A second prescription is LI-4 *(Hegu)*, TB-6 *(Zhigou)*. Needle points on affected side with electro-acupuncture.

8) Transplantation of pterygium: The first prescription is ear points Eye, Liver. Needle affected side. A second prescription is ear points Neurogate, Eye, Vision. Needle affected side.

9) Removal of lacrimal sac, pus drainage from lacrimal sac: The first prescription is LI-4 *(Hegu)*, Li-3 *(Taichong)*. Needle points on affected side. A second prescription is LI-4 *(Hegu)*, B-2 *(Zanzhu)*, LI-20 *(Yingxiang)*. Needle points on affected side.

10) Removal of foreign matter from eye: LI-4 *(Hegu)* on both sides, TB-6 *(Zhigou)* on affected side only; points on ear: join Forehead to Vision, and Neurogate to Sympathetic. For ear points, needle both sides.

Surgery of the mouth, jaw and face

1) Excision of parotid tumor: S-40 *(Fenglong)*, GB-38 *(Yangfu)*, B-59 *(Fuyang)*, S-43 *(Xiangu)*, Li-3 *(Taichong)*, GB-43 *(Xiaxi)*. Needle both sides. After Qi is obtained, cease further needle manipulation.

2) Surgery on submaxillary region: S-40 *(Fenglong)*, GB-38 *(Yangfu)*, B-59 *(Fuyang)*, Li-3 *(Taichong)*, Sp-4 *(Gongsun)*. Needle affected side.

3) Surgery on the mandible: S-40 *(Fenglong)*, GB-38 *(Yangfu)*, B-59 *(Fuyang)*, Li-3 *(Taichong)*, Sp-4 *(Gongsun)*, P-6 *(Neiguan)*. Needle affected side.

4) Surgery on the temporo-maxillary joint: S-40 *(Fenglong)*, GB-38 *(Yangfu)*, B-59 *(Fuyang)*, Li-3 *(Taichong)*. Needle these points on both sides. Sp-4 *(Gongsun)*, LI-4 *(Hegu)*. Needle these two points on affected side only.

5) Excision of mixed tumor in palatine region: LI-4 *(Hegu)*, P-6 *(Neiguan)*, Sp-4 *(Gongsun)*. Needle affected side.

Surgery of the ear, nose and throat

1) Mastoidectomy: The first prescription is TB-5 *(Waiguan)*, GB-34 *(Yanglingquan)*. Needle both sides, using electro-acupuncture. A second prescription is LI-4 *(Hegu)*, TB-6 *(Zhigou)*, and ear points Neurogate, Lung, and Kidney. Needle affected side. Manipulate needles for 10-20 minutes before surgery begins.

2) Myringotomy: LI-4 *(Hegu)*, SI-3 *(Houxi)*, TB-5 *(Waiguan)*. Needle both sides.

3) Tympanotomy: LI-4 *(Hegu)*. Needle one or both sides.

4) Laryngectomy: LI-4 *(Hegu)*, TB-6 *(Zhigou)*, and ear points Neurogate joined to Sympathetic, and Forehead joined to Stop Wheezing, Adrenal. Needle all points on left side.

5) Tonsillectomy: The first prescription is ear points Throat, Tonsils. Needle both sides. A second prescription is LI-4 *(Hegu)*. Needle both sides.

6) Incision at outside of nose: LI-4 *(Hegu)*, TB-6 *(Zhigou)*, S-3 *(Juliao)* joined to S-2 *(Sibai)*. Needle affected side.

7) Radical resection of maxillary sinus: LI-4 *(Hegu)*, TB-6 *(Zhigou)*. During pre-op needle manipulation, join S-3 *(Juliao)* to S-4 *(Dicang)*. Needle affected side.

8) Radical research of frontal sinus: LI-4 *(Hegu)*, TB-6 *(Zhigou)*, GB-14 *(Yangbai)* joined to B-2 *(Zanzhu)*, and S-3 *(Juliao)* joined to S-2 *(Sibai)*. Needle affected side.

9) Excision of nasal polyp: The first prescription is LI-4 *(Hegu)* or LI-20 *(Yingxiang)*. Needle one or both sides. A second prescription is ear point External Nose. Needle one or both sides.

10) Excision of thyroid tumor: LI-4 *(Hegu)*, P-6 *(Neiguan)*. Needle affected side.

Chest surgery

1) Dilatation and separation of bicuspid (mitral) valve: P-6 *(Neiguan)*, LI-4 *(Hegu)*, TB-6 *(Zhigou)*. Needle affected side.

2) Resection of pericardium: LI-4 *(Hegu)*, P-6 *(Neiguan)*. Needle both sides.

3) Pneumonectomy: The first prescription is LI-14 *(Binao)*. Needle affected side. A second prescription is TB-5 *(Waiguan)* joined to P-6 *(Neiguan)*. Needle affected side. Combine with breathing exercises.

Abdominal surgery

1) Stomach surgery: S-36 *(Zusanli)*, S-37 *(Shangjuxu)*. Needle one or both sides.

2) Splenectomy: LI-4 *(Hegu)*, P-6 *(Neiguan)*, S-36 *(Zusanli)*, Sp-6 *(Sanyinjiao)*, Li-3 *(Taichong)*. Needle affected side.

3) Appendectomy: The first prescription is S-37 *(Shangjuxu)*, M-LE-13 *(Lanweixue)*, Li-3 *(Taichong)*. Needle both sides. A second prescription is LI-4 *(Hegu)*, P-6 *(Neiguan)*, Sp-4 *(Gongsun)*. Needle both sides.

4) Repair of inguinal hernia: S-36 *(Zusanli)*, GB-28 *(Weidao)*. Needle both sides.

5) Caesarian section: S-36 *(Zusanli)*, Sp-6 *(Sanyinjiao)*, GB-26 *(Daimai)*, and the 'medial anesthetic point' midway between Sp-9 *(Yinlingquan)* and the inner malleolus. Needle both sides.

6) Complete hysterectomy: Gv-2 *(Yaoshu)*, Gv-4 *(Mingmen)*, GB-26 *(Daimai)*, S-36 *(Zusanli)*, Sp-6 *(Sanyinjiao)*, B-33 *(Zhongliao)* or B-32 *(Ciliao)*. Needle both sides.

7) Tubal ligation: S-36 *(Zusanli)*, Li-6 *(Zhongdu)*. Needle both sides.

8) Surgery in the perineal region: The first prescription is B-25 *(Dachangshu)*, and points in the sacral canal. Needle affected side using electro-acupuncture. A second prescription is ear points Lung, Distal Segment of Rectum. Needle affected side using electro-acupuncture.

Back and waist surgery

1) Spinal fusion: The first prescription is LI-4 *(Hegu)*, P-6 *(Neiguan)*, TB-7 *(Huizong)*, S-36 *(Zusanli)*, B-57 *(Chengshan)*, B-60 *(Kunlun)*, GB-38 *(Yangfu)*. Needle both sides. A second prescription is ear points Neurogate, Lung, Kidney, Thoracic Vertebrae, Lower Back. Needle affected side.

2) Removal of kidney: The first prescription is LI-4 *(Hegu)*, P-6 *(Neiguan)*, Sp-6 *(Sanyinjiao)*, Li-3 *(Taichong)*, S-36 *(Zusanli)*. Needle affected side. A second prescription is ear points Neurogate, Lung, Lumbar Vertebrae, Ureter. Needle affected side.

Limb surgery

1) Closed reduction of shoulder joint: The first prescription is ear points Neurogate, Sympathetic, Kidney, Shoulder joined to Shoulder Joint. Needle points on affected side. A second prescription is LI-4 *(Hegu)*, M-UE-30 *(Bizhong)*. Needle both sides. Also ear point, Shoulder. Needle affected side.

2) Amputation of forearm: L-5 *(Chize)*, H-2 *(Qingling)*, N-UE-14 *(Naoshang)*, join point one unit above anterior axillary crease with same in back. Needle both sides.

3) Three-nail fixation of fracture of femoral neck: S-36 *(Zusanli)*, S-40 *(Fenglong)*, B-59 *(Fuyang)*, GB-36 *(Waiqiu)*, GB-39 *(Juegu)*, Sp-6 *(Sanyinjiao)*, GB-40 *(Qiuxu)*, S-43 *(Xiangu)*. Needle affected side using electro-acupuncture.

4) Amputation of lower section of the leg: ear points Neurogate, Lung, Kidney, Sciatic Nerve joined to Sympathetic. Needle affected side using electro-acupuncture.

Chapter 3

Emergency Acupuncture

[Editors' introduction to acupuncture prescriptions. In the following chapters we will use a common format. Beneath the name of a disease will appear a short description of the illness according to traditional Chinese medicine, together with its associated principles of treatment. In the original Chinese text, a description of the disease according to Western medicine was also included, but we have chosen to omit this from the translation on the assumption that the reader is already familiar with the Western etiology of the disease, or may readily obtain this information from standard reference works in English. Modern Chinese medical textbooks frequently include both traditional and Western etiologies.

The introductory paragraph is followed by prescriptions for treatment. In some cases only needling is recommended. In most, however, several modes of acupuncture therapy are provided. The practitioner may choose among them. Now and then, the original authors of the text have recommended one method over another.

Two kinds of points appear in the prescriptions: principal and supplementary. Principal points are those used to treat the disease generally, while supplementary points are indicated for specific symptoms. Occasionally, a specified number of points among those in the prescription will be recommended, but more often not. Rather, the points in a prescription represent several appropriate loci from which the discerning practitioner may select. This is where a basic understanding of traditional theory is useful. An experienced acupuncturist can look at a list of points and see immediately that there are some which merely duplicate other points with similar characteristics. The practitioner may desire a balance between points neighboring the source of the disease and those further away, between those on the front of the body and those on the back, etc. (See chapter 1 of this Section.) From experience, the practitioner would know that one point may provide more stimulation than another, or that a related point not listed in the prescription could be substituted. Usually, only a few of the preferred points are actually used in any single session of treatment.

Often, an explanation of the traditional functions of certain points follows the needling prescription. This can be particularly helpful to the beginner. Reference should be made to the Introduction for an explanation of traditional medical terms and concepts. The index may be helpful.

In addition to the prescriptions recommended for each disease by the authors, several prescriptions from other sources, both ancient and modern, are gathered under the heading **Other prescriptions**. The name of each source has been abbreviated. The abbreviations are fully explained in the Table of Abbreviated Titles at the back of the book. (Appendix I)

Finally, items of importance in the diagnosis and treatment of the disease, including advice with respect to the suitability of methods other than acupuncture, are listed under the heading **Remarks**. Because the dosages given for injection therapy were often confusing and inconsistent, we have elected to omit them from this Section. Usually, 0.5-1 cc. was prescribed for each injection.]

567

DROWNING

In traditional terms, treatment is directed toward opening the Heart orifice to revive from unconsciousness, and clearing the obstruction from the Lungs and Heart.

Needling

Principal points: Co-1 *(Huiyin)*, Gv-25 *(Suliao)*, P-6 *(Neiguan)*, K-1 *(Yongquan)*
Supplementary points: L-9 *(Taiyuan)*, SI-3 *(Houxi)*, S-36 *(Zusanli)*

Method: At Co-1 *(Huiyin)* use a short, thick needle for strong stimulation. At Gv-25 *(Suliao)* and P-6 *(Neiguan)* manipulate needle continuously for maximum stimulation.

Discussion of points: Co-1 *(Huiyin)* is the point of intersection of the Conception, Governing and Penetrating channels. Yin (Conception channel) joins with Yang (Governing channel) at this point, and stimulation here can clear the obstruction from the Heart orifice. Gv-25 *(Suliao)*, a point on the Governing channel which communicates with the brain, is stimulated to clear the mind. P-6 *(Neiguan)*, the Connecting point on the Pericardium channel, can 'open' the Heart orifice. Stimulation of K-1 *(Yongquan)*, the Well point on the Kidney channel, can revive the patient from unconsciousness. L-9 *(Taiyuan)* is both the Source point on the Lung channel and the Meeting point of the blood vessels. It is therefore used to facilitate circulation in the vessels of the Lungs. SI-3 *(Houxi)* is the Transporting point on the Small Intestine channel and the Meeting point on the Governing channel. In combination with P-6 *(Neiguan)*, this point assists in clearing obstruction from the Heart. In combination with S-36 *(Zusanli)*, it calms the Stomach to regulate the Qi.

Other prescriptions

1. Co-1 *(Huiyin)*, Gv-25 *(Suliao)*, LI-4 *(Hegu)*, P-6 *(Neiguan)*, S-40 *(Fenglong)*, Li-3 *(Taichong)*. (Source: HIM)
2. Moxa at Co-8 *(Qizhong)*. (Source: GOA)

Remarks
Acupuncture is used in cases of drowning both to revive the victim from unconsciousness and to restore normal body function. However, before giving acupuncture, the water should be drained from the victim's lungs and stomach, and artificial respiration, as well as heart massage if necessary, should be given.

HEAT EXHAUSTION OR SUNSTROKE

Traditional medicine describes these illnesses as arising from excessive Heat, or a mixture of Heat and Dampness, which gives rise to feverishness, injury to the Normal Qi of the body, and sudden obstruction of the Qi circulating in the channels. The patient experiences disorientation, fainting and perhaps convulsions. If the body fluids become exhausted, the functioning of the Organs will decline (a Deficient condition).

Treatment is directed primarily at clearing and draining Heat from the body. In mild cases, the Stomach should be calmed. In severe cases, the Heart orifice must be cleared of obstruction and the Deficient condition stabilized.

Needling
Superficial condition
Principal points: Gv-14 *(Dazhui)*, LI-11 *(Quchi)*, LI-4 *(Hegu)*, S-43 *(Xiangu)*, Li-3 *(Taichong)*
Supplementary points: S-36 *(Zusanli)*, P-6 *(Neiguan)*, Co-12 *(Zhongwan)*, Sp-4 *(Gongsun)*

Method: First needle Gv-14 *(Dazhui)*, moderate to strong stimulation. Then needle the points on the limbs, retaining the needles in place for 15-30 minutes.

Severe condition

Principal points: Gv-26 *(Renzhong)*, M-UE-1 *(Shixuan)*, the Well points on the Primary channels, P-3 *(Quze)*, B-54 *(Weizhong)*

Supplementary points: Gv-20 *(Baihui)*, P-8 *(Laogong)*, K-1 *(Yongquan)*, P-6 *(Neiguan)*, M-HN-13 *(Yiming)*, S-36 *(Zusanli)*, SI-3 *(Houxi)*, GB-34 *(Yanglingquan)*, B-57 *(Chengshan)*, B-56 *(Chengjiu)*, M-HN-20 *(Jinjin/Yuye)*, Co-6 *(Qihai)*, Co-8 *(Qizhong)*, L-9 *(Taiyuan)*, K-7 *(Fuliu)*

Method: Rely primarily on the principal points, needling Gv-26 *(Renzhong)* but only pricking the others to let a few drops of blood. As for the supplementary points, if there is fainting, add Gv-20 *(Baihui)*, P-8 *(Laogong)* or K-1 *(Yongquan)*. For dizziness and nausea, add P-6 *(Neiguan)*, M-HN-13 *(Yiming)* or S-36 *(Zusanli)*. For convulsions, add SI-3 *(Houxi)*, GB-34 *(Yanglingquan)*. For spasms in the muscles of the calf, add B-57 *(Chengshan)*, B-56 *(Chengjiu)* or GB-34 *(Yanglingquan)*. For excessive thirst, add M-HN-20 *(Jinjin/Yuye)*, which is pricked to let blood. If excessive sweating exhausts the patient, use moxibustion at Co-6 *(Qihai)* or Co-8 *(Qizhong)*, or needle L-9 *(Taiyuan)* or K-7 *(Fuliu)*.

Discussion of points: The four points, Gv-14 *(Dazhui)* on the Governing channel, LI-11 *(Quchi)* and LI-4 *(Hegu)* on the Large Intestine channel, and S-43 *(Xiangu)* on the Stomach channel, all of which are situated on channels with 'much Qi and Blood', are well matched for clearing and draining Heat from the body. Li-3 *(Taichong)*, the Source point on the Liver channel, which is connected to the Stomach and Governing channels and a branch of which crosses the diaphragm, may be used to suppress the rebellious Qi, calm the Stomach and expand the chest. S-36 *(Zusanli)*, the Source point on the Stomach channel, and Sp-4 *(Gongsun)*, the Connecting point on the Spleen channel, are ideally matched for calming the Stomach and suppressing vomiting. Similar properties are shared by P-6 *(Neiguan)*, the Meeting point of the Yin Heel channel which enters the abdomen and traverses the region between the Stomach, Heart and Lungs, and Co-12 *(Zhongwan)*, the Alarm point of the Stomach.

Among the points used for severe cases of sunstroke, Gv-26 *(Renzhong)* is used for clearing obstructions from the Heart orifice. M-UE-1 *(Shixuan)* and the Well points, in addition to being points of intersection between the Yin and Yang channels which they help regulate, may also be stimulated to clear the Heart orifice and revive the patient from unconsciousness. P-3 *(Quze)* and B-54 *(Weizhong)*, the Uniting points on the Pericardium and Bladder channels, drain Heat from the body when pricked to let blood. In the event of coma, Gv-20 *(Baihui)* may be used to awaken the brain, P-8 *(Laogong)* to clear the Heart, and K-1 *(Yongquan)* to revive from unconsciousness. M-HN-13 *(Yiming)* has proven effective in recent experience for treating dizziness. SI-3 *(Houxi)*, the Meeting point on the Governing channel which connects with the brain, is stimulated to treat convulsions. GB-34 *(Yanglingquan)* is the Meeting point for the muscles and is therefore needled to relax the Muscle channels. Pricking the point M-HN-20 *(Jinjin/Yuye)* for excessive thirst generates fluid in the body by clearing Heat therefrom. The cessation of sweating, when Heat remains, is a dangerous symptom indicating that the Source Qi is nearing exhaustion. Co-6 *(Qihai)* is selected to 'nourish the Source and stabilize the Root', while L-9 *(Taiyuan)*, the Meeting point of the vessels, and K-7 *(Fuliu)*, the Penetrating point on the Kidney channel, are effective in restoring Qi to the vessels.

Ear acupuncture

Points: Neurogate, Subcortex, Sympathetic, Heart, Adrenal, Occiput, Ear Apex (prick to let blood)

Method: Strong stimulation. After manipulating needles for 5 minutes, retain in place for 30 minutes. Other points may be added according to associated symptoms.

Manipulation

Press Gv-26 *(Renzhong)* with the fingernail. Using the thumb, press with force against LI-4 *(Hegu)*, P-6 *(Neiguan)* and GB-21 *(Jianjing)*.

Other prescriptions
1. LI-4 *(Hegu)*, Li-3 *(Taichong)*, Gv-14 *(Dazhui)*, GB-20 *(Fengchi)*, S-36 *(Zusanli)* with moderate stimulation. (Source: HIM)
2. M-UE-1 *(Shixuan)* (bleed first), Gv-20 *(Baihui)*, Gv-26 *(Renzhong)*, K-1 *(Yongquan)*. For tremors of the upper extremities, add LI-4 *(Hegu)* and LI-11 *(Quchi)*. For those of the lower extremities, add B-54 *(Weizhong)* and B-57 *(Chengshan)*. For Fever, add Gv-14 *(Dazhui)* and LI-11 *(Quchi)*. (Source: CCMHCD)
3. Gv-26 *(Renzhong)*, Co-12 *(Zhongwan)*, Co-6 *(Qihai)*, LI-11 *(Quchi)*, LI-4 *(Hegu)*, P-9 *(Zhongchong)*, S-36 *(Zusanli)*, S-44 *(Neiting)*. (Source: MSAM)
4. Co-9 *(Shuifen)*, Gv-14 *(Dazhui)*, P-7 *(Daling)*, B-54 *(Weizhong)*. (Source: GCAM)

Remarks
• This illness occurs rather suddenly, and if not treated properly can become dangerous and even fatal. In serious cases, a combination of Chinese and Western methods is indicated.
• Acupuncture is effective in treating this illness.
• Preventative measures are stressed to avoid overheating the body.

CONVULSIONS

In traditional medicine, this condition is usually thought to be caused by Wind or Heat Excesses of external origin. The Qi in the Primary channels becomes rebellious and dysfunction results. Many problems can lead to convulsions. Among them are a high fever that injures the Yin and gives rise to Wind in the Liver (primarily in children), or an excess of Phlegm which obstructs the cavities and vessels causing a loss of function in the Muscle channels.

Treatment is based on dispersing the Excess from, and regulating the Governing channel. Where fever accompanies the convulsions, supplementary points are recommended to eliminate Heat from the body.

Needling
Febrile convulsions
Principal points: M-HN-3 *(Yintang)*, M-HN-9 *(Taiyang)*, M-UE-9 *(Sifeng)*, M-UE-1 *(Shixuan)* (prick to let blood), Gv-14 *(Dazhui)*, Gv-12 *(Shenzhu)*, LI-11 *(Quchi)*, LI-4 *(Hegu)*
Supplementary points: P-8 *(Laogong)*, TB-5 *(Waiguan)*, K-1 *(Yongquan)*

Non-febrile convulsions
Principal points: Gv-14 *(Dazhui)*, Gv-8 *(Jinsuo)*, SI-3 *(Houxi)*, GB-34 *(Yanglingquan)*
Supplementary points: Gv-12 *(Shenzhu)*, LI-4 *(Hegu)*, N-HN-54 *(Anmian)*, Li-3 *(Taichong)*, Gv-26 *(Renzhong)*

Method: First choose among the principal points. If no clear effect, add supplementary points according to symptoms. Generally, use strong stimulation.

Ear acupuncture
Points: Subcortex, Occiput, Heart, Liver, Neurogate. If there is high fever, prick Ear Apex.

Other prescriptions
1. Principal points: Gv-26 *(Renzhong)*, LI-4 *(Hegu)*, GB-34 *(Yanglingquan)*. Supplementary points: P-6 *(Neiguan)*, GB-20 *(Fengchi)*, K-1 *(Yongquan)*. (Source: BDH)
2. L-10 *(Yuyi)*, B-57 *(Chengshan)*, B-60 *(Kunlun)*. (Source: OXH)
3. Infantile convulsions: SI-4 *(Wangu)* (Source: GOA); prick L-11 *(Shaoshang)*, Gv-26 *(Renzhong)*, K-1 *(Yongquan)*. (Source: SPMD)

Remarks
- To avoid suffocation and injury, lie the patient down, loosen his clothes and be sure that the respiratory tract is clear.
- Acupuncture is only used to treat the symptoms of this condition, so it is important that the physician examine the patient to get at the cause. It may be necessary to use oral medication for reducing fever, strengthening the Heart and sedating the patient, in addition to acupuncture.
- In cases of infantile convulsions, the physician may consider combining acupuncture with finger massage up and down the spine.
- In emergencies, the fingertips can be used in place of needles, pressing against the points with force.

SHOCK

Traditional medicine associates shock with fainting, the exhaustion of vital body functions, or diseases in which the strength of Yin and Yang is depleted. Exhausted Yin refers to an excessive loss of body fluids through sweating, vomiting, bleeding, diarrhea, etc. Because of the close reciprocal relationship between Yin and Yang, a depletion of one, e.g., the Blood (Yin), may cause depletion of the other, e.g., Qi (Yang). Or, if the Yang element is itself weakened, it may be unable to withstand an attack of the Cold Excess externally, further injuring and depleting the Yang and resulting in shock.

Acute treatment is directed toward dispersing the fainting condition and restoring the Yang.

Needling
Principal points: Gv-25 *(Suliao),* P-6 *(Neiguan)*
Supplementary points: Gv-26 *(Renzhong),* P-9 *(Zhongchong),* K-1 *(Yongquan),* S-36 *(Zusanli)*

Method: Needle the principal points continuously, with moderate stimulation, until the blood pressure rises to a stable level. Retain needles, or needle intermittently for several minutes. If blood pressure does not rise significantly, either supplementary points or electro-acupuncture may be added.

Moxibustion
Principal Points: Gv-20 *(Baihui),* Co-8 *(Qizhong),* Co-6 *(Qihai),* Co-4 *(Guanyuan)*
Method: Burn moxa sticks or cones until local sweating appears.

Ear acupuncture
Principal points: Adrenal, Raise Blood Pressure Point, Subcortex, Heart
Supplementary points: Thyroid, Hormone, Neurogate, Lung, Liver, Sympathetic
Method: First choose from among the principal points, two to four points on both ears. Needle intermittently, retaining the needles for 1-2 hours. If there is no significant effect, add supplementary points.

Other prescriptions
1. First needle Gv-26 *(Renzhong),* P-9 *(Zhongchong)* with intermittent stimulation. If the effect is not satisfactory, add P-6 *(Neiguan),* and if the blood pressure remains low, add Gv-25 *(Suliao).* Moderate to strong stimulation. (Source: HNMT)
2. Needle Gv-26 *(Renzhong)* and K-1 *(Yongquan)* with strong stimulation intermittently for 15 minutes. If there is no significant improvement in symptoms or blood pressure, add Gv-25 *(Suliao)* and P-6 *(Neiguan),* stimulating continuously, or moxi Co-6 *(Qihai)* and Co-4 *(Guanyuan)* until the symptoms have disappeared. (Source: CCMHCD)

Remarks
- The cause of shock must be carefully determined so as to select the best method of treatment. Some cases will require a combination of Chinese and Western methods.
- Acupuncture has been particularly effective in treating septic shock.

COMA

Most symptoms associated with coma, according to traditional medicine, are caused by penetration of Heat from without. After invading the body, the Phlegm and Fire from this 'Hot poison' obstruct the body cavities and obscure the 'light of the Spirit', i.e., they induce coma. In its initial stages, coma is referred to as a 'closed' condition. If, however, the body cannot recover sufficiently, the illness may deteriorate to the point that vital Organs cease to function and a so-called 'abandoned' condition ensues, resulting in death. [See discussion of 'closed' and 'abandoned' conditions under Cerebrovascular Accident in chapter 5 of this Section.]

For coma in the 'closed' stage, treatment is aimed at opening the cavities to drain the Heat. In the 'abandoned' stage, treatment is directed at restoring the Yang and stabilizing those functions that are being 'abandoned'.

Needling
'Closed' condition
Principal points: Gv-26 *(Renzhong)*, M-UE-1 *(Shixuan)*, LI-4 *(Hegu)*, Li-3 *(Taichong)*
Supplementary points: Gv-14 *(Dazhui)*, P-6 *(Neiguan)*, S-40 *(Fenglong)*, K-1 *(Yongquan)*

Method: Needle Gv-26 *(Renzhong)* intermittently, and prick M-UE-1 *(Shixuan)* to let a few drops of blood. If necessary, add supplementary points according to symptoms.

'Abandoned' condition
Principal points: Gv-20 *(Baihui)*, Co-6 *(Qihai)*, Co-4 *(Guanyuan)*, Gv-25 *(Suliao)*, L-9 *(Taiyuan)*, K-7 *(Fuliu)*
Supplementary points: LI-4 *(Hegu)*, P-8 *(Laogong)*, S-36 *(Zusanli)*

Method: Use moxibustion on points Gv-20 *(Baihui)*, Co-6 *(Qihai)* and Co-4 *(Guanyuan)*. Needle K-7 *(Fuliu)*, Gv-25 *(Suliao)* and L-9 *(Taiyuan)*. If the result is not satisfactory, add supplementary points.

Ear acupuncture
Points: Heart, Subcortex, Neurogate, Brain, Sympathetic
Method: Choose two to three points on both ears. Retain needles for 30 minutes with strong stimulation every 5 minutes.

Remarks
Careful examination of the patient is essential to determine and treat the root cause of the coma.

FAINTING

Traditional Chinese medicine regards this symptom as generally being caused by a disruption in the flow of Qi through the channels, which temporarily prevents the Blood and Qi from circulating to the head, and the Yang Qi from reaching the extremities. The Protective and Nourishing Qi become rebellious in the channels. Weakness, emotional stress and exhausting labor are among the causes which give rise to this condition.

Treatment is based upon the principles of dispersing the fainting and calming the Middle Burner (i.e., Spleen and Stomach).

Needling
Principal points: Gv-26 *(Renzhong)*, P-9 *(Zhongchong)*, S-36 *(Zusanli)*
Supplementary points: L-11 *(Shaoshang)*, LI-4 *(Hegu)*, SI-3 *(Houxi)* joined to P-8 *(Laogong)*, K-1 *(Yongquan)*

Method: Needle Gv-26 *(Renzhong)* with short, rapid thrusts (strong stimulation). Then needle P-9 *(Zhongchong)* and S-36 *(Zusanli)*. If the result is unsatisfactory, select supplementary points.

Moxibustion

Points: Gv-20 *(Baihui)*, Co-6 *(Qihai)*

Method: Use moxa stick, warming Gv-20 *(Baihui)* first. If result is unsatisfactory, add Co-6 *(Qihai)*.

Ear acupuncture

Points: Heart, Subcortex, Adrenal, Neurogate

Method: Use strong stimulation for a short period of time.

Remarks

• It is imperative to thoroughly examine the patient to determine the cause of the fainting. In many cases, for example if the fainting is associated with cardiac arrhythmias, hypoglycemia or cerebrovascular spasm, it is necessary to combine Chinese with Western methods of treatment in order to cure the underlying condition.

• Prior to beginning treatment, lie the patient down with the head slightly lower than the feet, loosen the clothing and keep the patient warm.

• Acupuncture is definitely effective in treating fainting due to functional problems.

Chapter 4

Infectious Diseases

COMMON COLD

Traditional medicine considers this illness to be caused by Wind attacking the body from without, preventing the Lung Qi from being properly distributed. It is because the Qi of the Lungs passes through the nose and is intimately related to the skin that the Wind Excess usually attacks the Lungs first.

This disease is distinguished according to its symptoms as Wind Cold or Wind Hot, either one of which may become transformed into the other. Wind Cold symptoms include headache, fever, absence of sweating, chills, soreness in the limbs, congested and drippy nose, thin white fur on the tongue, and a floating, tight pulse. Wind Hot symptoms include a feeling of distension in the head, sore throat, coughing yellow and thick phlegm, high fever with only slight chills (if any), dryness of the mouth, thin and yellow fur on the tongue, and a floating, rapid pulse.

Wind Cold type colds are treated according to the principle of dispersing the Exterior condition and scattering the Wind. Wind Hot colds are treated by dispersing the Exterior condition and cooling the Heat.

Needling

Principal points: GB-20 *(Fengchi)*, L-7 *(Lieque)*, and TB-5 *(Waiguan)* for Wind Cold; GB-20 *(Fengchi)*, Gv-14 *(Dazhui)*, LI-11 *(Quchi)*, and LI-4 *(Hegu)* for Wind Hot.

Supplementary points: LI-20 *(Yingxiang)*, M-HN-14 *(Bitong)*, M-HN-3 *(Yintang)*, M-HN-9 *(Taiyang)*, Co-22 *(Tiantu)*, S-40 *(Fenglong)*, B-12 *(Fengmen)*, B-13 *(Feishu)* and the vertebral points M-BW-35 *(Jiaji)* from the 5th cervical to the 4th thoracic vertebra.

Method: When needling GB-20 *(Fengchi)*, it is best if the needle sensation can be felt all the way to the frontal region of the head. This is particularly effective in treating nasal congestion and headache. If the nose remains congested, LI-20 *(Yingxiang)* can be joined to M-HN-14 *(Bitong)*; if the headache persists, add M-HN-3 *(Yintang)* and M-HN-9 *(Taiyang)*. If there is coughing with phlegm, use Co-22 *(Tiantu)*, S-40 *(Fenglong)*, and one or two of the M-BW-35 *(Jiaji)* vertebral points. Cups can be applied at B-12 *(Fengmen)* and B-13 *(Feishu)* if there is soreness in the upper back and neck, or the moving cup method may be applied along the Governing channel from about Gv-14 *(Dazhui)* to the lumbar vertebrae and back up again, stopping in the region of B-13 *(Feishu)*.

Discussion of points: GB-20 *(Fengchi)* is the point of intersection of the Gall Bladder and the Yang Linking channels. Because the Yang Linking channel controls the Exterior Yang, it is useful in dispersing Exterior conditions. This point may be used for both Wind Cold and Wind Hot colds. For Wind Cold type colds, TB-5 *(Waiguan)*, the Connecting point of the Triple Burner and the Yang Linking channels, strengthens the effect of dispersing the Exterior condition. This point combined with

574

the Connecting point of the Lung channel, L-7 *(Lieque)*, which aids the Lungs is distributing the Qi downward and disperses Wind, makes a particularly effective combination. For Wind Hot colds, Gv-14 *(Dazhui)*, the point of intersection of all the Yang channels on the Governing channel, is recommended for cooling the Heat. Combined with it are two points of the Large Intestine channel, LI-11 *(Quchi)* and LI-4 *(Hegu)*, which drain Heat by dispersing the Exterior condition. (The Large Intestine channel has abundant Qi and Blood, and is well suited for draining.) Points LI-20 *(Yingxiang)*, M-HN-14 *(Bitong)*, M-HN-3 *(Yintang)*, and M-HN-9 *(Taiyang)* are local points for congested nose and headache. For coughing, Co-22 *(Tiantu)* is needled to help free the passage of Lung Qi, S-40 *(Fenglong)* to transform Phlegm, and the vertebral points M-BW-35 *(Jiaji)* are selected according to the spinal segment parallel to the location of the symptoms.

Injection therapy
Points: GB-20 *(Fengchi)* or N-BW-5 *(Waidingchuan)*
Method: Inject either Vitamin B1 or a 5% extract solution of *Angelica sinesis (danggui)* at each point.

Ear acupuncture
Points: Lungs, Bronchi, Inner Nose, Throat, Forehead

Foot acupuncture
Points: #46, #47

Other prescriptions
1. Wind Cold: Gv-14 *(Dazhui)* and L-7 *(Lieque)*. Wind Hot: Gv-14 *(Dazhui)* and L-11 *(Shaoshang)*. (Source: NOCM)
2. GB-20 *(Fengchi)*, Gv-16 *(Fengfu)*, Gv-14 *(Dazhui)*, GB-1 *(Tongziliao)*, LI-11 *(Quchi)*, S-36 *(Zusanli)*, TB-6 *(Zhigou)*, S-44 *(Neiting)*, B-36 *(Fufen)*, B-37 *(Pohu)*. (Source: NAM)
3. For common cold: B-13 *(Feishu)* and Gv-13 *(Taodao)*. (Source: OHS)

Remarks
• Cold symptoms are similar to those of more serious illnesses. Further examination is therefore necessary, particularly of children when contagious diseases are prevalent.
• The methods above can be supplemented by massage at M-HN-3 *(Yintang)*, M-HN-9 *(Taiyang)*, GB-20 *(Fengchi)*, GB-21 *(Jianjing)*, LI-11 *(Quchi)*, and LI-4 *(Hegu)*.

WHOOPING COUGH (Pertussis)

This illness is said to result from Wind and Heat, which render the Lungs incapable of carrying out their cleansing and descending functions. The air passages are closed and obstructed by Phlegm and the Lung Qi cannot pass freely downward. After a long time (the Chinese term for this disease is the 'Hundred-Day Cough'), the Lung's passageways become damaged and the disease is difficult to cure.

Treatment is based on quieting the cough and transforming the Phlegm.

Needling
Principal points: M-UE-9 *(Sifeng)*, P-6 *(Neiguan)*, LI-4 *(Hegu)*
Supplementary points: Gv-14 *(Dazhui)*, Gv-12 *(Shenzhu)*, L-9 *(Taiyuan)*, S-40 *(Fenglong)*

Method: Needle one or two of the M-UE-9 *(Sifeng)* points, and squeeze fingers so that a small amount of yellow or white liquid is exuded. Then needle P-6 *(Neiguan)* and LI-4 *(Hegu)* with moderate to strong stimulation for a few minutes, and withdraw the needles. Do not retain. If results are unsatisfactory, add supplementary points.

Discussion of points: In recent experience, M-UE-9 *(Sifeng)* has proven effective in treating this disease. P-6 *(Neiguan)*, the Meeting point on the Yin Linking channel, is capable of expanding the chest and regulating the Qi. LI-4 *(Hegu)*, the Source point of the Large Intestine channel, can spread the Lung Qi and overcome the Wind and Heat Excesses. Gv-14 *(Dazhui)*, the point of intersection of all the Yang channels on the Governing channel, is needled to disperse the Exterior condition and eliminate the Excesses. Gv-12 *(Shenzhu)* is located parallel to the Associated point of the Lungs, B-13 *(Feishu)*. This point, combined with the Lung Source point, L-9 *(Taiyuan)*, and the Stomach Connecting point, S-40 *(Fenglong)*, can restore order to the Lungs, still the cough, eliminate Wind and transform Phlegm.

Cupping

Cups are applied on the upper back and neck around such points as B-12 *(Fengmen)* and B-13 *(Feishu)*. Treat daily or on alternating days.

Ear acupuncture

Points: Bronchi, Lungs, Stop Wheezing, Neurogate, Sympathetic
Method: Select 2-3 points on one ear, rotate with other ear on alternating days.

Cutaneous acupuncture

Principal points: B-13 *(Feishu)*, B-12 *(Fengmen)*, Co-12 *(Zhongwan)*, LI-2 *(Erjian)*, S-40 *(Fenglong)*, L-5 *(Chize)*, and M-BW-35 *(Jiaji)* from the 1st to the 4th thoracic vertebrae.
Supplementary points: S-36 *(Zusanli)*, Co-6 *(Qihai)*, Co-22 *(Tiantu)*, Gv-12 *(Shenzhu)*, LI-4 *(Hegu)*

Other prescriptions

1. B-13 *(Feishu)* and L-7 *(Lieque)* once daily. (Source: HIM)
2. Cup B-13 *(Feishu)*, B-38 *(Gaohuangshu)*, and L-1 *(Zhongfu)*. Alternate chest and back, 2-3 cups per treatment, for 5-8 minutes. (Source: NOCM)
3. GB-20 *(Fengchi)*, Gv-14 *(Dazhui)*, B-12 *(Fengmen)*, Co-22 *(Tiantu)*, Co-13 *(Shangwan)*, L-9 *(Taiyuan)*, S-36 *(Zusanli)*, B-10 *(Tianzhu)*, Gv-12 *(Shenzhu)*, B-13 *(Feishu)*, K-27 *(Shufu)*, Co-12 *(Zhongwan)*, L-8 *(Jingqu)*, and S-40 *(Fenglong)*. Shallow insertion with moderate stimulation once daily. (Source: CAM)
4. Needle Sp-5 *(Shangqiu)* and moxi B-13 *(Feishu)*; needle LI-4 *(Hegu)* and moxi B-38 *(Gaohuangshu)*; use warm needle method at LI-11 *(Quchi)*; moxi S-12 *(Quepen)*; moxi B-18 *(Ganshu)* and B-21 *(Weishu)*, needle Sp-5 *(Shangqiu)*, LI-11 *(Quchi)*. Rotate point groups. For needling, use shallow insertion with strong stimulation and quick removal of needle. Use moxa stick for 10-15 minutes. (Source: NAM)

CONTAGIOUS PAROTITIS (Mumps)

Traditional medicine regards this disease as being caused either by seasonal Heat (literally, Warm Poison) or the Wind and Heat Excesses which, acting in concert, attack the body through the Lesser Yang and Yang Brightness channels, and the parotid glands with Phlegm and Heat. If the disease penetrates to the Absolute Yin channels (connected to the Lesser Yang channels) it may lead to inflammation of the testicles.

The principle of treatment is to disperse the Wind and clear the Heat so as to open the channels.

Needling

Principal points: TB-17 *(Yifeng)*, S-6 *(Jiache)*, LI-4 *(Hegu)*
Supplementary points: LI-11 *(Quchi)*, L-11 *(Shaoshang)*, LI-1 *(Shangyang)*, Sp-10 *(Xuehai)*, Sp-6 *(Sanyinjiao)*, Li-8 *(Ququan)*, Li-2 *(Xingjian)*

Method: First needle the principal points. If there is fever, add LI-11 *(Quchi)*. If the swelling and pain is severe, prick L-11 *(Shaoshang)* and LI-1 *(Shangyang)* for a few drops of blood. In cases where the testicles are affected, Sp-10 *(Xuehai)*, Li-8 *(Ququan)*, Sp-6 *(Sanyinjiao)*, and Li-2 *(Xingjian)*.

Discussion of the points: Needling TB-17 *(Yifeng)* and S-6 *(Jiache)* clears local obstruction to the passage of Qi and Blood. LI-4 *(Hegu)*, the Source point of the Large Intestine channel, helps to alleviate conditions in areas traversed by that channel, including the area of the parotid glands. LI-11 *(Quchi)* may be added to reduce fever, and to clear and drain Heat from the Yang Brightness channels. Pricking points L-11 *(Shaoshang)* and LI-1 *(Shangyang)* clears and drains the Heat. Needling Sp-10 *(Xuehai)* for inflammation of the testicles clears the Heat in the Blood. Li-8 *(Ququan)* and Li-2 *(Xingjian)* spread and drain the Qi from the Liver channel. As the point of intersection of the three Yin channels of the Leg, Sp-6 *(Sanyinjiao)*, like Sp-10 *(Xuehai)*, clears the Blood, and spreads and regulates the Qi in the Absolute Yin Liver channel which penetrates the groin.

Barefoot doctor acupuncture
Points: Barefoot Doctor point, Thoracic #5

Ear acupuncture
Points: Parotid Gland, Face Area, Subcortex, point of tenderness
Method: Strong stimulation. Retain needles for 20 minutes with intermittent manipulation. Treat once daily.

Foot acupuncture
Points: #19, #26, #27

Cutaneous acupuncture
Principal points: LI-4 *(Hegu)*, S-6 *(Jiache)*, LI-2 *(Erjian)*, TB-17 *(Yifeng)*, L-7 *(Lieque)*, TB-5 *(Waiguan)*, M-BW-35 *(Jiaji)* from the 1st to the 4th thoracic vertebra
Supplementary points: LI-10 *(Shousanli)*, S-44 *(Neiting)*, and GB-43 *(Xiaxi)*

Other prescriptions
1. Moxi M-HN-10 *(Erjian)* until it becomes red. (Source: NOCM)
2. GB-20 *(Fengchi)*, B-11 *(Dashu)*, LI-11 *(Quchi)*, TB-10 *(Tianjing)*, TB-5 *(Waiguan)*, LI-4 *(Hegu)*, TB-2 *(Yemen)*. Daily with strong stimulation. (Source: CAM)
3. S-6 *(Jiache)*, LI-4 *(Hegu)*, S-5 *(Daying)*, TB-17 *(Yifeng)*, GB-20 *(Fengchi)*, S-36 *(Zusanli)*, S-8 *(Touwei)*, S-7 *(Xiaguan)*, GB-12 *(Wangu)*, B-11 *(Dashu)*, SI-13 *(Quyuan)*. (Source: NAM)
4. LI-4 *(Hegu)*, L-7 *(Lieque)*, S-4 *(Dicang)*, S-6 *(Jiache)*, Co-24 *(Chengjiang)*, LI-10 *(Shousanli)*, M-HN-20 *(Jinjin)*. (Source: GCAM)

BACTERIAL DYSENTERY

Traditional medicine regards this illness as resulting from Dampness and Heat collecting in the Stomach and Intestines through ingestion of unclean food or drink. It is treated according to the principle of clearing the Dampness and Heat so as to facilitate the stabilization of the Stomach and Intestines.

Needling
Principal points: S-37 *(Shangjuxu)* or S-36 *(Zusanli)*, S-25 *(Tianshu)*
Supplementary points: N-CA-3 *(Zhixie)*, LI-11 *(Quchi)*, P-6 *(Neiguan)*, Co-4 *(Guanyuan)*

Method: P-6 *(Neiguan)* can be added to the principal points for nausea or vomiting; Co-4 *(Guanyuan)* for tenesmus; N-CA-3 *(Zhixie)* for frequent bowel movements; and LI-11 *(Quchi)* for fever. Use strong stimulation and do not retain needles. Alternatively, the needles can be retained for 30 minutes with intermittent manipulation. Electro-acupuncture may be used. In the beginning, treat 1-3 times daily. As the symptoms improve, once a day is sufficient.

Discussion of the points: S-37 *(Shangjuxu),* the Lower Uniting point of the Large Intestine, is effective in draining that Organ when needled. Together with S-25 *(Tianshu),* the Alarm point of the Large Intestine, Dampness and Heat can be drained from the Intestines. P-6 *(Neiguan)* is used for nausea and vomiting because of its ability to calm the Stomach. Co-4 *(Guanyuan)* is the Alarm point of the Small Intestine, and can eliminate the obstruction from the Intestines, making it a useful point in treating tenesmus. Needling LI-11 *(Quchi)* drains Heat. N-CA-3 *(Zhixie)* has proven effective in recent experience in treating this disease.

Ear acupuncture
Points: Large Intestine, Small Intestine, Subcortex, Sympathetic, Neurogate
Method: Needle 1-2 times daily with moderate to strong stimulation, retaining the needles for 15-20 minutes.

Injection Therapy
Points: S-25 *(Tianshu)*
Method: Inject a 25% solution of glucose, or vitamin B1. Inject each day, bilaterally.

Moxibustion
Points: Co-8 *(Shenque),* Co-12 *(Zhongwan),* S-25 *(Tianshu),* Co-4 *(Guanyuan),* B-20 *(Pishu),* B-23 *(Shenshu).* Use only in chronic cases.

Foot Acupuncture
Points: #8, #5.

Other Prescriptions
1. Chronic dysentery: Co-4 *(Guanyuan),* Co-6 *(Qihai),* B-23 *(Shenshu),* B-20 *(Pishu),* B-25 *(Dachangshu),* Sp-6 *(Sanyinjiao),* S-36 *(Zusanli).* Use moxibustion at 2-3 points daily for 10-15 minutes. (Source: NOCM)
2. Diarrhea with blood and pus (for children): moxi M-BW-35 *(Jiaji).* (Source: CNLAM)
3. LI-4 *(Hegu),* S-36 *(Zusanli).* If severe, add B-29 *(Zhonglushu).* (Source: SPMD)
4. Damp Hot dysentery: S-44 *(Neiting),* S-25 *(Tianshu),* Sp-1 *(Yinbai),* Co-6 *(Qihai),* K-6 *(Zhaohai),* P-6 *(Neiguan).* Cold dysentery: TB-5 *(Waiguan),* Co-12 *(Zhongwan),* Sp-1 *(Yinbai),* S-25 *(Tianshu),* B-62 *(Shenmai).* (Source: GCAM)
5. Red and white dysentery (moxibustion at all points): Gv-1 *(Changqiang),* Gv-4 *(Mingmen).* If abdominal cramps increase after bowel movements, add Co-10 *(Xiawan),* S-25 *(Tianshu).* For chronic diarrhea: Co-12 *(Zhongwan),* B-20 *(Pishu),* S-25 *(Tianshu),* B-22 *(Sanjiaoshu),* B-25 *(Dachangshu),* S-36 *(Zusanli),* Sp-6 *(Sanyinjiao).* (Source: PDM)

Remarks
●Acupuncture is effective in treating this disease. If the symptoms improve, but stool cultures remain positive, antibiotics should be used.
●Moxibustion is more effective in chronic cases.

INFECTIOUS HEPATITIS

A variety of traditional disease patterns are associated with the symptoms of this condition. Possible causes for some of these patterns, as noted in the *Inner Classic,* include stagnation of the Nourishing and Protective Qi in the Liver, a struggle between the Normal Qi and abnormal factors , and swelling of the Liver with accompanying pain in the sides and abdomen. Jaundice is a manifestation of Heat and Dampness creating an imbalance between the Liver and the Spleen.

Treatment is directed toward clearing the Dampness and cooling the Heat, supporting the spreading functions of the Liver and the transportive functions of the Spleen.

Needling

First prescription: Gv-14 *(Dazhui)*, Gv-9 *(Zhiyang)*, B-18 *(Ganshu)*, B-19 *(Danshu)*, and B-20 *(Pishu)*. The corresponding vertebral points M-BW-35 *(Jiaji)* may also be used.

Second prescription: GB-34 *(Yanglingquan)* and S-36 *(Zusanli)*.

Third prescription: Sp-9 *(Yinlingquan)* and Sp-6 *(Sanyinjiao)*.

Method: When jaundice appears, Gv-14 *(Dazhui)* and Gv-9 *(Zhiyang)* are the principal points. The remaining points in the first prescription are supplementary and may be used in rotation. When the jaundice has disappeared, the second and third prescriptions may be alternated. Use moderate to strong stimulation. Six treatments constitute one course. During the first course of treatment, needle once daily. Thereafter, treat on alternating days.

Discussion of points: As the point of intersection of all the Yang channels on the Governing channel, Gv-14 *(Dazhui)* is an excellent choice for draining Heat from the body. Gv-9 *(Zhiyang)*, also on the Governing channel, has traditionally been effective in treating jaundice. The three points B-18 *(Ganshu)*, B-19 *(Danshu)*, and GB-34 *(Yanglingquan)* all drain Dampness and Heat from the Liver and Gall Bladder. B-20 *(Pishu)* and S-36 *(Zusanli)* strengthen the Spleen to help transform the Dampness. Finally, Sp-9 *(Yinlingquan)* and Sp-6 *(Sanyinjiao)* facilitate urination and, through the passage of excess urine, drain Dampness from the body.

Injection therapy

Points: B-18 *(Ganshu)*, N-BW-8 *(Ganre)*, Li-14 *(Qimen)*, Li-6 *(Zhongdu)*, GB-24 *(Riyue)*.

Method: 1) For acute hepatitis, first inject vitamin B1. When the jaundice has receded, use *Radix isatidis (banlangen)*. For chronic hepatitis, inject Glucurolactonum once daily at each point. 10-15 treatments constitute a course. 2) Inject *Artemesia capillaris glyclrrhiza* extract *(yinchen gancao ye)* daily. Three weeks of treatment constitute one course. 3) Inject extract of *Angelica sinesis (danggui)* at each point daily. 10-15 treatments constitute one course.

Barefoot doctor acupuncture

Points: Barefoot Doctor point, Thoracic #8, #12

Ear acupuncture

Points: Hepatitis, Liver, Triple Burner, Sympathetic, Pancreas/Gall Bladder, Liver Yang

Other prescriptions

1. B-19 *(Danshu)*, Li-3 *(Taichong)*, GB-34 *(Yanglingquan)*; B-18 *(Ganshu)*, S-36 *(Zusanli)*, Gv-9 *(Zhiyang)*; B-20 *(Pishu)*, Li-14 *(Qimen)*, B-10 *(Tianzhu)*. Rotate point groups. Strong stimulation, once daily. 10 treatments to a course for acute cases; 14 treatments to a course for chronic cases. (Source: HNMT)

2. "In Liver diseases . . . there is a feeling of fullness below the ribs or occasional vertigo. Needle Li-1 *(Dadun)*, and burn 100 cones of moxa on Li-2 *(Xingjian)*, Li-3 *(Taichong)*, Li-8 *(Ququan)*, Li-6 *(Zhongdu)*, and Li-14 *(Qimen)*. Burn 50 cones of moxa above the 9th [thoracic] vertebra. When the Excess resides in the Liver, both sides hurt. When there is Cold . . . choose Li-2 *(Xingjian)* to move things beneath the ribs and strengthen; S-36 *(Zusanli)* to warm the Stomach." (Source: TDP)

3. Pain in the sides: GB-39 *(Xuanzhong)*, GB-11 *(Qiaoyin)*, TB-5 *(Waiguan)*, S-36 *(Zusanli)*, TB-6 *(Zhigou)*, Li-13 *(Zhangmen)*, Li-4 *(Zhongfeng)*, GB-34 *(Yanglingquan)*, Li-2 *(Xingjian)*, Li-6 *(Zhongdu)*, Li-14 *(Qimen)*, GB-40 *(Qiuxu)*, K-1 *(Yongquan)*. Pain and fullness in the chest and sides: Sp-4 *(Gongsun)*, S-36 *(Zusanli)*, Li-3 *(Taichong)*, Sp-6 *(Sanyinjiao)*. (Source: OM)

4. Insufferable pain in the chest and sides: Li-14 *(Qimen)*, Li-13 *(Zhangmen)*, Li-2 *(Xingjian)*, GB-40 *(Qiuxu)*, K-1 *(Yongquan)*. (Source: PUB)

5. For jaundice with occassional, slight fevers use Li-4 *(Zhongfeng)* and LI-13 *(Wuli)*; for jaundice with abdominal fullness and inability to eat, use Gv-6 *(Jizhong)*; for jaundice, frequent sighing, inability to swallow, fullness in the flanks, desire to vomit, and a feeling of lethargy and heaviness, use B-20 *(Pishu)*. (Source: CNLAM)

Remarks

• Needles that have been used on patients with hepatitis must be sterilized according to the most rigorous standards.

• In a minority of severe, acute hepatitis cases, acupuncture is only a supplementary mode of therapy which must be combined with other modes of Chinese and Western medicine in order to save the patient.

SEQUELAE OF INFANTILE PARALYSIS (Polio)

This condition falls within the traditional pattern of 'atrophy'. Wind, Dampness, and Heat invade the Lungs and Stomach through the nose and mouth. Where they collect, Heat is formed. This injures the channels and disrupts the Qi and Blood, leaving the Muscle channels malnourished. The muscles and tendons become soft and shortened, while smaller connective tissues become flaccid and elongated. If the Heat grows excessive such that it penetrates the Heart and Lungs, the chest cavity will become obstructed and the condition perilous.

Treatment is based on the principle of expanding and regulating the channels.

Needling
Paralysis of the lower limb

Principal points: Gv-4 *(Mingmen)*, Gv-3 *(Yangguan)*, vertebral points M-BW-35 *(Jiaji)* from the 1st to the 5th lumbar vertebra. On the affected side, add B-31 *(Shangliao)*, B-32 *(Ciliao)*, GB-30 *(Huantiao)*, B-51 *(Yinmen)*, S-32 *(Futu)*, S-36 *(Zusanli)*, GB-34 *(Yanglingquan)*

Supplementary points: B-49 *(Zhibian)*, N-LE-18 *(Jianxi)*, M-LE-24 *(Linghou)*, B-53 *(Weiyang)*, B-54 *(Weizhong)*, S-41 *(Jiexi)*, N-LE-4 *(Naoqing)*

Paralysis of the upper limb

Principal points: Gv-14 *(Dazhui)*, LI-15 *(Jianyu)*, TB-14 *(Jianliao)*, SI-9 *(Jianzhen)*, LI-11 *(Quchi)*, LI-10 *(Shousanli)*, LI-4 *(Hegu)*

Supplementary points: SI-8 *(Xiaohai)*, TB-5 *(Waiguan)*, TB-10 *(Tianjing)*, and the vertebral points M-BW-35 *(Jiaji)* from the 5th to the 7th cervical vertebra

Paralysis of the face

Points: S-7 *(Xiaguan)*, S-6 *(Jiache)*, N-HN-20 *(Qianzheng)*, LI-4 *(Hegu)*

Paralysis of the neck

Points: B-10 *(Tianzhu)*, N-HN-47 *(Xinyi)*, SI-17 *(Tianrong)*, and M-BW-35 *(Jiaji)* from the 2nd to the 6th cervical vertebra

Paralysis of the abdomen

Points: Co-12 *(Zhongwan)*, S-21 *(Liangmen)*, S-25 *(Tianshu)*, Co-6 *(Qihai)*, S-37 *(Shangjuxu)*

Method: Begin treatment as soon as possible after the onset of paralysis. This will help control the development of the paralysis and bring about a speedier recovery. Several (rather than a few) points should be selected, needle penetration should be relatively superficial, and the needles should either not be retained at all, or for only a short time. For cases which are less recent, needle penetration can be deeper, the stimulation more intense, and the needle may be retained for a longer period of time.

Great needle acupuncture

Points: At GB-30 *(Huantiao)* the needle is inserted downward; at M-UE-30 *(Bizhong)*, insert needle in all four directions consecutively; at S-31 *(Biguan)* insert downward; at S-32 *(Futu)* insert in all four directions consecutively; at N-LE-25 *(Weishang)* insert downward, to the left and right, into the semitendinous and semimembranous tendon, and the biceps femoris muscle (especially for knee deformity); at B-54 *(Weizhong)* insert upward or downward; at Sp-9 *(Yinlingquan)* insert downward; at S-36 *(Zusanli)* insert downward; at N-LE-3 *(Genping)* especially for atrophy of the Achilles' tendon. Needling may also be used at K-3 *(Taixi)*, or B-60 *(Kunlun)* pointed in all directions, the ankle wriggled and the foot flexed during treatment. At K-6 *(Zhaohai)* or K-3 *(Taixi)*, insert toward B-60 *(Kunlun)*, especially for in-turned foot. While needling, rotate the ankle outward. At B-62 *(Shenmai)* or B-60 *(Kunlun)*, insert toward B-63 *(Jinmen)* and the Achilles' tendon, especially for out-turned foot. While needling, rotate the ankle inward.

Method: Choose one or two points in the affected area. Treat on alternating days. Electro-acupuncture may be used for points above the knee.

Injection therapy

1. Inject 10% glucose solution into B-51 *(Yinmen)* in the biceps femoris muscle, S-32 *(Futu)* in the quadriceps femoris muscle, S-36 *(Zusanli)* in the tibialis anterior muscle, and GB-30 *(Huantiao)* in the gluteus maximus and medius muscles.

2. Inject long-acting vitamin B1 at or near the nerve trunk at each of 2 to 4 points. Treat daily or on alternating days. Common sites include GB-30 *(Huantiao)*, B-25 *(Dachangshu)*, N-LE-58 *(Waiyinlian)* and S-36 *(Zusanli)*.

Cutaneous acupuncture

Paralysis of the upper limb

Principal points: LI-11 *(Quchi)*, LI-15 *(Jianyu)*, TB-5 *(Waiguan)*, LI-4 *(Hegu)*, TB-4 *(Yangchi)*, Co-6 *(Qihai)*, M-BW-35 *(Jiaji)* from the 5th to the 9th thoracic vertebra

Supplementary points: GB-31 *(Fengshi)*, S-41 *(Jiexi)*, Gv-4 *(Mingmen)*, B-57 *(Chengshan)*, B-54 *(Weizhong)*

Paralysis of the face

Use the points listed under 'Facial Paralysis' in this Section.

Paralysis of abdominal muscles

Principal points: Co-12 *(Zhongwan)*, S-21 *(Liangmen)*, Co-6 *(Qihai)*, S-30 *(Qichong)*, S-25 *(Tianshu)*, S-27 *(Daju)*, S-29 *(Guilai)*, M-BW-35 *(Jiaji)* from the 8th to the 14th thoracic vertebra

Supplementary points: Co-4 *(Guanyuan)*, Co-10 *(Xiawan)*, Sp-16 *(Fuai)*, Sp-15 *(Daheng)*, Sp-14 *(Fujie)*

Paralysis of the neck

Points: B-10 *(Tianzhu)*, M-HN-30 *(Bailao)*, N-HN-47 *(Xinyi)*, LI-17 *(Tianding)*, SI-17 *(Tianrong)*, Gv-16 *(Fengfu)*, M-HN-31 *(Chonggu)*, GB-20 *(Fengchi)*, SI-15 *(Jianzhongshu)*, TB-16 *(Tianyou)*, M-HN-35 *(Jiaji)* from the 1st to the 5th thoracic vertebra

Method: Select points according to the location of the paralysis. Needle daily or on alternating days, 10 to 15 treatments to one course of treatment.

Electro-acupuncture

Method: Choose points along nerves innervating affected muscle groups.

Lower back

1) M-BW-35 *(Jiaji)* at the second lumbar vertebra and B-32 *(Ciliao)*
2) B-25 *(Dachangshu)*, M-BW-33 *(Tunzhong)*

581

Lower limb

1) GB-30 *(Huantiao)* on the sciatic nerve combined with B-51 *(Yinmen)* in the biceps femoris muscle, or B-50 *(Chengfu)*, GB-31 *(Fengshi)*, N-LE-26 *(Zhili)*, or B-49 *(Zhibian)*

2) N-LE-58 *(Waiyinlian)* on the femoral nerve, combined with S-32 *(Futu)* in the quadriceps femoris, Sp-10 *(Xuehai)*, or S-34 *(Liangqiu)*

3) N-LE-58 *(Waiyinlian)* and N-LE-18 *(Jianxi)*

4) B-54 *(Weizhong)* on the fibial nerve, and a point just medial to the Achilles' tendon and the superior margin of the calcaneous

5) B-54 *(Weizhong)* on the tibial nerve and N-LE-9 *(Genjin)* on the sural nerve, or N-LE-10 *(Jiuwaifan)*

6) M-LE-24 *(Linghou)* on the common peroneal nerve, and S-36 *(Zusanli)* on the tibial anterior muscle, or N-LE-11 *(Jiuneifan)*

7) GB-30 *(Huantiao)* and B-54 *(Weizhong);* or GB-30 *(Huantiao)* and B-49 *(Zhibian);* or B-54 *(Weizhong)* and M-LE-24 *(Linghou)*

8) M-LE-24 *(Linghou)* and S-41 *(Jiexi)*, or GB-39 *(Juegu)*, GB-40 *(Qiuxu)*, or N-LE-4 *(Naoqing)*

Upper limb

1) SI-9 *(Jianzhen)* on the axillary and radial nerves and the center of the deltoid muscle

2) LI-15 *(Jianyu)* in the deltoid muscle and LI-11 *(Quchi)* on the radial nerve with superficial insertion, median nerve with deep insertion

3) LI-15 *(Jianyu)* in the deltoid muscle and LI-10 *(Shousanli)* on the median nerve

4) SI-8 *(Xiaohai)* on the ulnar nerve and P-6 *(Neiguan)* on the median nerve, or LI-4 *(Hegu)* and SI-3 *(Houxi)*

Threading, embedding, and loop-tying

Method: Choose points along nerves innervating affected muscle groups.

Buttocks

N-BW-16 *(Tiaoyue)*, GB-30 *(Huantiao)*, N-LE-56 *(Kuanjiu)*, M-BW-33 *(Tunzhong)*, and B-49 *(Zhibian)*

Lower back

B-23 *(Shenshu)*, B-26 *(Guanyuanshu)*, B-25 *(Dachangshu)*, Gv-3 *(Yaoyangguan)*, B-32 *(Ciliao)*. Only embed thread at these points.

Anterior thigh

N-LE-23 *(Maibu)*, S-31 *(Biguan)*, S-32 *(Futu)*, N-LE-19 *(Siqiang)*, N-LE-18 *(Jianxi)*, and points one unit below Sp-10 *(Xuehai)* and S-34 *(Liangqiu)*

Posterior thigh

N-LE-26 *(Zhili)*, N-LE-29 *(Yinkang)*, N-LE-46 *(Yangkang)*, B-50 *(Chengfu)*, B-51 *(Yinmen)*, N-LE-25 *(Weishang)*. (To correct 'back knee', the tendon of the biceps femoris is tied to the semimembranous tendons.)

Medial aspect of the thigh

N-LE-31 *(Jiejian)*

Lateral aspect of the thigh

N-LE-35 *(Qianjin)* and GB-31 *(Fengshi)*

Anterior lower leg

At the superior and inferior margins of the patella, and S-36 *(Zusanli)*. Points to be threaded.

Posterior lower leg

B-57 *(Chengshan)* and N-LE-9 *(Genjin).* Points to be threaded.

Foot

The Achilles' tendon can either be threaded or tied. Commonly used for atrophy of the Achilles' tendon.

Upper limb

N-UE-11 *(Taijian),* N-UE-10 *(Jubi),* and LI-14 *(Binao)*

Loop-tying method: A semi-circular pattern is most common; a horizontal "8" is also used, most often at Gv-3 *(Yaoyangguan).* For lateral rotation of the lower limb, loop the points N-LE-56 *(Kuanjiu),* N-LE-46 *(Yangkang)* and N-LE-35 *(Qianjin).* For 'back knee', loop the points N-LE-56 *(Kuanjiu),* N-LE-25 *(Weishang)* and B-51 *(Yinmen).* If one side of the pelvis is abnormally low, B-25 *(Dachangshu)* or B-26 *(Guanyuanshu)* on that side can be tied; if abnormally high, B-25 *(Dachangshu)* should be embedded with thread only.

Important: The threading method should be used at points along the side of the spine or lower leg, or points in severely atrophied muscle. Points on the bellies of muscles and tendons should first be stroked with forceps and then loop-tied. Flaccid muscle should be tied a little tighter than less flaccid muscle. Points on contracted muscle should be stroked more with the forceps to loosen them, then embedded without tying.

Other prescriptions

1. GB-20 *(Fengchi),* Gv-14 *(Dazhui),* Gv-7 *(Zhongshu),* B-23 *(Shenshu),* S-25 *(Tianshu),* S-36 *(Zusanli),* B-10 *(Tianzhu),* Gv-12 *(Shenzhu),* Gv-4 *(Mingmen),* B-22 *(Sanjiaoshu),* Co-6 *(Qihai),* GB-34 *(Yanglingquan).* (Source: CAM)

2. Acute stage: Gv-20 *(Baihui),* Gv-16 *(Fengfu),* GB-20 *(Fengchi),* Gv-14 *(Dazhui),* B-11 *(Dashu),* B-12 *(Fengmen),* Gv-4 *(Mingmen),* Gv-3 *(Yaoyangguan),* LI-15 *(Jianyu),* LI-11 *(Quchi),* P-6 *(Neiguan),* GB-30 *(Huantiao),* S-36 *(Zusanli),* Sp-6 *(Sanyinjiao).*

Sequelae: Upper extremity paralysis: Gv-14 *(Dazhui),* GB-21 *(Jianjing),* LI-15 *(Jianyu),* LI-11 *(Quchi),* LI-4 *(Hegu).* Lower extremity paralysis: Gv-4 *(Mingmen),* B-23 *(Shenshu),* Gv-3 *(Yaoyangquan),* B-31 to 34 *(Shangliao to Xialiao),* GB-30 *(Huantiao),* GB-31 *(Fengshi),* GB-34 *(Yanglingquan),* S-34 *(Liangqiu),* S-36 *(Zusanli),* B-57 *(Chengshan),* B-62 *(Shenmai).* (Source: HAM)

Remarks

• During the course of treatment, both physical therapy and manipulation should be used in addition to acupuncture.

• During the early and recovery stages of this disease, needling should be the principal method of acupuncture treatment, and the other techniques supplementary. For the sequelae, embedding and loop-tying the points with thread can be added.

• For serious deformity of the joints, corrective surgery may be considered.

• During the acute and recovery stages, Chinese herbal medicine, both internal and external, may be used in conjunction with acupuncture.

MALARIA

In Chinese medicine, this disease is believed to invade the body and reside in an intermediate position between Exterior and Interior conditions. (According to the six channel diagnostics, this is one type of Lesser Yang condition.) This disease pattern, which is used to describe almost any kind of tidal fever, shares certain of the pathological characteristics of both Exterior and Interior conditions. The Yin and Yang are divided and struggle against each other.

The principle of treatment is to spread the Yang Qi through the Governing channel, and regulate the Yin and Yang.

Needling

Principal points: Gv-14 *(Dazhui)*, Gv-13 *(Taodao)*, P-6 *(Neiguan)*, P-5 *(Jianshi)* and M-BW-35 *(Jiaji)* at points of tenderness from the 3rd to the 12th thoracic vertebra

Supplementary points: LI-11 *(Quchi)*, Sp-10 *(Xuehai)*, GB-34 *(Yanglingquan)* and K-7 *(Fuliu)*

Method: Generally, treatment should be given 2-3 hours before an attack. Use strong stimulation without retaining the needles, or retain the needles for 15-30 minutes with intermittent needling. Treat daily for 3 to 6 days.

Discussion of the points: Needling Gv-14 *(Dazhui)* and Gv-13 *(Taodao)* spreads the Yang Qi through the Governing channel which 'governs' the Yang Qi of the whole body. P-6 *(Neiguan)* and P-5 *(Jianshi)* are both on the Absolute Yin Pericardium channel which is paired with the Lesser Yang Triple Burner channel in a Yin/Yang relationship. Needling these points drains the Triple Burner, thereby restoring the balance between the Interior (Yin) and Exterior (Yang). The vertebral points M-BW-35 *(Jiaji)* lie on a Divergent branch of the Governing channel which joins with the Leg Greater Yang Bladder channel. These points share therapeutic properties in common with points along the Governing channel. Stimulating the vertebral points routes the Excess through the Bladder channel. LI-11 *(Quchi)*, the Uniting point of the Arm Yang Brightness Large Intestine channel, and GB-34 *(Yanglingquan)*, the Uniting point of the Leg Lesser Yang Gall Bladder channel, regulates the Yang Qi in these channels. Sp-10 *(Xuehai)* on the Leg Greater Yin Spleen channel and K-7 *(Fuliu)* on the Leg Lesser Yin Kidney channel, together with the points already mentioned on the Arm Absolute Yin Pericardium channel, collectively regulate the Qi in these three Yin channels.

Ear acupuncture

Points: Adrenal, Subcortex, Endocrine, Neurogate, Spleen

Method: Needle 1-2 hours before an attack, retaining the needles for 1 hour. Treat daily for 3 days. The Spleen point is used for patients who suffer repeated attacks.

Cupping

Cutaneous acupuncture

Principal points: Gv-14 *(Dazhui)* (prick to let blood), Gv-13 *(Taodao)*, Gv-16 *(Fengfu)*, Gv-12 *(Shenzhu)*, P-5 *(Jianshi)*, K-3 *(Taixi)*, LI-4 *(Hegu)*, Li-3 *(Taichong)*, B-11 *(Dashu)* (prick to let blood) and M-BW-35 *(Jiaji)* from the 5th thoracic to the 5th sacral vertebra

Supplementary points: P-6 *(Neiguan)*, K-7 *(Fuliu)*, S-31 *(Biguan)*, Li-13 *(Zhangmen)*, GB-39 *(Xuanzhong)*, B-38 *(Gaohuang)*, Gv-10 *(Lingtai)*, Gv-4 *(Mingmen)*, M-HN-31 *(Chonggu)*

Other prescriptions

1. M-HN-31 *(Chonggu)*, Gv-14 *(Dazhui)*, Gv-13 *(Taodao)*, K-3 *(Taixi)*, SI-3 *(Houxi)*, P-5 *(Jianshi)*, K-7 *(Fuliu)*, H-7 *(Shenmen)*, Li-13 *(Zhangmen)*, B-20 *(Pishu)*. (Source: NAM)

2. Gv-14 *(Dazhui)* or Gv-13 *(Taodao)*, P-5 *(Jianshi)*, SI-3 *(Houxi)*, K-7 *(Fuliu)*. Use moderate stimulation. (Source: CAM)

3. Place a bit of mashed *Eclipta prostrada L. (hanliancao)* on the palmar surface of the forearm between two tendons [P-5 *(Jianshi)*]. Press with an ancient coin and wrap in silk. Before long a blister will arise. This is called 'heavenly moxibustion' and is used in the treatment of tidal fevers. (Source: TDP)

4. Gv-20 *(Baihui)*, L-8 *(Jingqu)*, SI-2 *(Qiangu)*. (Source: CDR)

5. Moxi at Gv-14 *(Dazhui)* and Gv-12 *(Shenzhu)*; needle B-40 *(Yixi)* for profuse sweating, Li-13 *(Zhangmen)*, P-5 *(Jianshi)* for chronic tidal fever, SI-3 *(Houxi)* for chills before fever, GB-30 *(Huantiao)*, B-57 *(Chengshan)*, B-60 *(Kunlun)*, K-3 *(Taixi)*, Sp-4 *(Gongsun)*, B-67 *(Zhiyin)*, LI-4 *(Hegu)*. For chronic tidal fevers that resist treatment, burn 7 cones of moxa at B-20 *(Pishu)*. (Source: IACC)

6. Chills followed by fever: GB-39 *(Xuanzhong)*, Gv-20 *(Baihui)*, B-38 *(Gaohuang)*, LI-4 *(Hegu)*. Fever followed by chills: LI-11 *(Quchi)*, GB-39 *(Xuanzhong)*, B-38 *(Gaohuang)*, M-HN-30 *(Bailao)*. Fever longer than chills: SI-3 *(Houxi)*, P-5 *(Jianshi)*, M-HN-30 *(Bailao)*, LI-11 *(Quchi)*. Chills longer than fever: SI-3 *(Houxi)*, M-HN-30 *(Bailao)*, LI-11 *(Quchi)*. (Source: GCAM)

Remarks
- If, after needling, the symptoms are still not under control, treatment should be supplemented with medication.
- Careful attention must be given to patients with malignant malaria. When necessary, other Chinese and Western modes of treatment should be used.

FILARIAL ELEPHANTIASIS

Chinese medicine regards this illness as resulting from a collection of Heat and Dampness which obstructs the Vessels, congeals the Blood and stagnates the Qi.

Treatment is directed toward activating the Blood to eliminate congealed Blood and open the channels.

Letting blood and cupping
Points: S-36 *(Zusanli)*, S-39 *(Xiajuxu)*, Sp-9 *(Yinglingquan)*, Sp-6 *(Sanyinjiao)* and the point of greatest swelling

Method: Tap the points with a cutaneous needle until they begin to bleed, or use a pyramid needle or surgical instrument to the same effect. Then apply cups for five to ten minutes. Remove cups and bandage. Treat once daily.

Remarks
- Do not use this method on ulcerated areas.

CHYLURIA

According to tradition, this illness is caused by Dampness and Heat collecting and 'steaming' the Triple Burner, thereby disrupting its distribution of water. The Yin is said to be Deficient in the Kidneys, which prevents that Organ from processing fatty liquids. Alternatively, because of insufficient Kidney Yang, the Middle Qi sinks and there is a general sagging, both literally and functionally, of the Organs in the abdomen.

Treatment is based on clearing the water passageways and regulating the Spleen and Kidneys.

Needling
Points: Co-4 *(Guanyuan)*, Sp-6 *(Sanyinjiao)*

Method: Use moderate stimulation. Treat daily or on alternating days, 15-20 treatments constituting one course.

Discussion of points: Co-4 *(Guanyuan)* is the Alarm point of the Small Intestine and is the point of intersection of the three Leg Yin channels on the Conception channel. It also has a close relationship with the Source Qi. Because the Small Intestine has the function of separating the clean (nutrients) from the unclean (waste) in food, and because the Conception channel circulates within the Abdomen, needling Co-4 *(Guanyuan)* regulates and strengthens the Kidney Qi, facilitates the digestive and excretory functions of the abdominal Organs, and opens the water passageways. Sp-6 *(Sanyinjiao)* is the point of intersection of the three Leg Yin channels. Its effect on these channels is to relieve Dampness in the Spleen and Damp Heat in the Lower Burner while facilitating the passage of urine.

Moxibustion

Points: Co-8 *(Qizhong)*, Co-9 *(Shuifen)*, Co-5 *(Shimen)*, Co-17 *(Shanzhong)*, Co-7 *(Yinjiao)*, Gv-4 *(Mingmen)*, Co-11 *(Jianli)*, Co-4 *(Guanyuan)*, Co-6 *(Qihai)*, K-27 *(Shufu)*, GB-26 *(Daimai)*, S-13 *(Qihu)*, Sp-21 *(Dabao)*, and other points of tenderness.

Method: Select 2-3 points in rotation. Treat once daily. Burn moxa sticks for 10-15 minutes, or 5-7 cones of moxa on a slice of ginger.

Other prescriptions

1. The Five Urinary Dysfunctions: 7 cones of moxa on salt at Co-8 *(Qizhong)* and moxa at Sp-6 *(Sanyinjiao)*. (Source: GOA)

2. The Five Urinary Dysfunctions: B-17 *(Geshu)*, B-20 *(Pishu)*, B-23 *(Shenshu)*, Co-6 *(Qihai)*, Co-5 *(Shimen)*, Co-4 *(Guanyuan)*, P-5 *(Jianshi)*, Sp-10 *(Xuehai)*, Sp-6 *(Sanyinjiao)*, K-7 *(Fuliu)*, K-2 *(Rangu)*, Li-1 *(Dadun)*. (Source: IACC)

Remarks

• Needling and moxibustion can be alternated or used together, if preferred. The patient should be encouraged to rest and reduce intake of fatty foods.

SCHISTOSOMIASIS

Chinese medicine recognizes that this disease is caused by a worm whose poison forms an obstruction which impedes the circulation of Qi and Blood through the vessels, and causes the passage of water and food to stagnate.

Treatment is based on dispersing and draining the Qi of the Triple Burner so as to eliminate the worms' poison.

Electro-acupuncture

Points: N-BW-22 *(Zhongjiaoshu)* and N-BW-38 *(Xiajiaoshu)*

Method: Insert the needle at N-BW-22 *(Zhongjiaoshu)* toward the spine at a 75° angle to the surface of the skin. At this angle the needle should be inserted to a depth of 2.5-2.8 units, reaching beneath the transverse processes of the 12th thoracic and 1st lumbar vertebrae. A needle should be inserted only on the left side, to avoid penetrating the inferior vena cava on the right. Attach one electrode to the needle and place the other in the middle of the upper abdomen. When needling N-BW-38 *(Xiajiaoshu)* the doctor should try to penetrate to the anterior margin of the sacrum, inserting the needle bilaterally to a depth of 3 units. The electrodes should then be attached to each. Needle N-BW-22 *(Zhongjiaoshu)* in the morning and N-BW-38 *(Xiajiaoshu)* in the afternoon for 15 minutes each. Ten treatments constitute one course. When needling N-BW-22 *(Zhongjiaoshu)*, there may be some distension on the left side of the lower abdomen or around the umbilicus. When needling N-BW-38 *(Xiajiaoshu)*, the patient may experience the sensation of defecation or urination. Generally, after several days of treatment these phenomena disappear.

Discussion of the points: Both of these points are new. N-BW-22 *(Zhongjiaoshu)* is located on the celiac plexus, along the course of the Bladder channel, and its stimulation can affect the activities of the Liver, Gall Bladder, Spleen, Stomach, Kidneys, and Intestines, as well as the functioning of the blood vessels in the abdomen. It was therefore given the name Associated point of the Middle Burner. N-BW-38 *(Xiajiaoshu)*, on the other hand, is located on the pelvic plexus along the course of the Governing and Bladder channels. Stimulating this point can affect activities of the lower abdominal organs. Its name is translated as the Associated point of the Lower Burner. Needling both points regulates the Qi along the course of the Triple Burner, and expels the worms.

Other prescriptions

1. Moxibustion for the toxin of poisonous worms: 3 cones of moxa on the tip of the little toe. (Source: TDP)

2. If the body is jaundiced and emaciated, there is no strength in the extremities, the abdomen is swollen like a drum, and in the flanks there is accumulated Qi like stone eggs, use Li-13 *(Zhangmen)*. When there is edema and the skin of the lower abdomen is thick, use Sp-6 *(Sanyinjiao)* and Co-5 *(Shimen)*. When there is ascites, use S-36 *(Zusanli)*. When the upper abdomen is swollen and distended and the area around the umbilicus is uncomfortable, use Li-1 *(Dadun)*. (Source: CNLAM)

3. Simple distension due to poisonous worm: apply moxa to B-18 *(Ganshu)*, B-20 *(Pishu)*, B-22 *(Sanjiaoshu)*, Co-9 *(Shuifen)*, Sp-4 *(Gongsun)*, Li-1 *(Dadun)*. (No reference)

4. Liver Accumulation (Fat Qi): apply 7 cones of moxa at B-18 *(Ganshu)*, 21 cones at Li-13 *(Zhangmen)*, 7 cones at Li-2 *(Xingjian)*. (No reference)

5. Method for the toxin of poisonous worm: Co-12 *(Zhongwan)* and K-6 *(Zhaohai)*. (Source: IACC)

Remarks

• Electro-acupuncture is a new method for treating schistosomiasis in the advanced stage. The rate at which this method eliminates worms is still too low. Further progress is needed.

PULMONARY TUBERCULOSIS

In traditional medicine, pulmonary tuberculosis is referred to by a variety of names, most of which are types of 'Deficient Consumption'. In the Sui Dynasty book, *Discussion of the Origins of Symptoms of Disease,* it is related that this condition is contagious. The disease focuses primarily in the Lungs but also involves the Spleen and Kidneys.

Traditionally, this disease is divided into two categories: Deficient Yin and Deficient Yang.

In the case of Deficient Yin, the Yin of the Lungs is depleted, Fire destroys the body fluids, and the vessels in the Lungs are injured. This results in afternoon fevers (sometimes low grade), night sweats, flushed cheeks, hacking cough, yellow phlegm, coughing blood or blood in the phlegm, emaciation, dry mouth and throat, irritability, insomnia, dark red tongue or red at the edges and tip, and a fine, rapid pulse. If the coughing is prolonged the voice will become raspy.

With Deficient Yang, the Lung Qi is exhausted and the Yang of the Spleen and Kidneys is Deficient. Symptoms of Deficient Yang include prolonged coughing, shortness of breath, acute sensitivity to cold, spontaneous sweating, alternating fever and chills, lack of appetite, loose stool, fine sputum, pale tongue with white fur, and a weak pulse. Sometimes there is also edema of the lower limb, lower back pain, lassitude, spermatorrhea, irregular menstruation or amenorrhea and other Deficient Kidney symptoms.

Based on the reciprocal relationship of Yin and Yang, Deficient Yin symptoms and Deficient Yang symptoms often coexist simultaneously or transform one to the other. This transformation process almost always occurs near the end of the illness.

Treatment is based upon the principles of strengthening the Lung Qi and invigorating the Spleen and Stomach Yang (the Middle Burner).

Needling

Principal points: B-13 *(Feishu)*, Gv-14 *(Dazhui)*, L-6 *(Kongzui)*, S-36 *(Zusanli)*, N-BW-6 *(Jiehexue)*

Supplementary points: Sp-4 *(Gongsun)*, L-9 *(Taiyuan)*, K-3 *(Taixi)*, L-1 *(Zhongfu)*, B-17 *(Geshu)*, H-6 *(Yinxi)*, H-7 *(Shenmen)*, Co-12 *(Zhongwan)*, S-25 *(Tianshu)*, Sp-6 *(Sanyinjiao)*, B-23 *(Shenshu)*, Co-4 *(Guanyuan)*, Co-17 *(Shanzhong)*

Method: Use principal points as basis of prescription, intermittent needling with moderate to strong stimulation. For coughing blood (Deficient Yin symptom), add B-17 *(Geshu)* and L-1 *(Zhongfu);* for cough, add L-9 *(Taiyuan);* night sweats, add H-6 *(Yinxi);* irritability and insomnia, add H-7

(Shenmen); suppressed appetite, use Sp-4 *(Gongsun)* and Co-12 *(Zhongwan);* loose stool, add S-25 *(Tianshu);* spermatorrhea or irregular menstruation, use K-3 *(Taixi)* and Sp-6 *(Sanyinjiao);* for sensitivity to cold and shortness of breath (Deficient Yang symptoms), use moxibustion at B-23 *(Shenshu),* Co-4 *(Guanyuan)* and Co-17 *(Shanzhong).* Moxibustion may also be used at points S-25 *(Tianshu),* B-13 *(Feishu)* and B-17 *(Geshu).*

Discussion of points: Gv-14 *(Dazhui),* the point of intersection of the three Leg Yang channels on the Governing channel, can be used to treat Deficient Yin symptoms of recurrent fever and hot sensation in the bones. Needling B-13 *(Feishu)* and L-6 *(Kongzui)* strengthens the Lungs and disperses the Fire lodged therein. S-36 *(Zusanli),* the Uniting point of the Stomach, is chosen to regulate and strengthen the Spleen and Stomach which support the Lung Qi. N-BW-6 *(Jiehexue)* is a new point which has proven effective in treating tuberculosis. For the Deficient Yin symptom of coughing blood, L-1 *(Zhongfu),* the Alarm point of the Lungs, cools the Lungs and B-17 *(Geshu),* the Meeting point of the Blood, channels the Blood back to the vessels. L-9 *(Taiyuan)* is the Source point of the Lung channel. Its stimulation can suppress the coughing by restoring order to the Lungs. Night sweats is another Deficient Yin symptom. Needling H-6 *(Yinxi),* the Accumulating point on the Arm Lesser Yin Heart channel, can eliminate the Heat and stop the sweating. H-7 *(Shenmen)* calms the Heart and pacifies the Spirit. It is selected for treating irritability and insomnia. Sp-4 *(Gongsun),* the Connecting point of the Spleen channel, is stimulated for lack of appetite. Co-12 *(Zhongwan),* the Alarm point of the Stomach, may be added to calm the Stomach and Spleen. S-25 *(Tianshu)* is the Alarm point of the Large Intestine. It regulates that Organ and is useful in treating diarrhea. For spermatorrhea or irregular menstruation, K-3 *(Taixi),* the Kidney Source point, is combined with Sp-6 *(Sanyinjiao)* to strengthen the Kidneys. Moxibustion is applied at B-23 *(Shenshu)* and Co-4 *(Guanyuan)* for patients with the Deficient Yang variety of this disease, so as to support and stabilize the Source (i.e., the Kidneys). Co-17 *(Shanzhong)* is added to warm and strengthen the Ancestral Qi.

Injection therapy
Principal points: N-BW-6 *(Jiehexue),* B-13 *(Feishu),* L-1 *(Zhongfu)*
Supplementary points: B-38 *(Gaohuangshu),* LI-11 *(Quchi),* L-6 *(Kongzui)*
Method: Inject either vitamin B1 or streptomycin. Insert needle .5 to .8 units at each point and inject fluid at a moderate rate.

Ear acupuncture
Points: Lung, Occiput, Sympathetic, Neurogate, Stop Wheezing

Embedding thread
1. N-BW-6 *(Jiehexue),* join B-14 *(Jueyinshu)* to B-13 *(Geshu),* join L-1 *(Zhongfu)* to L-2 *(Yunmen).*
2. B-38 *(Gaohuang),* N-BW-20 *(Feirexue).*
Method: The two prescriptions should be alternated, allowing 20-30 days between the first embedding and the second.

Other prescriptions
1. Coughing blood: L-10 *(Yuji),* L-5 *(Chize),* P-5 *(Jianshi),* H-7 *(Shenmen),* L-9 *(Taiyuan),* P-8 *(Laogong),* Li-8 *(Ququan),* K-3 *(Taixi),* K-2 *(Rangu),* Li-3 *(Taichong),* B-13 *(Feishu)* one hundred cones of moxa, B-18 *(Ganshu)* three cones of moxa, B-20 *(Pishu)* two cones of moxa. (Source: CDR)
2. Deficient consumption: up to 500 cones of moxa on Co-4 *(Guanyuan).* (Source: BBQS)
3. Coughing red sputum: M-HN-30 *(Bailao),* B-13 *(Feishu),* Co-12 *(Zhongwan),* S-36 *(Zusanli).* (Source: GCAM)
4. Hemoptysis with pulmonary tuberculosis: Principal points: L-7 *(Lieque),* L-9 *(Taiyuan),* L-5 *(Chize),* S-36 *(Zusanli).* Supplementary points: H-7 *(Shenmen),* L-10 *(Yuji),* P-7 *(Daling).* For cough add Gv-14 *(Dazhui),* B-13 *(Feishu),* and S-40 *(Fenglong).* Insomnia, add H-7 *(Shenmen),*

Sp-6 *(Sanyinjiao)*, and Li-3 *(Taichong)*. Chest pain, add TB-6 *(Zhigou)*, H-6 *(Yinxi)*. Night sweats, add SI-3 *(Houxi)* and LI-4 *(Hegu)*. (Source: SJTM)

Remarks
• The effectiveness of acupuncture treatment can be strengthened by the concurrent use of Chinese herbal and antituberculin drugs.
• The patient's nutrition is very important in strengthening his resistance to this disease. Eating utensils and other articles which the patient uses should be sterilized.
• Moxibustion was frequently recommended in ancient Chinese medical texts for the hot, 'steaming' sensation in the bones, recurrent fever, coughing and coughing blood symptoms associated with this disease.

SCROFULA

According to traditional etiology, this condition is caused by the stagnation of Liver Qi which generates Fire, transforming the body fluids into Phlegm which obstructs the channels. It may also arise from weakness in the Lungs and Kidneys generating Fire. This prevents the Lungs from distributing the fluids, which instead transform into Phlegm and congeal.

Treatment is directed at warming the Yang to open the channels.

Moxibustion
Points: Gv-20 *(Baihui)*, TB-10 *(Tianjing)*, M-UE-46 *(Zhoujian)* and the vicinity of the affected lymph node
Method: Burn 5 to 7 moxa cones directly on each of the points, in rotation. In the vicinity of the lymph node itself, the moxa can be placed on a ginger wafer and ignited.

Piercing method
1. Search for a 'point of reaction' near the 7th cervical vertebra, at the inferior angle of the shoulder blade and along the posterior axillary crease, bilaterally; or
2. Select B-31 *(Shangliao)*, B-32 *(Ciliao)* or B-33 *(Zhongliao)*, bilaterally, plus the point midway between each of the bilateral points. Each of these points, bilaterally, plus the midpoint constitutes a three point grouping. Pierce one three point grouping daily; or
3. Using the distance between the transverse crease of the distal and middle joints of the middle finger as one unit, measure 7 units down the spine from Gv-14 *(Dazhui)*. There are five pair of points. The first two points are one unit lateral to the spine from this location, on each side. One unit lateral to the first points, bilaterally, is the second pair of points. The third pair is one unit below the points in the second pair, and the fourth pair is yet another unit below the third. The fifth pair is comprised of LI-14 *(Binao)*, bilaterally. Pierce one pair of points per treatment.

Hot needle acupuncture
Insert a heated needle into the center of each affected node. Allow 2-3 days between treatments.

Incision method
1st prescription: B-17 *(Geshu)*, B-18 *(Ganshu)*
2nd prescription: Co-15 *(Jiuwei)*
Method: Make an incision 1 to 2 cm. in length at the point, and remove a small amount of fatty tissue. Treat once weekly.

Injection method
Points: N-BW-6 *(Jiehexue)*, B-13 *(Feishu)* and the affected lymph node
Method: Inject streptomycin into each point. Treat once daily.

Barefoot doctor acupuncture
Points: Barefoot Doctor point, Thoracic #5

Other prescriptions

1. Take a clove of garlic and make a hole in the center. Take a small moxa cone, insert in garlic, and place over the scrofula. Light the moxa. Warm but don't burn the area. Each time use 7 cones. Perform 3 times daily until scrofula disappears. (Source: TDP)

2. Apply 100 cones of moxa at Li-13 *(Zhangmen)*, GB-41 *(Linqi)*, TB-6 *(Zhigou)*, GB-38 *(Yangfu)*. Apply as many cones of moxa at each of the four corners of the lesion. (Source: CNLAM)

3. Apply 7-9 cones of moxa at LI-15 *(Jianyu)*; 14 cones each at LI-11 *(Quchi)*, P-1 *(Tianchi)*, and TB-10 *(Tianjing)*; 21 cones at LI-3 *(Sanjian)*. Scrofula that extends to the back of the neck: Apply 7 moxa cones at LI-15 *(Jianyu)*, M-UE-46 *(Zhoujian)*, and S-9 *(Renying)*; 14 cones at SI-14 *(Jianwaishu)* and TB-10 *(Tianjing)*. (Source: IACC)

4. Scrofula tubercles: GB-21 *(Jianjing)*, LI-11 *(Quchi)*, TB-10 *(Tianjing)*, TB-8 *(Sanyangluo)*, Sp-9 *(Yinlingquan)*. (Source: GCAM)

Remarks

- Do not directly needle a lymph node which has pustulated.
- Acupuncture is effective in treating this condition, but if ulceration has already occurred, it is necessary to combine acupuncture with drugs, or consider surgery.

Chapter 5

Internal and Pediatric Diseases

BRONCHITIS

According to Chinese medicine, the Qi from the Lungs spreads to the pores of the skin and reaches upward to the nose and mouth. When an Excess of external origin (e.g., Wind) enters the body through the pores, nose or mouth, the spreading and cleansing functions of the Lung Qi are hindered. The onset of disease is abrupt, in the manner of acute bronchitis.

Chronic bronchitis, on the other hand, may be caused by weakness in the transportive and transformative functions of the Spleen, whereby Phlegm and Dampness collect and rise to the Lungs. It may also occur when prolonged coughing injures the Lungs, and the Kidneys, in a Deficient condition, are unable to take in the Lung Qi which therefore does not properly descend.

Treatment is based on the principles of spreading the Lung Qi and causing it to descend, eliminating the Wind and transforming the Phlegm.

Needling

Principal points: M-BW-1 *(Dingchuan)*, B-12 *(Fengmen)*, B-13 *(Feishu)*, LI-4 *(Hegu)*

Supplementary points: LI-11 *(Quchi)*, Gv-14 *(Dazhui)*, L-5 *(Chize)*, L-7 *(Lieque)*, S-40 *(Fenglong)* and the vertebral points M-BW-35 *(Jiaji)* from the 7th cervical to the 6th thoracic vertebra

Method: Strong stimulation without retaining the needles, or moderate stimulation, retaining the needles for 5-15 minutes with intermittent needling. For acute bronchitis, needle once or twice daily. When the symptoms improve, needle once daily or on alternating days until the symptoms disappear. For chronic bronchitis, needle once daily or on alternating days. Ten treatments constitute one course. In addition to the principal points, add LI-11 *(Quchi)* and Gv-14 *(Dazhui)* for chills and fever; M-BW-35 *(Jiaji)* for soreness in the muscles of the back; L-5 *(Chize)* and L-7 *(Lieque)* for persistant coughing; S-40 *(Fenglong)* for Phlegm.

Discussion of points: B-12 *(Fengmen)* is the point of intersection of the Governing channel on the Bladder channel, and LI-4 *(Hegu)* is the Source point of the Large Intestine channel. Combined, these points eliminate Wind and disperse the Exterior condition. B-13 *(Feishu)*, as the Associated point of the Lung, is a site at which the Lung Qi accumulates. Needling this point helps spread the Lung Qi to treat coughing. Needling M-BW-1 *(Dingchuan)*, situated on a Divergent branch of the Governing channel, spreads the Lung Qi to relieve the wheezing symptoms. Gv-14 *(Dazhui)*, the point of intersection of the Yang channels on the Governing channel, and LI-11 *(Quchi)*, the Uniting point of the Large Intestine channel, are both useful for dispersing Heat. Stimulating L-5 *(Chize)* and L-7 *(Lieque)* spreads the Lung Qi so as to treat coughing, while S-40 *(Fenglong)* is effective for coughing

Phlegm because it stabilizes the Stomach and eliminates the Phlegm. Needling the vertebral points M-BW-35 *(Jiaji)* facilitates the free circulation of Qi through the Governing and Bladder channels.

Injection therapy
This method is generally used for chronic bronchitis only.

Points: vertebral points M-BW-35 *(Jiaji)* from the 7th cervical to the 6th thoracic vertebra

Method: Inject vitamin B1, or placental tissue extract, or *Angelica sinesis (danggui)*. Begin with the 7th cervical vertebra and move downward injecting one point, bilaterally, daily or on alternating days. E.g., inject the 7th cervical vertebral point on the first day, the 1st thoracic vertebral point the second day, etc. Twenty treatments constitute one course.

Ear acupuncture
Points: Lung, Kidney, Stop Wheezing

Method: Needle once daily or on alternating days, retaining needles from 30 minutes to 1 hour. For chronic bronchitis, ten treatments constitute one course.

Cutaneous acupuncture
Tap along the upper back until the skin is red or there is slight bleeding.

Moxibustion
Use for chronic bronchitis.

Method: 1. 'Grain of wheat' moxa. Points: Gv-14 *(Dazhui)*, B-13 *(Feishu)* or B-12 *(Fengmen)*, B-38 *(Gaohuang)*. Burn moxa once every 3-5 days. Five treatments constitute one course. 2. Moxa stick. Same points as above. Treat daily, 5-10 minutes or until the skin becomes red. This method is frequently used in conjunction with needling, first needling and then warming with the moxa stick.

Cupping
Method: 1. Place cups at Gv-14 *(Dazhui)*, B-12 *(Fengmen)*, B-13 *(Feishu)*, B-38 *(Gaohuang)* and SI-13 *(Quyuan)*. Treat once every 3-4 days, depending on the skin reaction. Five treatments constitute one course. This method is often used in conjunction with needling, inserting the needles first then placing the cups over them. 2. Moving the cups. Slide the cups along the upper back and both sides of the spine. Treat once every 3-5 days. Five treatments constitute one course. 3. Let blood and apply cups at same locations as #2.

Embedding thread
Points: M-BW-1 *(Dingchuan)*, B-13 *(Feishu)*, Co-17 *(Shanzhong)*

Method: Using a suture needle, embed sheep-gut thread in the muscle below the point. (See embedding thread method under bronchial asthma.)

Other prescriptions
1. GB-12 *(Wangu)*, B-10 *(Tianzhu)*, GB-20 *(Fengchi)*, Gv-12 *(Shenzhu)*, B-11 *(Dazhu)*, B-12 *(Fengmen)*, B-13 *(Feishu)*, B-17 *(Geshu)*, B-19 *(Danshu)*, P-3 *(Quze)*, LI-4 *(Hegu)*, Co-22 *(Tiantu)*. (Source: NAM)

2. B-11 *(Dazhu)*, B-13 *(Feishu)*, Co-22 *(Tiantu)*, L-5 *(Chize)*, TB-5 *(Waiguan)*, L-8 *(Jingqu)*, Sp-6 *(Sanyinjiao)*. Needle daily. (Source: CAM)

3. Co-17 *(Shanzhong)*, Co-22 *(Tiantu)*, M-BW-1 *(Dingchuan)*, S-40 *(Fenglong)*, LI-11 *(Quchi)*, S-36 *(Zusanli)*. (Source: HNMT)

4. For cough: S-12 *(Quepen)*, Co-17 *(Shanzhong)*, Co-14 *(Juque)*, L-10 *(Yuji)*, L-7 *(Lieque)*, SI-1 *(Shaoze)*, B-15 *(Xinshu)*, S-14 *(Kufang)*. (Source: CNLAM)

5. For chronic cough: moxi B-38 *(Gaohuang)* and moxi B-13 *(Feishu)*. (Source: CNLAM)

6. For cough with Phlegm: moxi Co-22 *(Tiantu)* and B-13 *(Feishu)*. (Source: SCCM)

7. For cough: moxi at Co-22 *(Tiantu)*, B-13 *(Feishu)*, GB-21 *(Jianjing)*, L-11 *(Shaoshang)*, K-2 *(Rangu)*, B-18 *(Ganshu)*, Li-14 *(Qimen)*, Li-2 *(Xingjian)*, Co-23 *(Lianquan)*, LI-18 *(Futu)*; needle

P-3 *(Quze)*, SI-2 *(Qiangu)*. For Hot cough with flushed face, use TB-6 *(Zhigou)*. For nausea, use S-36 *(Zusanli)*. (Source: GOA)

8. For cough: 7 cones of moxa on Co-22 *(Tiantu)* and K-27 *(Shufu)*, 3 cones of moxa on Co-20 *(Huagai)* and S-18 *(Rugen)*, 7 cones of moxa on B-12 *(Fengmen)*, 14 cones of moxa on B-13 *(Feishu)*, Gv-12 *(Shenzhu)*, and Gv-9 *(Zhiyang)*. Needle L-7 *(Lieque)*. (Source: IACC)

9. Chronic cough resistant to treatment: B-13 *(Feishu)*, S-36 *(Zusanli)*, Co-17 *(Shanzhong)*, S-18 *(Rugen)*, B-12 *(Fengmen)*, S-12 *(Quepen)*. (Source: GCAM)

Remarks

• Acupuncture treatment for acute and chronic bronchitis is basically the same. If bronchitis is accompanied by other conditions, such as emphysema, care should be taken to treat them both.

BRONCHIAL ASTHMA

The panting and wheezing symptoms with which this condition is associated in Chinese medicine are related to the Lungs, Spleen and Kidneys. Usually, this disease is caused when Wind and Cold invade the Lungs which become obstructed with Phlegm and Dampness, thus preventing the Qi from descending. Because the Lung Qi is 'rooted' in the Kidneys, when asthma is prolonged the Kidneys become weakened and may be unable to take in the Qi from the Lungs. A condition of Excess in the Lungs may also exist alongside a Deficient condition in the Kidneys.

Treatment is directed toward relieving the wheezing by causing the 'rebellious' Qi to descend, and spreading the Lung Qi to eliminate the Phlegm. Acupuncture is often used during an asthma attack.

Needling

Principal points: M-BW-1 *(Dingchuan)*, Co-22 *(Tiantu)*, Co-21 *(Xuanji)*, Co-17 *(Shanzhong)*
Supplementary points: S-40 *(Fenglong)*, Gv-14 *(Dazhui)*, LI-4 *(Hegu)*, Co-4 *(Guanyuan)*, S-36 *(Zusanli)*

Method: Moderate to strong stimulation. Retain needle at M-BW-1 *(Dingchuan)* after a few minutes' needling. Do not retain needle at Co-22 *(Tiantu)*. Use transverse insertion at points Co-21 *(Xuanji)* and Co-17 *(Shanzhong)*, extending the needle about one inch toward the left, right, above and below the point in succession. Retain needles at these points after manipulation. If much Phlegm, add S-40 *(Fenglong); respiratory* infection, add Gv-14 *(Dazhui)* and LI-4 *(Hegu)*. For those patients whose wheezing has persisted for a considerable time, add Co-4 *(Guanyuan)* and S-36 *(Zusanli)*.

Discussion of points: M-BW-1 *(Dingchuan)* has been effective in recent experience for stopping the wheezing. Co-22 *(Tiantu)* and Co-17 *(Shanzhong)* cause the 'rebellious' Lung Qi to descend properly. Needling Co-21 *(Xuanji)* spreads the Lung Qi. S-40 *(Fenglong)* transforms and disperses Phlegm. Co-4 *(Guanyuan)* and S-36 *(Zusanli)* both strengthen the Spleen and Kidneys, nourishing the 'source'. Gv-14 *(Dazhui)* and LI-4 *(Hegu)* disperse the Exterior condition by scattering the Excesses, Wind and Cold.

Injection therapy

This method is ordinarily used between asthma attacks, when the symptoms are temporarily in abeyance.
Points: M-BW-35 *(Jiaji)* from the 7th cervical to the 6th thoracic vertebra
Method: Use placental tissue extract, or vitamin B1, or vitamin B2. For each treatment, daily or on alternating days, choose one point, bilaterally. Begin with the vertebral point outside the 7th cervical vertebra and progress downward. Twenty treatments constitute one course of treatment.

Ear acupuncture

This method is generally used during an asthma attack.
Points: Lung, Kidney, Adrenal, Sympathetic, Stop Wheezing

Method: Select 2-3 points for each treatment, or use electric probing device to locate points of tenderness on the auricle. Retain needles for 30 minutes to 1 hour after manipulation.

Cutaneous acupuncture

This method is generally used during an asthma attack.

Method: Tap needle along the upper back and nape of neck, particularly in the area between the left and right paths of the Bladder channel. Tapping should continue until the skin feels hot and the patient is breathing more freely.

Moxibustion

This method is generally used between asthma attacks, when the symptoms are temporarily in abeyance.

Points: Gv-14 *(Dazhui)*, B-12 *(Fengmen)*, B-13 *(Feishu)*, Co-17 *(Shanzhong)*

Method: Use either the 'grain of wheat' or small cone method of direct moxibustion. For each treatment, apply 3-5 grains (or cones) at each point. Treat once every ten days. Three treatments constitute one course.

Cupping

1. Using 'moving the cups' method, slide the cups along the upper back and both sides of the spine; or 2. Let blood and then apply cups at points within this area.

Embedding thread

Method: Eight points are selected on each side of the spine. Each point is approximately one unit beside the successive spinous processes from the 7th cervical to the 7th thoracic vertebrae. Using a suture needle, a piece of sheep-gut thread is embedded between consecutive points on the same side of the spine. I.e., the needle is inserted at the first point and emerges at the second, inserted at the third point and emerges at the fourth, etc.

Incision method

Points: M-BW-1 *(Dingchuan)*, Co-17 *(Shanzhong)*

Method: After rigorous sterilization of the area surrounding the points and the injection of a local anesthetic, an incision .5-1 cm. in length and .4-.5 cm. in depth is made at each point. A small amount of fatty tissue is removed and the inside of the wound stroked with hemostatic forceps to provide further stimulation. Apply pressure to stop bleeding. Generally, it is unnecessary to stitch the wound closed; it need only be dressed and secured with tape. The wound should heal within a week. If effective, this procedure can be repeated a second and third time. If repeated, the incision should be made about .5 cm. beside the first.

Head acupuncture

Point: Thoracic cavity area (bilaterally)

Hand acupuncture

Points: Cough and Wheeze point
Method: Strong stimulation, retaining the needle 3-5 minutes.

Other prescriptions

1. B-10 *(Tianzhu)*, GB-20 *(Fengchi)*, S-13 *(Qihu)*, SI-14 *(Jianwaishu)*, B-11 *(Dazhu)*, B-12 *(Fengmen)*, B-13 *(Feishu)*, B-14 *(Jueyinshu)*, B-15 *(Xinshu)*, B-36 *(Fufen)*, B-38 *(Gaohuang)*, LI-4 *(Hegu)*. (Source: NAM)

2. B-13 *(Feishu)*, B-16 *(Dushu)*, Co-22 *(Tiantu)*, Co-17 *(Shanzhong)*, GB-21 *(Jianjing)*, Co-12 *(Zhongwan)*, Co-6 *(Qihai)*, L-7 *(Lieque)*, S-36 *(Zusanli)*, Sp-6 *(Sanyinjiao)*. (Source: CAM)

3. M-BW-1 *(Dingchuan)*, Co-17 *(Shanzhong)*, P-6 *(Neiguan)*, Gv-14 *(Dazhui)*, N-BW-8 *(Ganrexue)*, S-40 *(Fenglong)*. (Source: HNMT)

4. Burn 3 cones of moxa at Co-21 *(Xuanji)*, Co-6 *(Qihai)*, Co-17 *(Shanzhong)*, Li-14 *(Qimen)*, Gv-9 *(Zhiyang)* and wheezing immediately stops. (Source: CBZJ)

5. The point B-13 *(Feishu)* will be sore to the touch on all asthmatics. Those patients who have received acupuncture at B-13 *(Feishu)* with no result will be cured if moxibustion is performed there. (Source: CNLAM)

6. L-2 *(Yunmen)*, S-9 *(Renying)*, and K-25 *(Shencang)* for severe coughing and wheezing that won't stop; Co-22 *(Tiantu)* and Co-20 *(Huagai)* for explosive wheezing; B-37 *(Pohu)* and L-1 *(Zhongfu)* for wheezing when exercising; Co-17 *(Shanzhong)* for coughing and wheezing; Co-21 *(Xuanji)* for coughing and wheezing with throat sounds; LI-3 *(Sanjian)* for wheezing. (Source: CNLAM)

7. For wheezing: apply moxa at L-1 *(Zhongfu)*, L-2 *(Yunmen)*, L-3 *(Tianfu)*, Co-20 *(Huagai)*, and B-13 *(Feishu)*. (Source: GOA)

8. For wheezing, use Co-22 *(Tiantu)*, Co-21 *(Xuanji)*, Co-20 *(Huagai)*, Co-17 *(Shanzhong)*, S-18 *(Rugen)*, Li-14 *(Qimen)*, Co-6 *(Qihai)*, and a point beneath the seventh [cervical] vertebra. For asthma, use moxa at Co-21 *(Xuanji)*, Co-20 *(Huagai)*, Co-17 *(Shanzhong)*, GB-21 *(Jianjing)*, SI-15 *(Jianzhongshu)*, L-9 *(Taiyuan)*, and S-36 *(Zusanli)*. (Source: IACC)

9. Severe asthma: K-27 *(Shufu)*, Co-22 *(Tiantu)*, Co-17 *(Shanzhong)*, B-13 *(Feishu)*, S-36 *(Zusanli)*, Co-12 *(Zhongwan)*, B-38 *(Gaohuang)*, Co-6 *(Qihai)*, Co-4 *(Guanyuan)*, and S-18 *(Rugen)*. (Source: GCAM)

Remarks
- Acupuncture has been used with relatively good results in treating simple bronchial asthma.
- Normal precautions for asthma patients apply. It is recommended that physical exercise be encouraged to strengthen the body's resistance to disease.

CHRONIC HEART FAILURE

In Chinese medicine, this disease is considered to be part of a condition in which the Yang Qi of the Heart and Kidneys is Deficient. Because the Yang functions of the Heart are weak, Blood congeals in the blood vessels. Because the Kidney Qi is Deficient, it lacks the strength to take in the Lung Qi. As a result, the normal transformation of Qi is disrupted and water and Dampness overflow.

Treatment is therefore based on the principles of aiding and securing the Source (i.e., the Kidneys) as well as strengthening the Heart and Spirit.

Previously, it was thought that heart disease should not be treated with acupuncture. During the Cultural Revolution, however, acupuncture and moxibustion were used to treat chronic heart failure caused by rheumatic valve damage. This experience showed that acupuncture can improve the functioning of the heart and has since opened the way for the use of acupuncture in the treatment of heart disease.

Needling
Principal points: 1st group includes P-6 *(Neiguan)*, P-5 *(Jianshi)*, H-8 *(Shaofu)*; 2nd group includes P-6 *(Neiguan)*, P-4 *(Ximen)*, P-3 *(Quze)*

Supplementary points: To regulate gastro-intestinal function, use Co-12 *(Zhongwan)*, S-25 *(Tianshu)*, Co-6 *(Qihai)* and S-36 *(Zusanli)*. To strengthen the Source, (i.e., the source of vitality in the Kidneys) and facilitate movement in the Lower Burner (which includes the Kidneys), use Co-4 *(Guanyuan)*, S-29 *(Guilai)* and Co-6 *(Qihai)*. To facilitate urination and eliminate edema (i.e., to circulate the Yang so as to benefit the water), add Co-9 *(Shuifen)*, S-28 *(Shuidao)*, K-7 *(Fuliu)*, K-5 *(Shuiquan)*, B-58 *(Feiyang)*, Sp-9 *(Yinlingquan)*, join Co-3 *(Zhongji)* to Co-2 *(Qugu)*. To treat distension of the Liver (i.e., to remove stasis or congealed Blood), use Li-3 *(Taichong)*, Li-13 *(Zhangmen)* and B-18 *(Ganshu)*. To relieve panting (by suppressing the 'rebellious Qi'), suppress the coughing and eliminate Phlegm, add B-13 *(Feishu)*, Co-22 *(Tiantu)*, K-27 *(Shufu)*, Co-17 *(Shanzhong)*, H-8 *(Shaofu)* and LI-4 *(Hegu)*.

Method: Select one of the two groups of principal points and no more than six or seven of the supplementary points according to symptoms. Needles should be inserted deeply (within the specific limitations set for each point) and strong stimulation should be applied. Needles need not be retained, but can be withdrawn when the patient feels the characteristic needle sensation. Treat once daily for 7-10 days. Thereafter, allow a few days rest before treatment is resumed. Although daily treatment is preferred, treatment on alternating days is also acceptable.

Discussion of points: H-8 *(Shaofu)*, the Gushing point on the Heart channel, is recommended for heart-related conditions. The functions of the remaining principal points, all on the Pericardium channel, are similar to those of points on the Heart channel. Stimulation of points on both channels helps strengthen the Heart and calm the Spirit.

The Middle Burner (Spleen/Stomach) is the root of nourishment after birth. The lack of appetite associated with chronic heart conditions is caused by a Deficiency in the Spleen/Stomach, brought on by exhaustion of the Heart Yang. This condition is treated by needling Co-12 *(Zhongwan)*, the Alarm point of the Stomach, S-25 *(Tianshu)*, the Alarm point of the Large Intestine, and S-36 *(Zusanli)*, the Lower Uniting point of the Stomach. Needling Co-6 *(Qihai)*, the so-called 'sea of Qi', benefits the Qi. The region below the navel is the seat of the Source Qi and the Kidneys. Needling Co-4 *(Guanyuan)* and Co-6 *(Qihai)* strengthens the Source and nourishes the Kidney Yang. These points may be matched with S-29 *(Guilai)* to reduce abdominal distension, and Co-9 *(Shuifen)* and Co-3 *(Zhongji)* to open the water passages. K-7 *(Fuliu)* is the Penetrating point and K-5 *(Shuiquan)* is the Gushing point of the Kidney channel, while B-58 *(Feiyang)* is the Connecting point of the Bladder channel with the Kidney channel. The use of points on these two connected channels strengthens the functioning of the Kidneys. Adding Sp-9 *(Yinlingquan)*, the Uniting point of the Spleen channel, removes the Dampness to treat edema. The Liver is enlarged in patients with chronic heart failure, causing discomfort in the flanks. Therefore, Li-13 *(Zhangmen)* is combined with Li-3 *(Taichong)*, the Source point of the Liver channel, so as to spread the Liver Qi and disperse congealed Blood. For respiratory symptoms, B-13 *(Feishu)*, K-27 *(Shufu)*, Co-17 *(Shanzhong)*, Co-22 *(Tiantu)* and LI-4 *(Hegu)* are used. H-8 *(Shaofu)* is stimulated to strengthen the Heart so as to spread Blood through the vessels.

Injection therapy

Points: P-6 *(Neiguan)*, P-5 *(Jianshi)*, M-BW-1 *(Dingchuan)*, B-13 *(Feishu)*, B-15 *(Xinshu)*

Method: Inject *Angelica sinesis (danggui)* at each point.

Remarks

• Where possible, encourage the patient to engage in suitable physical exercise to increase strength. For severe cases, however, the patient will definitely require a thorough rest for a period of time.

• Acupuncture treatment can improve the functioning of the heart, reducing the need for Digitalis. However, for those patients whose heart function has suffered rather severe damage, it is improper to cease using this medicine too early. And when there is infection, extreme fatigue or other added burden on the heart, it is essential to continue the use of this medicine over the short run, in addition to acupuncture.

• After the patient has recovered sufficiently to resume normal activity, P-6 *(Neiguan)*, S-36 *(Zusanli)* and related points can be needled 2-3 times each week to secure the effectiveness of the treatment.

HYPERTENSION

In Chinese medicine, this condition is related to an imbalance of the Yin and Yang functional aspects of the Kidneys and Liver, or to an over-abundance of Phlegm and Dampness.

The Liver is dependent on the Kidney Yin to 'moisten and soften' it. If the Kidney Yin becomes Deficient, it may cause the Liver Yang to grow Excessive, which in turn may further exhaust the

Kidney Yin. If the imbalance continues to escalate in this manner, the Excess of Liver Yang generates Fire which may stir up Interior Wind. Unless held in check, the condition known as 'penetrating Wind', or stroke, may ultimately result.

The condition of Excessive Liver Yang is associated with such symptoms as headache, dizziness, insomnia and tinnitus and is often accompanied by the appearance of Phlegm. Because of the mutual dependency of Yin and Yang, should the Yin functions be adversely affected as described above, the Yang functions may soon follow, leaving both Yin and Yang in a Deficient state.

What in Western medicine is called hypertension usually corresponds to one of five distinct patterns in Chinese medicine. (See the Introduction for explanation of the rationale of these patterns.)

1. Liver Fire Ascendant: Headache, irritability, occassional stiffness in the neck, flushed face, red eyes, dry mouth, constipation, yellow fur on tongue, chordlike strong or rapid pulse.

2. Deficient Yin/Excessive Yang: Dizziness, blurred vision, tinnitus, a sensation of weakness and irritability in the Heart, insomnia, excessive dreaming, numb sensation in the limbs, red tongue, chordlike fine pulse (possibly rapid).

3. Obstruction of Phlegm and Dampness: Congested feeling in the chest, palpitations, dizziness, nausea, vomiting, limbs heavy and numb with clumsy movement, heavy and greasy fur on the tongue, chordlike slippery pulse.

4. Interior movement of Liver Wind: Severe headache and dizziness, fainting, asphasia, convulsions, stroke.

5. Deficient Yin and Yang: Dizziness, shortness of breath, tinnitus, mental fatigue, numbness in feet and hands, legs weak, frequent urination (especially at night in some cases), possibly impotence, tongue slightly pale, sunken fine pulse.

Needling

Principal points: GB-20 *(Fengchi)*, LI-11 *(Quchi)*, S-36 *(Zusanli)*, Li-3 *(Taichong)*

Supplementary points: Li-2 *(Xingjian)*, M-HN-9 *(Taiyang)*, TB-17 *(Yifeng)*, H-7 *(Shenmen)*, N-HN-22(b) *(Anmian #2)*, Sp-6 (Sanyinjiao), K-3 *(Taixi)*, GB-34 *(Yanglingquan)*, Sp-9 *(Yinglingquan)*, S-40 *(Fenglong)*, P-6 *(Neiguan)*, Co-4 *(Guanyuan)*, Co-6 *(Qihai)*

Method: LI-11 *(Quchi)* may be needled separately or joined to H-3 *(Shaohai)*. Use moderate to strong stimulation, retaining needle 10-15 minutes. If there is severe headache and dizziness, flushed face and red eyes, Li-2 *(Xingjian)*, GB-34 *(Yanglingquan)*, M-HN-9 *(Taiyang)* and TB-17 *(Yifeng)* should be considered. If there are symptoms of Excessive Phlegm and Dampness (lumps and a feeling of fullness and depression in the chest, nausea or vomiting, palpitations and dizziness) add P-6 *(Neiguan)*, S-40 *(Fenglong)* and Sp-9 *(Yinlingquan)*. For symptoms of Empty Kidney Yin (dizziness, blurred vision, tinnitus, irritability and insomnia) add K-3 *(Taixi)*, Sp-6 *(Sanyinjiao)*, H-7 *(Shenmen)*, and N-HN-22(b) *(Anmian #2)*. Empty Yang symptoms (rapid, shallow breathing, fatigue and lassitude, frequent urination) can be treated with moxibustion (separately or in conjunction with acupuncture) at points Co-6 *(Qihai)* and Co-4 *(Guanyuan)*.

Discussion of points: GB-20 *(Fengchi)*, the Meeting point of the Yang Linking channel on the Gall Bladder channel, clears out and contains the Excessive Yang Qi. LI-11 *(Quchi)* and S-36 *(Zusanli)*, both on Yang channels, drain Excesses from the Yang channels. Li-3 *(Taichong)* on the Liver channel balances the forces in the Liver and extinguishes Liver Wind. When Yang is Excessive, needling M-HN-9 *(Taiyang)*, TB-17 *(Yifeng)* and GB-20 *(Fengchi)* contains the Excess. Li-2 *(Xingjian)*, the Gushing point on the Liver channel, and GB-34 *(Yanglingquan)*, the Uniting point on the Gall Bladder channel, are needled to cleanse the Fire from the Liver and Gall Bladder. For Phlegm and Dampness, use P-6 *(Neiguan)* and S-40 *(Fenglong)* to transform the Phlegm and pacify the Stomach/Spleen, and Sp-9 *(Yinlingquan)*, the Uniting point of the Spleen channel, to assist the Spleen in disposing of the undesirable fluids and cause them to descend. For Deficient Kidney Yin, select K-3 *(Taixi)*, the Source point of the Kidney channel, and Sp-6 *(Sanyinjiao)*, the point of intersection of the three Leg Yin channels, to strengthen and regulate those channels. To calm the Spirit, add H-7 *(Shenmen)* and N-HN-22(b) *(Anmian #2)*. For Deficient Yang, apply moxibustion at Co-6 *(Qihai)*, the 'sea' of Qi, and Co-4 *(Guanyuan)*, the 'root' of the Source Qi, so as to warm the 'fire at the gate of life', i.e., the Yang function of the Kidneys.

597

Ear acupuncture
Points: Subcortex, Lower Blood Pressure Groove, Neurogate, Heart, Sympathetic
Method: Generally, retain needles 1-2 hours.

Injection therapy
Points: S-36 *(Zusanli)* and P-6 *(Neiguan);* or LI-4 *(Hegu)* and Sp-6 *(Sanyinjiao);* or Li-3 *(Taichong)* and LI-11 *(Quchi)*
Method: The three prescriptions above can be rotated, using one pair of points for each treatment. Inject .25% procaine hydrochloride solution into each point daily. Ten treatments constitute one course.

Embedding thread
Points: N-BW-2 *(Xueyadian)* and B-15 *(Xinshu);* or LI-11 *(Quchi)* and S-36 *(Zusanli)*
Method: Alternate the two pair of points, embedding thread at one pair for each treatment. Allow 15-20 days between treatments.

Cutaneous acupuncture
Points: Tap along both sides of the spine, particularly stresssing the lumbar-sacral region. Other areas which may also be tapped include the cervical vertebrae, forehead and occipital regions, the perimeter of the orbit of the eyes, the palms of hands and soles of feet.
Method: Use a very mild method of stimulation, beginning close to the spine, and tapping from bottom. Repeat procedure further from the spine. Afterward, areas on the head and extremities may be tapped.

Cupping
Points: Along the medial course of the Bladder channel. Also LI-15 *(Jianyu)*, LI-11 *(Quchi)*, LI-4 *(Hegu)*, B-50 *(Chengfu)*, B-54 *(Weizhong)*, B-56 *(Chengjin)*, N-LE-25 *(Weishang)*, B-60 *(Kunlun)*, K-1 *(Yongquan)*, B-62 *(Shenmai)*, S-36 *(Zusanli)*
Method: Select points according to specific symptoms. Except for the points on the head, medium or large cups may be used. Generally, about 10 cups should be applied during each treatment, for 10-15 minutes.

Head acupuncture
Points: Leg motor and sensory area (bilaterally), Thoracic cavity area, Blood vessel dilation and constriction area, other areas depending upon symptoms

Other prescriptions
1. Hypertension: S-36 *(Zusanli)*, P-6 *(Neiguan)*, Sp-6 *(Sanyinjiao)*, Gv-20 *(Baihui)*, LI-4 *(Hegu)*, Li-2 *(Xingjian)*. (Source: JTM)
2. Hypertension: LI-11 *(Quchi)*, S-9 *(Renying)*, S-36 *(Zusanli)*. Usually the blood pressure falls within thirty minutes of needling LI-11 *(Quchi)*. If the appetite is reduced, add S-36 *(Zusanli)*. (Source: RAT)
3. Dizziness: Gv-20 *(Baihui)*, GB-19 *(Naokong)*, B-10 *(Tianzhu)*. (Source: CNLAM)
4. Dizziness: GB-15 *(Linqi)*, SI-5 *(Yanggu)*, SI-4 *(Wangu)*, B-62 *(Shenmai)*. Headache with red face and eyes: H-5 *(Tongli)* and S-41 *(Jiexi)*. (Source: CDR)
5. Headache and dizziness: Needle GB-20 *(Fengchi)* and burn 21 cones of moxa on GB-19 *(Naokong)* and GB-16 *(Muchuang)*. (Source: BBQS)

Remarks
- Acupuncture is definitely effective in treating primary hypertension.
- In persistent cases, combine acupuncture with Chinese and Western medicine for better results.
- In the past, moxibustion has not been used to treat this condition. However, recent clinical experience has shown that applying moxibustion at points S-36 *(Zusanli)*, GB-39 *(Juegu)*, P-6 *(Neiguan)*, Gv-20 *(Baihui)* and other sites is effective.

- The patient should avoid emotional excitement. If he or she has little physical activity, appropriate physical excercise should be encouraged.
- If the blood pressure exceeds 200/120, strong acupuncture stimulation should be avoided.

STOMACH-ACHE

Generally speaking, Chinese medicine regards stomach-ache as resulting from obstruction of the Stomach Qi. This condition may arise from Cold or Heat in the Stomach, or it may occur when emotional depression causes the Liver Qi to 'encroach' upon the Stomach. Other etiological factors include irregular eating habits, which cause an interruption in the flow of Stomach Qi; Phlegm and Dampness in the Spleen/Stomach, which causes food and liquids to remain in and obstruct the Stomach; or Congealed Blood.

Treatment is directed toward facilitating the movement of Qi and harmonizing the Stomach.

Needling
Principal points: P-6 *(Neiguan),* S-36 *(Zusanli)*

Supplementary points: Co-12 *(Zhongwan),* B-21 *(Weishu),* Co-14 *(Juque),* S-40 *(Fenglong),* Sp-6 *(Sanyinjiao),* Li-3 *(Taichong),* Co-11 *(Jianli),* Sp-4 *(Gongsun),* B-20 *(Pishu),* B-17 *(Geshu),* Co-4 *(Guanyuan),* S-43 *(Xiangu),* S-44 *(Neiting),* Sp-9 *(Yinlingquan),* M-BW-35 *(Jiaji)* from the 8th to the 12th thoracic vertebra

Method: Needle principal points with moderate to strong stimulation, retaining needles with or without intermittent manipulation. Treat once daily or on alternating days. If the stomach pains are particularly severe, needle 2-3 times daily.

For Liver-related symptoms (stomach pain that changes location, fullness or distension which is temporarily relieved by belching, sour taste in mouth or vomiting sour fluids), add Co-12 *(Zhongwan)* and Li-3 *(Taichong).* For Deficiency and Cold in the Spleen/Stomach (pain which diminishes when the Stomach is warmed and rubbed, but increases when cold beverages or food are consumed; vomiting clear fluids, undigested food; loose stool), use moxibustion at B-20 *(Pishu),* B-21 *(Weishu)* and Co-4 *(Guanyuan).* For symptoms of Phlegm and Dampness (frothing vomit, dizziness, palpitations, lumpy feeling in the chest region), use moxibustion at Co-14 *(Juque)* and needle S-40 *(Fenglong)* and Sp-9 *(Yinlingquan).* For symptoms of Congealed Blood (Stomach pain increases upon pressure, localized Stomach pain or lumps, dark stool or vomiting blood), add B-17 *(Geshu),* Sp-6 *(Sanyinjiao)* and Sp-4 *(Gongsun).* For Heat and Depressed Qi in the Stomach (rather intense pain, fever, bitter taste, thirst, dark and yellow urine, constipation), use S-43 *(Xiangu)* and S-44 *(Neiting).* If food collects in and obstructs the Stomach (fullness, distension and pain, patient desiring but unable to belch, vomiting sour, partially digested food, patient cannot bear the thought of food or drink, possibly diarrhea), add Co-11 *(Jianli).* The vertebral points M-BW-35 *(Jiaji)* are used only in chronic cases.

Discussion of points: P-6 *(Neiguan),* on the Pericardium channel which is linked with the Yin Linking channel, is used to treat diseases of the Stomach, Heart and chest. S-36 *(Zusanli),* the Uniting point of the Stomach, is particularly effective in treating diseases of that Organ. For imbalance between the Liver and Stomach, Co-12 *(Zhongwan)* and B-21 *(Weishu)* may be needled to harmonize the Stomach Qi and Li-3 *(Taichong),* the Source point on the Liver channel, to pacify the Liver Qi. When the Spleen/Stomach are Deficient and Cold, moxibustion is applied at B-20 *(Pishu)* and B-21 *(Weishu)* so as to warm the Middle Burner, and at Co-4 *(Guanyuan)* to warm the Kidney Yang (the basis of the transformative and transportive functions of the Spleen/Stomach). Needling Co-14 *(Juque)* and S-40 *(Fenglong)* transforms the Phlegm and facilitates movement in the Middle Burner. Needling Sp-9 *(Yinlingquan)* strengthens the Spleen and moves fluids. To treat Congealed Blood, it is necessary to move the Blood and disperse obstruction. B-17 *(Geshu),* the Meeting point of the Blood, Sp-6 *(Sanyinjiao),* at the juncture of the three Leg Yin channels, and Sp-4 *(Gongsun),* the Connecting point of the Spleen channel which is linked to the Penetrating channel (the 'sea of Blood') are selected for this purpose. For Heat and constrained Stomach Qi, S-43 *(Xiangu)* and S-44 *(Neiting)* are used to drain the Heat from the Stomach channel. Finally, to treat the condition of food which collects in and obstructs the Stomach, add Co-11 *(Jianli)* to expand the Middle and harmonize the Stomach.

Ear acupuncture
Points: Stomach, Sympathetic, Subcortex, Duodenum
Method: Select 2-3 points each treatment, retaining needles for 20-30 minutes.

Injection therapy
Points: S-36 *(Zusanli)*, M-BW-35 *(Jiaji)* from the 8th to the 12th thoracic vertebra
Method: Select one point, bilaterally, and inject 0.5-1% procaine. Treat once daily, alternating points; or
Point: B-45 *(Weicang)*
Method: Insert needle to a depth of 0.8-1 unit then inject vitamin B1. Treat once daily; or
Points: S-36 *(Zusanli)*, Co-12 *(Zhongwan)*, B-20 *(Pishu)*
Method: Inject atropine hydrochloride. Treat once daily.

Head acupuncture
Point: Stomach area, bilaterally

Embedding thread
Points: Join B-21 *(Weishu)* to B-20 *(Pishu)* and Co-12 *(Zhongwan)* to Co-13 *(Shangwan)*; or join S-21 *(Liangmen)* to S-20 *(Chengman)* and B-45 *(Weicang)* to B-44 *(Yishe)*; or join S-21 *(Liangmen)* to N-BW-13 *(Kuiyangxue)*.
Method: Select points in one of the groups above and embed with sheepgut thread. If the result is unsatisfactory, after a suitable interval of time try another point group. This method is appropriate for stomach-ache related to ulcers.

Cupping
Place cups on the upper abdomen and back, e.g., at points Co-12 *(Zhongwan)*, S-21 *(Liangmen)*, K-21 *(Youmen)*, B-18 *(Ganshu)*, B-21 *(Weishu)*, B-22 *(Sanjiaoshu)*, etc. Points S-36 *(Zusanli)* and P-6 *(Neiguan)* are also appropriate. Use large or medium cups, treating from 10-15 minutes.

Remarks
• Because there are many causes of upper abdominal pain, a careful examination is necessary to establish its source.
• When needling points Co-12 *(Zhongwan)* or Co-13 *(Shangwan)* with deep needle insertions, care must be taken not to point the needle toward the left or right where it might puncture blood vessels in the stomach.
• Acupuncture is relatively effective in treating this condition. After needling, the pain is generally relieved.

PROLAPSED STOMACH

Traditional Chinese medicine attributes this condition to weakness of the Spleen and Stomach Qi (Middle Burner) which consequently sinks, leaving the Stomach unsupported. The Spleen supports the muscles of the body by providing nourishment through its digestive function. If this function is severely impaired, the muscles, particularly in the upper abdomen, lack strength and the Stomach prolapses.

Treatment is primarily directed toward supporting the Qi of the Middle Burner, strengthening the Spleen and calming the Stomach.

Needling
    Points: N-CA-18 *(Weishangxue),* Co-4 *(Guanyuan),* Co-6 *(Qihai),* S-36 *(Zusanli)*

    Method: When needling N-CA-18 *(Weishangxue),* a #26 gauge, 5-inch needle may be inserted transversely so as to penetrate the abdominal muscles, joining this point to Co-6 *(Qihai)* or Co-4 *(Guanyuan).* If the stomach has prolapsed less than 6 cm., needle Co-6 *(Qihai)* separately; if more than 6 cm., needle Co-4 *(Guanyuan).* After needling is finished, continue with the 'support stomach' method set out below. Treat on alternating days with strong stimulation. Ten to twenty treatments constitute one course.
    'Support stomach' method: Place the right hand in a firm supporting position below the stomach and slowly but firmly push the stomach upward. Repeat several times.

    As an alternative prescription, the physician should feel the patient's skin along the course of the Conception channel between Co-14 *(Juque)* and Co-13 *(Shangwan)* for any pea-sized nodules, either superficially or in deeper tissue. Repeat this procedure between Co-13 *(Shangwan)* and the umbilicus. If such nodules are discovered, insert a needle of appropriate length joining one nodule to another. Rotate and agitate the needle, gradually withdrawing it from the skin. The needle sensation should be perceived as far as the lower abdomen, and the patient may feel that the stomach is lifting. Some patients may experience pain in the lower abdomen. One to two treatments constitute a course, allowing 15 days to 1 month between treatments. If, after one course of treatment, there is no improvement, this method should be abandoned.

Embedding thread
    Points: Join B-21 *(Weishu)* to B-20 *(Pishu),* and Co-12 *(Zhongwan)* to Co-13 *(Shangwan);* or join a point 4 units lateral to Co-11 *(Jianli)* to Co-8 *(Shenque),* and join M-LE-13 *(Lanweixue)* to S-36 *(Zusanli).*
    Method: Embed thread at the points in the first point group. After 20-30 days, embed the points in the second group.

Other prescriptions
    1. B-10 *(Tianzhu),* B-11 *(Dazhu),* B-17 *(Geshu),* B-18 *(Ganshu),* B-22 *(Sanjiaoshu),* S-20 *(Chengman),* S-21 *(Liangmen).* Warm needle method once daily. Medicinal moxa sticks can also be used. (Source: CAM)
    2. First needle the principal points Co-6 *(Qihai)* and S-36 *(Zusanli).* In severe cases, add Co-4 *(Guanyuan)* and Co-12 *(Zhongwan).* (Source: RAT)
    3. Group 1: P-6 *(Neiguan),* Sp-6 *(Sanyinjiao),* and Li-13 *(Zhangmen)* joined to Sp-14 *(Fujie).* Group 2: Sp-15 *(Daheng)* joined to Co-8 *(Qizhong),* S-37 *(Shangjuxu),* M-UE-32 *(Zeqian).* Needle each group on alternating days for 10 days. Retain needles in abdominal points for 20 minutes. Separate courses of treatment by three days. (Source: HCNMT)

Remarks
    • Persons suffering from this condition often have underdeveloped abdominal muscles. They should be encouraged to strengthen these muscles through physical exercise, though not too vigorously at first.
    • Patients should be discouraged from over-eating. Small amounts of nutritious food are preferred, so as to lighten the burden on the stomach. Meals should be eaten slowly and followed by a rest period.

SIMPLE GOITER

    As early as the Sui Dynasty (late 6th century), it was recognized that goiter was associated with habitation in the mountains. From a modern perspective, this may be because of the limited amount of iodine found in the spring water of that environment. It was also believed related to emotional causes.

Emotional distress may impede the flow of Qi allowing Dampness and Phlegm to coagulate and obstruct the channels.

Treatment is therefore directed toward opening the channels and stimulating the Blood, so as to move the Qi and eliminate the obstruction.

Needling

Principal points: N-HN-43 *(Qiying)*, LI-4 *(Hegu)*, M-BW-35 *(Jiaji)* from the 3rd to the 5th cervical vertebra

Supplementary points: Co-22 *(Tiantu)*, LI-11 *(Quchi)*, GB-20 *(Fengchi)*, TB-3 *(Zhongzhu)*

Method: Depending on the size of the goiter, the position of N-HN-43 *(Qiying)* may vary somewhat. The needle should be inserted at the margin of the thyroid gland at a 45° angle into the center of the mass. Use strong stimulation at LI-4 *(Hegu)*. Treat on alternating days. Do not retain the needles. If N-HN-43 *(Qiying)* cannot be needled repeatedly, use the vertebral points M-BW-35 *(Jiaji)* instead. If the swelling on the neck is of a non-nodular nature, after checking the extent of the swelling, 1-2 needles can generally be inserted at acupuncture points contiguous to the affected side. After insertion, the needles should be raised and thrust 2-6 times. If the result is unsatisfactory, increase the number of thrusts or use thicker needles. Use supplementary points in rotation.

Moxibustion

Points: Co-22 *(Tiantu)*, L-2 *(Yunmen)*, LI-14 *(Binao)*, LI-11 *(Quchi)*, Li-4 *(Zhongfeng)*, Co-17 *(Shanzhong)*, GB-20(Fengchi), Gv-14 *(Dazhui)*, S-11 *(Qishe)*, TB-13 *(Naohui)*, L-3 *(Tianfu)*, S-42 *(Chongyang)*

Method: If direct or indirect moxibustion is used, burn 7 cones at Co-17 *(Shanzhong)*, 18 cones at each of the other points.

Piercing method

Hold the mass firmly with the left hand. Using a relatively thick needle (#26-#28 gauge), quickly pierce the center of the mass and withdraw the needle, letting a few drops of blood. Treat once daily. Seven treatments constitute one course. Caution must be exercised to avoid puncturing the artery.

Ear acupuncture

Points: Endocrine, Thyroid and other appropriate points

Cutaneous acupuncture

Tap around both the front and back of the neck and over the shoulder blades. This method is appropriate for patients whose neck skin is rather loose, or after the mass has been reduced somewhat. It may also be used in conjunction with ordinary needling.

Other prescriptions

1. Growth on the front of the neck: Gv-17 *(Naohu)*, B-7 *(Tongtian)*, TB-12 *(Xiaoluo)*, Co-22 *(Tiantu)*. (Source: CNLAM)

2. Goiter: The peak of the goiter, Co-22 *(Tiantu)*, LI-11 *(Quchi)*. Strong stimulation without retaining the needles. Needle daily, 7-10 days constituting one course of treatment. (Source: HCNMT)

3. Goiter: M-UE-32 *(Zeqian)*, Co-22 *(Tiantu)*, LI-4 *(Hegu)*, LI-11 *(Quchi)*, S-9 *(Renying)*, S-10 *(Shuitu)*. Add cutaneous needle method in the affected area. (Source: NCM)

4. Growth on front of neck: Apply up to 100 cones of moxa at GB-20 *(Fengchi)*, at the hairline above the ear, and at Gv-14 *(Dazhui)*; 30 cones of moxa at 1.5 units lateral to Gv-14 *(Dazhui)*, and a cone of moxa for each year of patient's age at LI-14 *(Binao)*. (Source: ATDP)

Remarks

- The physician should be careful to avoid piercing the trachea, larynx or blood vessels of the neck.
- Acupuncture therapy is definitely effective in treating this disease. For the best results, however,

602

oral dosages of iodine should also be taken. If both methods are ineffective, surgery should be considered.

HYPERTHYROIDISM

Chinese medicine regards this condition as arising from emotional distress or frustration, which prevents the Qi of the Liver and Spleen from flowing through the channels. Instead, Fire is generated which depletes the Heart Yin. This causes Phlegm to accumulate and gradually obstruct the channels in the neck.

Treatment is directed toward spreading the Liver Qi and draining Fire so as to break up the accumulation.

Needling

Principal points: P-5 *(Jianshi)*, Sp-6 *(Sanyinjiao)*, N-HN-43 *(Qiying)*, M-BW-35 *(Jiaji)* from the 3rd to the 5th cervical vertebra

Supplementary point: H-6 *(Yinxi)*, K-7 *(Fuliu)*, N-HN-44 *(Shangtianzhu)*, P-6 *(Neiguan)*, LI-4 *(Hegu)*, Li-3 *(Taichong)*, H-7 *(Shenmen)*, N-HN-54 *(Anmian)*, B-2 *(Zanzhu)*, S-2 *(Sibai)*, GB-20 *(Fengchi)*

Method: First needle P-5 *(Jianshi)*, rotating the needle several times. Add Sp-6 *(Sanyinjiao)*, retaining both needles 15 minutes. Insert at N-HN-43 *(Qiying)* to proper depth, then withdraw needle without retaining. Avoid the blood vessel. If multiple use of N-HN-43 *(Qiying)* is thought unsuitable, the vertebral points M-BW-35 *(Jiaji)* may be substituted. In this event, choose one point, bilaterally, for each treatment, rotating the needle vigorously. For excessive sweating, add H-6 *(Yinxi)* and K-7 *(Fuliu)*. For palpitations or insomnia, add H-7 *(Shenmen)* and N-HN-54 *(Anmian)*. For sexual irritability and flushed face, add Li-3 *(Taichong)* and GB-20 *(Fengchi)*. For protruding eyes, use N-HN-44 *(Shangtianzhu)*, B-2 *(Zanzhu)* and S-2 *(Sibai)*. For tachycardia, add P-6 *(Neiguan)*.

Discussion of points: Needling Sp-6 *(Sanyinjiao)* regulates the three Leg Yin channels (Liver, Spleen and Kidney). P-5 *(Jianshi)* drains Fire from the Heart. N-HN-43 *(Qiying)* is chosen to break up the accumulating Qi in the channels of the neck. For excessive sweating, H-6 *(Yinxi)*, the Gushing point on the Heart channel, and K-7 *(Fuliu)*, the Traversing point on the Kidney channel, are selected to clear the Heart, nourish the Kidneys and stop the sweating. H-7 *(Shenmen)*, the Source point on the Heart channel, is combined with N-HN-54 *(Anmian)* to calm the Spirit in the treatment of palpitations and insomnia. Li-3 *(Taichong)* pacifies the Liver and GB-20 *(Fengchi)* drains Excessive Yang; together, they are used to treat flushed face and irritability. P-6 *(Neiguan)* calms the Heart. Points N-HN-44 *(Shangtianzhu)*, B-2 *(Zanzhu)* and S-2 *(Sibai)* are selected because of their proximity to the eyes.

Ear acupuncture

Principal points: Neurogate, Subcortex, Endocrine, Thyroid, Stop Wheezing

Supplementary points: Heart, Lung

Method: Choose 2-3 points at which to imbed the needles (either ear tacks or small needles secured with tape) for each treatment. Retain needles for one week during which time the patient should be encouraged to massage those points in which the needles are embedded. At the end of the week, remove the needles and place 2-3 more in other points.

Moxibustion

For direct or indirect moxibustion, burn approximately 50 cones at L-3 *(Tianfu)*. Other points listed under moxibustion treatment for goiter may be chosen as well.

Cutaneous acupuncture

Tap in the vicinity of the disease and points M-BW-35 *(Jiaji)* between the 5th to the 10th thoracic vertebrae, B-18 *(Ganshu)*, Li-3 *(Taichong)*, Sp-3 *(Taibai)*, Co-22 *(Tiantu)*, S-36 *(Zusanli)*, LI-11 *(Quchi)*, LI-4 *(Hegu)* and TB-17 *(Yifeng)*.

Other prescriptions

1. The five neck growths: LI-18 *(Futu)*, Co-22 *(Tiantu)*, SI-16 *(Tianchuang)*, S-12 *(Quepen)*, K-27 *(Shufu)*, L-1 *(Zhongfu)*, Co-17 *(Shanzhong)*, LI-4 *(Hegu)*, M-UE-1 *(Shixuan)* (prick), L-7 *(Lieque)* (needle this point first). (Source: CCAM)

2. Neck growth with swollen throat: L-3 *(Tianfu)*, TB-13 *(Naohui)*, S-11 *(Qishe)*. (Source: CNLAM)

3. Enlarged thyroid. Group 1: GB-20 *(Fengchi)*, Gv-14 *(Dazhui)*, B-11 *(Dazhu)*, Co-22 *(Tiantu)*, S-10 *(Shuitu)*, Gv-4 *(Mingmen)*, TB-3 *(Zhongzhu)*. Group 2: B-10 *(Tianzhu)*, Gv-12 *(Shenzhu)*, B-12 *(Fengmen)*, Co-23 *(Lianquan)*, S-9 *(Renying)*, Gv-3 *(Yaoyangguan)*, GB-26 *(Daimai)*. Rotate each group on alternating days with moderate stimulation. (Source: CAM)

4. Enlarged thyroid. Principal points: S-9 *(Renying)* joined to Co-22 *(Tiantu)*. Supplementary points: LI-4 *(Hegu)*, S-36 *(Zusanli)*, M-UE-32 *(Zeqian)*, K-3 *(Taixi)*, Sp-6 *(Sanyinjiao)*, P-6 *(Neiguan)*. This treatment is suitable for hyperthyroid patients. When joining S-9 *(Renying)* to Co-22 *(Tiantu)*, penetrate the enlarged thyroid, being careful to avoid the superficial veins and trachea. Use moderate stimulation and retain needles for 20 minutes with occassional manipulation. Use 1-2 supplementary points daily. These are especially useful in slowing the heart rate. For insomnia, select N-HN-54 *(Anmian)*, GB-20 *(Fengchi)*, and M-HN-9 *(Taiyang)*. Needle daily, 15 treatments constituting a course. (Source: HCNMT)

5. Enlarged thyroid: Gv-14 *(Dazhui)*, B-15 *(Xinshu)*, GB-21 *(Jianjing)*, LI-11 *(Quchi)*, S-36 *(Zusanli)*, Sp-6 *(Sanyinjiao)*, Co-22 *(Tiantu)*, SI-14 *(Jianwaishu)*, B-13 *(Feishu)*, B-23 *(Shenshu)*, H-7 *(Shenmen)* in rotation. After obtaining needle sensation, retain the needle for 20 minutes. Apply indirect moxa at the enlarged thyroid for 5 minutes. (Source NCM #6)

Remarks

• Acupuncture therapy is effective in treating this disease, but significant results are generally slow in coming. Acupuncture may be combined with other methods.

• If the disease develops into a thyroid storm (high fever, vomiting and nausea, irritability or even coma), combined Chinese and Western emergency methods should be used to save the patient.

• The occurrence and development of this disease is closely related to the emotional condition of the patient, whose anxieties must be allayed and who must be encouraged to adopt a positive, optimistic attitude. This will definitely contribute to the effectiveness of the treatment.

• Appropriate rest and a nutritious diet are important considerations.

DIABETES MELLITUS

This disease corresponds to what in traditional medicine is called 'thirsting and wasting disease'. Its origin is believed to be related to eating fatty or sweet foods in excess, and to emotional factors. In chapter 47 of *Simple Questions,* it is explained that ". . . fat causes Interior Heat while sweetness causes fullness in the Middle Burner. The Qi therefore rises and overflows and the condition changes into that of thirsting and wasting." A passage from chapter 46 of the *Spiritual Axis* elaborates: "The five inner [Yin] Organs are soft and weak and prone to symptoms of wasting Heat . . . When there is something soft and weak there must be something hard and strong. Frequent anger is hard and strong, and the soft and weak are thereby easily injured."

This condition arises when Heat exhausts the body fluids, injuring the Yin. It may also occur when there is Deficiency of the Kidney Yang, whose Essence is unable to transform the Qi. Depending on the pattern, the disease is classified as upper, middle and lower wasting. These conditions are intimately related to the Lungs, Spleen and Kidneys respectively. The first is characterized by great thirst, the second by great hunger, and the third by frequent urination and/or lumbar pain.

Treatment is directed toward draining the Heat which has collected in the Triple Burner.

Needling

Principal points: M-BW-12 *(Yishu)*, B-13 *(Feishu)*, B-20 *(Pishu)*, B-23 *(Shenshu)*, S-36 *(Zusanli)*, K-3 *(Taixi)*

Supplementary points: L-11 *(Shaoshang)*, L-10 *(Yuji)*, B-17 *(Geshu)*, B-21 *(Weishu)*, Co-12 *(Zhongwan)*, N-BW-10 *(Pirexue)*, Co-4 *(Guanyuan)*, K-7 *(Fuliu)*, K-5 *(Shuiquan)*

Method: The principal points on the back should be needled with only mild stimulation and without retaining the needles. The remaining points can be needled with moderate stimulation, retaining the needles from 10-15 minutes. Treat on alternating days, ten treatments constituting one course.

For excessive thirst, add L-11 *(Shaoshang)*, L-10 *(Yuji)* and B-17 *(Geshu)*. For increased appetite accompanied by emaciation of the muscles, add M-BW-10 *(Pirexue)*, B-21 *(Weishu)* and Co-12 *(Zhongwan)*. For frequent urination, add Co-4 *(Guanyuan)*, K-7 *(Fuliu)* and K-5 *(Shuiquan)*.

Discussion of points: N-BW-12 *(Yishu)* has proven effective in recent experience for controlling the function of the pancreas. B-13 *(Feishu)*, B-20 *(Pishu)*, and B-23 *(Shenshu)*, the Associated points of the Lung, Spleen and Kidneys, are useful in draining the Heat from the three Burners. S-36 *(Zusanli)*, the Uniting point of the Stomach, and K-3 *(Taixi)*, the Source point of the Kidneys, are selected to regulate the Qi of the Lung, Spleen and Kidney channels. When Heat has injured the Lung Yin, causing thirst, L-11 *(Shaoshang)* and L-10 *(Yuji)* are used to drain Fire from the Lungs. Needling B-17 *(Geshu)*, the Meeting point of the Blood, helps the Blood generate fluids. When there is Heat in the Spleen and Stomach resulting in hunger and emaciation, N-BW-10 *(Pirexue)*, B-21 *(Weishu)*, Co-12 *(Zhongwan)* and other Alarm and Associated points are needled to drain the Excess. When there is frequent urination and Deficient Kidney Yang, Co-4 *(Guanyuan)* may be used to strengthen the Source Qi, and K-7 *(Fuliu)* together with K-5 *(Shuiquan)* to stabilize the Kidney Qi.

Ear acupuncture

Points: For thirst, use Endocrine, Lung, Thirst. For hunger, choose Endocrine, Stomach. For frequent urination, choose Endocrine, Kidney, Bladder.

Method: Insert and retain needles for about 15 minutes. Ten treatments constitute one course. Intradermal needles (or ear tacks) may also be used.

Cutaneous acupuncture

Tap along both sides of the spine, emphasizing the region between the 7th to the 10th thoracic vertebrae. Each treatment should last about 5-10 minutes daily, or on alternating days. Fifteen to thirty treatments constitute one course.

Moxibustion

For dryness in the mouth, burn 100 cones at B-27 *(Xiaochangshu)*. For frequent urination, moxa can be burned at the tips of the little finger and toe, as well as at points along the cervical vertebrae (e.g., Gv-14 *(Dazhui)*.

Other prescriptions

1. Thirst and emaciation: Co-24 *(Chengjiang)*, B-44 *(Yishe)*, TB-1 *(Guanchong)*, K-2 *(Rangu)*. (Source: PUB)

2. Thirst and emaciation: Use up to 200 cones of moxa (cumulative) at Co-4 *(Guanyuan)*. (Source: BBQS)

Remarks

• Acupuncture is to be used only as a supplementary method for treating this disease, and must be combined with other medication.

• Among diabetic patients, the body's resistance to disease is usually very low, rendering it more easily subject to infection. Therefore, sterilization of the needles must be particularly rigorous.

• Normal dietary restrictions for diabetics apply.

ARTHRITIS

The various types of arthritis, as that word is understood in Western medicine, are contained under the singular rubric of Blockage (or Obstruction) in Chinese medicine. This condition occurs when the circulation of Qi and Blood through the channels is hindered by Wind, Cold and/or Dampness. The disease is classified according to the Excess that predominates. E.g., if Heat accompanies Wind and Dampness, or if at a certain stage of the disease Cold becomes Heat, then Heat Blockage can occur. If the disorder is prolonged, it may enter the internal Organs, often resulting in coagulated Blood and circulatory disturbances. This is known as Heart Blockage.

In Chinese medicine, there are five principal Blockages or Obstructions:

1. Moving (Wind) Blockage: Pain in the joints is widespread and moves from one area of the body to another. There is often fever and chills, rapid pulse and yellow fur on the tongue.

2. Stationary (Damp) Blockage: The pain is localized and does not move. The body and limbs feel heavy and there is numbness, edema, greasy fur on the tongue and a moderate pulse.

3. Painful (Cold) Blockage: Severe pain in one part, or over one half of the body which becomes worse when the patient encounters cold and diminishes when the patient is warm. The fur on the tongue is thin and white, the pulse wiry and tight.

4. Heat Blockage: The flesh is hot, the area of pain is red and swollen, and the pain increases upon contact. Mouth and tongue are parched, urine dark. There is constipation, the fur on the tongue is yellow and greasy, and the pulse rapid.

5. Heart Blockage: Uncomfortable and congested feeling about the chest, palpitations, asthmatic panting, irritability.

Treatment is directed toward restoring balance by opening the channels to spread the Qi and Blood.

Needling

Points: Select both contiguous and distant points on channels which traverse the area of pain. For arthritis associated with Wind, needling is the primary method. For arthritis associated with Dampness or Cold, a combination of needling and moxibustion is recommended. For arthritis associated with Heat, let a few drops of blood at related points. The points recommended for arthritis at specific joints are set forth below.

Jaw: S-7 *(Xiaguan)*, SI-19 *(Tinggong)*, TB-17 *(Yifeng)*, LI-4 *(Hegu)*

Vertebrae: The vertebral points M-BW-35 *(Jiaji)* corresponding to the area of pain, B-51 *(Yinmen)*, B-54 *(Weizhong)*, Gv-26 *(Renzhong)*

Shoulder: LI-15 *(Jianyu)*, TB-14 *(Jianliao)*, M-UE-48 *(Jianneiling)*, SI-11 *(Tianzong)*, TB-3 *(Zhongzhu)*, GB-34 *(Yanglingquan)*

Elbow: LI-11 *(Quchi)*, TB-10 *(Tianjing)*, LI-4 *(Hegu)*

Wrist, metacarpal, fingers: TB-5 *(Waiguan)*, LI-10 *(Shousanli)*, LI-5 *(Yangxi)*, TB-4 *(Yangchi)*, SI-4 *(Wangu)*, P-7 *(Daling)*, M-UE-50 *(Shangbaxie)*, M-UE-9 *(Sifeng)*

Lumbosacral: Gv-3 *(Yaoyangguan)*, M-BW-25 *(Shiqizhuixia)*, B-30 *(Baihuanshu)*, B-26 *(Guanyuanshu)*, B-54 *(Weizhong)*, B-60 *(Kunlun)*

Sacroiliac: B-27 *(Xiaochangshu)*, B-28 *(Pangguangshu)*, local point of pain

Hip: GB-30 *(Huantiao)*, GB-29 *(Juliao)*, GB-34 *(Yanglingquan)*, GB-39 *(Juegu)*

Knee: M-LE-27 *(Heding)*, M-LE-15 *(Xixia)*, S-35 *(Xiyan)*, S-34 *(Liangqiu)*, S-36 *(Zusanli)*, GB-34 *(Yanglingquan)*, Sp-9 *(Yinlingquan)*

Ankle: S-41 *(Jiexi)*, GB-40 *(Qiuxu)*, K-3 *(Taixi)*, B-60 *(Kunlun)*, GB-35 *(Yangjiao)*, K-8 *(Jiaoxin)*

Metatarsophalangeal: M-LE-41 *(Shangbafeng)*, Sp-4 *(Gongsun)*, B-65 *(Shugu)*, GB-38 *(Yangfu)*, Sp-5 *(Shangqiu)*

For symptoms associated with Heart Blockage, add P-4 *(Ximen)*, P-6 *(Neiguan)*, H-7 *(Shenmen)*. In addition, consult treatment for rheumatic heart disease.

Method: Select among the points listed above according to the area of pain. Some points can be joined to others, e.g., LI-11 *(Quchi)* to H-3 *(Shaohai)*, or GB-34 *(Yanglingquan)* to Sp-9

(Yinlingquan). Some points may require stronger stimulation than others, e.g., GB-30 *(Huantiao)* or B-51 *(Yinmen).* For rather severe cases, treat once daily. For most cases, however, treating on alternating days is sufficient. Ten treatments constitute one course. Points on channels traversing the area of pain, although not listed in the specific prescriptions above, may also be selected. For chronic or stubborn cases of the Cold or Damp varieties of arthritis, moxibustion should be used more often. However, moxibustion is counter-indicated for arthritis associated with Heat. Electro-acupuncture may also be used at the same points. Treat 5-15 minutes. Ten treatments constitute one course.

Injection therapy

Points: Choose from among the points listed above, points of pain, and the origins and insertions of related muscles. Among these, points of pain are most commonly selected.

Method: Inject *Angelica sinesis (danggui)* at each point. Alternatively, inject .5% procaine, 5-10% glucose or saline solution, or vitamin B1. Inject once every 1-3 days. Ten treatments constitute one course. Do not inject too many points at one session. If several joints are affected, inject a point at the joint with the most severe pain, alternating with other joints at successive sessions.

Ear acupuncture

Points: Sympathetic, Neurogate, point of tenderness on the ear associated with the location of pain on the body

Method: Ear acupuncture is generally used for arthritis whose primary characteristic is pain. Depending on the severity of pain, needle daily or on alternating days. Ten treatments constitute one course.

Cupping

Select a point or points near the affected joint and leave the cups in place for 10-15 minutes. This method may be combined with cutaneous acupuncture, applying the cups after tapping with the cutaneous needle. When the cups are removed, the skin should be red and there may be a small amount of bleeding. Apply the cups once every 2-4 days. Five treatments constitute one course.

Cutaneous acupuncture

This method is generally used for arthritis whose primary characteristic is swelling. Tap in the vicinity of the swollen joint, as well as the back of the head and neck. Tap along the sides of the spine at the spinal segment corresponding to the location of the affected joint. Treat once every three days. Five treatments constitute a course.

Other prescriptions

1. Wind Blockage: TB-10 *(Tianjing),* L-5 *(Chize),* H-3 *(Shaohai),* B-54 *(Weizhong),* and GB-38 *(Yangfu).* (Source: CDR)

2. Shoulder pain [so severe that the patient] wants to break it off: SI-6 *(Yanglao)* and B-10 *(Tianzhu).* (Source: TDP)

3. Cold Wind-caused arm pain: First needle GB-21 *(Jianjing),* LI-11 *(Quchi),* LI-10 *(Shousanli),* LI-8 *(Xialian).* Then needle LI-13 *(Wuli),* LI-9 *(Shanglian),* and L-8 *(Jingqu).* (Source: GCAM)

4. Moving Wind in the joints when the fingers and toes cannot be flexed or extended, accompanied by vertigo and belching: B-58 *(Feiyang).* (Source: CNLAM)

5. Blockage with pain while walking or spasm of the arm, waist, foot, elbow, or knee: 50 cones of moxa at the site of pain. If low back pain due to Damp Cold, burn 50 cones of moxa at Gv-2 *(Yaoshu).* (Source: BBQS)

6. Rheumatoid arthritis. Principal points: LI-15 *(Jianyu),* LI-11 *(Quchi),* M-UE-30 *(Bizhong),* LI-4 *(Hegu),* GB-30 *(Huantiao),* S-36 *(Zusanli).* Supplementary points: For fingers, M-UE-22 *(Baxie);* wrist, LI-5 *(Yangxi),* P-7 *(Daling);* elbow, P-3 *(Quze);* shoulder, TB-14 *(Jianliao);* hip, GB-31 *(Fengshi);* knee, S-35 *(Xiyan);* ankle, B-60 *(Kunlun);* toes, M-LE-8 *(Bafeng);* spine, Gv-14 *(Dazhui)* and Gv-15 *(Yamen).* (Source: HCNMT)

Remarks

• If procaine is injected, an allergy test should be given beforehand. When injecting any fluid into points contiguous to the joints, care must be exercised to avoid penetrating the joint cavity itself. *Injections should not be given in the lumbosacral region on pregnant women.*

• For rheumatoid arthritis, anti-inflammatory medicine may be combined with acupuncture.

• Manipulation and physical therapy may be used in conjunction with acupuncture to increase its effectiveness.

• Acupuncture is relatively effective in treating this condition. Needling is considered the primary method of therapy. During the acute stage, cutaneous acupuncture can be used in conjunction with cupping so as to cause a small amount of bleeding. During the chronic stage, when the Cold variety of arthritis is particularly evident, needling should be combined with moxibustion.

TRIGEMINAL NEURALGIA

According to Chinese medicine this condition is caused by an attack of Wind and Heat from without which obstructs the flow of Qi and Blood in the channels. Alternatively, it may arise from an Excessive Hot condition in the Liver and Stomach penetrating upward; or from a Deficient Yin/Excessive Yang condition; or from weak Kidney Yin (fluids) unable to check the Fire which rages upward out of control.

Treatment is directed at spreading the Qi through the channels in the affected area.

Needling

Principal points: M-HN-9 *(Taiyang)*, B-2 *(Zanzhu)*, S-2 *(Sibai)*, S-7 *(Xiaguan)*, and M-HN-18 *(Jiachengjiang)*

Supplementary points: LI-4 *(Hegu)*, S-44 *(Neiting)*, Li-3 *(Taichong)*, S-36 *(Zusanli)*, TB-5 *(Waiguan)*, K-3 *(Taixi)*, and GB-20 *(Fengchi)*

Method: For pain along the opthalmic branch, use M-HN-9 *(Taiyang)* or B-2 *(Zanzhu)*. When needling the latter point, the needle should be directed laterally and downward, so that the needle sensation radiates throughout the forehead. For pain along the mandibular branch, use S-2 *(Sibai)* pointing the needle laterally and upward so that the needle sensation reaches the upper lip. For pain along the maxillary branch, use S-7 *(Xiaguan)* and M-HN-18 *(Jiachengjiang)* pointing the needle in a medial, downward direction so that the needle sensation reaches the lower lip. Use mild to moderate stimulation, retaining the needles about 15 minutes with intermittent manipulation.

For symptoms associated with Wind (wandering pain, sensitivity to cold), use LI-4 *(Hegu)*, the Source point of the Large Intestine channel, and TB-5 *(Waiguan)*, the Meeting point of the Triple Burner channel with the Yang Linking channel. For symptoms associated with Fire ascending from the Liver and Stomach (irritability, thirst, constipation), use Li-3 *(Taichong)*, the Source point of the Liver channel, S-44 *(Neiting)*, the Gushing point of the Stomach channel, and S-36 *(Zusanli)*, the Lower Meeting point of the Stomach. For Deficient Yin/Excessive Yang (fatigue, emaciation, flushed cheeks), use K-3 *(Taixi)*, the Source point of the Kidney channel, to nourish the Yin, and GB-20 *(Fengchi)*, the Meeting point of the Gall Bladder channel with the Yang Linking channel, to clear the Yang.

Discussion of points: All the principal points are situated on branches of the trigeminal nerve, and are selected according to the method of using contiguous points to treat a local disease so as to spread the Qi through the channels in the affected area.

Injection therapy

Points: Inject B-2 *(Zanzhu)* for pain along the first branch, S-2 *(Sibai)* for pain along the second branch, and S-7 *(Xiaguan)* or M-HN-18 *(Jiachengjiang)* for pain along the third branch of the trigeminal nerve.

Method: Inject procaine hydrochloride, or vitamin B12. Treat once every 2-3 days.

Ear acupuncture

Points: Forehead, Mandible, Maxilla, and Sympathetic

Method: After twirling the needle for a short time, and finding the effective analgesic point, insert an intradermal needle (ear tack) at the point.

Cutaneous acupuncture

Tap in the vicinity of numbness or pain. The area around the ears at the temple, the nose, palms of the hands and tips of the fingers may also be tapped with the cutaneous needle. Tap with greater firmness at the situs of the pain or numbness than at other locations.

Head acupuncture

Points: Facial area in the Sensory area on the opposite side of the head from the pain

Foot acupuncture

Points: #49, #13

Other prescriptions

1. Principal points: LI-3 *(Sanjian)* and LI-4 *(Hegu)*. Supplementary points: opthalmic branch, M-HN-9 *(Taiyang)*, GB-3 *(Shangguan)*, GB-14 *(Yangbai)* and B-2 *(Zanzhu)*; maxillary branch, GB-1 *(Tongziliao)*, S-2 *(Sibai)*, S-7 *(Xiaguan)*, SI-18 *(Quanliao)*, and S-3 *(Juliao)*; mandibular branch, S-6 *(Jiache)*, S-5 *(Daying)*, and GB-2 *(Tinghui)*. Method: Each time pick one principal point and one supplementary point. Needle once or twice daily with moderate to strong stimulation. (Source: HCNMT)

2. Principal points: GB-1 *(Tongziliao)*, LI-4 *(Hegu)*, and M-HN-9 *(Taiyang)*. Supplementary points: M-HN-3 *(Yintang)*. Method: Use 2-3 principal points together with the supplementary point. Retain needles for one-half hour after obtaining needle sensation. Treat every other day. (Source: JTM)

Remarks

• If the efficacy of acupuncture is not apparent, this method can be combined with other modes of Chinese and Western medicine. A procaine bloc may also be utilized. If necessary, surgery may be considered, but here there is still a possibility of recurrence.

FACIAL PARALYSIS

Chinese medicine ascribes this condition to Wind and Cold of external origin which invade the channels traversing the face and disrupt the flow of Qi and Blood, preventing the vessels and muscles from receiving the necessary moistening and nourishment.

Treatment is directed toward spreading the Qi through the channels of the face.

Needling

Principal points: GB-20 *(Fengchi)*, GB-14 *(Yangbai)*, S-4 *(Dicang)*, S-2 *(Sibai)*, and LI-4 *(Hegu)*

Supplementary points: Gv-26 *(Renzhong)*, M-HN-18 *(Jiachengjiang)*, M-HN-9 *(Taiyang)*, S-7 *(Xiaguan)*, S-36 *(Zusanli)*, S-44 *(Neiting)*, LI-19 *(Heliao)*

Method: Needle S-2 *(Sibai)* with either a straight or transverse insertion, pointed downward. GB-14 *(Yangbai)* may be joined to M-HN-6 *(Yuyao)*, and S-4 *(Dicang)* may be joined to S-6 *(Jiache)*. If the mouth is 'awry' due to the neuralgia, add Gv-26 *(Renzhong)* and LI-19 *(Heliao)*. M-HN-9 *(Taiyang)* may be joined to S-6 *(Jiache)*. The other points can be added in rotation—the best method being a mixture of contiguous points on the face and distant points on the limbs. Superficial insertion of the needles with moderate stimulation is recommended. Treat daily or on alternating days. With the exception of LI-4 *(Hegu)*, needle points on the affected side only.

Discussion of points: All of the facial points are situated in muscles innervated by the facial nerve. Needling these points will help spread the Qi through the channels in the face. Needling GB-20 *(Fengchi)* disperses Wind and Cold. The Large Intestine and Stomach channels both traverse the face. Needling LI-4 *(Hegu)*, S-44 *(Neiting)* and S-36 *(Zusanli)* on these channels opens them to the circulation of Qi.

Electro-acupuncture

Points: TB-17 *(Yifeng)*, N-HN-9 *(Tingling)*, and S-4 *(Dicang)* joined to S-6 *(Jiache)*

Method: Choose 1-2 points each session and stimulate for several seconds. Treat daily or on alternating days. Ten treatments constitute one course. If after electric stimulation the muscles twitch, it is a sign that recovery will be relatively rapid. On the other hand, if the teeth clench more tightly together it means that the needles have been inserted too deeply into the masseter muscle. The needles should be withdrawn and reinserted.

Injection therapy

Points: N-HN-20 *(Qianzheng)*, LI-7 *(Wenliu)*, M-HN-9 *(Taiyang)*, and TB-17 *(Yifeng)*

Method: Insert needles and retain for 5-10 minutes until the needle sensation is obtained. Inject vitamin B1. Treat once daily. Points S-4 *(Dicang)*, LI-20 *(Yingxiang)* and LI-4 *(Hegu)* may also be used in rotation as substitutes for the points above.

Embedding thread

Points: Join S-6 *(Jiache)* to a point .5 unit below the earlobe; join S-2 *(Sibai)* to SI-18 *(Quanliao)*; join S-4 *(Dicang)* to M-HN-17 *(Sanxiao)*; join GB-14 *(Yangbai)* to M-HN-5 *(Touguangming)*. The distant points LI-4 *(Hegu)*, L-7 *(Lieque)* and Sp-10 *(Xuehai)* may also be embedded.

Method: Depending upon the location of the paralysis, select (in rotation) a pair of points from the list above, embedding fine sheep-gut thread. (Ordinarily, there will be no need to use a local anesthetic.) Combine with one or two of the distant points. This method is suitable for patients whose symptoms are prolonged.

Cutaneous acupuncture and cupping

Points: S-4 *(Dicang)*, LI-19 *(Heliao)*, M-HN-18 *(Jiachengjiang)*, S-6 *(Jiache)*, S-7 *(Xiaguan)*, GB-14 *(Yangbai)*, S-2 *(Sibai)*, TB-17 *(Yifeng)*, M-HN-9 *(Taiyang)*

Method: Use points on affected side only. Apply the cutaneous needle at a few points listed above so as to cause a small amount of bleeding. If desired, after tapping the points with the cutaneous needle, apply small cups for 5-10 minutes. Treat on alternating days. This method is recommended for the stage of this disease when symptoms such as facial muscle spasms and mouth awry appear.

Head acupuncture

Points: Facial area in the Motor area on either the affected or opposite side of the head

Other prescriptions

1. TB-17 *(Yifeng)*, SI-17 *(Tianrong)*, GB-2 *(Tinghui)*, S-3 *(Juliao)*, S-2 *(Sibai)*, B-2 *(Zanzhu)*, TB-23 *(Sizhukong)*, GB-7 *(Qubin)*, S-6 *(Jiache)*, GB-1 *(Tongziliao)*, S-4 *(Dicang)*, and LI-19 *(Heliao)*. (Source: NAM)

2. Mouth and eyes awry: S-6 *(Jiache)*, Gv-26 *(Renzhong)*, L-7 *(Lieque)*, L-9 *(Taiyuan)*, LI-4 *(Hegu)*, LI-2 *(Erjian)*, S-4 *(Dicang)*, and TB-23 *(Sizhukong)*. (Source: CDR)

3. Mouth and eyes awry: GB-2 *(Tinghui)*, S-6 *(Jiache)*, and S-4 *(Dicang)*. If the face is pulled to the right, apply moxa on the left. If it is pulled to the left, apply moxa on the right. Make the cones of moxa the size of wheat grains and burn 14 cones at each point. (Source: CNLAM)

4. Mouth and eyes awry: First needle S-4 *(Dicang)*, S-6 *(Jiache)*, Gv-26 *(Renzhong)*, and LI-4 *(Hegu)*. If after cure there is remission in 2-4 weeks, needle GB-2 *(Tinghui)*, Co-24 *(Chengjiang)*, and TB-17 *(Yifeng)*. (Source: GCAM)

5. Mouth awry: LI-7 *(Wenliu)*, LI-6 *(Pianli)*, LI-2 *(Erjian)*, and S-44 *(Neiting)*. (Source: PUB)

610

Remarks

• This condition should be distinguished as either peripheral or central nervous system facial paralysis. If it is related to the central nervous system, the number of points on the face should be reduced, and the treatment should proceed according to the method discussed under the title Cerebrovascular Accident later in the Section.

• In the beginning, do not use strong stimulation. Electro-acupuncture is ordinarily reserved until after the first or second week of treatment.

• Acupuncture is relatively effective in treating this disease. More rapid results may be obtained when acupuncture is combined with manipulation, hot compresses, or Chinese and Western oral medication.

Appendix: Facial Muscular Spasm

Needle S-2 *(Sibai)*, pointing the needle toward the infraorbital foramen to a depth of approximately .5 inch. After the characteristic needle sensation has been obtained, retain the needle for 30 minutes. Treat once or twice daily.

Alternatively, join M-HN-9 *(Taiyang)* to S-6 *(Jiache)*, or join S-4 *(Dicang)* to TB-17 *(Yifeng)*, or join S-2 *(Sibai)* to S-7 *(Xiaguan)* and needle LI-4 *(Hegu)* separately. Use strong stimulation for both alternatives.

SCIATICA

Like arthritis, sciatica falls within the traditional domain of Blockage (or Obstruction). It is said to arise when Wind and Cold or Wind and Dampness lodge in the channels and impede the flow of Qi, resulting in pain. If Wind is predominant, the pain is characterized by its wandering nature. If Cold predominates, the pain is particularly intense. If the illness is prolonged the Qi congeals and may cause the Blood to congeal. At this point the disease is established and will be very difficult to cure.

Treatment is directed toward opening the channels so as to facilitate the flow of Qi.

Needling

Principal points: B-23 *(Shenshu)*, B-30 *(Baihuanshu)*, GB-30 *(Huantiao)*, B-50 *(Chengfu)*, B-51 *(Yinmen)*, B-54 *(Weizhong)*, GB-34 *(Yanglingquan)*

Supplementary points: B-31 *(Shangliao)*, B-32 *(Ciliao)*, B-49 *(Zhibian)*, B-57 *(Chengshan)*, GB-39 *(Xuanzhong)*, B-60 *(Kunlun)*, GB-41 *(Zulinqi)*, the vertebral points M-BW-35 *(Jiaji)* from the 2nd to the 5th lumbar vertebra, as well as the points of pain

Method: Choose 3-5 points each session. Use moderate to strong stimulation, projecting the numb sensation down the leg. If the pain arises from the nerve root, the vertebral points M-BW-35 *(Jiaji)* may be used. During the acute stage, needle once daily. As the symptoms improve, needle every second or third day. The principal points are, by definition, the foundation of the needling prescription. The supplementary points are added according to the particular situs of pain.

Ear acupuncture

Points: Ischium, Adrenal, Buttocks, Neurogate, Lumbar Vertebrae, Sacrum

Method: Moderate to strong stimulation, retaining the needles from 10-30 minutes with intermittent manipulation. Needle daily or on alternating days. Intradermal needles may also be embedded for 3-7 days.

Electro-acupuncture

Points: For pain arising from the nerve root, use the vertebral points M-BW-35 *(Jiaji)* from the 4th to the 5th lumbar vertebra, GB-34 *(Yanglingquan)*, B-54 *(Weizhong)*. For nerve trunk or primary sciatica, use B-49 *(Zhibian)* or GB-30 *(Huantiao)*, and GB-34 *(Yanglingquan)* or B-54 *(Weizhong)*.

Method: Use relatively strong, high frequency stimulation for 5-10 minutes.

Cutaneous acupuncture and cupping

Points: M-BW-35 *(Jiaji)* from the 2nd to the 5th lumbar vertebra, the lumbosacral region, along the course of the channel that traverses the area of pain, and points of tenderness

Method: Tap with the cutaneous needle with sufficient firmness to cause slight bleeding, then apply cups. For sciatica at the nerve roots, tap most forcefully along the sides of the spine at the vertebral points M-BW-35 *(Jiaji)*. For sciatica along the nerve trunk, give more attention to points of tenderness in the lumbosacral region.

Injection therapy

1. Inject a 10% glucose solution into M-BW-35 *(Jiaji)* from the 2nd to the 4th lumbar vertebra, *or* 2. inject a solution made from vitamin B1 and vitamin B12 into either B-49 *(Zhibian)* or GB-30 *(Huantiao); or* 3. inject a 10% procaine solution into either GB-30 *(Huantiao)* or the point of pain. For particularly painful symptoms, inject procaine along the lumbar vertebrae and at point GB-30 *(Huantiao)*. If the pain extends down the leg, raise the needle slightly and quickly when injecting the medicine, so as to provide a bloc at the point.

Head acupuncture

Points: Lower limbs sensory area, and the Leg motor and sensory area on the side of the head opposite the affected limb

Hand acupuncture

Point: Sciatic Nerve

Method: Use strong stimulation. When needling, the affected area may be simultaneously massaged. If the pain is on the left side, needle the right hand, and vice versa. If the pain extends to both sides, needle both hands. Retain needles 15-20 minutes.

Foot acupuncture

Points: #3, #35

Other prescriptions

1. Pain in the lower back and legs: GB-30 *(Huantiao)*, GB-31 *(Fengshi)*, S-33 *(Yinshi)*, B-54 *(Weizhong)*, B-57 *(Chengshan)*, B-60 *(Kunlun)*, and B-62 *(Shenmai)*. (Source: CDR)

2. Pain in the lower back and legs: B-54 *(Weizhong)* and Gv-26 *(Renzhong)*. (Source: GCAM)

3. Weak lower back and legs: B-31 *(Shangliao)*, GB-30 *(Huantiao)*, GB-34 *(Yanglingquan)*, and S-39 *(Xiajuxu)*. (Source: PUB)

4. Pain in the low back and knees: GB-30 *(Huantiao)*, B-60 *(Kunlun)*, GB-34 *(Yanglingquan)*, and SI-6 *(Yanglao)*. Use moxibustion. (Source: PDM)

5. Low back and hip pain: 100 cones of moxa at Co-4 *(Guanyuan)*. (Source: BBQS)

6. Sciatica. Commonly used points: GB-30 *(Huantiao)*, GB-34 *(Yanglingquan)*, B-54 *(Weizhong)*, GB-31 *(Fengshi)*, B-23 *(Shenshu)*, B-60 *(Kunlun)*, GB-39 *(Juegu)*, and B-25 *(Dachangshu)*. Supplementary points: B-50 *(Chengfu)*, B-57 *(Chengshan)*, Gv-2 *(Yaoshu)*, B-31-34 *(Shangliao-Xialiao)*, GB-43 *(Xiaxi)*, S-36 *(Zusanli)*, S-32 *(Futu)*, S-34 *(Liangqiu)*, S-31 *(Biguan)*, M-BW-24 *(Yaoyan)*, M-BW-33 *(Tunzhong)*, S-41 *(Jiexi)*, and B-58 *(Feiyang)*. (Source: JTM)

7. Sciatica. Principal points: GB-30 *(Huantiao)* and GB-34 *(Yanglingquan)*; Lumbosacral area, add B-23 *(Shenshu)*, B-25 *(Dachangshu)*, and B-31-34 *(Shangliao-Xialiao)*; Lower extremities, add B-50 *(Chengfu)*, GB-31 *(Fengshi)*, B-51 *(Yinmen)*, S-32 *(Futu)*, B-54 *(Weizhong)*, S-36 *(Zusanli)*, B-57 *(Chengshan)*, GB-39 *(Juegu)*, and B-60 *(Kunlun)*. Twist and turn the needles until the patient feels a numb, sore, distended sensation throughout the area. Retain the needles for 20-30 minutes or longer. Twist the needles once every 3-5 minutes. Needle daily or every other day. (Source: FCM)

612

Remarks

- If the pain is caused by slipped disc, manipulation may be combined with acupuncture.
- In order to cure the problem at its source, it is important to determine the origin of the sciatic pain.
- Acupuncture is definitely effective in treating this condition. If combined with other therapeutic methods, e.g., ultraviolet radiation, the results are even more pronounced. For severe cases, a combination of Chinese and Western medicine may be appropriate.

MULTIPLE NEURITIS

Traditional Chinese medicine teaches that this condition is caused by Dampness moving to the limbs, where it obstructs the channels and coagulates the Qi and Blood within them. Because the Spleen, by providing nourishment, controls the movement of the limbs, only when the Spleen's transportive and transformative functions are impaired will Dampness succeed in lodging in the limbs. First pain, then numbness, and finally debility mark the stages of its pathological development.

Treatment is directed toward opening the channels so as to facilitate the circulation of Qi and Blood.

Needling

Principal points: For the upper limb, use LI-15 *(Jianyu)*, LI-11 *(Quchi)*, TB-5 *(Waiguan)*, and LI-4 *(Hegu)*. For the lower limb, select GB-30 *(Huantiao)*, GB-34 *(Yanglingquan)*, GB-39 *(Xuanzhong)*, Sp-6 *(Sanyinjiao)*

Supplementary points: M-UE-22 *(Baxie)*, TB-4 *(Yangchi)*, SI-6 *(Yanglao)*, SI-3 *(Houxi)*, H-3 *(Shaohai)* and other related points on the upper limb; Sp-3 *(Taibai)*, Sp-7 *(Lougu)*, S-36 *(Zusanli)*, S-41 *(Jiexi)*, and M-LE-8 *(Bafeng)* on the lower limb

Method: Treat once daily. For mild cases, treat every other day. Continue treatment for 2-4 weeks. Use moderate stimulation. The points above may be joined to one another where appropriate.

Ear acupuncture

Points: Neurogate, Sympathetic, and points associated with affected area

Injection therapy

Points: LI-11 *(Quchi)*, TB-5 *(Waiguan)*, GB-34 *(Yanglingquan)*, GB-39 *(Xuanzhong)*, LI-4 *(Hegu)*, and Li-3 *(Taichong)*

Method: Inject 2-4 of the points listed above with vitamin B1, B6 or B12. Treat on alternating days. Ten treatments constitute a course.

Cutaneous acupuncture

Tap with firmness at the fingertips, toes, and affected areas. Tap with less force at contiguous and distant points along related channels, and at the back of the head. Treat daily or on alternating days. Thirty treatments constitute a course.

Barefoot doctor acupuncture

Points: Barefoot Doctor point, Thoracic #5, Lumbar #1, Posterior *Hegu*, Ankle

Head acupuncture

Depending on which symptoms are most significant, select corresponding part of Motor or Sensory area.

Other prescriptions

1. Numb hands: LI-11 *(Quchi)*, TB-6 *(Zhigou)*, TB-13 *(Naohui)*, SI-4 *(Wangu)*, and LI-12 *(Zhouliao)*. (Source: CNLAM)

2. Numb feet: GB-38 *(Yangfu)*, GB-35 *(Yangjiao)*, GB-39 *(Juegu)*, Li-2 *(Xingjian)*, B-60 *(Kunlun)*, and GB-40 *(Qiuxu)*. (Source: GCAM)

3. Multiple neuritis. Group 1: LI-11 *(Quchi)* joined to H-3 *(Shaohai)*, TB-3 *(Zhongzhu)*, GB-30 *(Huantiao)*, GB-34 *(Yanglingquan)* joined to Sp-9 *(Yinglingquan)*, and S-41 *(Jiexi)* joined to B-62 *(Shenmai)*. Group 2: P-6 *(Neiguan)* joined to TB-5 *(Waiguan)*, LI-4 *(Hegu)* joined to P-8 *(Laogong)*, lumbar section of M-BW-35 *(Jiaji)*. Group 3: LI-10 *(Shousanli)*, SI-6 *(Yanglao)*, B-31 *(Shangliao)*, B-54 *(Weizhong)*, GB-39 *(Juegu)* joined to Sp-6 *(Sanyinjiao)*. Use strong stimulation. Needle daily. Rotate the three groups of points. Ten to fifteen treatments constitute one course of treatment. (Source: HCNMT)

4. Multiple neuritis: In addition to local points, use Gv-14 *(Dazhui)*, Gv-12 *(Shenzhu)*, Gv-9 *(Zhiyang)*, B-14 *(Jueyinshu)*, B-16 *(Dushu)*, LI-11 *(Quchi)*, TB-5 *(Waiguan)*, GB-34 *(Yanglingquan)*, and B-60 *(Kunlun)*. Moderate stimulation. (Source: CAM)

Remarks

• When treating this illness, attention should be given to the source of the problem, and medication or preventative measures prescribed accordingly.

• Care must be taken to ensure that the patient is receiving proper nutrition.

• Acupuncture is definitely effective in treating this condition. If supplemented by physical exercise and appropriate medication, the result will be better.

PARAPLEGIA

In Chinese medicine this condition falls within the realm of Atrophy. It is caused by an injury to either the Governing or Girdle channels of the back, which prevents the Qi and Blood from circulating through them.

Treatment is directed primarily toward opening and regulating the Governing channel. Points along the nerves and muscles affected by the paralysis are also selected for local stimulation.

Needling

Principal points: Select vertebral points M-BW-35 *(Jiaji)* or Associated points 1 to 2 vertebrae above and below the spinal injury, bilaterally.

Supplementary points: 1. Select points located on nerves supplying paralyzed muscle groups. For example, on the brachial plexus, use M-HN-41 *(Jingbi)*, M-UE-40 *(Yeling)*, SI-9 *(Jianzhen)*, etc. On the radial nerve, use L-5 *(Chize)*, LI-11 *(Quchi)*. On the median nerve, select P-3 *(Quze)*, P-6 *(Neiguan)*. On the femoral nerve, use Li-11 *(Yinlian)*, Sp-12 *(Chongmen)*. On the sciatic nerve, use B-49 *(Zhibian)*, B-51 *(Yinmen)*. On the common peroneal nerve, select N-LE-32 *(Houyangguan)*. On the superficial peroneal nerve, use N-LE-17 *(Lingxia)*. On the deep peroneal nerve, use S-36 *(Zusanli)*. On the tibial nerve, use B-54 *(Weizhong)*, B-57 *(Chengshan)*.

2. Select points located in paralyzed muscle groups.

Shoulder: For paralysis of the muscles of abduction of the arm (deltoid, supraspinatus), use N-UE-14 *(Naoshang)*, LI-15 *(Jianyu)*, etc. For paralysis of the muscles which lift the arm forward, (anterior insertion of the deltoid, coracobrachialis, etc.), use M-UE-48 *(Jianneiling)*. For paralysis of the muscles which raise the arm backward (latissimus dorsi, teres major, posterior insertion of the deltoid, etc.), use B-17 *(Geshu)*, B-19 *(Danshu)*, SI-9 *(Jianzhen)*, TB-14 *(Jianliao)*.

Elbow: For paralysis of the muscles which flex the lower arm at the elbow (biceps brachii, brachialis), use N-UE-9 *(Gongzhong)*, etc. For paralysis of the muscles which extend the lower arm at the elbow (triceps brachii), use N-UE-12 *(Yingshang)*.

Wrist: For paralysis of the muscles used to extend the wrist (ulnar and radial extensors), use N-UE-7 *(Yingxia)*, TB-9 *(Sidu)*, LI-10 *(Shousanli)*, LI-8 *(Xialian)*, etc. For paralysis of the muscles which flex the wrist (ulnar and radial flexors), use M-UE-30 *(Bizhong)*.

Fingers: For paralysis of the muscles which control the fingers, join LI-4 *(Hegu)* to P-8 *(Laogong)*.

Hip: For paralysis of the flexor muscles (psoas major, etc.), needle GB-27 *(Wushu)* with a straight insertion along the surface of the hip and N-CA-6 *(Shuxi)*. For paralysis of the extensor muscles (gluteus maximus, biceps femoris, semimembranosus, semitendonosus, etc.), use B-51 *(Yinmen)*, N-LE-26 *(Zhili)*, and join B-49 *(Zhibian)* to GB-30 *(Huantiao)*. For paralysis of the muscles of abduction (gluteus medius and minimus), use N-BW-16 *(Tiaoyue)*, etc. For paralysis of the muscles of adduction (adductor magnus, longus and brevis, etc.), use N-LE-31 *(Jiejian)*, N-LE-20 *(Jixia)*, Li-9 *(Yinbao)*.

Knee: For paralysis of the extensor muscles (quadriceps femoris, etc.), use S-32 *(Futu)*, N-LE-23 *(Maibu)*, N-LE-18 *(Jianxi)*. For paralysis of the flexor muscles (biceps femoris, semitendinosus, semimembranosus, etc.), use B-51 *(Yinmen)*, N-LE-26 *(Zhili)*.

Foot: For paralysis of the plantar flexor muscles (gastrocnemius, soleus, etc.), use B-55 *(Heyang)*, B-57 *(Chengshan)*, N-LE-9 *(Luodi)*. For paralysis of the dorsal extensor muscles (tibialis anterior, etc.), use S-36 *(Zusanli)*, N-LE-8 *(Lishang)*, N-LE-5 *(Jingxia)*. For paralysis of muscles of medial deviation (posterior tibialis, flexor digitorum longus, etc.), use B-57 *(Chengshan)*, N-LE-10(b) *(Jiuwaifan #2)*. For paralylsis of the muscles of lateral deviation (peroneus longus and brevis, etc.), use GB-34 *(Yanglingquan)*, N-LE-11 *(Jiuneifan)*, GB-39 *(Xuanzhong)*.

3. Select points on the fingers and toes: M-UE-1 *(Shixuan)*, M-UE-49 *(Shiwang)*, M-LE-6 *(Qiduan)* and the Well points of each of the 12 Primary channels.

4. Select 'Relieve Spasm' points: Certain sites on the limbs and elsewhere on the bodies of patients with spastic paralysis are points which, when pressed, will often relieve muscle spasm. These points are used only for this purpose.

5. Select points for functional impairment of organs in the pelvic cavity: For disruption of bladder function, use B-30 *(Baihuanshu)*, Co-3 *(Zhongji)*, and N-CA-17 *(Yinbian)*. For disruption of rectal function, use Sp-15 *(Daheng)*, N-CA-11 *(Tongbian)* and TB-6 *(Zhigou)*.

Method: 1. Generally, the principal points should be the basis of the prescription. The physician may also select 1-2 of the supplementary points on the affected nerve or muscle groups, bilaterally. Paralyzed nerves or muscles, corresponding to higher segments or locations on the body, should be treated first. Then gradually move downward to treat lower positions on the body. If necessary, points located on the ends of the fingers and toes may be used as well. When needling the vertebral points M-BW-35 *(Jiaji)* or Associated points near the spinal cord, slant the needle toward the spinal column. It is best if the spinal nerves can be stimulated.

2. When the nerves are stimulated directly, it is best to use a relatively fine needle, and to limit needle manipulation. When points in muscles are needled, contiguous points may be joined with a single needle.

3. When treating patients with spastic paralysis, in addition to the points for relieving spasms listed above, regular acupuncture points on the paralyzed muscles may also be used. However, attention should be given to balance complementary muscle groups. For example, if there are spasms in a flexor muscle, points may be needled in that muscle with strong stimulation for a relatively lengthy period of time. Needle points in the related extensor muscles for a shorter period of time. In this way, relative muscle strength will be balanced.

Great needle acupuncture

Principal points: The great needle may be inserted at Gv-14 *(Dazhui)* with a transverse insertion, and joined just below the skin with a point further down the spinal column corresponding to the site of the spinal injury. Because manipulation and insertion of the neeedle in such shallow tissue is difficult, the less experienced physician may prefer to insert two or three shorter needles in successive points down the spine. Alternatively, the great needle may be inserted with a transverse insertion at the vertebral points M-BW-35 *(Jiaji)* corresponding to the level of spinal injury, bilaterally, and joined just below the skin to the sacro-iliac.

Supplementary points: Select according to the affected muscle or joint function.

Upper Limb: For abduction of the arm and shoulder, insert at LI-15 *(Jianyu)* downward into the deltoid muscle. For flexion of the elbow, join N-UE-10 *(Jubi)* to N-UE-9 *(Gongzhong)*. For dropped wrist, join LI-11 *(Quchi)* to LI-6 *(Pianli)*. For extension of the elbow, join LI-15 *(Jianyu)* to N-UE-12 *(Yingshang)*. For curled fingers, join LI-4 *(Hegu)* to P-8 *(Laogong)* or SI-3 *(Houxi)*.

Lower Limb: For flexion at the hip, join GB-27 *(Wushu)* to N-LE-58 *(Waiyinlian)*. For extension at the hip, join B-49 *(Zhibian)* to GB-30 *(Huantiao)*. For adduction of the leg, join N-LE-30

(Houxuehai) to N-LE-31 *(Jiejian)*. For abduction of the leg, join N-BW-16 *(Tiaoyue)* to GB-29 *(Juliao)*, or GB-33 *(Xiyangguan)* to GB-31 *(Fengshi)*. For extension at the knee, join N-LE-18 *(Jianxi)* to S-32 *(Futu)*. For flexion at the knee, join B-54 *(Weizhong)* to B-51 *(Yinmen)*. For 'drop' foot, join S-36 *(Zusanli)* to S-39 *(Xiajuxu)*. For 'raised' foot, join B-54 *(Weizhong)* to B-57 *(Chengshan)*. For inward club foot, join GB-34 *(Yanglingquan)* to GB-39 *(Juegu)*. For outward club foot, join B-58 *(Feiyang)* to K-8 *(Jiaoxin)*.

Method: When needling points on the back, it is best to have the patient in a sitting position, with his lower back straight and head slightly bowed. For needling other points, the patient should be lying either supine or prone. Treat daily or on alternating days. If needling daily, it is best to select a few groups of points on the back and limbs that can be used in rotation.

Injection therapy
1. Spinal cord stimulants: Inject dimeflilnum at point Gv-2 *(Yaoshu)*; or inject galanthamine at M-BW-35 *(Jiaji)*; or inject GABA into the appropriate vertebral points M-BW-35 *(Jiaji)* or Associated points of the back.
2. Nerve nutrients: Select one or two of the following: vitamin B1, vitamin B2, vitamin B12 or nicotinamide. Inject at selected points on the back and limbs.
3. Chinese herbs: Inject 3% *Angelica sinesis (danggui)* solution, or a 15% *Angelica sinesis, ligusticum (chuanxiong)*, and *Carthamus (honghua)* solution at vertebral points M-BW-35 *(Jiaji)* and other points on the limbs.
4. To relieve spasms: Inject a magnesium sulphate solution plus a 2% procaine hydrochloride solution into the spastic muscle; or, inject phenobarbital or valium. Inject phenobarbital solution; or inject valium into the spastic muscle group.
5. Other medication: Inject adenosine triphosphate (ATP), or inosine into appropriate vertebral points M-BW-35 *(Jiaji)*. This method is used only in the early stages of the condition.

Other prescriptions
1. GB-21 *(Jianjing)*, LI-15 *(Jianyu)*, LI-11 *(Quchi)*, TB-3 *(Zhongzhu)*, LI-4 *(Hegu)*, GB-38 *(Yangfu)*, GB-34 *(Yanglingquan)*, S-36 *(Zusanli)*, B-60 *(Kunlun)*. (Source: IACC)

Remarks
• Acupuncture must be combined with physical exercise (with assistance if necessary) to prevent hardening of the joints and tendons.

INTERCOSTAL NEURALGIA

Chinese medicine usually ascribes this condition to a disorder of the Liver. Indeed, the Liver and Gall Bladder channels traverse this region of the body. Pent-up emotions or anger can injure the Liver and cause its Qi to rebel in a lateral direction. The normal passage of Qi through the channels is thereby obstructed. If this condition is prolonged, it may affect the flow of Blood as well, causing it to coagulate.

Another source of this condition is said to be the stagnation of body fluids and Phlegm in the area of the ribs, which prevents the circulation of Qi and causes pain.

Treatment is directed toward opening the channels to facilitate the flow of Qi.

Needling
Principal points: TB-6 *(Zhigou)*, Li-5 *(Ligou)*, GB-34 *(Yanglingquan)*, and the vertebral point M-BW-35 *(Jiaji)* corresponding to the level of pain

Supplementary points: Li-14 *(Qimen)*, GB-40 *(Qiuxu)*, Li-2 *(Xingjian)*, Li-3 *(Taichong)*, B-18 *(Ganshu)*, B-17 *(Geshu)*, Li-13 *(Zhangmen)*, S-40 *(Fenglong)*, Sp-9 *(Yinlingquan)*, and P-6 *(Neiguan)*

Method: First, needle the principal points with strong stimulation, retaining the needles from 10-15 minutes. For symptoms associated with stagnant Liver Qi and lateral rebellion (e.g., wandering pain, fullness in the chest and abdomen, belching, symptoms exacerbated when patient is angry or depressed, but diminish when patient's mood is cheerful), add the supplementary points Li-2 *(Xingjian)*, Li-3 *(Taichong)*, P-6 *(Neiguan)*, and GB-40 *(Qiuxu)*. For symptoms associated with coagulated Blood (e.g., sharp, fixed pain which increases at night, dark stool, etc.), add Li-14 *(Qimen)*, B-17 *(Geshu)*, and B-18 *(Ganshu)*. For symptoms associated with fluids collecting and forming Phlegm (e.g., intense pain in the ribs reaching as far as the shoulder blades, coughing thin sputum, fullness, wheezing and possibly lumps forming in the chest), add S-40 *(Fenglong)*, Li-13 *(Zhangmen)* and Sp-9 *(Yinlingquan)*.

Discussion of the points: Because the ribs are traversed by the Gall Bladder, Liver and Triple Burner channels, the points along these channels are needled so as to disperse the stagnant Qi and direct it properly through the vessels. When the Liver Qi is constrained, Li-2 *(Xingjian)* and Li-3 *(Taichong)* are needled to spread the Liver Qi. To strengthen this effect, add GB-40 *(Qiuxu)*, the Source point on the Gall Bladder channel, and P-6 *(Neiguan)*, the Connecting point on the Pericardium channel. The Liver channel's Alarm point, Li-14 *(Qimen)*, is combined with B-18 *(Ganshu)* and B-17 *(Geshu)* to eliminate coagulated Blood. When the fluids collect and form Phlegm, use S-40 *(Fenglong)* to transform the Phlegm, Li-13 *(Zhangmen)*, the Alarm point of the Spleen channel, and Sp-9 *(Yinlingquan)*, the Uniting point of the Spleen channel, to strengthen the Spleen so as to get the fluids moving.

Ear acupuncture
Points: Thorax, Neurogate, Sympathetic, Occiput, Lung and other points of tenderness in the ear
Method: Manipulate the needle at each point for 1-2 minutes, then retain for 15-20 minutes with intermittent manipulation.

Cutaneous acupuncture
Principal points: B-18 *(Ganshu)*, Li-6 *(Zhongdu)*, Li-14 *(Qimen)*, GB-34 *(Yanglingquan)*, TB-6 *(Zhigou)*, B-19 *(Danshu)*, GB-24 *(Riyue)* and the vertebral points M-BW-35 *(Jiaji)* from the 5th to the 10th thoracic vertebra
Supplementary points: B-17 *(Geshu)*, Sp-17 *(Shidou)*, GB-36 *(Waiqiu)*, Li-3 *(Taichong)*, B-14 *(Jueyinshu)*, and Li-13 *(Zhangmen)*
Method: Tap the cutaneous needle at the points listed above in the affected area until slight bleeding appears, then apply cups.

Hand acupuncture
Point: Chest
Method: Strong stimulation, retaining needles 15-20 minutes.

Barefoot doctor acupuncture
Points: Barefoot Doctor point, Thoracic #5 and #8

Injection therapy
Points: Select the vertebral point M-BW-35 *(Jiaji)* corresponding to the level of pain
Method: Inject 2% procaine hydrochloride; or, inject vitamin B12 or vitamin B1. Treat once daily or on alternating days.

Other prescriptions
1. Rib pain: SI-5 *(Yanggu)*, SI-4 *(Wangu)*, TB-6 *(Zhigou)*, B-17 *(Geshu)*, B-62 *(Shenmai)*. (Source: CDR)
2. Rib pain: B-29 *(Zhonglushu)*, B-17 *(Geshu)*, GB-11 *(Qiaoyin)*, SI-5 *(Yanggu)*, and TB-19 *(Luxi)*. (Source: PUB)

3. Rib pain: Use moxa at Co-6 *(Qihai)*, Co-4 *(Guanyuan)*, Li-14 *(Qimen)*, and GB-11 *(Qiaoyin)*. Suitable for rib pain so severe that the patient is barely breathing. (Source: PDM)

4. Li-2 *(Xingjian)*, S-18 *(Rugen)*. Supplementary points: LI-11 *(Quchi)*, Co-17 *(Shanzhong)*, Sp-20 *(Zhourong)*. Use mild stimulation. The needles are inserted just deep enough to obtain a numb, sore, distended sensation and are retained for half an hour. Treat every other day. (Source: JTM)

5. Intercostal neuralgia: B-11 *(Dazhu)*, B-12 *(Fengmen)*, B-13 *(Feishu)*, B-15 *(Xinshu)*, B-18 *(Ganshu)*, K-22 *(Bulang)*, K-25 *(Shencang)*, L-5 *(Chize)*, L-9 *(Taiyuan)*. Use moderate stimulation. (Source: CAM)

Remarks

• The cutaneous acupuncture and cupping method is counter-indicated for cases involving herpes zoster.

• The origins of this condition are many. To thoroughly eliminate the source of pain, the primary cause must be diagnosed and treated.

• Acupuncture is definitely effective in treating this condition. If results are unsatisfactory, supplement with manipulation and physical therapy.

SPASM OF THE DIAPHRAGM (Hiccough)

According to traditional medicine, this condition is caused by a disorder of the Qi, which rebels upward. There are two kinds, Excessive and Deficient. If the patient is otherwise in robust health, with a clear, resonant hiccough, a feeling of fullness or even lumps in the chest and abdominal regions, constipation, belching a putrid smelling gas, etc., the condition is regarded as Excessive. If, on the other hand, the patient's general condition is weak, the sound of the hiccough very low and slight, with rapid breathing and a cold sensation in the limbs, the condition is Deficient and more serious.

Treatment is directed toward stabilizing the Qi and suppressing its rebelliousness.

Needling

Principal points: Co-22 *(Tiantu)*, B-17 *(Geshu)*, and P-6 *(Neiguan)*

Supplementary points: Co-12 *(Zhongwan)*, Co-17 *(Shangzhong)*, S-36 *(Zusanli)*, Co-14 *(Juque)*, Li-2 *(Xingjian)*, S-44 *(Neiting)*, Co-4 *(Guanyuan)*, Co-6 *(Qihai)*, and S-25 *(Tianshu)*

Method: The principal points are the basis of the prescription. Use moderate to strong stimulation with intermittent needle manipulation. For Excessive condition (see above), add Co-14 *(Juque)*, S-25 *(Tianshu)*, Li-2 *(Xingjian)*, and S-44 *(Neiting)*. For Deficient condition, add Co-4 *(Guanyuan)*, Co-12 *(Zhongwan)*, Co-6 *(Qihai)* and S-36 *(Zusanli)*. The point Co-17 *(Shanzhong)* may be used for either the Deficient or Excessive condition.

Discussion of points: Co-22 *(Tiantu)* is the point of intersection of the Yin Linking channel on the Conception channel, and is used for suppressing rebellious Qi. P-6 *(Neiguan)* also joins with the Yin Linking channel, and is needled to expand the chest so as to facilitate the function of the diaphragm. B-17 *(Geshu)* is the Associated point of the diaphragm on the back. Through this point, diseases of the membranes of the diaphragm may be treated. Co-17 *(Shanzhong)* is the Meeting point of Qi, and is called the 'upper sea of Qi'. Needling this point stabilizes the Qi. For Excessive conditions, Co-14 *(Juque)* is added to clear the chest, S-25 *(Tianshu)* to provide a connection with the Yang Organs' Qi, Li-2 *(Xingjian)* to drain Fire from the Liver, and S-44 *(Neiting)* to cool the Stomach. For Deficient conditions, Co-4 *(Guanyuan)* and Co-6 *(Qihai)* are used to strengthen the Kidneys, and Co-12 *(Zhongwan)* and S-36 *(Zusanli)* to strengthen the Qi of the Middle Burner.

Ear acupuncture

Points: Neurogate, Diaphragm, Subcortex

Method: Needle points bilaterally, using strong stimulation and retaining needles for one hour.

Moxibustion

Points: Co-17 *(Shanzhong)*, Co-12 *(Zhongwan)*, Co-4 *(Guanyuan)*

Method: Using the direct or indirect methods, burn five to nine cones of moxa. If the hiccoughs continue, burn moxa at B-23 *(Shenshu)*. Generally, the hiccoughs will cease after moxibustion treatment. If not, continue with more moxibustion.

Hand acupuncture

Point: Vertex

Method: Use straight insertion and strong stimulation without retaining the needle.

Injection therapy

Principal points: B-21 *(Weishu)*, or B-45 *(Weicang)* and P-6 *(Neiguan)*

Supplementary points: Co-15 *(Jiuwei)*, LI-10 *(Shousanli)*

Method: Use *Angelica sinesis (danggui)* or other appropriate medication. Treat daily or on alternating days. Seven to twelve treatments constitute one course. Allow 3-5 days rest between courses of treatment.

Cupping

Points: B-17 *(Geshu)*, B-41 *(Geguan)*, B-18 *(Ganshu)*, Co-12 *(Zhongwan)*, S-18 *(Rugen)*

Method: Use medium size cups. Apply for 10-15 minutes.

Other prescriptions

1. Principal point: Co-22 *(Tiantu)*. Supplementary points: P-6 *(Neiguan)*, Co-12 *(Zhongwan)*. If strong stimulation to the principal point is ineffective, add one of the supplementary points. (Source: RAT)

2. Sudden hiccoughs: Apply many moxa cones at Co-17 *(Shanzhong)*, L-1 *(Zhongfu)*, and other points on abdomen. Apply 7 cones of moxa at L-5 *(Chize)* and Co-14 *(Juque)*. (Source: PUB)

3. Belching: Apply moxa at Li-14 *(Qimen)*, Co-17 *(Shanzhong)*, and Co-12 *(Zhongwan)*. (Source: OM)

4. Belching: Apply 3 cones of moxa at S-18 *(Rugen)*, axilla point (on the rib below the hairline of the axilla), L-1 *(Zhongfu)*, B-12 *(Fengmen)*, GB-21 *(Jianjing)*, Co-24 *(Chengjiang)*, Co-17 *(Shanzhong)*, Co-12 *(Zhongwan)*, Li-14 *(Qimen)*, Co-6 *(Qihai)*, S-36 *(Zusanli)*, and Sp-6 *(Sanyinjiao)*. When moxa burns down to the skin, remove cones. (Source: PDM)

Remarks

• For chronic cases, not only must the hiccoughs themselves be treated, but the origin must be diagnosed and treated as well.

• For mild cases, the nose can be pinched to cause sneezing. For more serious cases, moxibustion may be used. The results are generally good.

• In addition to acupuncture, other common methods for treating hiccoughs include having the patient close his or her eyes while the physician 'tweaks' the nose closed for a couple minutes; or, pressure may be applied to the eyeball until it feels sore and swollen.

CEREBROVASCULAR ACCIDENT (Stroke)

In Chinese medicine this condition is known by different names, the most common of which is Penetrating Wind. Its etiology is generally related to an imbalance of Yin and Yang, such that Deficient Kidney or Liver Yin is unable to restrain the Liver Yang which flares upward, like Fire. This Fire in the Liver then transforms into Interior Wind, causing the Qi and Blood to rebel upward. Phlegm is formed, which obstructs the cavities and vessels. Loss of consciousness ensues.

Wind may also be generated by Phlegm and Heat which can form when a person has eaten too many sweet and fatty foods. Or, the body may become vulnerable to Wind of external origin when it is in a weak and Deficient condition.

Traditional medicine distinguishes between acute symptoms affecting the internal Organs, and symptoms of sequelae of stroke which are associated with the channels. The acute symptoms affecting the Organs are further distinguished as 'closed' and 'abandoned'.

Acute symptoms include sudden loss of consciousness, disorientation, coma, shortness of breath, facial paralysis, hemiplegia. A 'closed' acute conditon is further evidenced by tightly clenched hands, inability to move the bowels or urinate, clenched teeth, flushed face, rough breathing and the presence of Phlegm. An 'abandoned' condition is one in which the eyes are closed, mouth flaccid, hands loose, cheeks reddened, and there is snoring. If an 'abandoned' condition persists, the face becomes pale, there is no control over excretory function, and the limbs feel cold. The 'abandoned' condition is the more serious of the two and frequently is the stage toward which a 'closed' condition deteriorates.

Symptoms associated with the channels, i.e., the sequelae of stroke, include hemiplegia, facial paralysis, difficult, broken speech, saliva dribbling from the mouth, and difficulty in swallowing. Some of these symptoms may appear without the patient suffering coma, and may be accompanied by numbness in the hands, feet and face, tremors in the fingers, a heavy sensation in the hands and feet, dizziness, excessive Phlegm, etc.

For the 'closed' condition, treatment is directed toward clearing the orifices, draining the Heat, and suppressing the rebellious Qi. For the 'abandoned' condition, treatment proceeds according to the principle of stabilizing the Yang. For sequelae of stroke, treatment is directed toward clearing the channels so as to facilitate the circulation of Qi, thus activating the Blood and eliminating the Wind.

Needling
'Closed' acute condition

Principal points: Gv-26 *(Renzhong)*, K-1 *(Yongquan)*, P-8 *(Laogong)*, GB-20 *(Fengchi)*, P-6 *(Neiguan)*, LI-4 *(Hegu)*, and the Well points of the 12 Primary channels

'Abandoned' acute condition

Principal points: In addition to the points above, use Co-4 *(Guanyuan)*, Co-6 *(Qihai)*, and S-36 *(Zusanli)*

Supplementary points: The following points may be used to supplement the principal points for both the 'closed' and 'abandoned' conditions: P-7 *(Daling)*, Li-2 *(Xingjian)*, S-25 *(Tianshu)*, S-37 *(Shangjuxu)*, Co-17 *(Shanzhong)*, B-23 *(Shenshu)*, Gv-4 *(Mingmen)*, Li-3 *(Taichong)*, GB-34 *(Yanglingquan)*, Co-22 *(Tiantu)*, and S-40 *(Fenglong)*

Method: For the 'closed' condition, use relatively strong stimulation, and for the 'abandoned' condition, use mild stimulation. In the early stages, before the condition becomes 'abandoned', needling is appropriate. However, in the later stages burn moxa for relatively long periods of time at points Co-4 *(Guanyuan)*, Co-6 *(Qihai)* and S-36 *(Zusanli)*. For flushed face, thirst, irritability, constipation (symptoms associated with Fire), select from among P-7 *(Daling)*, Li-2 *(Xingjian)*, S-25 *(Tianshu)*, and S-37 *(Shangjuxu)*. For coldness in the limbs, sweating, shortness of breath and panting (symptoms associated with exhausted Source Qi), use Co-17 *(Shanzhong)*, B-23 *(Shenshu)*, and Gv-4 *(Mingmen)*, combining moxibustion and acupuncture. For severe headache, dizziness, spasm of the hands and feet, convulsions (symptoms associated with Wind rising from the Liver), select Li-3 *(Taichong)* and GB-34 *(Yanglingquan)*. For Phlegm, fullness or lumps in the chest or upper abdomen, heaviness in the limbs (symptoms associated with Phlegm), choose Co-22 *(Tiantu)*, S-40 *(Fenglong)* and P-6 *(Neiguan)*.

Sequelae of cerebrovascular accident
Choose points according to the location of the symptoms.

Principal points for the upper limb: LI-15 *(Jianyu)*, LI-11 *(Quchi)*, LI-4 *(Hegu)*, TB-5 *(Waiguan)*, N-UE-27 *(Zhitan #1)*, and M-UE-30 *(Bizhong)*.

Supplementary points: TB-14 *(Jianliao)*, LI-10 *(Shousanli)*, TB-4 *(Yangchi)*, and TB-3 *(Zhongzhu)*

Method: LI-11 *(Quchi)* may be joined to H-3 *(Shaohai)* and LI-4 *(Hegu)* to SI-3 *(Houxi)*. Needle the affected side with strong stimulation. If desired, the healthy side may be needled later with mild stimulation.

Principal points for the lower limb: GB-30 *(Huantiao)*, GB-31 *(Fengshi)*, GB-34 *(Yangling-quan)*, M-LE-13 *(Lanweixue)*, GB-39 *(Xuanzhong)*, S-41 *(Jiexi)*, N-LE-11 *(Jiuneifan)*, N-LE-10(a) *(Jiuwaifan #1)*, N-LE-10(b) *(Jiuwaifan #2)*, and S-36 *(Zusanli)*.

Supplementary points: N-LE-40 *(Tanli)*, N-LE-9 *(Luodi)*, B-60 *(Kunlun)*, Li-3 *(Taichong)*, GB-41 *(Zulinqi)*, and B-64 *(Jinggu)*

Method: Needle affected side with strong stimulation. If desired, the healthy side may be needled with mild stimulation.

Principal points for facial paralysis: TB-17 *(Yifeng)*, S-4 *(Dicang)*, S-2 *(Sibai)*, S-6 *(Jiache)*, LI-4 *(Hegu)*, and N-HN-20 *(Qianzheng)*

Supplementary points: B-2 *(Zanzhu)*, GB-14 *(Yangbai)*, Gv-26 *(Renzhong)*, SI-18 *(Quanliao)*, and M-HN-18 *(Jiachengjiang)*

Method: Needle S-2 *(Sibai)* with either a straight or transverse insertion, pointing the needle downward. S-4 *(Dicang)* can be joined to S-6 *(Jiache)*, and GB-14 *(Yangbai)* to M-HN-6 *(Yuyao)*. Insert needles superficially. Use moderate stimulation. Treat daily or on alternating days.

Principal points for impaired speech due to paralysis of tongue: M-HN-21 *(Shanglianquan)*, H-5 *(Tongli)*, Co-22 *(Tiantu)*

Supplementary points: Gv-15 *(Yamen)*, K-6 *(Zhaohai)*

Method: Care must be taken not to insert needle too deeply at Co-22 *(Tiantu)*. At Gv-15 *(Yamen)*, the needle should be slanted slightly downward. Treat daily or on alternating days. The points in this prescription may also be used for difficulty in swallowing.

Electro-acupuncture

Points used for hemiplegia: LI-15 *(Jianyu)*, LI-11 *(Quchi)*, TB-5 *(Waiguan)*, LI-4 *(Hegu)*, GB-30 *(Huantiao)*, GB-31 *(Fengshi)*, GB-34 *(Yanglingquan)*, and GB-39 *(Xuanzhong)*

Method: Select 2-3 points, bilaterally, depending on the location of the paralysis. After the needle is inserted, manipulate until the characteristic needle sensation is obtained. Apply electrodes to the needles, and gradually increase the level of electric current. After about 30 seconds, turn off the current momentarily. Then turn it on again for another 30 seconds. This process may be repeated 3 or 4 times, or until the patient feels soreness, numbness, distension or a burning sensation in the vicinity of the point, and the muscles show rhythmic contractions.

Injection therapy

In the early stages of hemiplegia, inject a 5% solution of ganimalonum, or andenosine triphosphate (ATP) into GB-20 *(Fengchi)* on the affected side. In the later stages, inject vitamin B1 and nicotinamide. Caution: do not insert the needle too deeply into GB-20 *(Fengchi)*.

Ear acupuncture

Points: Kidney, Brain Stem, Neurogate, Heart, Occiput, Subcortex

Head acupuncture

For hemiplegia, first select the corresponding Motor area on the side of the head opposite the paralysis. Combine with stimulation of the Sensory area and Leg motor and sensory area. For sensory impairment on one side, select the corresponding Sensory area on the opposite side of the head. For motor (Broca's) aphasia, use the Facial area on the opposite side. For sensory (Wernicke's) aphasia, use the Speech #3 area on the opposite side. For compulsive aphasia, select the Speech #2 area on the opposite side. For edema of the paralyzed limbs, stimulate the Blood vessel dilation and constriction area on the opposite side of the head.

Cutaneous acupuncture

Points for hemiplegia: B-18 *(Ganshu)*, B-23 *(Shenshu)*, B-31-34 *(Shangliao, Ciliao, Zhongliao and Xialiao)*, the vertebral points M-BW-35 *(Jiaji)* from the 5th to the 21st vertebra, LI-11 *(Quchi)*, L-9 *(Taiyuan)*, GB-34 *(Yanglingquan)*, GB-31 *(Fengshi)*, GB-39 *(Xuanzhong)*, and Li-1 *(Dadun)*

Points for slurred speech: P-4 *(Ximen)*, Gv-15 *(Yamen)*, H-6 *(Yinxi)*, H-5 *(Tongli)*, P-6 *(Neiguan)*, Co-23 *(Lianquan)*, and the vertebral points M-BW-35 *(Jiaji)* from the 3rd to the 6th thoracic vertebra, and from the 8th thoracic to the 5th sacral vertebra. These points may be supplemented with K-6 *(Zhaohai)*, Co-14 *(Juque)*, K-1 *(Yongquan)*, and Li-5 *(Ligou)*.

Cupping
Points: LI-15 *(Jianyu)*, LI-11 *(Quchi)*, TB-4 *(Yangchi)*, B-49 *(Zhibian)*, GB-30 *(Huantiao)*, GB-34 *(Yanglingquan)*, and GB-40 *(Qiuxu)*
Method: For each treatment, select 1-2 points on both the upper and lower limbs.

Other prescriptions
1. Upper extremity: LI-4 *(Hegu)* joined to P-8 *(Laogong)*, SI-6 *(Yanglao)*, H-7 *(Shenmen)*, P-6 *(Neiguan)* joined to TB-5 *(Waiguan)*, M-UE-30 *(Bizhong)*, LI-10 *(Shousanli)*, N-UE-11 *(Taijian)*, LI-15 *(Jianyu)* with the needle inserted in all directions, N-UE-7 *(Yingxia)*. Lower extremity: N-BW-15 *(Shenji)*, GB-30 *(Huantiao)*, B-51 *(Yinmen)*, S-32 *(Futu)*, B-57 *(Chengshan)*, GB-34 *(Yanglingquan)* joined to Sp-9 *(Yinglingquan)*, GB-31 *(Fengshi)*, N-LE-18 *(Jianxi)*, S-36 *(Zusanli)*, Sp-6 *(Sanyinjiao)*, GB-39 *(Juegu)*, B-60 *(Kunlun)*, K-3 *(Taixi)*, and N-LE-8 *(Lishang)*. Head: N-HN-54 *(Anmian)* and GB-20 *(Fengchi)*. Method: Select points in rotation. A course of treatment is from 10-15 days, allowing 3-5 days between courses. For hypertension, add LI-11 *(Quchi)*. (Source: HCNMT)
2. Paralysis: LI-11 *(Quchi)*, LI-5 *(Yangxi)*, LI-4 *(Hegu)*, TB-3 *(Zhongzhu)*, GB-38 *(Yangfu)*, S-36 *(Zusanli)* and B-60 *(Kunlun)*. (Source: GCAM)
3. Inability to speak, hemiplegia: Apply 3 cones of moxa at Gv-20 *(Baihui)*, hairline anterior to the ear, GB-21 *(Jianjing)*, GB-31 *(Fengshi)*, S-36 *(Zusanli)*, GB-39 *(Juegu)*, and LI-11 *(Quchi)*. For right-sided problems moxi the left side, and vice versa. (Source: CNLAM)
4. Penetrating Wind when the patient falls down and is suddenly unconscious with jaws clenched, due to stagnation of Phlegm: Using a pyramid needle, prick the twelve Well points letting the bad Blood out. (Source: MQK)
5. Penetrating Wind with hemiplegia: LI-4 *(Hegu)*, LI-10 *(Shousanli)*, LI-11 *(Quchi)*, GB-21 *(Jianjing)*, GB-30 *(Huantiao)*, Sp-10 *(Xuehai)*, GB-34 *(Yanglingquan)*, Sp-9 *(Yinlingquan)*, S-36 *(Zusanli)*, GB-39 *(Juegu)*, and B-60 *(Kunlun)*. First strengthen the healthy side, then drain the diseased side. (Source: JDC)

Remarks
• During the acute stage while the patient is in a coma, Chinese herbal medicine may be used in addition to acupuncture. If the condition is perilous, Chinese and Western methods should be combined to save the patient.
• A paralyzed patient should be encouraged to exercise the limbs so as to hasten recovery of motor function.
• If the patient's blood pressure exceeds 200/120, strong needle stimulation should be avoided, and electro-acupuncture used only with the utmost caution.
• If the patient has lost feeling in a limb, moxibustion should be used only with great care, so as to avoid inadvertent burns.
• Except in emergencies, needling must be used sparingly on patients suffering from acute cerebral or subarachnoid hemorrhage.
• Acupuncture definitely has a therapeutic effect in treating cerebrovascular accident.
• Manipulation and physical therapy may be used in conjunction with acupuncture to strengthen the result in treating hemiplegia.

SEIZURES (Epilepsy)

According to traditional Chinese medicine, this condition is usually related to Deficient Kidney and Liver Yin. Injury to the Kidney Yin causes Interior Wind to arise in the Liver and Phlegm to rebel upward, disrupting the Qi in the channels and confusing the mind and senses.

A book of the Ming dynasty, *Outline of Medicine,* explains: "In epilepsy the Phlegm Excess rebels upward. Because the Phlegm Excess rebels upward, the Qi in the head becomes disorderly. Because the Qi in the head is disorderly, the vessels close and the orifices [senses] become disconnected with the result that the ears do not hear sounds, the eyes do not recognize people and the victim becomes dizzy and collapses."

Treatment is directed toward clearing the orifices of the head (senses), transforming the Phlegm, and calming the Liver by extinguishing the Wind.

Needling

Principal points: Gv-16 *(Fengfu),* GB-20 *(Fengchi),* Gv-26 *(Renzhong),* Gv-14 *(Dazhui),* M-BW-29 *(Yaoqi)*

Supplementary points: B-62 *(Shenmai),* K-6 *(Zhaohai),* P-6 *(Neiguan)* or P-5 *(Jianshi),* H-7 *(Shenmen)* or H-5 *(Tongli),* LI-4 *(Hegu),* Li-3 *(Taichong),* Sp-6 *(Sanyinjiao),* GB-34 *(Yanglingquan),* Co-14 *(Juque),* Co-12 *(Zhongwan),* S-40 *(Fenglong),* Gv-24 *(Shenting)*

Method: Use principal points first. For grand mal type epilepsy, add K-6 *(Zhaohai)* if the seizure occurs during the day, B-62 *(Shenmai)* if at night. Other supplementary points may be used where appropriate. For petit mal type epilepsy, P-6 *(Neiguan),* H-7 *(Shenmen)* and Gv-24 *(Shenting)* may be added to tranquilize the mind. For psychomotor type epilepsy, add P-5 *(Jianshi)* and H-7 *(Shenmen)* to awaken the Spirit, and S-40 *(Fenglong),* Co-14 *(Juque)* or Co-12 *(Zhongwan)* to clear the chest and cause the Phlegm to descend. For focal epilepsy, add LI-4 *(Hegu)* and Li-3 *(Taichong)* to open the 'Four Gates', GB-34 *(Yanglingquan)* to relax the muscles and tendons, and Sp-6 *(Sanyinjiao)* to regulate the Leg Yin channels. In addition to the points above, Gv-20 *(Baihui),* which awakens the brain, B-15 *(Xinshu),* which calms the Spirit, and B-18 *(Ganshu),* which pacifies the Liver may be added as desired. Between seizures, Co-4 *(Guanyuan)* and K-3 *(Taixi)* may be treated either with needling or moxibustion. During a seizure, use strong needle stimulation. Treat one or more times daily. Ten treatments constitute a course.

Discussion of principal points: GB-20 *(Fengchi),* Gv-16 *(Fengfu)* and Gv-14 *(Dazhui)* are used to drain the Wind, cleanse the Yang which has been obscured by Phlegm, pacify the Spirit, and clear the brain. Gv-26 *(Renzhong)* may be needled to regulate the Yin and Yang and open the orifices of the head (senses) so as to revive the patient from unconsciousness. M-BW-29 *(Yaoqi)* is a point which has traditionally been effective in treating epileptic seizures.

Ear acupuncture

Points: Neurogate, Heart, Kidneys, Occiput, Stomach, Subcortex, Brain

Injection therapy

Points: H-7 *(Shenmen),* B-15 *(Xinshu),* B-44 *(Yishe),* Co-15 *(Jiuwei),* Gv-15 *(Yamen),* P-6 *(Neiguan),* S-36 *(Zusanli)*

Method: Inject vitamin B1 or vitamin B12. Select a few of the above points for injection at each treatment.

Electro-acupuncture

Points: Gv-24 *(Shenting),* P-6 *(Neiguan);* or M-HN-9 *(Taiyang),* S-36 *(Zusanli);* or GB-20 *(Fengchi),* B-61 *(Pushen)*

Method: Use a moderate level of electrical stimulation for 5-10 minutes. The three prescriptions above may be used in rotation, one pair of points per treatment.

Moxibustion

Points: Gv-20 *(Baihui),* Co-15 *(Jiuwei),* Co-13 *(Shangwan),* H-7 *(Shenmen)* and B-62 *(Shenmai)* for seizures during the day, or K-6 *(Zhaohai)* for seizures occurring at night.

Barefoot doctor acupuncture

Points: Barefoot Doctor point, Thoracic #5 and #8, Posterior *Hegu*

Head acupuncture
Points: Motor area, Sensory area, Leg motor and sensory area. Other areas may be added as the situation requires.

Foot acupuncture
Points: #2, #34

Embedding thread
Principal points: Gv-14 *(Dazhui)*, Gv-15 *(Yamen)*
Supplementary points: M-HN-13 *(Yiming)*, H-7 *(Shenmen)*
Method: Select 2-3 points for each treatment, allowing 20 days between treatments.

Other prescriptions
1. Seizures: B-2 *(Zanzhu)*, TB-10 *(Tianjing)*, H-3 *(Shaohai)*, H-7 *(Shenmen)*, B-63 *(Jinmen)*, Sp-5 *(Shangqiu)*, Li-2 *(Xingjian)*, B-66 *(Tonggu)*, B-15 *(Xinshu)* (burn 100 cones of moxa), and SI-3 *(Houxi)*. (Source: CDR)

2. Seizures: K-1 *(Yongquan)*, B-15 *(Xinshu)*, S-36 *(Zusanli)*, Co-15 *(Jiuwei)*, Co-12 *(Zhongwan)*, L-11 *(Shaoshang)*, and Co-14 *(Juque)*. (Source: GCAM)

3. Seizures: Burn 50 cones of moxa at Co-12 *(Zhongwan)*. (Source: BBQS)

4. Seizures: Co-15 *(Jiuwei)*, SI-3 *(Houxi)*, K-1 *(Yongquan)*, B-15 *(Xinshu)*, GB-35 *(Yangjiao)*, S-36 *(Zusanli)*, Li-3 *(Taichong)*, P-5 *(Jianshi)*, and Co-13 *(Shangwan)*. (Source: OM)

5. Seizures. Principal points: GB-20 *(Fengchi)* and Gv-16 *(Fengfu)*. Supplementary points: H-5 *(Tongli)*, Sp-6 *(Sanyinjiao)*, P-6 *(Neiguan)*, and Li-3 *(Taichong)*. Needle one principal point and two supplementary points daily. Courses of treatment are 10 days, separated by 3 days. During a seizure, needle Gv-26 *(Renzhong)* and K-1 *(Yongquan)*. (Source: HCNMT)

6. Seizures. Principal points: Gv-15 *(Yamen)* and SI-3 *(Houxi)*. Supplementary points: GB-20 *(Fengchi)*, M-BW-29 *(Yaoqi)*, Gv-26 *(Renzhong)*, and P-6 *(Neiguan)*. During seizures, needle Gv-26 *(Renzhong)*. Between seizures, needle the principal points. If this is not effective (in reducing seizures), use the supplementary points. When needling M-BW-29 *(Yaoqi)*, the needle should point upward. (Source: RAT)

Remarks
- Acupuncture therapy is only a supplementary method of treating this condition. Appropriate oral medication must be used in addition and, in some cases, surgery.

HEADACHE

Traditional Chinese medicine ascribes headache to a variety of factors, among them Wind, Heat, Excessive Liver Yang, Phlegm, Dampness and Deficiency, especially of the Kidney Qi.

Treatment varies according to the source of the problem. The particular channels affected by this condition can be determined on the basis of which part of the head hurts.

Needling
Principal points: GB-20 *(Fengchi)*, M-HN-9 *(Taiyang)*, Gv-20 *(Baihui)*, Li-3 *(Taichong)*, GB-8 *(Shuaigu)*, TB-3 *(Zhongzhu)*
Supplementary points: LI-4 *(Hegu)*, L-7 *(Lieque)*, TB-5 *(Waiguan)*, Gv-16 *(Fengfu)*, Li-2 *(Xingjian)*, GB-40 *(Qiuxu)*, K-3 *(Taixi)*, SI-3 *(Houxi)*, GB-41 *(Zulinqi)*, B-65 *(Shugu)*, B-2 *(Zanzhu)*, GB-14 *(Yangbai)*, S-8 *(Touwei)*, Co-12 *(Zhongwan)*, S-40 *(Fenglong)*, Co-6 *(Qihai)*, Co-4 *(Guanyuan)*, B-10 *(Tianzhu)*

Method: First, needle GB-20 *(Fengchi)* until the needle sensation extends to the fronto-temporal region. For headache at the vertex, add Gv-20 *(Baihui)* and Li-3 *(Taichong)*. For temporal headache, add M-HN-9 *(Taiyang)* joined to GB-8 *(Shuaigu)* and TB-3 *(Zhongzhu)*. For frontal headache, add GB-14 *(Yangbai)* joined to B-2 *(Zanzhu)* and LI-4 *(Hegu)*. For occipital headache, add B-10 *(Tianzhu)* and SI-3 *(Houxi)*. Needle with small amplitude until the Qi sensation is obtained. Then needle vigorously for 5-15 minutes. Some of the points above, among them M-HN-9 *(Taiyang)*, Gv-20 *(Baihui)*, TB-3 *(Zhongzhu)* and Li-3 *(Taichong)* may be used regardless of the location of the headache.

If the headache is caused by Wind, add Gv-16 *(Fengfu)*, L-7 *(Lieque)* and TB-5 *(Waiguan)*. Acute symptoms associated with Wind of an external origin include sudden onset, fever and chills, stuffy nose, aching body and possibly coughing. Chronic symptoms which accompany the prolonged presence of Wind in the body, include frequent headaches, shivering and sensitivity to wind, body fatigue.

If the headache is due to Excessive Liver Yang, add K-3 *(Taixi)*, B-23 *(Shenshu)* and P-5 *(Xingjian)*. Symptoms associated with this condition include dizziness, insomnia, emotional fatigue, soreness in the lower back, spermatorrhea, palpitations, tinnitus, blurred vision, amnesia.

If the headache arises from Deficient Kidney Qi, add Co-4 *(Guanyuan)*, Co-6 *(Qihai)* and S-36 *(Zusanli)*. Symptoms associated with this condition include fatigue and lowered voice. Moxibustion may also be applied at these points.

If the headache is associated with Heat in the Stomach or Fire in the Liver and Gall Bladder, add GB-40 *(Qiuxu)*, Li-3 *(Taichong)*, S-43 *(Xiangu)*, S-8 *(Touwei)*. Symptoms of these conditions include burning fever, severe headache, bloodshot eyes, pain in the ribs, thirst, constipation, vomiting or lumps in the upper abdomen and chest, etc.

If the headache is caused by Dampness and Phlegm, add Co-12 *(Zhongwan)* and S-40 *(Fenglong)*. Symptoms associated with this condition include fullness or lumps in the upper abdomen or chest, vomiting frothy fluids, vertigo, etc. If these symptoms are accompanied by Deficient Qi, add S-36 *(Zusanli)*, Co-4 *(Guanyuan)* and Co-6 *(Qihai)*. Apply moxibustion at these points for Deficient Qi.

Ear acupuncture

Points: Subcortex, Forehead, Occiput, Kidneys, Pancreas/Gall Bladder and other points of tenderness on the ear

Method: After inserting the needles, manipulate intermittently. For persistent headache, use strong stimulation for about 5 minutes. Intradermal needles may also be embedded for periods of 1-7 days.

Cutaneous acupuncture and cupping

Principal points: From the 1st lumbar to the 4th sacral vertebra

Supplementary points: GB-20 *(Fengchi)*, M-HN-9 *(Taiyang)*, GB-14 *(Yangbai)*

Method: Tap along the vertebrae, then at the site of pain on the head, as well as the palms and finger tips. If the headache is severe, also tap supplementary points until there is slight bleeding, then apply cups.

Injection therapy

Points: GB-20 *(Fengchi)*, B-10 *(Tianzhu)*, GB-14 *(Yangbai)*, B-2 *(Zanzhu)*

Method: Inject, on the affected side, either *Angelica sinesis (danggui)*, vitamin B1 and B12, a 10% glucose solution, or saline. Insert needle 0.3-0.5 inch, withdraw slightly, then inject the medicine. This will cause the sensation to extend outward from the point. Treat once every other day.

Head acupuncture

Points: For frontal headache, use the Facial area in the Sensory area on either the affected side, or both sides of the head. For occipital headache, use the Lower limb, head and trunk area in the Sensory area.

Hand acupuncture

Points: Forehead, Vertex, and supplement with M-HN-3 *(Yintang)*. Or, Side of Head, Occiput, and supplement with LI-11 *(Quchi)* or M-HN-9 *(Taiyang)*

Method: Select one of the two prescriptions above according to the location of the headache. Use strong stimulation, retaining the needles for 15-20 minutes with intermittent needle manipulation. Seven to ten treatments constitute one course.

Foot acupuncture
Points: #20, #46, #47, #48

Other prescriptions
1. Head Wind: Gv-23 *(Shangxing)*, Gv-21 *(Qianding)*, Gv-20 *(Baihui)*, SI-5 *(Yanggu)*, LI-4 *(Hegu)*, TB-1 *(Guanchong)*, B-60 *(Kunlun)* and GB-43 *(Xiaxi)*. (Source: CDR)
2. Head Wind with vertex pain: Gv-20 *(Baihui)*, Gv-19 *(Houding)*, and LI-4 *(Hegu)*. (Source: GCAM)
3. Lateral or midline headache: Moxibustion at GB-19 *(Naokong)*, GB-20 *(Fengchi)*, L-7 *(Lieque)*, L-9 *(Taiyuan)*, LI-4 *(Hegu)*, and S-41 *(Jiexi)*. (Source: PDM)
4. If lateral head Wind includes the eyes and teeth, burn 21 cones of moxa at GB-19 *(Naokong)* and GB-16 *(Muchuang)*. For pain on left side, apply moxa on the right, and vice versa. (Source: BBQS)
5. Headache with dizziness: LI-17 *(Tianding)*, B-12 *(Fengmen)*, B-60 *(Kunlun)*, Co-4 *(Guanyuan)*, and TB-1 *(Guanchong)*. (Source: PUB)

Remarks
• Avoid deep insertion at Gv-16 *(Fengfu)*. If necessary, use a slanted insertion. Caution must also be observed if the physician chooses to join two points here with a transverse insertion.
• If the headache is due to hypertension, strong needle stimulation should be avoided.
• Acupuncture is relatively effective in treating this condition. However, the causes of headache are complex, and acupuncture treatment should be preceded by careful diagnosis to determine the source of the problem. Other modes of Chinese and Western medicine may therefore be needed in addition to acupuncture, in order to treat the root cause.
• Manipulation and breathing exercises *(Qigong)* have proven effective in the treatment of chronic headache and are therefore recommended in conjunction with acupuncture therapy.

NEURASTHENIA

In Chinese medicine, the symptoms associated with this condition include depression, palpitations, insomnia, lassitude, spermatorrhea and others. It is attributed to weakness or disruption of the Heart, Liver, Spleen or Kidney Qi. The depletion of Kidney Yin may cause Fire in the Heart to flare upward and the Liver Yang to become Excessive. Alternatively, because of repressed emotions, the Liver may be unable to perform its spreading function. This, in turn, harms the digestive and transportive functions of the Spleen.

Treatment is directed toward calming the Heart's Spirit, strengthening the Kidneys and regulating the Liver and Spleen.

Needling
Principal points: P-6 *(Neiguan)*, H-7 *(Shenmen)*, M-HN-3 *(Yintang)* (transverse insertion downward), N-HN-54 *(Anmian)*, S-36 *(Zusanli)*, K-3 *(Taixi)*
Supplementary points: GB-20 *(Fengchi)*, Gv-20 *(Baihui)*, TB-23 *(Sizhukong)*, Co-12 *(Zhongwan)*, B-20 *(Pishu)*, B-18 *(Ganshu)*, Sp-6 *(Sanyinjiao)*, B-15 *(Xinshu)*, B-23 *(Shenshu)*, Gv-4 *(Mingmen)*, Co-4 *(Guanyuan)*, Co-6 *(Qihai)*, Li-2 *(Xingjian)*, P-4 *(Ximen)*

Method: Use the principal points as the basis of the prescription. For dysfunction of the Liver and Spleen, select from among Li-2 *(Xingjian)*, Co-12 *(Zhongwan)*, B-18 *(Ganshu)*, and B-20 *(Pishu)*. Symptoms associated with these Organs include depression, irritability, periodic feeling of depression in the chest and pain in the ribs, nausea or vomiting, repressed belching, constricted sensation in the throat, lumps, distension or pain in the abdomen, reduced capacity of the stomach. For depleted Kidney Yin and its attendant Liver Yang Excess or Fire in the Heart, use B-15 *(Xinshu)*, P-4 *(Ximen)*, B-23 *(Shenshu)*, GB-20 *(Fengchi)*, and TB-23 *(Sizhukong)*. Associated symptoms include insomnia, frequent dreams, spermatorrhea, irritability, disorientation, dizziness, tinnitus, palpitations and nervous fright. For diminished Kidney function (Yang), select from Gv-4 *(Mingmen)*, Co-4 *(Guanyuan)*, and Co-6 *(Qihai)*. Symptoms associated with this pattern include impotence, premature ejaculation, soreness in the lower back, spermatorrhea, cold hands and feet, dizziness and blurred vision, emotional and physical lassitude, etc. For all of these conditions, needle with mild stimulation, retaining needles for about 10 minutes. Moxibustion may also be applied at Co-4 *(Guanyuan)*, Gv-4 *(Mingmen)*, Co-6 *(Qihai)*, and S-36 *(Zusanli)*.

Ear acupuncture
   Points: Subcortex, Sympathetic, Heart, Kidneys, Spleen, Endocrine, Neurogate
   Method: Select a few points from those listed. Retain needles about 10 minutes.

Injection therapy
   Points: N-HN-54 *(Anmian)*, B-15 *(Xinshu)*, Co-14 *(Juque)*, Co-12 *(Zhongwan)*, S-36 *(Zusanli)*, B-18 *(Ganshu)*, B-20 *(Pishu)*, B-23 *(Shenshu)*, B-14 *(Jueyinshu)*
   Method: Select 2-3 points according to symptoms. Inject either a 10% glucose solution, *Angelica sinesis (danggui)* or vitamin B1 and B12. For persistent insomnia, a sedative may also be injected.

Embedding thread
   Points: Join B-23 *(Shenshu)* to B-22 *(Sanjiaoshu)*; or N-HN-22(b) *(Anmian #2)*, Gv-14 *(Dazhui)*, S-36 *(Zusanli)*
   Method: Use these two point groupings in rotation. Allow 20-30 days between treatments.

Barefoot doctor acupuncture
   Points: Barefoot Doctor point, Thoracic #5 and #8, Posterior *Hegu*

Head acupuncture
   Points: Motor area, Sensory area, Leg motor and sensory area. Depending on the symptoms, additional areas may be added to the prescription.

Foot acupuncture
   Points: #2, #46, #48

Other prescriptions
   1. N-HN-22(a) *(Anmian #1)*, H-7 *(Shenmen)*, and P-6 *(Neiguan)*. Use moderate to strong stimulation. Treat once daily, preferably just before bedtime. If results are not satisfactory, add M-HN-13 *(Yiming)*, S-36 *(Zusanli)*, and SP-6 *(Sanyinjiao)*. (Source: HCNMT)
   2. First group: GB-20 *(Fengchi)*, B-11 *(Dashu)*, B-15 *(Xinshu)*, B-22 *(Sanjiaoshu)*, Co-4 *(Guanyuan)*, P-6 *(Neiguan)*, and S-36 *(Zusanli)*. Second group: B-10 *(Tianzhu)*, Gv-12 *(Shenzhu)*, B-14 *(Jueyinshu)*, B-23 *(Shenshu)*, Co-6 *(Qihai)*, H-5 *(Tongli)*, and Sp-6 *(Sanyinjiao)*. Use mild stimulation, alternating the first and second point groups every other day. Or, tap cutaneous needle around each of the points daily. Use moxibustion at Co-4 *(Guanyuan)*. (Source: CAM)
   3. For chest pains and irritability: L-10 *(Yuji)*, L-11 *(Shaoshang)*, Sp-4 *(Gongsun)*, S-41 *(Jiexi)*, B-67 *(Zhiyin)*, and GB-12 *(Wangu)*. For spermatorrhea or impotence: use moxibustion at Li-4 *(Zhongfeng)*, B-47 *(Zhishi)*, and B-38 *(Gaohuangshu)*. (Source: PUB)
   4. For amnesia, palpitation, insomnia: P-6 *(Neiguan)*, H-7 *(Shenmen)*, and H-3 *(Shaohai)*.
   5. For disorientation: GB-16 *(Muchuang)*, B-8 *(Luoque)*, Gv-20 *(Baihui)*, B-62 *(Shenmai)*, and B-67 *(Zhiyin)*. (Source: CDR)
   6. Burn 50 cones of moxa at Co-12 *(Zhongwan)*, 100 cones at Co-4 *(Guanyuan)*. (Source: BBQS)

Remarks

• This condition is related to a functional disorder of the cerebrum. There are many causes, and the physician should make a careful diagnosis before treatment begins.

• The patient should be encouraged both to have a positive mental attitude and to engage in suitable physical exercise. These factors will contribute to a more rapid recovery.

• Acupuncture is definitely effective in treating this condition. The result will be strengthened if acupuncture is combined with appropriate Chinese and Western medicine.

HYSTERIA

What is known in the West as hysteria often falls within the traditional Chinese category of 'irritated Organ'. Manifestations of hysteria are sometimes regarded as symptoms of either 'depression pattern' or 'spasm pattern'.

Hysteria is understood to be an imbalance of the Heart and Spirit brought about by emotional excess. A writing of the Qing dynasty, entitled *The Golden Mirror of Medicine,* explains the term 'irritable Organ' in these words: "Organ refers to the Heart. When the Heart is calm it stores the Spirit. When it is injured by the seven emotions, the Heart cannot remain calm and the Spirit becomes irritable and unsettled."

This disorder may arise from a variety of factors, among them rebellious or Excessive Qi, hyperactive Yang, and Phlegm, all of which obscure and obstruct the senses.

Treatment is directed toward clearing the Heart and calming the Spirit, draining Fire (created by obstructed Qi) and eliminating Phlegm. Other points are chosen according to particular symptoms.

Needling

Principal points: P-6 *(Neiguan),* H-7 *(Shenmen),* Gv-26 *(Renzhong),* SI-3 *(Houxi)*

Supplementary points: LI-4 *(Hegu),* Li-3 *(Taichong),* L-11 *(Shaoshang),* Li-1 *(Dadun),* K-1 *(Yongquan),* Sp-6 *(Sanyinjiao),* LI-11 *(Quchi),* GB-34 *(Yanglingquan),* GB-30 *(Huantiao),* N-HN-15 *(Yilong),* TB-21 *(Ermen),* TB-17 *(Yifeng),* K-4 *(Dazhong),* Co-22 *(Tiantu),* B-1 *(Jingming),* TB-23 *(Sizhukong),* Gv-20 *(Baihui),* K-6 *(Zhaohai)*

Method: Use moderate to strong stimulation. Do not retain needles. The principal points are the basis of the prescription. As for supplementary points, if there are epileptic type seizures or convulsions, use LI-11 *(Quchi),* L-11 *(Shaoshang),* GB-34 *(Yanglingquan),* GB-30 *(Huantiao),* LI-4 *(Hegu)* and Li-3 *(Taichong).* For symptoms of stiffness and insomnia, add Li-1 *(Dadun),* K-1 *(Yongquan),* and Gv-20 *(Baihui).* For constricted throat, use K-6 *(Zhaohai)* and Co-22 *(Tiantu).* For obstructed vision, use B-1 *(Jingming)* and TB-23 *(Sizhukong).* For impaired hearing, add TB-21 *(Ermen),* TB-17 *(Yifeng)* and N-HN-15 *(Yilong).* For hysterical aphasia, add Co-22 *(Tiantu).* For sudden laughing/crying, use P-7 *(Daling),* L-11 *(Shaoshang),* K-4 *(Dazhong)* and Sp-6 *(Sanyinjiao).* Select 3-5 points for each treatment. Treat once daily or on alternating days.

Ear acupuncture

Principal points: Heart, Kidneys, Subcortex, Brain Stem, Neurogate

Supplementary points: Stomach, Sympathetic

Method: Select 2-3 points for each treatment, using both principal and supplementary points in rotation. Strong stimulation is recommended. (If there is constriction of the throat, add the Throat and Esophagus points.)

Barefoot doctor acupuncture

Points: Barefoot Doctor point, Thoracic #5 and #8, Posterior *Hegu*

Foot acupuncture

Points: #4, #34, #46

Other prescriptons

1. For sudden laughing/crying: Gv-20 *(Baihui)* and Gv-26 *(Renzhong).* (Source: CDR)

2. For sleepiness: K-3 *(Taixi),* K-4 *(Dazhong),* K-6 *(Zhaohai),* LI-2 *(Erjian),* and Li-10 *(Wuli).* (Source: PUB)

3. For hysterical seizure: First group: B-60 *(Kunlun)* and SI-3 *(Houxi).* Second group: Gv-26 *(Renzhong)* and LI-4 *(Hegu)* joined to P-8 *(Laogong).* Third group: Gv-20 *(Baihui)* and P-6 *(Neiguan)* joined to TB-5 *(Waiguan).* Select one group for each treatment and use strong stimulation. (Source: HCNMT)

4. For 'spasm pattern' hysteria: Burn 50 cones of moxa at Co-12 *(Zhongwan).* (Source: BBQS)

Remarks

• During acupuncture treatment the physician should calm and assure the patient, as well as encourage him or her to take a positive attitude.

• Acupuncture is definitely effective in treating this condition. It may be used in conjunction with other modes of Chinese and Western medicine. The patient should be encouraged to participate in appropriate physical exercise so as to maintain good physical and mental health.

PSYCHOSIS (Schizophrenia)

Generally speaking, this condition falls within the traditional realms or 'madness' and 'insanity'. The first is more active and manic in nature (Yang), and has traditionally been characterized by such behavior as climbing to high places and singing, stripping naked and running, berating others, inexplicable singing and crying, going without sleep, etc. The second is quiet and depressive (Yin), and is associated with such symptoms as blank expression, constant sleeping, sitting woodenly, talking to oneself, depression, awkward and slow movement, etc.

Madness is caused by depression and anger which transforms into Fire in the Liver and Gall Bladder. Accompanied by Phlegm, it disrupts the Spirit in the Heart.

Insanity results from excessive anxiety which impedes the circulation of Qi and causes the fluids to congeal and form Phlegm. When Phlegm rises, the senses become obscured and consciousness disrupted.

Treatment is directed toward clearing the Heart and senses by eliminating Phlegm. For symptoms associated with madness, the Yang channels must be cleared by draining the Heat. For symptoms of insanity, the channels must be opened to vent the repressed emotions. Hallucinations are treated according to the particular symptoms.

Needling

Principal points: For madness, use N-HN-32 *(Dingshen),* Gv-14 *(Dazhui),* GB-20 *(Fengchi),* join Co-15 *(Jiuwei)* to Co-13 *(Shangwan),* join P-5 *(Jianshi)* to TB-6 *(Zhigou),* S-40 *(Fenglong).* For insanity, use Gv-15 *(Yamen),* Co-11 *(Jianli),* P-6 *(Neiguan),* H-5 *(Tongli),* Sp-6 *(Sanyinjiao),* join Gv-20 *(Baihui)* to M-HN-1 *(Sishencong),* M-HN-3 *(Yintang)* (transverse insertion pointed downward)

Supplementary points: SI-19 *(Tinggong),* TB-17 *(Yifeng),* B-1 *(Jingming),* N-HN-54 *(Anmian),* B-39 *(Shentang),* B-18 *(Ganshu),* LI-4 *(Hegu),* N-UE-15 *(Hubian),* GB-34 *(Yanglingquan),* Li-5 *(Ligou),* Li-3 *(Taichong),* L-11 *(Shaoshang),* P-8 *(Laogong),* K-4 *(Dazhong),* H-7 *(Shenmen)*

Method: For manic psychosis (madness), select from among the first group of principal points. In addition, use P-8 *(Laogong),* L-11 *(Shaoshang),* LI-4 *(Hegu),* Li-3 *(Taichong)* and N-HN-54 *(Anmian).* For depressive psychosis (insanity), select from among the second group of principal points. In addition, use K-4 *(Dazhong),* GB-34 *(Yanglingquan),* Li-5 *(Ligou),* H-7 *(Shenmen)* and other supplementary points as the symptoms warrant. For visual hallucinations, add B-1 *(Jingming);* for auditory hallucination, add TB-17 *(Yifeng).* Needle N-HN-32 *(Dingshen)* with a slanted insertion upward to a depth of about 1.5 units. Points Gv-15 *(Yamen)* and Gv-14 *(Dazhui)* should be needled to a depth of no more than 1.5 units.

Ear acupuncture

Points: Sympathetic, Neurogate, Heart, Liver, Subcortex, Endocrine, Stomach, Occiput

Method: Select 1-2 points for each treatment. Ear acupuncture may be used in conjunction with needling points on the body.

Injection therapy

Points: B-15 *(Xinshu),* Co-14 *(Juque),* B-17 *(Geshu),* P-5 *(Jianshi),* S-36 *(Zusanli),* H-7 *(Shenmen)*

Method: Inject chlorpromazine daily in 1-2 of the points. Rotate points. This method is suitable for manic psychosis.

Moxibustion

Points: For manic psychosis, use Gv-20 *(Baihui);* for depressive psychosis, use Li-1 *(Dadun);* for hallucinations, use SI-16 *(Tianchuang)*

Method: Burn 7 moxa cones at each point, 14 cones for severe cases.

Other prescriptions

1. Madness: H-3 *(Shaohai),* P-5 *(Jianshi),* H-7 *(Shenmen),* LI-4 *(Hegu),* SI-3 *(Houxi),* K-7 *(Fuliu),* and TB-23 *(Sizhukong).* For stupor: H-7 *(Shenmen),* L-11 *(Shaoshang),* K-1 *(Yongquan),* and B-15 *(Xinshu).* (Source: CDR)

2. Thirteen points for psychosis (madness and insanity): Gv-26 *(Renzhong),* L-11 *(Shaoshang),* Sp-1 *(Yinbai),* P-7 *(Daling),* B-62 *(Shenmai)* (use hot needle acupuncture), Gv-16 *(Fengfu),* S-6 *(Jiache)* (use warming the needle method), Co-24 *(Chengjiang),* P-8 *(Laogong),* Gv-23 *(Shang-xing),* Co-1 *(Huiyin)* for males (for females, use a point at the opening of the vagina), LI-11 *(Quchi)* (use hot needle acupuncture), and prick M-HN-37 *(Haiquan).* Needle thirteen points in order. (Source: TDP)

3. Madness: LI-11 *(Quchi),* GB-39 *(Juegu),* M-HN-30 *(Bailao),* and K-1 *(Yongquan).* (Source: GCAM)

4. Psychosis (madness and insanity): B-58 *(Feiyang),* S-23 *(Taiyi),* and S-24 *(Huaroumen).* (Source: PUB)

5. Madness: Burn 20-30 moxa cones at Co-14 *(Juque)* and 5 moxa cones at B-15 *(Xinshu),* bilaterally. (Source: BBQS)

6. For severe manic psychosis: Principal points include Gv-14 *(Dazhui),* Gv-13 *(Taodao).* The first group of supplementary points includes: M-HN-28 *(Fengyan),* Gv-26 *(Renzhong),* and Sp-6 *(Sanyinjiao).* The second group includes: M-HN-13 *(Yiming),* LI-4 *(Hegu)* joined to P-8 *(Laogong),* and S-36 *(Zusanli).* Treat daily. Rotate supplementary point groups. (Source: HCNMT)

Remarks

• Acupuncture and moxibustion are definitely effective in treating this condition. However, results vary according to the type of psychosis. Other modes of Chinese and Western medicine may be used in conjunction with acupuncture.

• Some patients will exhibit signs before a recurrence of psychosis such as insomnia, restlessness, etc. If used at this time, acupuncture may effectively prevent such recurrence.

• Psychiatric counseling should accompany treatment so as to resolve, as far as possible, those factors which caused the condition, and to encourage a confident attitude in the patient.

INDIGESTION

Traditional medicine regards this condition as a disorder of the Spleen and Stomach. It may arise from a variety of sources. The body may be affected by the Excesses of Heat and Dampness common to summer and fall, or Wind and Cold common to spring and winter. Irregular eating habits may lead to stagnation and obstruction in the Middle Burner (Stomach and Spleen). If Deficient Spleen Yang produces Cold, the Qi in the Middle may become Deficient, which will disrupt the digestive and transportive functions of the Stomach and Spleen. If the body fluids become exhausted after prolonged diarrhea or vomiting, Heat may prevail, causing confusion of the Spirit and Wind in the Liver. If the Yin (fluids) is sufficiently injured, it could affect the Yang such that it too is weakened and unable to secure the fluids in the body. Thus, body fluids become even more depleted and the condition deteriorates as both Yin and Yang become perilously Deficient.

Treatment is directed toward strengthening the transportive functions of the Stomach and Spleen. Other points are selected according to symptoms.

Needling
Principal points: S-36 *(Zusanli)*, S-25 *(Tianshu)*, Co-12 *(Zhongwan)*, M-UE-9 *(Sifeng)*
Supplementary points: P-6 *(Neiguan)*, LI-4 *(Hegu)*, Li-3 *(Taichong)*, Sp-9 *(Yinlingquan)*, Sp-6 *(Sanyinjiao)*, LI-11 *(Quchi)*, GB-34 *(Yanglingquan)*, Co-4 *(Guanyuan)*, Co-6 *(Qihai)*, B-20 *(Pishu)*, B-23 *(Shenshu)*, L-11 *(Shaoshang)*, L-5 *(Chize)*, B-54 *(Weizhong)*

Method: Needle the principal points with moderate stimulation, daily or on alternating days. If, after 3-5 treatments, the result is unsatisfactory, apply moxibustion at Co-6 *(Qihai)*, Co-12 *(Zhongwan)* and S-25 *(Tianshu)*. The supplementary points may be used as follows: For vomiting, add P-6 *(Neiguan)*. For chronic diarrhea, a symptom associated with Deficient Spleen, add B-20 *(Pishu)*, Sp-9 *(Yinlingquan)* and Sp-6 *(Sanyinjiao)*. For disorientation, add Gv-26 *(Renzhong)*. For spasm of the hands and feet, add LI-4 *(Hegu)*, Li-3 *(Taichong)*, GB-34 *(Yanglingquan)* and LI-11 *(Quchi)*. For coldness in the limbs, add B-23 *(Shenshu)* and Co-4 *(Guanyuan)*. If the fever continues, use L-11 *(Shaoshang)*, L-5 *(Chize)* or B-54 *(Weizhong)* by pricking the points to let a few drops of blood. When needling M-UE-9 *(Sifeng)*, prick the point to draw a small amount of yellow fluid.

Moxibustion
Points S-25 *(Tianshu)*, Co-4 *(Guanyuan)*, Co-8 *(Shenque)*
Method: Moxibustion is suitable for diarrhea, a symptom associated either with Deficient Spleen or the presence of Cold or Dampness in the Spleen. Although direct moxibustion is recommended, the indirect method can be used if physician or patient prefers. Burn 5-7 cones at each of 2 of the 3 points in the prescription. Rotate the points. Treat daily or on alternating days. Needling the same points prior to moxibustion is permitted.

Injection therapy
Points: S-25 *(Tianshu)*, S-36 *(Zusanli)* or S-37 *(Shangjuxu)*
Method: Select 2 of the 3 points each treatment, rotating them the following session. Inject vitamin B1 or distilled water, once daily for 3-5 days.

Ear acupuncture
Principal points: Sympathetic, Neurogate, Stomach, Large Intetine, and other points of tenderness on the ear
Supplementary points: Small Intestine, Pancreas/Gall Bladder

Incision method
Make an incision at either Palm #5 or beside the spinous process of the 11th thoracic vertebra.

Cutaneous acupuncture
Principal points: M-UE-9 *(Sifeng)*, which should be pricked only to draw a small amount of yellow fluid, B-20 *(Pishu)*, B-21 *(Weishu)*, B-22 *(Sanjiaoshu)*, S-36 *(Zusanli)*, LI-4 *(Hegu)*, M-BW-35 *(Jiaji)* from the 6th to the 10th thoracic vertebra

Supplementary points: Gv-12 *(Shenzhu)*, Co-4 *(Guanyuan)*, Co-12 *(Zhongwan)*, Co-6 *(Qihai)*, Sp-6 *(Sanyinjiao)*

Hand acupuncture

Points: The mid-point between P-8 *(Laogong)* and P-7 *(Daling)*

Method: Use strong stimulation. While needling, ask the patient to massage the affected area vigorously.

Other prescriptions

1. Chronic diarrhea (accompanying Deficient Cold condition): Co-4 *(Guanyuan)*, Co-3 *(Zhongji)*, Co-12 *(Zhongwan)*, and S-21 *(Liangmen)*. For abdominal pain, cold feet and hands, add S-25 *(Tianshu)*; for fullness in abdomen, add Sp-6 *(Sanyinjiao)*; for cold feet and hands, add Co-6 *(Qihai)*. Use moxibustion. (Source: PDM)

2. Infantile vomiting and diarrhea: If accompanied by a sunken, fine pulse and cold hands and feet, burn 150 moxa cones (cumulatively) below the umbilicus. (Source: BBQS)

3. Infantile indigestion: Principal point is S-36 *(Zusanli)*; supplementary points are B-25 *(Dachangshu)* or LI-4 *(Hegu)*. If accompanied by vomiting, add P-6 *(Neiguan)*. Manipulate needles for 10-20 minutes. As a supplementary method, burn moxa stick in circular pattern above S-25 *(Tianshu)* for 3-4 minutes at a time. (Source: JTM)

4. Infantile emaciation: Burn three moxa cones within the 3 units above the coccyx. (Source: GCAM)

Remarks

• Manipulation has proven effective in treating this condition. It may be used in conjunction with acupuncture.

ENURESIS

In Chinese medicine, this condition is associated with the Lungs, Spleen, Kidneys and Bladder. If the Kidney Yang is Deficient, it may be unable to properly secure the body fluids, and the Bladder may be unable to restrain them. Alternatively, if the Spleen function is weakened, or the fluid regulating function of the Lungs disrupted, fluids will pass through the body at an abnormal rate. Finally, if a child who wets his bed is not corrected, it may become an habitual practice resulting in this condition.

Treatment is directed toward warming and strengthening the Kidney Yang and Qi so as to secure the excessive fluids. Other points are chosen according to the particular symptoms.

Needling

Principal points: Co-4 *(Guanyuan)*, Sp-6 *(Sanyinjiao)*

Supplementary points: Gv-20 *(Baihui)*, Co-6 *(Qihai)*, Co-3 *(Zhongji)*, Sp-9 *(Yinlingquan)*, B-23 *(Shenshu)*, B-20 *(Pishu)*, S-36 *(Zusanli)*, L-7 *(Lieque)*

Method: Use moderate to strong stimulation. When needling points in the abdominal region, try to get the needle sensation to extend to the area of the genitals by pointing the needles with a slanted insertion downward. For points on the lower limb, however, it is best if the needle sensation is conducted upward. Treat once daily, 10-15 treatments constituting one course. Allow 3-5 days between courses of treatment. For enuresis due to Deficient Spleen, add to the principal points the supplementary points B-20 *(Pishu)* and S-36 *(Zusanli)*. Symptoms associated with Deficient Spleen include indigestion, fullness in the abdomen, intestinal noises and diarrhea. For enuresis associated with Deficient Kidneys, add B-23 *(Shenshu)*, Gv-20 *(Baihui)* and Co-6 *(Qihai)*. These points strengthen the Kidneys and raise the Qi. Points Co-4 *(Guanyuan)*, Co-6 *(Qihai)* and Co-3 *(Zhongji)* can be needled in rotation or joined to each other with the transverse insertion of a single needle.

Discussion of principal points: Co-4 *(Guanyuan)* is the point of intersection of the three Leg Yin channels on the Conception channel. Needling this point can strengthen the Kidney Yang so as to secure the fluids. Needling Sp-6 *(Sanyinjiao)* can strengthen the Qi in the three Leg Yin channels and thereby assist the Bladder in restraining the fluids.

Ear acupuncture
Points: Sympathetic, Brain, Kidney, Bladder, Occiput, Urethra, and other points of tenderness on the ear

Method: Needle daily or on alternating days, retaining the needles for half an hour. Some effects should be seen after 3-5 treatments. Continue treating once every five days to secure the result.

Moxibustion
Points: Gv-20 *(Baihui)*, Gv-4 *(Mingmen)*, Co-4 *(Guanyuan)*, B-33 *(Zhongliao)*

Method: Use 2-3 points in rotation, treating once daily. Burn 7 small moxa cones at each point or heat with moxa stick.

Injection therapy
Principal points: B-23 *(Shenshu)*, B-28 *(Pangguangshu)*

Supplementary points: Co-3 *(Zhongji)*, Co-9 *(Shuifen)*, Co-4 *(Guanyuan)*, Sp-6 *(Sanyinjiao)*

Method: Inject either *Angelica sinesis (danggui)*, vitamin B1, vitamin B12 or placental extract. For weaker patients with chronic enuresis, the medicine should be injected very slowly. Injection may also be made at points of tenderness found during palpation diagnosis.

Embedding thread
Points: Sp-6 *(Sanyinjiao)*, B-23 *(Shenshu)*, B-28 *(Pangguangshu)*, join Co-3 *(Zhongji)* to Co-2 *(Qugu)*

Cutaneous acupuncture
Principal points: Co-4 *(Guanyuan)*, Co-6 *(Qihai)*, Co-2 *(Qugu)*, B-23 *(Shenshu)*, Sp-6 *(Sanyinjiao)*, M-BW-35 *(Jiaji)* from the 4th thoracic to the 2nd lumbar vertebra

Supplementary points: Co-3 *(Zhongji)*, K-3 *(Taixi)*, B-33 *(Zhongliao)*, B-32 *(Ciliao)*, B-28 *(Pangguangshu)*

Method: Tap lightly over these points, then apply cups if desired.

Head acupuncture
Points: Leg motor and sensory area, Reproduction area

Foot acupuncture
Point: #44

Other prescriptions
1. H-7 *(Shenmen)*, L-10 *(Yuji)*, Li-3 *(Taichong)*, Li-1 *(Dadun)*, Co-4 *(Guanyuan)*. (Source: CDR)

2. Co-6 *(Qihai)*, Co-4 *(Guanyuan)*, Sp-9 *(Yinlingquan)*, Li-1 *(Dadun)*, Li-2 *(Xingjian)*. (Source: IACC)

3. Co-4 *(Guanyuan)*, L-1 *(Zhongfu)*, H-7 *(Shenmen)*. (Source: PUB)

4. Principal points: Co-3 *(Zhongji)*, Co-4 *(Guanyuan)*, B-23 *(Shenshu)*, B-28 *(Pangguangshu)*, Sp-6 *(Sanyinjiao)*. Supplementary points: Co-6 *(Qihai)*, B-26 *(Guanyuanshu)*, B-32 *(Ciliao)*, S-36 *(Zusanli)*, Li-1 *(Dadun)*, H-7 *(Shenmen)*, K-6 *(Zhaohai)*. Generally, use acupuncture and moxibustion together. Apply mild needle stimulation, inserting to a depth at which Qi is obtained. Retain needles 15-20 minutes, unless the patient is a child who can't sit still. For moxibustion, the use of a moxa stick is recommended, utilizing the 'sparrow pecking' method until the skin is red. For weak patients, more moxibustion than acupuncture is appropriate. Treat on alternating days, five treatments constitute one course. (Source: JCM)

5. Principal points: Co-4 *(Guanyuan)*, Co-3 *(Zhongji)*, and Sp-6 *(Sanyinjiao)*. Supplementary points: LI-4 *(Hegu)*, Co-2 *(Qugu)*, Gv-14 *(Dazhui)*, and B-28 *(Pangguangshu)*. Select 3-5 points each treatment. After inserting and manipulating the needle, it is important that the patient feels the characteristic Qi sensation. If the needle sensation is felt to radiate in the direction of the perineum when points Co-4 *(Guanyuan)* and Co-3 *(Zhongji)* are needled, the result will be better. Moxa stick

may also be applied for 10-15 minutes. Treat once daily, six treatments constitute one course. (Source: JTM)

Remarks
- When points on the lower abdomen are to be needled, be sure that the patient has urinated beforehand.
- During the period of treatment, the patient should avoid drinking beverages in the evening, and should be awakened at fixed times to use the toilet.
- Acupuncture is relatively effective in treating this condition.
- The patient should be encouraged to overcome emotional factors like fear and nervousness.
- Patients whose health is particularly weak should avoid strenuous and exhausting activities. Other medication in addition to acupuncture should be prescribed to strengthen such patients.
- If enuresis is related to some other functional disorder, the other must be treated as well.

Chapter 6

Surgical and Dermatological Diseases

ERYSIPELAS

According to Chinese medicine, this disease is caused by Heat and Poison which collects in the skin, blocks the channels, and causes the Qi and Blood to stagnate.

Treatment is directed toward activating the Blood to eliminate the stagnation, and dispersing the Heat and Poison.

Cupping and letting blood
Use a cutaneous needle or surgical instrument to prick the skin over the affected area, causing a small amount of bleeding. Apply cups. Treat once or twice daily.

Needling
Principal points: Gv-14 *(Dazhui)*, LI-11 *(Quchi)*, S-43 *(Xiangu)*, B-54 *(Weizhong)*
Supplementary points: M-HN-9 *(Taiyang)*, P-6 *(Neiguan)*, S-36 *(Zusanli)*
Method: Needling may be used in conjunction with the cupping and letting blood method. Use straight needle insertions at Gv-14 *(Dazhui)*, LI-11 *(Quchi)* and S-43 *(Xiangu)* with strong stimulation. Direct the needles so that the sensation extends in all directions. Prick B-54 *(Weizhong)* and its vicinity to let a little blood. For headache, add M-HN-9 *(Taiyang)*. For nausea, add P-6 *(Neiguan)* and S-36 *(Zusanli)*.

Barefoot doctor acupuncture
Points: Barefoot Doctor point, Thoracic #5

Ear acupuncture
Points: Neurogate, Adrenal, Subcortex, Occiput
Method: Select 2-3 points each session. Use moderate to strong stimulation, retaining the needles from thirty minutes to one hour. This method is effective in eliminating the pain and inflammation.

Injection therapy
Select 1-2 lymph nodes from either a contiguous area that drains the affected tissue or along the inguinal canal. Inject Ringer's solution.

Other prescriptions
1. Wash the affected area with warm water. Then use a pyramid needle to prick the area 20-30 times. (Source: CBCA)
2. Generalized 'red cinnabar' (rash): Gv-20 *(Baihui)*, LI-11 *(Quchi)*, S-36 *(Zusanli)*, and B-54 *(Weizhong)*. (Source: GCAM)

Remarks

- Acupuncture is inappropriate for erysipelas in the region of the eyes.
- For erysipelas complicated by infection, combined Chinese and Western methods of treatment should be considered.
- Acupuncture therapy is effective in treating this condition, particularly for erysipelas on the lower limb.

FURUNCLE (Boil)

According to traditional medicine, excessive consumption of alcoholic beverages or greasy foods may cause Heat to collect in the Organs, producing internally the Poison which manifests as this disease. Alternatively, the Poison may be of external origin, invading the body through contamination of the skin. Such contamination obstructs the passage of Qi and Blood which collects and generates Heat in the skin.

Treatment is directed toward draining the Governing channel and eliminating Heat from the Blood.

Needling and letting blood

Principal points: Gv-12 *(Shenzhu),* Gv-10 *(Lingtai),* LI-4 *(Hegu),* B-54 *(Weizhong)* (prick to let blood)

Supplementary points: Select 1-3 common points along the channel adjoining the site of the furuncle; or for 'red line furuncle' (acute lymphangitis), a relatively thick needle or surgical instrument may be inserted at the end of the 'line' toward the site of the infection so as to let blood and incise the head of the furuncle. If accompanied by high fever, add LI-11 *(Quchi)* and Gv-14 *(Dazhui).* For disorientation or delirium, add Gv-26 *(Renzhong),* M-UE-1 *(Shixuan),* SI-8 *(Xiaohai)* and P-4 *(Ximen).*

Method: Needle once or twice daily with strong stimulation. It is best if the needle sensation expands outward from the point.

Piercing method

Search for nodules on either side of the spine. Pierce these with a thick needle. Treat once daily.

Barefoot doctor acupuncture

Points: Barefoot Doctor point, Thoracic #5

Hot needle acupuncture

This method is appropriate for purulent furuncle. Insert thick needle into the head of the furuncle. This method may be used as an alternative to surgical incision.

Cupping

After the furuncle has been surgically incised, or pierced with a hot needle, apply a large cup to aid in removing the pus.

Ear acupuncture

Points: Neurogate, Adrenal, Subcortex, Occiput, and the point associated with the affected site
Method: Select 2-3 points each session. Use moderate to strong stimulation, retaining the needles for thirty minutes to one hour. Treat once or twice daily.

Injection therapy

Select 1-2 lymph nodes from either an adjoining area that drains the affected tissue, or along the inguinal canal. Inject Ringer's solution.

Other prescriptions

1. For all carbuncular swellings, puncture the center with needle and make at least 10 punctures

around the circumference. This will cause bleeding. Wipe the blood away and apply medicine. If the medicine goes through the holes caused by acupuncture, the results will be excellent. If not, the results will be uncertain. (Source: TDP)

2. Carbuncles (those that can be bled are curable, those that can't, aren't): LI-4 *(Hegu)*, LI-11 *(Quchi)*, S-36 *(Zusanli)*, B-54 *(Weizhong)*. (Source: GCAM)

3. Carbuncles on the back: GB-21 *(Jianjing)*, S-36 *(Zusanli)*, B-54 *(Weizhong)*, GB-41 *(Linqi)*, Li-2 *(Xingjian)*, H-5 *(Tongli)*, H-3 *(Shaohai)*, Li-3 *(Taichong)*. (Source: GCAM)

4. For carbuncles on the face and around the mouth, apply moxa at LI-4 *(Hegu)* and the carbuncle will disappear. If they appear on the hands, apply moxa at LI-11 *(Quchi)*. If they appear above the scapulae, apply moxa at S-36 *(Zusanli)*, B-54 *(Weizhong)*, and GB-41 *(Linqi)*, and you cannot go wrong. Apply moxa at Li-2 *(Xingjian)*, H-5 *(Tongli)*, H-3 *(Shaohai)*, and Li-3 *(Taichong)* and the disease will not get worse. (Source: GOA)

5. If there are carbuncles on both flanks, the Poison can run toward the Heart. This is an emergency. Burn 3-5 cones of moxa on the tip of the carbuncle and bleed above, below, to the left, and to the right of where the moxa is burnt. (Source: GS)

6. Put garlic paste around the base of the carbuncle and burn moxa on the tip until the carbuncle bursts. (Source: TLM)

Remarks
- Squeezing or incising the furuncle too early may cause infection.
- If the furuncle develops into septicemia, other Chinese and Western medication should be used.
- Acupuncture therapy is regarded as a supplementary method to lancing in the treatment of this condition.

ACUTE MASTITIS

According to Chinese medicine, the sources of this condition are several. It may be caused by a nursing baby blowing wind against the breast, or by Heat collecting there. Alternatively, repressed Liver Qi may become stagnant and cause the Blood to coagulate, impeding circulation through the vessels in the breast and suppressing lactation. This in turn causes Dampness and Heat to collect, forming Poison.

Treatment is directed toward opening the vessels in the breast by clearing and draining the Heat and Poison.

Needling
Principal points: Co-17 *(Shanzhong)*, SI-1 *(Shaoze)*, S-18 *(Rugen)*
Supplementary points: P-6 *(Neiguan)*, TB-10 *(Tianjing)*

Method: Treat 1-3 times daily with moderate stimulation, retaining needles for 30 minutes with occasional manipulation.

Discussion of points: The nipples are within the domain of the Liver channel and the breasts are traversed by a branch of the Stomach channel. S-18 *(Rugen)* is selected to drain Heat from the Stomach channel, P-6 *(Neiguan)* and TB-10 *(Tianjing)* are needled to spread the Qi in the Pericardium and Triple Burner channels, and Co-17 *(Shanzhong)* can be added to regulate the Qi in the chest. Experience has shown that SI-1 *(Shaoze)* is also effective in treating this disease.

Barefoot doctor acupuncture
Points: Barefoot Doctor point, Thoracic #5

Moxibustion
In the early stages of this condition apply a paste of either crushed white onion or garlic on the affected tissue. Then warm with the moxa stick for 10-20 minutes. Treat once or twice daily.

Ear acupuncture

Points: Mammary Glands, Neurogate, Occiput, Adrenal, Subcortex

Method: Select 2-3 points each session. Use moderate to strong stimulation, retaining needles for thirty minutes to one hour. Treat once daily.

Injection therapy

Select 1-2 subaxillary or inguinal lymph nodes on the affected side. Inject Ringer's solution.

Cupping

This method is helpful in draining the pus in the later stage of mastitis. Apply cup over the affected tissue until the draining has ceased.

Other prescriptions

1. S-16 *(Yingchuang)*, Sp-18 *(Tianxi)*, S-18 *(Rugen)*, K-22 *(Bulang)*, B-18 *(Ganshu)*, H-1 *(Jiquan)*, P-2 *(Tianquan)*, B-38 *(Gaohuang)*, B-39 *(Shentang)*, GB-21 *(Jianjing)*, Co-17 *(Shanzhong)*, P-7 *(Daling)*, SI-1 *(Shaoze)*, B-54 *(Weizhong)*, S-36 *(Zusanli)*. (Source: NAM)

2. S-16 *(Yingchuang)*, S-18 *(Rugen)*, GB-21 *(Jianjing)*, LI-11 *(Quchi)*, S-37 *(Shangjuxu)*, Li-3 *(Taichong)*. Use strong stimulation. (Source: CAM)

3. Co-17 *(Shanzhong)*, LI-4 *(Hegu)*, LI-11 *(Quchi)*, and B-16 *(Dushu)*. Use moderate stimulation. (Source: HCNMT)

4. Abscessed breast: S-16 *(Yingchuang)*, GB-41 *(Linqi)*, K-23 *(Shenfeng)*, S-18 *(Rugen)*, S-36 *(Zusanli)*, S-39 *(Xiajuxu)*, LI-8 *(Xialian)*, Sp-18 *(Tianxi)*, GB-43 *(Xiaxi)*. (Source: CNLAM)

5. LI-8 *(Xialian)*, S-36 *(Zusanli)*, GB-43 *(Xiaxi)*, L-10 *(Yuji)*, B-54 *(Weizhong)*, SI-1 *(Shaoze)*. (Source: CDR)

6. 14 cones of moxa at LI-15 *(Jianyu)* and H-4 *(Lingdao)*; 7 (smaller people) or 14 (larger people) cones of moxa at LI-7 *(Wenliu)*; 14 cones of moxa at S-36 *(Zusanli)*, S-38 *(Tiaokou)*, and S-39 *(Xiajuxu)*. (Source: IACC)

7. Co-17 *(Shanzhong)*, P-7 *(Daling)*, B-54 *(Weizhong)*, SI-1 *(Shaoze)*, and K-27 *(Shufu)*. (Source: GCAM)

Remarks

• Acupuncture therapy is appropriate during the early stages of this condition and may be supplemented by hot compresses. If there is high fever, swelling and pain other methods of Chinese and Western medicine should be used in conjunction with acupuncture.

• If fully pustulated, the sore should be lanced.

TETANUS

There are records of this disease early in the history of Chinese medicine. It is believed to be caused by the Wind Excess invading the channels after injuries sustained from a fall, or lesion from a metal, bamboo or wooden instrument. After entering the channels, this Yang Excess increases, inducing Interior Wind. The functioning of the joints becomes abnormal and other symptoms associated with this disease appear. In severe cases, the Qi of the Organs is disturbed. Tetanus in newborns was known as 'umbilical Wind'.

Treatment is directed toward calming the Liver and extinguishing the Wind, cooling the Heat and suppressing convulsions.

Needling

Principal points: GB-20 *(Fengchi)*, Gv-26 *(Renzhong)*, Li-3 *(Taichong)*
Supplementary points: LI-4 *(Hegu)*, SI-3 *(Houxi)*, S-7 *(Xiaguan)*

Method: First, needle the principal points with moderate to strong stimulation and intermittent or continuous needle manipulation. If the result is unsatisfactory, add the supplementary points.

Between convulsions, the needles may be retained in place. Treat 1-3 times daily. When the symptoms are under control, intradermal needles may be embedded for periods of several hours or days. If continuous needle stimulation is required, high frequency electro-acupuncture may be used.

Discussion of points: GB-20 *(Fengchi)*, the point of intersection of the Yang Linking channel on the Gall Bladder channel, is needled to extinguish the Wind Excess and 'awaken' the brain from unconsciousness. Li-3 *(Taichong)*, the Source point of the Liver channel, is used to calm the Liver and extinguish the Wind so as to suppress convulsions. Gv-26 *(Renzhong)*, at the juncture of the Yin and Yang channels on the median line of the body (i.e., the Conception and Governing channels), is needled to regulate the rebellious Qi so as to clear the obscured senses. Because the Excess of this disease is found in the Large Intestine, Small Intestine and Governing channels (among others), LI-4 *(Hegu)*, the Source point of the Large Intestine channel, and SI-3 *(Houxi)*, the Transporting point of the Small Intestine channel and the Meeting point of the Governing channel are stimulated to cool the Heat and suppress convulsions. When the jaw is tightly shut, use the local point S-7 *(Xiaguan)*.

Ear acupuncture

Points: Subcortex, Occiput, Heart, Brain, Neurogate

Method: Select 2-3 points each session. Use moderate to strong stimulation, retaining needles for 30 minutes. Treat 1-3 times daily.

Injection therapy

Select 1-2 inguinal lymph nodes and inject Ringer's solution. In addition, tetanus antitoxin may be injected as a bloc around the focus of the disease.

Other prescriptions

1. Wind spasms with lockjaw: S-5 *(Daying)*; Cold Hot Wind spasms with hyperextension: Gv-15 *(Yamen)*; hyperextension: Gv-2 *(Yaoshu)*. (Source: CNLAM)

2. Hyperextension: B-18 *(Ganshu)*; lockjaw: S-6 *(Jiache)*, Co-24 *(Chengjiang)*, and LI-4 *(Hegu)*. (Source: GCAM)

3. Hyperextension with tonic-clonic seizures: B-5 *(Wuchu)*, Gv-12 *(Shenzhu)*, B-54 *(Weizhong)*, and B-60 *(Kunlun)*; lockjaw: Gv-28 *(Yinjiao)*, GB-3 *(Shangguan)*, S-5 *(Daying)*, and TB-17 *(Yifeng)*. (Source: TDP)

Remarks

• Acupuncture is only a supplementary method of treating tetanus and should be combined with conventional methods of eliminating the tetanus bacillus and dressing the wound.

ACUTE APPENDICITIS

In Chinese medicine, this condition is regarded as an abscess of the Intestines. Among its causes are irregular eating habits, strenuous activity too soon after eating, or an imbalance of cold and warmth in the abdomen which affects the digestive and transportive functions of the Stomach and Intestines. Such causes give rise to a combination of Dampness and Heat in the Intestines, where they obstruct the movement of Qi and Blood, and ultimately lead to this disorder.

Treatment is directed toward spreading the Qi in the Intestines and draining the Heat which has gathered there.

Needling

Principal points: M-LE-13 *(Lanweixue)*, S-37 *(Shangjuxu)*, S-36 *(Zusanli)*

Supplementary points: LI-4 *(Hegu)*, P-6 *(Neiguan)*, LI-11 *(Quchi)*, S-25 *(Tianshu)*

Method: Use strong stimulation and continuous needle manipulation for 2-3 minutes, then retain needles for 1-2 hours with intermittent manipulation. Treat 2-3 times daily until the symptoms disappear. If accompanied by high fever, add LI-4 *(Hegu)* and LI-11 *(Quchi)*. For abdominal pain, add S-25 *(Tianshu)*. For nausea or vomiting, electro-acupuncture may be used.

Discussion of points: S-37 *(Shangjuxu)* is the Lower Uniting point of the Large Intestine, and S-36 *(Zusanli)* the Lower Uniting point of the Stomach. M-LE-13 *(Lanweixue)* (literally, the 'appendix point'), has been effective in recent experience in treating this condition. All three points are located along the course of the Stomach channel, which is commonly chosen for treating diseases of the Intestines. (This practice dates from at least as early as the *Inner Classic*, in the 2nd century B.C.) The Alarm point of the Large Intestine, S-25 *(Tianshu)*, removes obstructions from the Intestines. LI-4 *(Hegu)* and LI-11 *(Quchi)* drain Heat from the Large Intestine channel and are therefore indicated for fever. P-6 *(Neiguan)*, the Meeting point of the Yin Linking channel on the Pericardium channel, harmonizes the Stomach and suppresses rebellious Qi. It is therefore indicated for nausea or vomiting.

Injection of lymph node
Select in inguinal lymph node and inject Ringer's solution once or twice daily.

Barefoot doctor acupuncture
Points: Barefoot Doctor point, Thoracic #5, Lumbar #1

Ear acupuncture
Points: Sympathetic, Neurogate
Method: Select 3-5 points each session, retaining needles 20-30 minutes. Treat once or twice daily.

Injection therapy
Points: M-LE-13 *(Lanweixue)* on the right side, and the point of tenderness on the abdomen
Method: Inject a 10% glucose solution into each point. Treat once daily.

Hand acupuncture
Point: Vertex
Method: Use strong stimulation. When the pain subsides, either remove the needle or retain for an additional 1-3 minutes.

Foot acupuncture
Point: #3
Method: Same as for Hand acupuncture above.

Other prescriptions
1. S-36 *(Zusanli)*, K-16 *(Huangshu)*, Sp-13 *(Fushe)*, P-6 *(Neiguan)*, LI-11 *(Quchi)*, B-24 *(Qihaishu)*, and B-25 *(Dachangshu)*. (Source: NAM)
2. Acute appendicitis: Sp-10 *(Xuehai)*, B-54 *(Weizhong)*, Sp-9 *(Yinlingquan)*, Sp-8 *(Diji)*, Sp-6 *(Sanyinjiao)*, Li-2 *(Xingjian)*, TB-10 *(Tianjing)*, LI-11 *(Quchi)*, and LI-4 *(Hegu)*. Use strong stimulation. Chronic appendicitis: B-24 *(Qihaishu)*, B-25 *(Dachangshu)*, S-3 *(Juliao)*, Sp-12 *(Chongmen)*, Sp-10 *(Xuehai)*, Sp-9 *(Yinglingquan)*, Sp-6 *(Sanyinjiao)*, and use moxa stick over the point of pain. (Source: CAM)
3. Pain from intestinal abscess: Sp-3 *(Taibai)*, S-43 *(Xiangu)*, and B-25 *(Dachangshu)*. (Source: GCAM)
4. Intestinal abscess: 100 cones of moxa on both tips of the elbows. (Source: TDP)

Remarks
• Acupuncture therapy is relatively effective in the treatment of simple acute appendicitis. For severe cases, where the white blood cell count indicates the possibility of abscessed or ruptured appendix, acupuncture alone is insufficient and the physician should consider surgical removal of the appendix.

• For chronic appendicitis, the same points may be used as for acute appendicitis. In addition, moxa sticks or indirect moxibustion may be used locally. Treat once daily or on alternating days.

ACUTE INTESTINAL OBSTRUCTION

According to traditional medicine, intestinal obstruction may be caused by the stagnation of Qi and Blood, Cold or Heat, or parasitic organisms collecting in the intestinal tract and blocking passage. Treatment is directed toward eliminating the blockage so as to open the intestinal passageways.

Needling

Principal points: S-37 *(Shangjuxu)*, S-39 *(Xiajuxu)*, Co-4 *(Guanyuan)*, S-25 *(Tianshu)*
Supplementary points: B-25 *(Dachangshu)*, P-6 *(Neiguan)*, S-36 *(Zusanli)*

Method: First, needle the principal points. If there is vomiting, add S-36 *(Zusanli)* and P-6 *(Neiguan)*. For constipation, add B-25 *(Dachangshu)*. Use strong stimulation, needling continuously for 2-3 minutes. Retain needles for 15-30 minute with periodic manipulation. Treat 3-4 times daily. Electro-acupuncture may be substituted for continuous needling.

Discussion of points: S-37 *(Shangjuxu)* is the Lower Uniting point of the Large Intestine. Co-4 *(Guanyuan)* is the Alarm point of the Small Intestine, and S-25 *(Tianshu)* the Alarm point of the Large Intestine. Together, these points can clear the obstruction from the Intestines. P-6 *(Neiguan)* and S-36 *(Zusanli)* are used to stabilize the Stomach so as to stop the vomiting.

Injection therapy

For paralytic intestinal obstruction, inject neostigmine into S-36 *(Zusanli)*. For vomiting (including that which follows the ingestion of medicine), inject atropine into S-36 *(Zusanli)*.

Ear acupuncture

Points: Large Intestine, Small Intestine, Stomach, Abdomen, Sympathetic, Neurogate, Subcortex
Method: Using moderate to strong stimulation, treat 1-3 times daily.

Other prescriptions

1. Principal points: Co-6 *(Qihai)* joined to Co-4 *(Guanyuan)*, S-36 *(Zusanli)*. Supplementary points: TB-6 *(Zhigou)*, B-25 *(Dachangshu)* (insert 2-3 units). Select one point from each group daily in rotation. Use moderate stimulation. (Source: HCNMT)
2. Abdominal pain: Co-12 *(Zhongwan)*, S-25 *(Tianshu)*, P-6 *(Neiguan)*, S-36 *(Zusanli)*, LI-4 *(Hegu)*, B-25 *(Dachangshu)*, B-20 *(Pishu)*, and B-32 *(Ciliao)*; vomiting: Co-13 *(Shangwan)*, Co-12 *(Zhongwan)*, S-36 *(Zusanli)*, LI-11 *(Quchi)*, and P-6 *(Neiguan)*. (Source: TAA)

Remarks

• If there is no improvement 6-24 hours after acupuncture therapy begins, surgery should be considered.
• Signs of improvement include diminished nausea or vomiting, reduction of abdominal pain, and passing gas or small bowel movements.

ACUTE PERFORATION OF GASTRIC AND DUODENAL ULCER

In its early stages, this condition is attributed to Phlegm lodging in the Stomach which, combined with irregular eating habits, emotional frustration, excessive fatigue, or the Cold Excess invading the body, leads to this disorder. Dysfunction ensues as Heat is generated, the blood vessels rupture and the coagulated Blood obstructs the Middle Burner, producing 'closure of the Interior and exhaustion of the Exterior'.

Needling

Points: Co-13 *(Shangwan)*, Co-12 *(Zhongwan)*, S-21 *(Liangmen)*, S-25 *(Tianshu)*, P-6 *(Neiguan)*, S-36 *(Zusanli)* and the point of pain

Method: Use strong stimulation, retaining the needles for thirty minutes to one hour with periodic needle manipulation. Treat once every 4-6 hours. Electro-acupuncture may also be utilized.

Injection therapy
Inject either a 2% *Angelica sinesis (danggui)* solution, or *Carthamus (honghua)* solution into 2-4 of the points listed above. Treat once or twice daily.

Ear acupuncture
Points: Stomach, Abdomen, Neurogate, Sympathetic, Subcortex

Method: Select 2-3 points each session. Use moderate to strong stimulation, retaining needles 20-30 minutes. Treat once every 4-6 hours.

Other prescriptions
1. B-17 *(Geshu)* for sudden severe stomach pain; Li-13 *(Zhangmen)* for chest pain and vomiting; and L-4 *(Xiabai)* for chest pain, dry heaves, and irritability. (Source: CNLAM)

Remarks
• Acupuncture is suitable for the early stages of this condition (i.e., when there is acute abdominal pain), and for simple perforated ulcer (the perforation is small and the general health and strength of the patient is good).

• During treatment, the patient should lie down.

• If, after acupuncture treatment, the patient becomes relaxed and intestinal noises are restored, such evidence indicates that acupuncture is working. If, on the other hand, after 6-12 hours there is no improvement or the condition worsens, other methods (including surgery) should be considered.

• The physician must be careful to distinguish this condition from pancreatitis, appendicitis and cholecystitis.

ACUTE DISEASE OF THE BILIARY TRACT

Under this heading are acute cholecystitis, gall stones and round worm in the biliary tract.

Cholecystitis and gall stones are attributed in traditional medicine to emotional problems, irregular eating habits or external Excesses. These factors may cause Dampness and Heat to collect, or allow parasitic organisms to gather, both of which may obstruct the spreading and draining functions of the Liver and Gall Bladder.

Symptoms associated with round worm in the biliary tract are due to the simultaneous presence of Cold in the Spleen and Heat in the Stomach, as well as movement of the round worm into the biliary tract which interferes with its functioning.

Treatment in all cases is directed toward spreading and draining the Gall Bladder Qi, expanding the Middle Burner (Spleen and Stomach) and calming the Stomach.

Needling
Prescription 1

This prescription is suitable for acute cholecystitis, gall stones or round worm in the biliary tract.

Principal points: M-LE-23 *(Dannangxue)*, P-6 *(Neiguan)*

Supplementary points: GB-34 *(Yanglingquan)*, S-36 *(Zusanli)*, GB-24 *(Riyue)* on the right side, and the vertebral points M-BW-35 *(Jiaji)* at the 8th and 9th thoracic vertebrae

Method: When an attack of pain occurs, first needle the principal points with strong stimulation until the pain is relieved. Thereafter, the needles may be retained, or intradermal needles substituted for a period of several hours to one or two days. If the results are not entirely satisfactory, add supplementary points. Needle GB-24 *(Riyue)* with a slanted insertion pointed downward. When needling the vertebral points M-BW-35 *(Jiaji)*, best results are obtained when the needle sensation extends toward the front of the body.

Discussion of points: GB-34 *(Yanglingquan)* is the Uniting point of the Gall Bladder channel, M-LE-23 *(Dannangxue)* (literally, the Gall Bladder point) has in recent experience proven effective in treating disorders of the Gall Bladder. GB-24 *(Riyue)* is the Alarm point of the Gall Bladder. Together, needling these three points spreads and drains the Gall Bladder Qi. P-6 *(Neiguan),* which connects with the Yin Linking channel, and S-36 *(Zusanli),* the Uniting point of the Stomach channel, are able to expand the Middle Burner and harmonize the Stomach.

Prescription 2
This method is suitable only for round worm in the biliary tract.

Principal points: Join LI-20 *(Yingxiang)* to S-2 *(Sibai)*
Supplementary points: S-36 *(Zusanli),* LI-11 *(Quchi),* Gv-26 *(Renzhong)*

Method: First needle the principal points with strong stimulation until the pain subsides, then withdraw the needles.

Ear acupuncture
Points: Pancreas/Gall Bladder, Liver, Sympathetic, Neurogate, Subcortex
Method: Select 2-3 points each session, in rotation. Retain needles for 20-30 minutes. During attack of pain use strong stimulation.

Barefoot doctor acupuncture
Points: Barefoot Doctor point, Thoracic #8 and #12

Hand acupuncture
Points: Gastro-intestinal
Method: Use strong stimulation during attacks of pain. Retain needles for 3-5 minutes.

Foot acupuncture
Points: #8, #25, #48
Method: Same as for hand acupuncture above.

Other prescriptions
1. Gallstones: B-22 *(Sanjiaoshu),* B-23 *(Shenshu),* B-24 *(Qihaishu),* B-25 *(Dachangshu),* Co-13 *(Shangwan),* Co-15 *(Jiuwei),* TB-5 *(Waiguan),* S-36 *(Zusanli),* right Li-13 *(Zhangmen),* and right GB-25 *(Jingmen).* (Source: NAM)
2. Biliary colic: B-18 *(Ganshu),* B-19 *(Danshu),* SI-4 *(Wangu),* GB-34 *(Yanglingquan),* GB-41 *(Zulinqi),* and Li-2 *(Xingjian).* Use strong stimulation. (Source: CAM)
3. Round worm in the biliary tract: Gv-10 *(Lingtai).* Use strong stimulation. Gallstone symptoms: B-19 *(Danshu),* Co-12 *(Zhongwan),* and S-36 *(Zusanli).* Use strong stimulation. Treat daily, ten treatments constituting one course. (Source: HCNMT)
4. Co-14 *(Juque)* treats chest pain due to round worm. (Source: ICAP)
5. Co-13 *(Shangwan)* treats chest pain with turbidity, excess saliva, and inability to lie on one's side. (Source: CNLAM)
6. Burning three cones of moxa over the intertarsal joint of the big toes will stop severe chest pain due to round worm. (Source: PUB)
7. Needle GB-40 *(Qiuxu)* and TB-3 *(Zhongzhu)* for rib pain. (Source: GOA)
8. Chest pain due to round worm: 14 cones of moxa at Co-14 *(Juque),* Sp-2 *(Dadu),* Sp-3 *(Taibai),* S-36 *(Zusanli),* and B-57 *(Chengshan).* (Source: IACC)

Remarks
• Acupuncture therapy is particularly effective in stopping the pain associated with these conditions. It is also suitable for treating acute cholecystitis and small gall stones.

HEMORRHOIDS

The traditional etiology of this condition parallels that of Western medicine. It is attributed to chronic difficulty in defecating, irregular eating habits, alcoholism, overindulgence in the consumption of spicy foods, sexual excess and general weakness.

Treatment is directed toward spreading the Qi which has collected and is obstructing the channels.

Needling
Points: B-30 *(Baihuanshu)*, Gv-1 *(Changqiang)*, B-57 *(Chengshan)*

Method: Insert needle at B-30 *(Baihuanshu)* pointed in a medial, downward direction. If possible, direct the needle sensation toward the anus. Insert needle perpendicularly at Gv-1 *(Changqiang)*, then direct the needle toward the left and then the right, at an oblique angle to the skin surface, causing the needle sensation to expand around the perimeter of the anus. Needle B-57 *(Chengshan)* with strong stimulation. Treat once daily.

Discussion of points: B-30 *(Baihuanshu)* and Gv-1 *(Changqiang)*, located in the vicinity of the anus, are local points. B-57 *(Chengshan)* is located on the Bladder channel, a Divergent branch of which enters the rectum. This point has traditionally been used to treat diseases associated with the rectum.

Piercing method
Select a point along a line one unit beside the spinous processes of the 2nd to the 5th lumbar vertebrae; or examine the lumbosacral region and above the frenulum labii superioris for the presence of pimple-like eruptions on the skin. Pierce these.

Ear acupuncture
Points: Distal Segment of Rectum, Neurogate, Subcortex
Method: Select 2-3 points each session, retaining needles for 20-30 minutes. Treat once daily.

Letting blood
Point: Co-7 *(Yinjiao)*
Method: Use a triangular needle to prick this point so as to let a few drops of blood.

Injection therapy
Points: Use both sides of the frenulum labii superioris
Method: Inject a 1% procaine hydrochloride solution in each side. Treat once daily.

Embedding thread
Points: Join B-26 *(Guanyuanshu)* to B-25 *(Dachangshu)*, and embed B-57 *(Chengshan)* separately.
Method: Embed thread bilaterally. Repeat after 20-30 days.

Other prescriptions
1. B-23 *(Shenshu)*, B-24 *(Qihaishu)*, B-25 *(Dachangshu)*, B-27 *(Xiaochangshu)*, Gv-4 *(Mingmen)*, Gv-1 *(Changqiang)*, Gv-20 *(Baihui)*, B-49 *(Zhibian)*, B-50 *(Chengfu)*, GB-39 *(Xuanzhong)*, Sp-6 *(Sanyinjiao)*, B-57 *(Chengshan)*, B-60 *(Kunlun)*, and B-35 *(Huiyang)*. (Source: NAM)
2. Gv-1 *(Changqiang)*, Gv-3 *(Yaoyangguan)*, B-32 *(Ciliao)*, M-UE-29 *(Erbai)*, Sp-6 *(Sanyinjiao)*. Use strong stimulation. For bleeding, add 5-7 cones of moxa at Gv-2 *(Yaoshu)*, Gv-3 *(Yaoyangguan)*, and Gv-20 *(Baihui)*. (Source: CAM)
3. B-58 *(Feiyang)* for sudden, severe hemorrhoidal pain; Sp-5 *(Shangqiu)* and K-7 *(Fuliu)* for feeling of urgency after bowel movements; P-8 *(Laogong)* for Hot hemorrhoids; Co-1 *(Huiyin)* for hemorrhoids; B-56 *(Chengjin)*, B-50 *(Chengfu)*, B-54 *(Weizhong)*, SI-5 *(Yanggu)* for painful

hemorrhoids with swelling under the armpits. (Source: TDP)

4. Place a slice of ginger over the hemorrhoid and burn 3 cones of moxa upon it. A yellow fluid will exude and the hemorrhoid will disappear. If there is more than one hemorrhoid, wait 3-5 days between treatments. (Source: IACC)

5. Hemorrhoids: Gv-4 *(Mingmen),* B-23 *(Shenshu),* Gv-1 *(Changqiang)* (one cone of moxa at this point for each year of life gives excellent results for bleeding symptom), Sp-6 *(Sanyinjiao)* (for bleeding), B-57 *(Chengshan)* (for chronic hemorrhoids). (Source: IACC)

6. The Five Hemorrhoids: B-54 *(Weizhong),* B-57 *(Chengshan),* B-58 *(Feiyang),* GB-38 *(Yangfu),* K-7 *(Fuliu),* Li-3 *(Taichong),* GB-43 *(Xiaxi),* Co-6 *(Qihai),* Co-1 *(Huiyin),* Gv-1 *(Changqiang).* (Source: GCAM)

7. Prolapsed rectum with chronic hemorrhoids: M-UE-29 *(Erbai),* Gv-20 *(Baihui),* B-47 *(Zhishi),* Gv-1 *(Changqiang).* (Source: GCAM)

Remarks

• Acupuncture is effective in relieving the pain and inflammation as well as the bleeding associated with hemorrhoids. However, surgery may be necessary in some cases to effect a fundamental cure.

PROLAPSED RECTUM

In Chinese medicine, this condition is attributed to a weak physical constitution, prolonged diarrhea or constipation, chronic cough, giving birth too often, or excessive exertion during childbirth. All of these factors may contribute to a weakening of the rectum which, like the Qi, sinks downward.

Treatment is directed toward lifting the sunken Qi from without.

Needling

Principal points: Gv-1 *(Changqiang),* B-57 *(Chengshan)*
Supplementary points: B-30 *(Baihuanshu),* Gv-20 *(Baihui)*

Method: First needle the principal points. After the needle has been inserted perpendicularly at Gv-1 *(Changqiang)* above the rectum, it can be partially withdrawn and redirected, first to the left, then to the right, so that the needle sensation expands throughout this region. Use strong stimulation at B-57 *(Chengshan).* If the result is unsatisfactory, add the supplementary points. B-30 *(Baihuanshu)* should be needled with a slanted insertion, the needle pointed in a medial, downward direction so that the sensation extends to the rectum. Use moxibustion at Gv-20 *(Baihui).* Treat once daily. Ten treatments constitute one course.

Discussion of the points: B-30 *(Baihuanshu)* and Gv-1 *(Changqiang)* are chosen to support the muscles around the rectum, B-57 *(Chengshan)* according to the principle of distant point selection. Applying moxibustion at Gv-20 *(Baihui)* raises the sunken Qi.

Piercing method

Select one point along a vertical line 1-1.5 units from the spine between the 3rd lumbar and 2nd sacral vertebrae for piercing.

Ear acupuncture

Points: Distal Segment of Rectum, Subcortex
Method: Use moderate to strong stimulation, retaining the needles for 30 minutes. Treat once daily. Ten treatments constitute one course.

Embedding thread

Points: B-57 *(Chengshan)* on one side only, Gv-1 *(Changqiang),* and any point .5 unit from the anus along an arc extending from the 3 o'clock to the 9 o'clock position.
Method: Embed thread at each of the three points. Repeat after 20-30 days.

Other prescriptions

1. B-22 *(Sanjiaoshu)*, B-23 *(Shenshu)*, B-24 *(Qihaishu)*, B-25 *Dachangshu)*, B-26 *(Guanyuanshu)*, S-25 *(Tianshu)*, Li-2 *(Xingjian)*, S-36 *(Zusanli)*. (Source: NAM)

2. Prolapsed rectum: Burn 7 cones of moxa on the coccyx and 1 cone for each year of life on the navel. (Source: ATDP)

3. Prolapsed rectum: Burn 7 cones of moxa on the xiphoid. (Source: NFO)

4. Prolapsed rectum: 3 cones of moxa on Gv-20 *(Baihui)*, B-21 *(Weishu)*, Gv-1 *(Changqiang)*. For Cold prolapsed rectum, burn 100 cones of moxa on Co-9 *(Shuifen)*. (Source: IACC)

5. Prolapsed rectum: B-25 *(Dachangshu)*, Gv-20 *(Baihui)*, Gv-1 *(Changqiang)*, GB-21 *(Jianjing)*, LI-4 *(Hegu)*, S-30 *(Qichong)*. (Source: OM)

Remarks

• Acupuncture is relatively effective in helping to restore the rectum in place, although surgery may still be necessary to effect a fundamental cure.

BUERGER'S DISEASE

Chinese medicine attributes this condition to an invasion by Cold and Dampness which lodge in the channels and obstruct the passage of Qi and Blood. Alternatively, it may arise from excessive use of tobacco and alcohol, whereby Fire is generated internally, the victim becomes angry and depressed, and the Qi and Blood become stagnant and coagulate. Finally, this condition may result from external trauma.

Treatment is directed toward activating the Blood so as to clear the channels.

Needling

Principal points: For the upper limb, join LI-11 *(Quchi)* to H-3 *(Shaohai)*, TB-5 *(Waiguan)* to P-6 *(Neiguan)*, and the vertebral points M-BW-35 *(Jiaji)* from the 6th cervical to the 3rd thoracic vertebra. For the lower limb, join GB-34 *(Yanglingquan)* to Sp-9 *(Yinlingquan)*, GB-39 *(Xuanzhong)* to Sp-6 *(Sanyinjiao)*, and the vertebral points M-BW-35 *(Jiaji)* from the 1st to the 3rd lumbar vertebra, or to N-BW-38 *(Xiajiaoshu)*.

Supplementary points: M-UE-50 *(Shangbaxie)*, M-LE-41 *(Shangbafeng)*

Method: First needle the principal points with strong stimulation for 2-3 minutes, retaining needles for 10-15 minutes thereafter. Electro-acupuncture may be used. For pain in the fingers or toes, use the appropriate supplementary points. Treat once daily. Fifteen to twenty treatments constitute one course.

Injection therapy

Points: B-15 *(Xinshu)*, B-17 *(Geshu)*, GB-34 *(Yanglingquan)*, Sp-6 *(Sanyinjiao)*, GB-39 *(Xuanzhong)*

Method: Select 2-3 points each session. Inject a 5% *Angelica sinesis (danggui)* solution at each point. Treat once daily. Ten treatments constitute one course.

Ear acupuncture

Points: Sympathetic, Kidneys, Adrenal, Liver, Endocrine, Occiput, Heart, Subcortex and the point corresponding to the affected limb

Method: Select 2-3 points each session. Treat once daily using moderate to strong stimulation. Alternatively, inject a .5% procaine solution at points Sympathetic and Adrenal, bilaterally, to establish a bloc.

Barefoot doctor acupuncture

Points: Barefoot Doctor point, Lumbar #1 and #4

Embedding thread and threading the points

Embedding thread
Points: Same as for injection therapy above
Method: Select 2-3 points each session and imbed thread. Allow 20-30 days between treatments.

Threading the points
Points: Sp-10 *(Xuehai)*, S-36 *(Zusanli)*, N-LE-19 *(Siqiang)*, B-57 *(Chengshan)*, S-40 *(Fenglong)*
Method: Use a suture needle to insert approximately 6 cm. of sheep gut thread into the points above. The needle should emerge about 3 cm. from the point of insertion. Re-insert the needle at the second hole so that it emerges again from the first. It is unnecessary either to make an incision or to tie the thread. Merely snip the ends and press under the skin. Select 2-3 points each session and allow 10-15 days between treatments. Four to five treatments constitute one course. Allow 2-3 months rest between courses of treatment.

Moxibustion
Warm the affected area with moxa sticks for 5-10 minutes daily.

Remarks
• Acupuncture effectively relieves pain in the early stages of this condition. In the latter stages, however, when ulcerations occur, acupuncture must be combined with surgery.

URINARY TRACT INFECTION

This condition falls within the traditional domain of urinary dysfunction. When the Kidneys are Deficient, Dampness and Heat may collect in the Lower Burner (Kidneys, Bladder and Intestines), and Bladder function (Qi) becomes disrupted. Because the Kidneys and Bladder are associated in a reciprocal Yin/Yang relationship, if the disease is prolonged it could damage either the Yin or Yang functions of the Kidneys, and possibly manifest itself both in Deficient and Excessive symptoms.

Treatment is directed toward spreading the Bladder Qi and clearing the Lower Burner of Heat and Dampness.

Needling
Principal points: B-23 *(Shenshu)*, B-28 *(Pangguangshu)*, Co-3 *(Zhongji)*, Sp-6 *(Sanyinjiao)*
Supplementary points: B-32 *(Ciliao)*, Li-8 *(Ququan)*

Method: Treat once daily with moderate to strong stimulation. Five to ten treatments constitute one course.

Discussion of points: B-23 *(Shenshu)* is the Associated point of the Kidneys and is used to regulate the Kidney Qi and water passageways. B-28 *(Pangguangshu)* is the Associated point of the Bladder; Co-3 *(Zhongji)* is the Alarm point of the Bladder and the point of intersection of the three Leg Yin channels on the Conception channel in the lower abdomen; Sp-6 *(Sanyinjiao)* is the point of intersection of the Leg Yin channels on the Spleen channel at the lower leg. Together, these three points can clear the Dampness and Heat from the Bladder and facilitate the functioning of the Lower Burner. Li-8 *(Ququan)* is the Uniting point of the Liver channel which traverses the genital region and lower abdomen. Needling this point drains the Lower Burner.

Ear acupuncture
Principal points: Kidney, Bladder, Urethra
Supplementary points: Subcortex, Sympathetic, Neurogate
Method: Needle daily or on alternating days with moderate to strong stimulation. Retain needles for 30 minutes with periodic needle manipulation. Five to ten treatments constitute one course.

Warm needle acupuncture

This method is appropriate in the treatment of chronic pyelonephritis or chronic cystitis.

Points: B-23 *(Shenshu)*, B-28 *(Pangguangshu)*, B-32 *(Ciliao)*, Co-3 *(Zhongji)*, Co-4 *(Guanyuan)*

Method: After inserting the needles, warm them with a moxa stick. Alternatively, moxibustion alone may be used at the points above, burning 3-5 moxa cones at each point.

Barefoot doctor acupuncture

Points: Barefoot Doctor point, Lumbar #1 and #4

Injection therapy

Select 1-2 inguinal lymph nodes and inject Ringer's solution into each.

Other prescriptions

1. B-23 *(Shenshu)*, K-9 *(Zhubin)*, S-29 *(Guilai)*, B-58 *(Feiyang)*, Co-3 *(Zhongji)*. Use 2-3 points with strong stimulation. (Source: HNMT)

2. Pyelonephritis: Acute—B-23 *(Shenshu)*, B-25 *(Dachangshu)*, B-54 *(Weizhong)*, Sp-10 *(Xuehai)*, S-36 *(Zusanli)*, Sp-6 *(Sanyinjiao)*, K-4 *(Dazhong)*. Strong stimulation. Chronic—B-22 *(Sanjiaoshu)*, B-16 *(Dushu)*, B-32 *(Ciliao)*. Mild stimulation. Moxa sticks can also be used. Other points: S-36 *(Zusanli)*, B-54 *(Weizhong)*. Cystitis: Acute—B-25 *(Dachangshu)*, B-28 *(Pangguangshu)*, B-31 *(Shangliao)*, B-33 *(Zhongliao)*, S-36 *(Zusanli)*, Sp-10 *(Xuehai)*, Sp-9 *(Yinlingquan)*, Sp-6 *(Sanyinjiao)*. Strong stimulation. Chronic—B-23 *(Shenshu)*, B-31 *(Shangliao)*, B-33 *(Zhongliao)*, Co-6 *(Qihai)*, Co-3 *(Zhongji)*. Treat daily with warm needle acupuncture. (Source: CAM)

3. The five urinary dysfunctions: Co-2 *(Qugu)* for yellow urine; Co-3 *(Zhongji)* for red, rough urine; K-7 *(Fuliu)* for diffuse, burning urine; B-32 *(Ciliao)* for red urine; Li-3 *(Taichong)* for urinary dysfunction. (Source: CNLAM)

4. For blood in the urine, use Co-6 *(Qihai)*, and Co-4 *(Guanyuan); for Hot urinary dysfunction, use Co-4 *(Guanyuan)* and S-30 *(Qichong)*. (Source: TWD)

Remarks

• During the period of treatment the patient should be encouraged to drink large amounts of water. However, if during chronic pyelonephritis renal failure develops, water intake should be controlled.

• If a high fever continues unabated, other methods of treatment should be considered in conjunction with acupuncture.

• Acupuncture therapy can help alleviate the irritation in the urinary tract.

RENAL COLIC

This condition is subsumed within the traditional category of 'stone urinary dysfunction.' It is said to be caused by Dampness and Heat collecting over a long period of time and forming a stone that obstructs the Bladder and flow of Qi, while preventing urine from being passed from the body.

Treatment is directed toward spreading and draining the contents of the water passageways by eliminating Dampness and Heat.

Needling

Principal points: B-23 *(Shenshu)*, Sp-6 *(Sanyinjiao)*
Supplementary points: B-47 *(Zhishi)*, K-3 *(Taixi)*

Method: First needle the principal points with moderate to strong stimulation for 3-5 minutes. If the result is unsatisfactory, add the supplementary points.

Discussion of points: B-23 *(Shenshu)*, the Associated point of the Kidney channel, and B-47 *(Zhishi)* spread and drain the obstructed Kidney Qi, facilitating flow through the water passageways.

Sp-6 *(Sanyinjiao)* is frequently used to treat diseases of the lower abdomen and urinary system. K-3 *(Taixi)* is the Source point of the Kidney channel.

Electro-acupuncture
Points: B-23 *(Shenshu)*, Sp-6 *(Sanyinjiao)*
Method: Use high frequency current for 5-10 minutes so as to provide strong stimulation at the points.

Injection therapy
Points: B-23 *(Shenshu)*, Sp-6 *(Sanyinjiao)*
Method: Inject a .5-1% procaine hydrochloride solution at each point. Administer allergy test beforehand.

Ear acupuncture
Points: Kidneys, Ureter, Subcortex, Sympathetic
Method: Manipulate needles for a few minutes after insertion.

Other prescriptions
1. Co-4 *(Guanyuan)*, S-36 *(Zusanli)*, B-58 *(Feiyang)*, Sp-6 *(Sanyinjiao)*, Co-3 *(Zhongji)*, B-23 *(Shenshu)*. Strong stimulation. (Source: HCNMT)

2. B-22 *(Sanjiaoshu)*, B-23 *(Shenshu)*, B-24 *(Qihaishu)*, B-46 *(Huangmen)*, B-47 *(Zhishi)*, B-25 *(Dachangshu)*, B-27 *(Xiaochangshu)*, B-26 *(Guanyuanshu)*, Sp-6 *(Sanyinjiao)*, Sp-9 *(Yinling-quan)*, K-3 *(Taixi)*. (Source: NAM)

3. Stone urinary dysfunction: 30 cones of moxa on either Co-4 *(Guanyuan)*, M-CA-15 *(Qimen)*, or Li-1 *(Dadun)*. (Source: CNLAM)

4. Painful urinary dysfunction: Moxi L-7 *(Lieque)*, Li-4 *(Zhongfeng)*, B-17 *(Geshu)*, B-18 *(Ganshu)*, B-20 *(Pishu)*, B-23 *(Shenshu)*, and Co-6 *(Qihai)*. (Source: PDM)

Remarks
• Acupuncture is definitely effective in alleviating the pain associated with this condition. If the result is unsatisfactory, however, other methods should be considered in conjunction with acupuncture.
• Jumping exercises are recommended, as this sometimes helps the body pass the stone.

PROSTATITIS

Chronic prostatitis is similar to the condition described as 'muddy urine' in traditional medical texts. Chinese medicine attributes this condition to Dampness and Heat which have collected in weakened Kidneys and moved downward thereafter. The disorder is closely associated with the Kidneys and Spleen.

Treatment is directed toward facilitating the passage of water and strengthening the Source Qi of the Kidneys.

Needling
Points: B-23 *(Shenshu)*, B-28 *(Pangguangshu)*, Co-4 *(Guanyuan)*, Sp-6 *(Sanyinjiao)*

Method: Use moderate to strong stimulation, treating once daily or on alternating days. Ten to fifteen treatments constitute one course.

Ear acupuncture
Points: Kidney, Bladder, Urethra, Pelvic Cavity
Method: Use strong stimulation, retaining the needles from 5-15 minutes. Treat once daily, or on alternating days. Ten to fifteen treatments constitute one course.

Therapy

Barefoot doctor acupuncture
Points: Barefoot Doctor point, Thoracic #5, Lumbar #1

Injection therapy
Select one inguinal lymph node and inject Ringer's solution.

Piercing method
Examine the vicinity of points B-28 *(Pangguangshu)* and B-25 *(Dachangshu)* for a point of response or tenderness. Pierce such point. Alternatively, pierce the aforementioned acupuncture points themselves. Allow 7-10 days rest before repeating treatment.

Cutaneous acupuncture
This method is suitable for chronic prostatitis.
Points: Sp-6 *(Sanyinjiao)*, Li-8 *(Ququan)*, Co-4 *(Guanyuan)*, Co-2 *(Qugu)*, S-29 *(Guilai)*, S-28 *(Shuidao)*. Also tap along the inguinal canal and the vertebral points M-BW-35 *(Jiaji)*, from the 7th thoracic to the 2nd lumbar vertebrae.

Other prescriptions
1. S-29 *(Guilai)*, M-CA-18 *(Zigong)*, Co-4 *(Guanyuan)*, K-9 *(Zhubin)*, Sp-6 *(Sanyinjiao)*. Moderate stimulation. (Source: HNMT)
2. Acute: Co-6 *(Qihai)*, Sp-10 *(Xuehai)*, Sp-9 *(Yinlingquan)*, Sp-6 *(Sanyinjiao)*, K-3 *(Taixi)*, K-6 *(Zhaohai)*. Strong stimulation. Chronic: Gv-2 *(Yaoshu)*, Co-3 *(Zhongji)*, Gv-20 *(Baihui)*, K-12 *(Dahe)*, Sp-6 *(Sanyinjiao)*. Mild stimulation and warm needle technique. Treat daily. (Source: CAM)

Remarks
• If this condition is accompanied by alternating chills and high fever, other methods of treatment should be used in conjunction with acupuncture therapy.

SPERMATORRHEA

In Chinese medicine a distinction is drawn between spermatorrhea which is accompanied by dreaming ('wet dreams'), and that which is not. The dreaming variety usually results from Deficient Kidney Yin, an abundance of Kidney Fire, or Dampness and Heat collecting in the Lower Burner (Kidneys, Bladder, Intestines) and disturbing the 'dwelling of semen'. The dreamless variety, on the other hand, results from the Kidney Qi being insufficient to retain the sperm which slips out involuntarily. In serious cases, this may even occur during the day. The latter condition is attributed to Deficiency in both the Kidneys and Heart which depletes the Essence and Qi.
Treatment is directed toward nourishing the Yin so as to strengthen the Base (Kidneys).

Needling
Principal points: Co-4 *(Guanyuan)*, Sp-6 *(Sanyinjiao)*
Supplementary points: P-5 *(Jianshi)*, B-23 *(Shenshu)*

Method: The principal points are the basis of the prescription and should be needled with moderate stimulation. If spermatorrhea is accompanied by dreams, add P-5 *(Jianshi)*. If no dreams, add B-23 *(Shenshu)*. Treat once daily or on alternating days. Five to seven treatments constitute one course. Low frequency electro-acupuncture may also be used.

Ear acupuncture
Points: Kidney, Bladder, Urethra, Pelvic Cavity
Method: Use moderate stimulation, retaining the needles for 5 minutes. Treat once daily or on alternating days. Five to ten treatments constitute one course.

Cutaneous acupuncture

Principal points: B-23 *(Shenshu)*, B-15 *(Xinshu)*, B-47 *(Zhishi)*, Co-4 *(Guanyuan)*, Sp-6 *Sanyinjiao)*, Co-3 *(Zhongji)*, Co-1 *(Huiyin)* and the vertebral points M-BW-35 *(Jiaji)* from the 4th thoracic to the 2nd lumbar vertebra

Supplementary points: K-3 *(Taixi)*, GB-25 *(Jingmen)*, Co-6 *(Qihai)*, K-12 *(Dahe)*, Li-4 *(Zhongfeng)*, Li-3 *(Taichong)*

Injection therapy

Points: Co-4 *(Guanyuan)*, Co-3 *(Zhongji)*

Method: Inject vitamin B1 or placental extract into each point. Treat once every 2-3 days. Five treatments constitute one course.

Moxibustion

Points: B-15 *(Xinshu)*, B-23 *(Shenshu)*, Gv-4 *(Mingmen)*, B-30 *(Baihuanshu)*, Co-3 *(Zhongji)*, Sp-6 *(Sanyinjiao)*, Li-4 *(Zhongfeng)*, K-2 *(Rangu)*

Other prescriptions

1. Co-4 *(Guanyuan)*, K-12 *(Dahe)*, Co-3 *(Zhongji)*, S-25 *(Tianshu)*, Co-2 *(Qugu)*, S-36 *(Zusanli)*, GB-20 *(Fengchi)*, B-10 *(Tianzhu)*, B-11 *(Dazhu)*, SI-14 *(Jianwaishu)*, Gv-14 *(Dazhui)*, Gv-12 *(Shenzhu)*, B-17 *(Geshu)*, B-31-34 *(Baliao)*, Gv-4 *(Mingmen)*, Sp-6 *(Sanyinjiao)*. (Source: NAM)

2. B-15 *(Xinshu)*, B-23 *(Shenshu)*, Gv-3 *(Yaoyangguan)*, Co-4 *(Guanyuan)*, Co-1 *(Huiyin)*, Sp-6 *(Sanyinjiao)*. Treat from once daily to once every third day. (Source: CAM)

3. For wet dreams with cloudy urine and difficulty urinating, burn 100 cones of moxa on B-23 *(Shenshu)*; for wet dreams, use B-38 *(Gaohuangshu)* or burn 50 cones of moxa on either Li-4 *(Zhongfeng)* or Sp-6 *(Sanyinjiao)*; for spermatorrhea, use Co-1 *(Huiyin)*, Li-8 *(Ququan)*, and Co-3 *(Zhongji)*. (Source: CNLAM)

4. Wet dreams: Li-8 *(Ququan)*—100 cones of moxa, Li-4 *(Zhongfeng)*, Li-3 *(Taichong)*, B-67 *(Zhiyin)*, B-17 *(Geshu)*, B-20 *(Pishu)*, Sp-6 *(Sanyinjiao)*. (Source: CDR)

5. Wet dreams: Not too much moxa on B-15 *(Xinshu)*; 1 cone of moxa for each year of age on B-38 *(Gaohuangshu)*, B-23 *(Shenshu)*, and Co-3 *(Zhongji)*; 5 cones of moxa on Gv-4 *(Mingmen)*; 50 cones of moxa on B-30 *(Baihuanshu)*; Sp-6 *(Sanyinjiao)*, Li-4 *(Zhongfeng)*, K-2 *(Rangu)*. (Source: IACC)

6. Spermatorrhea: B-15 *(Xinshu)*, B-23 *(Shenshu)*, Co-4 *(Guanyuan)*, Gv-4 *(Mingmen)*, B-30 *(Baihuanshu)*, Sp-6 *(Sanyinjiao)*. (Source: GCAM)

IMPOTENCE

Chinese medicine attributes this condition to the Heart and Spleen whose functions have been injured and suppressed, and to diminishment of the 'fire at the gate of life' (i.e., the Kidney Yang). Impotence is also closely associated with the Liver and Kidney channels. The Liver controls the muscles, and a Muscle channel is connected with the reproductive organs. Because of excessive anxiety, weakened Kidney Yang, or injury to and depletion of the Essence and Qi due to Cold, the patient is rendered incapable of obtaining an erection. Since it is the Kidney Yang which is weakened, impotence in Chinese is called 'withered Yang'. However, because the reproductive organs are considered Yin in nature, this condition is also referred to as 'withered Yin'.

Injury and suppression of the Heart and Spleen is associated with symptoms of irritability, restless sleep, waxy yellow complexion and loss of appetite. Symptoms associated with exhausted Kidney Yang include pallid complexion, dizziness, lassitude, low back pain and a sunken, fine and weak pulse.

Treatment is directed toward warming and strengthening the 'vital fire' (Kidney Yang).

Needling

Principal points: Co-4 *(Guanyuan)*, Sp-6 *(Sanyinjiao)*, Li-5 *(Ligou)*

Supplementary points: H-7 *(Shenmen)*, Gv-4 *(Mingmen)*

Method: First needle the principal points. For symptoms associated with injured and suppressed Heart and Spleen (see above), add H-7 *(Shenmen)*. For exhausted Kidney Yang, add Gv-4 *(Mingmen)*. Moxibustion may also be used at this point (either warm with moxa stick or burn 3-5 cones).

Discussion of points: Li-5 *(Ligou)* is the Connecting point on the Liver channel, which is linked with the penis. Co-4 *(Guanyuan)* is the point of intersection of the three Leg Yin channels on the Conception channel. Needling these two points strengthens the Yang at the Base (i.e., the Kidneys). Needling Sp-6 *(Sanyinjiao)* and H-7 *(Shenmen)* helps regulate the Heart and Spleen.

Electro-acupuncture
Points: B-31–34 *(Shangliao, Ciliao, Zhongliao* and *Xialiao)*, K-2 *(Rangu)*; or Co-4 *(Guanyuan)*, Sp-6 *(Sanyinjiao)*
Method: Use the two point groupings in rotation. Apply low frequency current for 3-5 minutes.

Ear acupuncture
Points: External Genitalia, Testicles, Endocrine, Subcortex, Neurogate
Method: Select 2-3 points each session. Use moderate stimulation, retaining the needles for 5-15 minutes. Treat once daily or on alternating days. Ten treatments constitute one course.

Barefoot doctor acupuncture
Points: Barefoot Doctor point, Thoracic #5, Lumbar #1 and #4

Injection therapy
Points: Co-4 *(Guanyuan)*, Co-3 *(Zhongji)*, B-23 *(Shenshu)*
Method: Inject vitamin B1, testosterone propionate, or HCG at the above points, in rotation. Treat once every 2-3 days. Four treatments constitute one course.

Other prescriptions
1. Co-4 *(Guanyuan)*, Sp-6 *(Sanyinjiao)*, B-23 *(Shenshu)*, S-36 *(Zusanli)*. Treat every other day. A needle can be buried at Sp-6 *(Sanyinjiao)* for 4-6 hours. (Source: HNMT)
2. Gv-20 *(Baihui)*, B-17 *(Geshu)*, B-21 *(Weishu)*, B-23 *(Shenshu)*, Gv-4 *(Mingmen)*, Gv-3 *(Yaoyangguan)*, Co-4 *(Guanyuan)*, Co-3 *(Zhongji)*. Moxi daily. (Source: CAM)
3. Inability to have an erection: Moxi on Gv-4 *(Mingmen)*, B-23 *(Shenshu)*, Co-6 *(Qihai)*, K-2 *(Rangu)*. (Source: IACC)
4. Impotence: Moxi on Gv-4 *(Mingmen)*, B-23 *(Shenshu)*, Co-6 *(Qihai)*, K-2 *(Rangu)*, SI-5 *(Yanggu)*. (Source: PDM)

Remarks
• The majority of impotence cases are functional in nature. It is important that the physician explain the condition to the patient so that he understands there is nothing to fear or be ashamed of. This should help speed recovery.
• Acupuncture is definitely effective in the treatment of this condition.

URINARY RETENTION AND INCONTINENCE

In Chinese medicine incontinence is attributed to a failure of the Bladder to retain urine. Retention of urine is ascribed to a functional impediment which prevents the urine from flowing. The latter arises when Fire or Dampness and Heat collect in the Lower Burner (Kidneys, Bladder, Intestines) and obstruct the channels, rendering the Bladder incapable of controlling the passage of fluids from the body. It is usually a condition of Excess. Incontinence, on the other hand, is due to unstable Kidney Qi, Deficient Bladder Qi or sinking Spleen Qi. It is commonly a Deficient condition.

Treatment in both cases is directed toward restoring circulation through the Lower Burner and regulating the Bladder.

Needling
Points: B-32 *(Ciliao),* B-53 *(Weiyang),* Co-3 *(Zhongji);* or Sp-6 *(Sanyinjiao),* B-23 *(Shenshu),* B-33 *(Zhongliao)*

Method: The two point groupings may be used in rotation. Apply moderate to strong stimulation. For retention of urine, continuously manipulate the needles, treating several times daily until micturation occurs. For incontinence, retain the needles in place for 15 minutes, treating once daily or on alternating days. Five to ten treatments constitute one course.

Discussion of points: B-32 *(Ciliao)* and B-33 *(Zhongliao)* serve the same function as the Associated point of the Bladder channel. B-53 *(Weiyang),* the Lower Uniting point of the Triple Burner, and Co-3 *(Zhongji),* the Alarm point of the Bladder, are both needled to stabilize Bladder function. B-23 *(Shenshu)* also facilitates Bladder function. Sp-6 *(Sanyinjiao)* is the point at which the three Leg Yin channels intersect. Needling this point helps restore circulation through the Lower Burner.

Electro-acupuncture
Points: Sp-6 *(Sanyinjiao),* B-28 *(Pangguangshu),* B-53 *(Weiyang),* N-BW-38 *(Xiajiaoshu);* or S-28 *(Shuidao)*
Method: Use the two point groupings in rotation. For incontinence, use low frequency current. For retention of urine, use high frequency current, and needle S-28 *(Shuidao)* bilaterally with the needle pointed in a medial direction and inserted to a depth just short of the walls of the bladder. *Caution must be exercised to avoid penetrating the bladder.* With strong current, micturation is usually obtained.

Moxibustion
Principal points: B-22 *(Sanjiaoshu),* B-27 *(Xiaochangshu),* Co-3 *(Zhongji),* B-67 *(Zhiyin)*
Supplementary points: Gv-28 *(Yinjiao),* Li-4 *(Zhongfeng),* Li-3 *(Taichong)*

Ear acupuncture
Principal points: Bladder, Urethra, Sympathetic, External Genitalia
Supplementary points: Kidney, Spleen, Triple Burner
Method: Select 2-3 points each session. Use moderate to strong stimulation, retaining needles 15-20 minutes.

Other prescriptions
1. Urinary retention: Co-4 *(Guanyuan),* Co-3 *(Zhongji),* Sp-6 *(Sanyinjiao),* Sp-9 *(Yinlingquan),* B-32 *(Ciliao).* (Source: HCNMT)
2. Paralysis of the bladder: Gv-3 *(Yaoyangguan),* B-32 *(Ciliao),* B-33 *(Zhongliao),* Co-4 *(Guanyuan),* Co-3 *(Zhongji),* Co-2 *(Qugu).* (Source: CAM)
3. Li-8 *(Ququan)* for urinary retention; Li-2 *(Xingjian)* for urinary retention with penile pain; B-48 *(Baohuang)* and B-49 *(Zhibian)* for inability to urinate; Co-24 *(Chengjiang)* for incontinence; Sp-9 *(Yinlingquan)* and GB-34 *(Yanglingquan)* for people who are unaware when they urinate. (Source: CNLAM)
4. Difficult urination: Sp-9 *(Yinlingquan),* Co-6 *(Qihai),* Sp-6 *(Sanyinjiao),* K-10 *(Yingu),* P-7 *(Daling).* (Source: GCAM)
5. Difficult urination: Moxi on B-22 *(Sanjiaoshu),* B-27 *(Xiaochangshu),* Sp-6 *(Sanyinjiao),* Co-3 *(Zhongji),* Li-4 *(Zhongfeng),* B-67 *(Zhiyin).* Incontinence: Moxi on Co-6 *(Qihai),* Co-4 *(Guanyuan),* Sp-9 *(Yinlingquan),* Li-1 *(Dadun),* Li-2 *(Xingjian).* (Source: PDM)

Remarks
- Acupuncture is definitely effective in treating both incontinence and retention of urine.
- It is important that the physician determine the underlying source of the condition.

ACUTE SPRAIN OF LOWER BACK

The traditional etiology of this condition parallels that of Western medicine. Treatment is based on the principles of clearing the obstruction from and regulating the Governing and Bladder channels which traverse the lower back.

Needling
Points: Gv-26 *(Renzhong)*, B-54 *(Weizhong)*, K-2 *(Rangu)*

Method: Needle Gv-26 *(Renzhong)* with strong stimulation. Prick B-54 *(Weizhong)* and K-2 *(Rangu)* to let a few drops of blood. Treat once daily.

Cutaneous acupuncture and cupping
Points: Points of tenderness
Method: Tap vigorously with the cutaneous needle, then apply cups and draw about 10 milliliters of blood.

Injection therapy
Points: Points of tenderness
Method: Inject a compound of 25% magnesium sulfate and 2% procaine hydrochloride into the muscle at the point of tenderness on the lower back; or, inject a compound of 10% glucose and 2% procaine hydrochloride into the points. Inject the medicine into different layers of sprained muscle tissue. Treat once every 2-5 days.

Air injection method
Points: Gv-4 *(Mingmen)*, B-54 *(Weizhong)*

Ear acupuncture
Points: Lumbar Vertebrae, Lumbago, Neurogate, Subcortex, Adrenal
Method: After inserting and manipulating needles for a few moments, retain in place for 15-20 minutes. Treat once daily. If this proves effective, intradermal needles may be embedded for 1-7 days.

Head acupuncture
Points: Lower limb area in Sensory area, Leg motor and sensory area (bilaterally)

Hand acupuncture
Point: Lumbar and Leg point

Foot acupuncture
Point: #25

Barefoot doctor acupuncture
Points: Barefoot Doctor point, Thoracic #5, Lumbar #1

Other prescriptions
1. Pain of strained lower back: L-5 *(Chize)*, B-54 *(Weizhong)*, Gv-26 *(Renzhong)*, GB-34 *(Yanglingquan)*, B-65 *(Shugu)*, B-60 *(Kunlun)*, B-34 *(Xialiao)*, Co-6 *(Qihai)*. (Source: OM)
2. Low back strain with difficulty in getting up: 3 cones of moxa on Gv-6 *(Jizhong)* and B-23 *(Shenshu)* and 7 cones of moxa on Gv-4 *(Mingmen)*, B-29 *(Zhonglushu)*, and Gv-2 *(Yaoshu)*. (Source: IACC)

3. Back strain with rib and low back pain: L-5 *(Chize)*, LI-11 *(Quchi)*, LI-4 *(Hegu)*, Sp-6 *(Sanyinjiao)*, Sp-9 *(Yinlingquan)*, Li-2 *(Xingjian)*, S-36 *(Zusanli)*, LI-10 *(Shousanli)*. (Source: GOA)

4. Low back strain: L-5 *(Chize)*, B-54 *(Weizhong)*, Gv-26 *(Renzhong)*, B-60 *(Kunlun)*, B-65 *(Shugu)*, TB-6 *(Zhigou)*, GB-34 *(Yanglingquan)*. (Source: GCAM)

CHRONIC LOW BACK PAIN

Chinese medicine refers to the lower back as the 'dwelling of the Kidneys'. The great majority of chronic low back pain conditions are therefore associated with Deficient Kidneys (which includes the reproductive organs). The Bladder is associated with the Kidneys in a Yin/Yang relationship. The Bladder channel traverses the lumbar region, and its Muscle channel embraces the waist as well as the upper spine. Thus, Deficient Kidneys and disrupted Qi along the Bladder channel, as well as injury to the Muscle channels in the lumbar region, attacks of Wind and Dampness (i.e., rheumatism) or other Excesses of external origin may all contribute to hindering the proper circulation of Qi and Blood in this region of the body, producing low back pain.

Treatment is directed toward spreading the Qi through the channels traversing this region, relaxing the muscles, and activating the Blood.

Needling
Principal points: points of tenderness, B-54 *(Weizhong)*, B-60 *(Kunlun)*
Supplementary points: B-22 *(Sanjiaoshu)*, B-23 *(Shenshu)*, M-BW-24 *(Yaoyan)*

Method: First, needle the principal points with moderate to strong stimulation. In areas of particular tenderness where there are muscle spasms, the needle may be inserted first in one direction, then partially withdrawn and reinserted in other directions. If necessary, supplementary points may be used, or the needles can be warmed with moxibustion. Electro-acupuncture may also be utilized. Either attach the electrodes to the handles of the needles or place directly on the points of tenderness. Finally, ultraviolet radiation can be directed at areas of tenderness and neighboring acupuncture points.

Cutaneous acupuncture and cupping
Points: Points of tenderness
Method: Tap with moderate force, then apply cups to draw out a small amount of blood.

Injection therapy
Points: Points of tenderness
Method: Inject a 10% glucose solution, or combine with vitamin B1; or inject glucose and tolazoline; or inject a 5% *Angelica sinesis (danggui)* solution.

If the first prescription is chosen, inject the medicine into areas of tenderness affected by muscle spasm, pointing the needle in different directions as the medicine is injected. With the second and third prescriptions, medicine can be injected directly into the most painful areas. Treat once every 3-4 days. Ten treatments constitute one course.

Moxibustion
Points: B-23 *(Shenshu)*, B-25 *(Dachangshu)*, M-BW-24 *(Yaoyan)*, Gv-4 *(Mingmen)*, M-BW-25 *(Shiqizhuixia)*, Gv-3 *(Yangguan)*
Method: Warm with moxa sticks for 5-10 minutes or burn 1-3 cones at the points using the indirect method. Treat once daily or on alternating days. Select 2-3 points each session.

Cupping
Prescription #1: Place cups at B-23 *(Shenshu)*, Gv-3 *(Yangguan)* and B-32 *(Ciliao)*. Treat once daily or on alternating days.

Prescription #2: Either place or move the cups along the course of the Bladder channel on the lower back. Treat once every 2-3 days.

Ear acupuncture
Points: Lumbar Vertebrae, Lumbago, Neurogate, Subcortex, Adrenal

Method: After inserting and manipulating needles for a few moments, retain in place for 15-20 minutes. Treat once daily. If this proves effective, intradermal needles may be embedded for 1-7 days.

Foot acupuncture
Points: #26, #30, #29, #35

Other prescriptions

1. Stiff back: Gv-11 *(Shendao)*, Gv-6 *(Jizhong)*, Gv-2 *(Yaoshu)*, Gv-1 *(Changqiang)*, B-11 *(Dazhu)*, B-17 *(Geshu)*, Co-9 *(Shuifen)*, B-20 *(Pishu)*, B-27 *(Xiaochangshu)*, B-28 *(Pangguangshu)*. Stiff and painful lower back: B-32 *(Ciliao)*, B-48 *(Baohuang)*, B-56 *(Chengjin)*, B-47 *(Zhishi)*, GB-25 *(Jingmen)*. (Source: TDP)

2. Low back pain: Gv-2 *(Yaoshu)*, B-28 *(Pangguangshu)*, Gv-1 *(Changqiang)*, S-30 *(Qichong)*, B-31 *(Shangliao)*, B-34 *(Xialiao)*, S-3 *(Juliao)*, B-13 *(Feishu)*. Low back pain with inability to straighten up: S-36 *(Zusanli)*, S-33 *(Yinshi)*, GB-38 *(Yangfu)*, Li-5 *(Ligou)*. Weak neck muscles in a hunchback: GB-20 *(Fengchi)*. (Source: CNLAM)

3. Five cones of moxa on B-23 *(Shenshu)*, B-29 *(Zhonglushu)*, and Gv-2 *(Yaoshu)*. (Source: TMLP)

4. Deficient Kidney low back pain: 14 cones of moxa on B-23 *(Shenshu)*, Gv-26 *(Renzhong)* and B-54 *(Weizhong)*. Stiff and painful low back: B-60 *(Kunlun)* and 14 cones of moxa on Gv-4 *(Mingmen)*. Sudden stagnant Qi with low back pain and inability to straighten up: B-47 *(Zhishi)* and Li-2 *(Xingjian)*. Pain in the spine with inability to flex or extend: if pain more in upper part of low back use LI-4 *(Hegu)*, if more in lower part use B-60 *(Kunlun)*, K-7 *(Fuliu)*. Insufferable low back pain: GB-20 *(Fengchi)*, LI-4 *(Hegu)*, B-60 *(Kunlun)*. (Source: OM)

5. Stagnant Blood low back pain: Moxi on B-23 *(Shenshu)* and B-60 *(Kunlun)*, prick to bleed B-54 *(Weizhong)*. Low back pain: GB-21 *(Jianjing)*, GB-30 *(Huantiao)*, S-33 *(Yinshi)*, S-36 *(Zusanli)*, B-54 *(Weizhong)*, B-57 *(Chengshan)*, GB-38 *(Yangfu)*, B-60 *(Kunlun)*, Gv-2 *(Yaoshu)*, B-23 *(Shenshu)*. Stiff and painful low back: Gv-2 *(Yaoshu)*, B-54 *(Weizhong)*, K-1 *(Yongquan)*, B-27 *(Xiaochangshu)*. (Source: GOA)

6. Back pain causing difficulty in walking: Li-13 *(Zhangmen)*, Gv-2 *(Yaoshu)*, prick B-54 *(Weizhong)*, apply 7 cones of moxa on B-60 *(Kunlun)*. (Source: IACC)

7. Deficient Kidney low back pain: B-23 *(Shenshu)*, B-54 *(Weizhong)*, K-3 *(Taixi)*, B-30 *(Baihuanshu)*. Stiff and painful low back: Gv-26 *(Renzhong)*, B-54 *(Weizhong)*. (Source: GCAM)

Remarks

- Hot packs may be used in conjunction with acupuncture to relieve the pain associated with either acute sprain or chronic strain of the lower back. Manipulation may also be useful in cases of chronic back strain.

DISEASES AFFECTING THE SOFT TISSUES OF THE SHOULDER

In Chinese medicine, most shoulder problems belong to the 'blockage' group of diseases. The Excesses of Wind, Cold and Dampness take advantage of persons who are exhausted, injured or even asleep, by attacking the body at the shoulder. Once lodged here, these Excesses obstruct the circulation of Qi and Blood through the channels, disrupting related muscle function.

Treatment is directed toward spreading the Qi and Blood, relaxing the muscles and clearing the channels of the shoulder.

Needling
Principal points: LI-15 *(Jianyu)*, SI-11 *(Tianzong)*, TB-14 *(Jianliao)*, M-UE-48 *(Jianneiling)*,

LI-16 *(Jugu)*

Supplementary points: LI-11 *(Quchi)*, LI-4 *(Hegu)*, L-5 *(Chize)*, L-9 *(Taiyuan)*, TB-9 *(Sidu)*, TB-4 *(Yangchi)*

Method: 1. Perifocal inflammation of the shoulder—use the local points LI-15 *(Jianyu)*, TB-14 *(Jianliao)* and M-UE-48 *(Jianneiling)*. Insert the needles in several different directions around each of the points.

2. Supraspinatus tendinitis—Use the local points LI-16 *(Jugu)* and LI-15 *(Jianyu)*. Insert needle perpendicularly at LI-16 *(Jugu)*, in a forward, lateral direction. Insert needle at LI-15 *(Jianyu)* level with the inferior margin of the acromion of the shoulder.

3. Bursitis of the shoulder (infra-acromial bursitis): After inserting a needle at LI-15 *(Jianyu)*, level with the inferior margin of the acromion, partially withdraw the needle and reinsert in a forward or backward direction.

(LI-11 *(Quchi)* and LI-4 *(Hegu)* may be added as distant points to all of the local point prescriptions above. Use moderate to strong stimulation at all of the points.)

4. Tenosynovitis of the biceps brachii longus muscle: Use the local point M-UE-48 *(Jianneiling)*, directing the needle first upward and then downward. Combine with L-5 *(Chize)* and L-9 *(Taiyuan)*. If the pain is concentrated at the back of the shoulder, use TB-14 *(Jianliao)* as the principal point, combined with TB-9 *(Sidu)* and TB-4 *(Yangchi)*.

For all prescriptions, needle once daily or on alternating days. Ten to fifteen treatments constitute one course. The needles can also be warmed with moxibustion, and electro-acupuncture may be applied.

Barefoot doctor acupuncture

Point: Three Needles at the Shoulder points

Injection therapy

Points: point(s) of tenderness

Method: Injection therapy is ordinarily used for perifocal inflammation of the shoulder and supraspinatus tendinitis. Inject a 10% glucose solution into each of the points. Treat once every other day. Ten treatments constitute one course.

For supraspinatus tendinitis, in addition to the glucose injection, slowly inject a 1% procaine hydrochloride solution into the most distinct point of tenderness at the greater tubercle of the humerus (approximately at LI-15 *(Jianyu)*. If injected correctly, the pain and functional impairment at the shoulder should almost immediately disappear. However, the patient should be cautioned that after a few hours the pain may return, perhaps more intensely than before. This pain may well diminish within a few days time and will not recur thereafter.

Ear acupuncture

Points: Point of tenderness in the Shoulder area of the ear, Subcortex, Neurogate, Adrenal

Method: Treat once daily or on alternating days. Ten treatments constitute one course. If preliminary result is satisfactory, intradermal needles can be embedded for 3-5 days.

Cutaneous acupuncture

Tap the needle in the shoulder region, particularly over the areas of tenderness. Treat once every 4-7 days. Five treatments constitute one course.

Moxibustion

Warm the affected area with moxa sticks for 10-20 minutes, once or twice daily. Ten treatments constitute one course.

Cupping

Place cups in the affected area, particularly at points of tenderness. Treat once every 2-4 days. Cupping may also be combined with cutaneous acupuncture to let a small amount of blood. Treat once every 4-7 days.

Head acupuncture

Point: Upper limb area of the Sensory area

Hand acupuncture

Point: Shoulder
Method: Use strong stimulation. Needle may be retained for 2-3 minutes.

Other prescriptions

1. SI-9 *(Jianzhen)* joined to H-1 *(Jiquan)*, SI-6 *(Yanglao)* joined to P-6 *(Neiguan)*, LI-15 *(Jianyu)* needled in three different directions, S-38 *(Tiaokou)* joined to B-57 *(Chengshan)*. (Source: HNMT)

2. Severe shoulder pain: SI-6 *(Yanglao)*, B-10 *(Tianzhu)*. (Source: TDP)

3. Painful shoulder that cannot be raised: LI-11 *(Quchi)*, TB-15 *(Tianliao)*. (Source: CNLAM)

4. Red, swollen, and painful posterior shoulder: TB-14 *(Jianliao)*, B-12 *(Fengmen)*, TB-3 *(Zhongzhu)*, B-11 *(Dazhu)*. (Source: GCAM)

Remarks

• The shoulder diseases above should be distinguished from arthritis.

• In the latter stages of perifocal inflammation of the shoulder, as the joint stiffens, exercise of the shoulder must be used in conjunction with acupuncture.

TENDINITIS OF THE ELBOW

Chinese medicine refers to this condition simply as 'elbow pain'. It is attributed to strain along the Muscle channels at the elbow which impedes the flow of Qi and Blood.

Treatment is directed toward relaxing the muscles and opening the channels.

Needling

Principal points: Point(s) of tenderness
Supplementary points: LI-4 *(Hegu)*, LI-10 *(Shousanli)*

Method: Insert needles at points of tenderness, then partially withdraw and reinsert in different directions so that the needle sensation extends around the points. Alternatively, several needles may be inserted in different directions at the same point. Use moderate to strong stimulation at the supplementary points. Treat once daily or on alternating days. Ten to fifteen treatments constitute one course.

Electro-acupuncture can be added, or the needles warmed with moxibustion.

Moxibustion

Warm the affected area with moxa sticks for 10-20 minutes, or burn 1-3 moxa cones utilizing the indirect method. Treat once or twice daily. If moxibustion is combined with acupuncture the result may be more satisfactory.

Cutaneous acupuncture and cupping

Points: Point(s) of tenderness
Method: First tap the affected area until there is slight bleeding, then apply cups. If difficulty is encountered keeping the cups in place, apply a layer of flour paste before attaching the cup. Treat once every 2-3 days.

Ear acupuncture

Points: The point of tenderness in the Elbow area of the ear, Subcortex, Neurogate, Adrenal
Method: Treat once daily or on alternating days. Ten to fifteen treatments constitute one course.

Other prescriptions

1. Painful elbow: S-42 *(Chongyang)*, LI-11 *(Quchi)*, TB-15 *(Tianliao)*. Inability to extend forearm: LI-10 *(Shousanli)*, GB-44 *(Qiaoyin)*. (Source: CNLAM)
2. Exhausted elbow: TB-10 *(Tianjing)*, LI-11 *(Quchi)*, P-5 *(Jianshi)*, LI-5 *(Yangxi)*, TB-3 *(Zhongzhu)*, L-9 *(Taiyuan)*, SI-4 *(Wangu)*, L-7 *(Lieque)*, TB-2 *(Yemen)*. (Source: GCAM)

Remarks

• During the course of treatment, the patient's elbow should be rested. If the joint becomes stiff due to inflammation, massage or surgery should be considered.

STENOSING-TENOSYNOVITIS OF THE
RADIAL STYLOID PROCESS

This condition, along with tenosynovitis of the flexor digitorum muscle, falls within the traditional domain of 'sinew blockage.' It is generally attributed to injury of the Muscle channels which obstructs the circulation of Qi and Blood.

Treatment is directed toward relaxing the muscles and facilitating the circulation through the channels.

Needling

Principal points: Point(s) of tenderness
Supplementary points: LI-5 *(Yangxi)*, L-7 *(Lieque)*, L-4 *(Hegu)*

Method: The most tender point is the most important in the prescription. Insert 2-4 needles at this point with transverse insertions pointed in different directions. Treat once daily or on alternating days. Ten to fifteen treatments constitute one course.

Injection therapy

Inject 5% *Angelica sinesis (danggui)* or cortisone acetate hydrocortisone, combined with 1% procaine, into the point of maximum tenderness. Treat once every 2-7 days.

Ear acupuncture

Points: Wrist, Neurogate, Subcortex
Method: Use moderate to strong stimulation, retaining needles 10-25 minutes. Ten to fifteen treatments constitute one course.

Cutaneous acupuncture

Tap the needle over the affected area until there is slight bleeding. This serves both an analgesic and anti-inflammatory function. Treat once daily or on alternating days.

Moxibustion

Warm the affected area with moxa sticks for 10-20 minutes. Treat 1-3 times daily.

Other prescriptions

1. Radial aspect of the wrist painful and immobile: LI-5 *(Yangxi)*. Exhausted wrist: L-7 *(Lieque)*. (Source: CNLAM)
2. Wrist pain: LI-5 *(Yangxi)*, LI-11 *(Quchi)*, SI-4 *(Wangu)*. (Source: OM)
3. Weak hand and wrist: L-7 *(Lieque)*. (Source: SPMD)

Remarks
- During the course of treatment, movement of the affected wrist should be kept to a minimum and the wrist itself kept warm.

TENOSYNOVITIS OF THE FLEXOR DIGITORUM MUSCLE

Needling
Points: Point(s) of tenderness
Method: Treat once daily or on alternating days.

Moxibustion
Warm the affected area with moxa sticks for 10-20 minutes, once or twice daily. Alternatively, burn 3-5 moxa cones at the point of tenderness using the indirect method, one to three times daily.

Injection therapy
Inject *Angelica sinesis (danggui),* hydrocortisone or predaisone acetate at the point of tenderness once every 2-7 days.

Remarks
- During the course of treatment, movement of the affected wrist should be limited, and the wrist kept warm.

TENOSYNOVIAL CYST

In Chinese medicine, treatment of this condition is directed toward relaxing the muscles and facilitating circulation through the channels.

Needling
Points: Locality of the cyst

Method: Use a thick needle to lance the cyst at its highest point, then manipulate the needle in and out so as to release some fluid. Thereafter, moxibustion may be used. If, after a week, the cyst has grown back to its original size, it may be lanced again.

Remarks
- After needling, the cyst should be dressed and bandaged for 3-5 days.

INJURIES TO THE SOFT TISSUES OF THE KNEE

Treated here are injuries to the tendons, ligaments and cartilage of the knee. In traditional medicine, treatment is directed toward relaxing the muscles and facilitating circulation through the channels.

Needling
Points: S-35 *(Yiyan)* both medial and lateral, B-54 *(Weizhong),* point(s) of tenderness

Method: For injury to the accessory ligaments of the knee, points of tenderness are most important. For injury to the fat cushion below the patella and the cruciform ligaments, needle S-35 *(Xiyan),* both medial and lateral, as well as B-54 *(Weizhong),* with moderate stimulation. Treat once daily or on alternating days. Ten to fifteen treatments constitute one course.

Remarks
- Injuries to the knee must be distinguished from arthritis.

INJURIES TO THE SOFT TISSUES OF THE ANKLE

In common with all injuries affecting connective tissues, treatment of this condition in Chinese medicine is directed toward relaxing the muscles and facilitating circulation through the affected channels.

Needling
Principal points: Point(s) of tenderness
Supplementary points: GB-39 *(Xuanzhong)*, Sp-6 *(Sanyinjiao)*

Method: First needle the point(s) of tenderness with moderate stimulation. If the result is unsatisfactory, add the supplementary points using strong stimulation. For injuries to the ligaments on the medial side, use Sp-6 *(Sanyinjiao)*; on the lateral side, use GB-39 *(Xuanzhong)*.

Cutaneous acupuncture and cupping
Tap along the affected area until there is slight bleeding, then apply cups for 3-5 minutes.

Moxibustion
Warm the affected area with moxa sticks for 10-15 minutes.

Remarks
• Acupuncture therapy is suitable for strained or sprained ankle. If the ligaments have torn, surgery must be considered.

STIFF NECK

Chinese medicine attributes this condition to an attack of Wind and Cold which enter the channels during sleep. Alternatively, the normal movement of Qi and Blood is disturbed and the muscle channels are strained when the sleeper assumes an awkward position.
Treatment centers on those channels which traverse the neck.

Needling
Principal points: M-UE-24 *(Luozhen)*, point(s) of pain
Supplementary points: SI-3 *(Houxi)*, GB-39 *(Xuanzhong)*

Method: First needle M-UE-24 *(Luozhen)* with moderate to strong stimulation. At the same time, ask the patient to exercise his neck by moving it around. If the pain is unabated, needle the points of pain. Use the supplementary points in rotation. Moxibustion may be applied to warm the needles at points of tenderness. Cups may be applied after needling. Electro-acupuncture may be used at points on the limbs.

Cutaneous acupuncture and cupping
Tap along the affected area until there is slight bleeding, then apply cups.
Alternatively, cutaneous acupuncture may be used independent of cupping at the following points:
Principal points: B-11 *(Dazhu)*, Gv-14 *(Dazhui)*, GB-21 *(Jianjing)*, SI-14 *(Jianwaishu)*, Gv-16 *(Fengfu)*, B-12 *(Fengmen)*, and the vertebral points M-BW-35 *(Jiaji)* from the 1st to the 4th cervical vertebra
Supplementary points: GB-20 *(Fengchi)*, B-64 *(Jinggu)*, SI-3 *(Houxi)*, TB-10 *(Tianjing)*

Injection therapy
Inject a 25% magnesium sulphate solution combined with 2% procaine hydrochloride into the point(s) of tenderness and affected muscle.

Air injection
Point: M-UE-24 *(Luozhen)* on the affected side

Ear acupuncture
Points: Neck, Cervical Vertebrae
Method: Use strong stimulation, retaining needles for 10-20 minutes.

Hand acupuncture
Point: Neck
Method: Use strong stimulation, retaining needle 3-5 minutes.

Foot acupuncture
Point: #23
Method: Same as hand acupuncture above

Other prescriptions
1. Immobile,severely painful neck: SI-1 *(Shaoze)*, SI-2 *(Qiangu)*, SI-3 *(Houxi)*, SI-5 *(Yanggu)*, GB-12 *(Wangu)*, B-60 *(Kunlun)*, H-3 *(Shaohai)*, B-2 *(Zanzhu)*. (Source: TDP)
2. Stiff neck: B-64 *(Jinggu)*, B-11 *(Dazhu)*, B-37 *(Pohu)*, GB-21 *(Jianjing)*, TB-16 *(Tianyou)*, SI-3 *(Houxi)*, B-10 *(Tianzhu)*. Sore neck that radiates into the back and shoulder: TB-10 *(Tianjing)*. (Source: CNLAM)
3. Stiff neck: Co-24 *(Chengjiang)*, Gv-16 *(Fengfu)*, SI-3 *(Houxi)*. (Source: OM)

Remarks
• The effect of acupuncture therapy is enhanced by the use of manipulation and hot packs after needling.

CARPAL TUNNEL SYNDROME

In traditional medicine, this disorder falls within the domain of 'blockage' or 'obstruction'. It is attributed to Cold, Dampness or Wind penetrating the muscles and sinews of the wrist, obstructing the circulation of Qi and Blood, and causing the Blood to coagulate.

Treatment is directed toward clearing the obstruction from the channels and activating the Blood.

Needling
Principal points: P-7 *(Daling)*, M-UE-50 *(Shangbaxie)*
Supplementary points: P-6 *(Neiguan)* or TB-5 *(Waiguan)*

Method: P-7 *(Daling)* is the most important point. Direct the needle into the carpal tunnel and use strong stimulation. Do not retain needle. If necessary, add the other points to strengthen the stimulation.

Cutaneous acupuncture
Tap along a band approximately 2 cm. in width, which encircles the affected wrist at 2 finger widths above the transverse crease. Tap until there is local congestion of blood.

Moxibustion
Warm with moxa stick for 10-20 minutes, twice daily.

Other prescriptions
1. Numb hand and forearm: TB-10 *(Tianjing)*, LI-11 *(Quchi)*, TB-5 *(Waiguan)*, L-8 *(Jingqu)*, TB-6 *(Zhigou)*, LI-5 *(Yangxi)*, SI-4 *(Wangu)*, LI-9 *(Shanglian)*, LI-4 *(Hegu)*. (Source: CDR)
2. Numb hand: L-11 *(Shaoshang)*. Hand pain: P-5 *(Jianshi)*. Hand blockage: P-8 *(Laogong)*. (Source: PUB)

3. Numb and painful hand: SI-3 *(Houxi)*, LI-3 *(Sanjian)*, M-UE-22 *(Baxie)*. (Source: ECAM)

Remarks
• The cutaneous acupuncture method in particular is definitely effective in reducing the inflammation and swelling during the early stages of this disease.

PAIN AT THE SOLE OF THE FOOT

Treated here is pain at the base of the calcaneus and metatarsal bones. Treatment is directed toward restoring circulation of Qi and Blood through the channels, the obstruction of which causes pain.

Needling
Principal points: Point(s) of pain
Supplementary points: B-57 *(Chengshan)*, K-3 *(Taixi)*, B-60 *(Kunlun)*

Method: First needle the point(s) of pain. If the pain does not abate, needle the supplementary points with moderate to strong stimulation.

Moxibustion
Warm the affected area with moxa stick for 10-20 minutes.

Remarks
• Acupuncture cannot be used to correct structural defects (e.g., bone deformity, spur, etc.) which may be the source of the pain. In such cases, surgery or other corrective measures may be necessary.

ECZEMA

In Chinese medicine, acute eczema is caused by Wind, Dampness and Heat penetrating the skin. Chronic eczema is attributed to Heat lodging in the Blood of persons suffering from Deficient Blood.
Treatment is directed toward clearing Heat and Dampness from the body.

Needling
Principal points: Gv-14 *(Dazhui)*, LI-11 *(Quchi)*, Sp-6 *(Sanyinjiao)*, H-7 *(Shenmen)*
Supplementary points: Sp-10 *(Xuehai)*, S-36 *(Zusanli)*

Method: First needle the principal points with moderate to strong stimulation. Treat once every other day. For chronic eczema, add Sp-10 *(Xuehai)* and S-36 *(Zusanli)*.

Discussion of points: Needling Gv-14 *(Dazhui)* and LI-11 *(Quchi)* drains the Wind and clears the Heat from the body. Sp-6 *(Sanyinjiao)*, at the junction of the three Leg Yin channels, can regulate those channels and eliminate the Dampness and Heat therein. H-7 *(Shenmen)* eliminates the itching by calming the Spirit. Sp-10 *(Xuehai)* harmonizes the Blood and S-36 *(Zusanli)* regulates the Spleen and Stomach which produce Blood.

Cutaneous acupuncture and cupping
Tap the affected area until there is slight bleeding, then apply cups.

Ear acupuncture
Principal points: Lung, Neurogate, Adrenal
Supplementary points: Liver, Subcortex
Method: Retain needles in place for 1-2 hours. For chronic eczema, add the supplementary points.

663

Moxibustion
Warm the affected area with moxa stick.

Barefoot doctor acupuncture
Points: Barefoot Doctor point, Thoracic #2 and #5

Head acupuncture
Points: The upper 2/5 of the Sensory area, bilaterally, or select an area in the Sensory area corresponding to the site of the eczema.

Remarks
• The cutaneous acupuncture and cupping method is particularly effective in the treatment of chronic eczema.

URTICARIA

Traditionally, this condition is attributed to Wind, Dampness and Heat penetrating the skin, or to Heat collecting in the Stomach and Intestines followed by an attack of Wind, which two Excesses settle in the pores of the skin. A bright red rash is a symptom of the Wind and Heat variety of urticaria, whereas a more dull colored rash, together with a heavy feeling in the body, indicate the Wind and Dampness variety.

Treatment is directed toward dispersing the Wind and activating the Blood.

Needling
Principal points: LI-11 *(Quchi)*, Sp-10 *(Xuehai)*, Sp-6 *(Sanyinjiao)*, S-36 *(Zusanli)*
Supplementary points: Gv-14 *(Dazhui)*, Sp-9 *(Yinlingquan)*

Method: The principal points form the basis of the prescription. Use moderate to strong stimulation with continuous needling for 1-3 minutes. For Wind/Heat urticaria, add Gv-14 *(Dazhui)*. For Wind/Dampness urticaria, add Sp-9 *(Yinlingquan)*.

Ear acupuncture
Points: The area on the ear corresponding to the site of the urticaria on the body, Endocrine, Lung, Adrenal
Method: Retain needles for 1 hour.

Barefoot doctor acupuncture
Points: Barefoot Doctor point, Thoracic #5

Head acupuncture
Needle the upper 2/5 of the Sensory area, bilaterally, or the area in the Sensory area corresponding to the site of the urticaria.

Cutaneous acupuncture
Principal points: GB-20 *(Fengchi)*, Sp-10 *(Xuehai)*, M-BW-35 *(Jiaji)* from the 2nd to the 5th thoracic and the 1st to the 4th sacral vertebrae
Supplementary points: LI-11 *(Quchi)*, B-12 *(Fengmen)*, Gv-16 *(Fengfu)*, B-54 *(Weizhong)*, B-13 *(Feishu)*, Sp-6 *(Sanyinjiao)*, LI-4 *(Hegu)*

Other prescriptions
1. Hot Wind rash: LI-11 *(Quchi)*, P-3 *(Quze)*, LI-4 *(Hegu)*, L-7 *(Lieque)*, B-13 *(Feishu)*, L-10 *(Yuji)*, H-7 *(Shenmen)*, P-6 *(Neiguan)*. (Source: COAM)
2. Wind rash: Sp-10 *(Xuehai)*, Sp-6 *(Sanyinjiao)*, LI-11 *(Quchi)*, LI-4 *(Hegu)*. (Source: ECAM)

3. Wind rash: LI-11 *(Quchi)*, GB-39 *(Xuanzhong)*, prick B-54 *(Weizhong)* to bleed. (Source: JDC)

Remarks
- If the symptoms include abdominal pain, diarrhea and (occasionally) difficult breathing, other methods of Chinese or Western medicine should be used.
- It is important to identify the source of this condition, which should be treated in addition to the external symptoms.
- Excellent results are obtained from treating this disease with acupuncture.

NEURODERMATITIS (Chronic Lichen Simplex)

In Chinese medicine, an analogous condition is known as 'ox-skin rash'.
Treatment is directed toward activating the Blood and clearing the channels.

Needling
Principal points: LI-11 *(Quchi)*, Sp-10 *(Xuehai)*
Supplementary points: LI-4 *(Hegu)*, Sp-6 *(Sanyinjiao)*, point of tenderness

Method: Use moderate to strong stimulation. Insert needles at the four 'corners' surrounding an area of dermatitis. Use transverse insertions such that the needles criss-cross the point of tenderness at the focus of the dermatitis.

Moxibustion
Warm the affected area with moxa stick for about 30 minutes.

Cutaneous acupuncture and cupping
Tap the affected area, then apply cups. Treat once daily.

Ear acupuncture
Points: Lung, Neurogate, Adrenal, Liver, Subcortex
Method: Retain needles for one hour. Treat once daily.

Letting Blood
Prick the posterior auricular vein to let a few drops of blood. This method may be combined with needling.

Barefoot doctor acupuncture
Points: Barefoot Doctor point, Thoracic #5

Head acupuncture
Points: Insert needle in the upper 2/5 of the Sensory area, bilaterally, or select an area in the Sensory area corresponding to the site of the neurodermatitis on the body.

Embedding thread
Thread the focus of the neurodermatitis with a cross (+) pattern, or a circular pattern. Allow 15 days between treatments.

Other prescriptions
1. GB-20 *(Fengchi)*, Gv-14 *(Dazhui)*, LI-11 *(Quchi)*, LI-4 *(Hegu)*, S-36 *(Zusanli)*, Sp-10 *(Xuehai)*, B-50 *(Chengfu)*, B-54 *(Weizhong)*, strong stimulation with a cutaneous needle over the affected area. (Source: HAM)

Remarks
- Acupuncture has been relatively effective in treating this disease in its early stages.

FROSTBITE

Treatment of this condition is directed toward activating the Blood and warming the channels.

Treatment
First needle around the perimeter of the frostbite with shallow pricking insertions, then warm with moxa stick. If large surfaces of the body are affected, needle Gv-14 *(Dazhui)*, Gv-26 *(Renzhong)* and K-1 *(Yongquan)* with strong stimulation. Treat once daily.

Remarks
- If the surface area of the frostbite is large and there is shock, combined Chinese and Western methods of emergency treatment are indicated.

LEPROSY

Chinese medicine attributes this disease to a pestilence or Poisonous Excess which penetrates the body when it is weak and lodges in the blood vessels. Since the Cultural Revolution, significant success has been achieved using this new medical therapy.

Incision therapy
Principal points: Sp-4 *(Gongsun)*, K-1 *(Yongquan)*, K-2 *(Rangu)*, S-36 *(Zusanli)*, S-21 *(Liangmen)*

Supplementary points: L-10 *(Yuji)*, LI-11 *(Quchi)*, LI-10 *(Shousanli)*, SI-8 *(Xiaohai)*, B-57 *(Chengshan)*, S-40 *(Fenglong)*, GB-34 *(Yanglingquan)*, Sp-9 *(Yinlingquan)*

Method: Select points according to the nature and location of associated symptoms (numbness, suppressed sweating, ulcerations, etc.). After sterilizing the affected tissue with alcohol and applying a local anesthetic, make a 1-1.5 cm. incision at the point(s) and insert hemostatic forceps into the wound to stimulate the underlying tissue. Once the needle sensation characteristic of acupuncture stimulation has been obtained, continue stimulation for 10-15 minutes. If, however, the needle sensation is not felt by the patient, the forceps may be inserted deeper beneath the connective tissue and manipulation resumed. For cases of long duration wherein the numbness is quite severe, stimulation should be strong. For less severe cases, stimulation should be correspondingly more mild. Treat once every 10-15 days.

Injection therapy
Points: Gv-23 *(Shangxing)*, LI-11 *(Quchi)*, P-6 *(Neiguan)*, S-36 *(Zusanli)*, Sp-6 *(Sanyinjiao)*, Sp-9 *(Yinlingquan)*

Method: Combine 12.5 grams each of the herbs *Phellodendrin amurense (huangbai)*, *Coptis japonica (huanglian)*, *Scutellaria baikalensis (huangqin)*, *Gardinia floride (shanzhi)*, *Paeonia suffructiccsa (danpi)* and *Salvia miltiovchizer (danshen)* with 900 milliliters of water. Boil this concoction down to 300 milliliters of liquid. This constitutes an anti-bacterial fluid that can be injected into the acupuncture points and leprous nodes. Select 1-3 points or nodes each session, injecting .3-.4 milliliters of the fluid into distant points and .1-.3 milliliters into local points or leprous nodes. Treat 2-3 times per week. Ten treatments constitute one course. After receiving the injections, the patient should feel local soreness, distension and numbness characteristic of injections at acupuncture points. Most patients will exhibit symptoms such as sensitivity to cold and low fever within 6-8 hours. No special measures need be taken for such symptoms.

Piercing the lymph nodes

This method is suitable for treating cases of leprosy which involve orchitis. Pierce the swollen lymph node through its center and retain needle for 15-20 minutes, manipulating needle only once during this time. Treat once every 1-2 days.

Remarks

- Patients with infectious leprosy must be treated in isolation so that the disease does not spread.

Chapter 7

Obstetric and Gynecological Diseases

IRREGULAR MENSTRUATION

In Chinese medicine, irregular menstruation is associated with the Kidney, Liver and Spleen channels. If the Kidneys are Deficient, the functions associated with the Penetrating and Conception channels are disrupted. If Heat collects in the Liver, that Organ cannot store Blood. Spleen Deficiency may prevent the Spleen from producing Blood. All of these disorders can affect the color, quantity and regularity of menstruation.

Early menstruation is usually a symptom of Heat in the Blood; late menstruation a symptom of Deficient and Cold conditions; and irregular menstrual flow (sometimes early, sometimes late) is a symptom related to depressed Liver Qi or Deficient Kidneys.

More particularly, symptoms associated with Heat in the Blood (early menstruation) include a large quantity of bright red blood, ordinarily accompanied by irritability, dark red complexion, fine and rapid or chord-like and rapid pulse, and a red tongue with yellow fur.

Symptoms associated with Deficient and Cold conditions (late menstruation) include a small quantity of blood which is thin in consistency and light in color, ordinarily a lack of strength, pallid complexion, sensitivity to cold and attraction to warmth, pale tongue and a slow, weak pulse.

Symptoms which accompany irregular menstruation associated with Deficient Kidneys include emaciation, dusty complexion, dizziness, lumbar pain and blood which varies in quantity and is pale in color. Symptoms which accompany depressed Liver Qi include a feeling of congestion in the chest, belching, pain in the lower abdomen before and/or after menstruation, and irregular menstrual flow which is dark purple in color.

Treatment is directed toward regulating the three Leg Yin channels as well as the Penetrating and Conception channels.

Needling

Principal points: Co-4 *(Guanyuan),* Sp-6 *(Sanyinjiao)*

Supplementary points: Sp-10 *(Xuehai),* Li-2 *(Xingjian),* S-36 *(Zusanli),* Sp-4 *(Gongsun),* Li-3 *(Taichong),* Gv-4 *(Mingmen),* P-6 *(Neiguan)*

Method: First needle the principal points. For early menstruation, add Sp-10 *(Xuehai),* Li-2 *(Xingjian).* For late menstruation, add S-36 *(Zusanli),* Sp-4 *(Gongsun).* For menstruation that is early one month and late the next, add Gv-4 *(Mingmen)* for Deficient Kidneys, and P-6 *(Neiguan),* Li-3 *(Taichong)* for depressed Liver Qi. Treat once every other day during the time when the woman is *not* menstruating. Ten treatments constitute one course.

Discussion of the points: Co-4 *(Guanyuan)* is on the Conception channel and is the point of intersection of the three Leg Yin channels on the abdomen. Sp-6 *(Sanyinjiao)* regulates the Qi of the three Leg Yin channels. The following supplementary points are selected according to the particular condition. Heat in the Blood: Sp-10 *(Xuehai)* cools the Blood and Li-2 *(Xingjian)* drains the Liver Fire. Deficient Spleen (lack of Blood): S-36 *(Zusanli)* strengthens the Spleen and Sp-4 *(Gongsun),* the Connecting point of the Spleen channel with the Penetrating channel, helps regulate the Spleen. Gv-4 *(Mingmen)* strengthens Deficient Kidneys. Li-3 *(Taichong)* spreads the Liver Qi and P-6 *(Neiguan)* expands the Middle Burner. Both points are therefore used to treat depressed Liver Qi.

Moxibustion

Point: Co-4 *(Guanyuan)*

Method: Begin treatment when menstruation has stopped. Burn 3-5 moxa cones on a ginger slice placed above this point. Treat on alternating days. Ten treatments constitute one course.

Embedding thread

Points: Join Co-3 *(Zhongji)* to Co-4 *(Guanyuan),* or embed single points B-20 *(Pishu),* B-23 *(Shenshu),* Sp-6 *(Sanyinjiao)*

Ear acupuncture

Points: Ovaries, Kidneys, Endocrine, Uterus

Method: Treat daily or on alternating days. Ten treatments constitute one course.

Head acupuncture

Points: Reproduction area, bilaterally

Other prescriptions

1. Irregular menstruation, amenorrhea, dysmenorrhea: Principal points: Co-4 *(Guanyuan),* Co-3 *(Zhongji).* Supplementary points: Sp-6 *(Sanyinjiao),* S-36 *(Zusanli),* Sp-10 *(Xuehai),* Sp-9 *(Yinlingquan).* Each treatment use one principal point and two supplementary points. Rotate points used. Treat once or twice a day, retaining needles for 15-20 minutes. Three weeks is one course of treatment. Separate courses by seven days. (Source: HCNMT)

2. Co-6 *(Qihai),* Li-1 *(Dadun),* K-10 *(Yingu),* Co-4 *(Guanyuan),* Li-3 *(Taichong),* K-2 *(Rangu),* Sp-6 *(Sanyinjiao),* Co-3 *(Zhongji),* Sp-2 *(Dadu),* S-12 *(Quepen),* S-10 *(Shuitu),* H-1 *(Jiquan),* P-3 *(Quze),* B-54 *(Weizhong).* (Source: NAM)

3. Irregular periods: Co-6 *(Qihai),* Co-3 *(Zhongji),* K-6 *(Zhaohai).* (Source: IACC)

4. Irregular periods: First needle Sp-4 *(Gongsun),* then Co-4 *(Guanyuan),* Co-6 *(Qihai),* S-25 *(Tianshu),* and Sp-6 *(Sanyinjiao).* Other: Co-3 *(Zhongji),* GB-26 *(Daimai)* (burn moxa), B-23 *(Shenshu).* (Source: GCAM)

Remarks

• Generally speaking, very good results are obtained with acupuncture therapy in the treatment of this condition.

AMENORRHEA

The principal causes of amenorrhea are dried and stagnant Blood. The first is a Deficient condition and is ordinarily related to an exhaustion of Kidney Qi, insufficient Blood in the uterus, and Deficiency in the Penetrating and Conception channels. The second is an Excessive condition which is generally related to depressed and stagnant Liver Qi which causes the Blood to coagulate and obstruct the channels, disrupting the functions of the Penetrating and Conception channels.

Symptoms associated with dried Blood include a gaunt appearance, dry skin, lassitude and occasionally low fever, night sweats, dizziness and palpitations. Stagnant Blood is associated with pain and distension in the lower abdomen, congestion in the chest, pain in the flanks or abdominal lumps, scaly skin.

Treatment is directed toward strengthening the Kidney Qi and clearing the obstruction from the Penetrating and Conception channels.

Needling

Principal points: B-23 *(Shenshu)*, Co-7 *(Yinjiao)*, Sp-6 *(Sanyinjiao)*

Supplementary points: B-17 *(Geshu)*, Sp-10 *(Xuehai)*, S-30 *(Qichong)*, Sp-8 *(Diji)*, Li-8 *(Ququan)*

Method: First needle the principal points. For dried Blood, add B-17 *(Geshu)* and Sp-10 *(Xuehai)*. For stagnant Blood, add S-30 *(Qichong)*, Sp-8 *(Diji)* and Li-8 *(Ququan)*. Use moderate stimulation. Treat on alternating days, ten treatments constituting one course. Electro-acupuncture may also be used, selecting one point on the trunk and another on the lower limb. Use moderate stimulation for 5-10 minutes.

Discussion of points: Needling B-23 *(Shenshu)* strengthens the Kidneys and is the Associated point of that Organ. Co-7 *(Yinjiao)*, the Meeting point of the Penetrating and Conception channels, clears the obstruction from those channels. Sp-6 *(Sanyinjiao)* regulates the functions of the three Leg Yin channels by keeping the Blood and Qi moving. B-17 *(Geshu)* and Sp-10 *(Xuehai)* benefit dried Blood. Li-8 *(Ququan)* spreads stagnant Liver Qi and Sp-8 *(Diji)* moves stagnant Blood. S-30 *(Qichong)* is the point of intersection of the Penetrating channel (the 'sea of blood') on the Stomach channel. Needling this point disperses the obstructed Qi, harmonizes the Blood, and eliminates coagulation.

Ear acupuncture

Points: Endocrine, Kidney, Liver, Spleen, Neurogate, Subcortex

Method: Use moderate stimulation. Treat on alternating days. Ten treatments constitute one course.

Cutaneous acupuncture

Principal points: B-18 *(Ganshu)*, B-23 *(Shenshu)*, B-20 *(Pishu)*, Li-3 *(Taichong)*, Sp-3 *(Taibai)*, S-36 *(Zusanli)*, Co-6 *(Qihai)*, Sp-6 *(Sanyinjiao)* and the vertebral points M-BW-35 *(Jiaji)* from the 11th thoracic to the 4th sacral vertebra

Supplementary points: Li-6 *(Zhongdu)*, K-5 *(Shuiquan)*, Sp-9 *(Yinlingquan)*, Li-2 *(Xingjian)*

Method: Use moderate to strong stimulation. Treat once daily or on alternating days. Ten treatments constitute one course.

Other prescriptions

1. Amenorrhea: B-23 *(Shenshu)*, Co-6 *(Qihai)*, Co-3 *(Zhongji)*, M-CA-24 *(Longmen)*, LI-4 *(Hegu)*, Sp-6 *(Sanyinjiao)*. (Source: HAM)

2. Cessation of menstruation: Gv-4 *(Mingmen)*, B-26 *(Guanyuanshu)*, B-32 *(Ciliao)*, Co-4 *(Guanyuan)*, GB-26 *(Daimai)*, Sp-8 *(Diji)*, Gv-3 *(Yaoyangguan)*, B-23 *(Shenshu)*, B-33 *(Zhongliao)*, Co-3 *(Zhongji)*, K-15 *(Zhongzhu)*, Sp-6 *(Sanyinjiao)*. (Source: CAM)

3. Cessation of menstruation: Gv-4 *(Mingmen)*, B-23 *(Shenshu)*, B-25 *(Dachangshu)*, Gv-1 *(Changqiang)*, LI-4 *(Hegu)*, Sp-6 *(Sanyinjiao)*, Sp-8 *(Diji)*, Sp-10 *(Xuehai)*, K-14 *(Siman)*, K-12 *(Dahe)*, Co-4 *(Guanyuan)*, Co-3 *(Zhongji)*, Co-2 *(Qugu)*, S-29 *(Guilai)*, B-60 *(Kunlun)*. (Source: NAM)

4. No periods: LI-11 *(Quchi)*, TB-6 *(Zhigou)*, S-36 *(Zusanli)*, Sp-6 *(Sanyinjaio)*. (Source: CDR)

5. Cessation of periods: Co-3 *(Zhongji)*, B-23 *(Shenshu)*, LI-4 *(Hegu)*, Sp-6 *(Sanyinjiao)*. (Source: GCAM)

6. If a woman is without periods or pregnancy and she has a yellowish complexion and vomits, use Sp-6 *(Sanyinjiao)* and LI-11 *(Quchi)*. TB-6 *(Zhigou)* and S-36 *(Zusanli)* may be used to treat women who are not catastrophically ill. (Source: GOA)

7. Cessation of periods: Moxa on Gv-2 *(Yaoshu)* and K-6 *(Zhaohai)*. (Source: PDM)

Remarks

• The possible relation of this condition to pregnancy or such diseases as anemia, tuberculosis,

670

nephritis, heart disease, tumors, etc., must be carefully determined by the physician and treated accordingly.

• Acupuncture is quite effective in the treatment of amenorrhea arising from emotional factors.

DYSMENORRHEA

Traditional medicine attributes menstrual pain to either congealed Blood or the Cold Excess which impede the circulation of Qi and obstruct the channels. Pain which precedes menstruation is usually a symptom of Excess associated with stagnant Qi and congealed Blood. Pain which follows menstruation is a Deficient symptom associated with Cold.

In addition to pain preceding menstruation, other symptoms associated with stagnant Qi and congealed Blood include distension and soreness in the flanks, chest and breasts, impeded menstrual flow, dark blood and occasionally clots.

Other symptoms associated with Cold include pallid complexion, lassitude, sensitivity to cold, abdominal pain which is alleviated when warmth is applied, scanty menstrual flow which is dull in color and clear.

Treatment is directed toward spreading the Qi through the uterus.

Needling
Principal points: Co-4 *(Guanyuan)*, Sp-6 *(Sanyinjiao)*
Supplementary points: S-29 *(Guilai)*, Co-7 *(Yinjiao)*, S-36 *(Zusanli)*, B-23 *(Shenshu)*, Co-6 *(Qihai)*

Method: Begin treatment one week prior to menstruation, treating once every other day. If the pain is severe, needle Sp-6 *(Sanyinjiao)* with strong stimulation for 20 minutes or until the pain is alleviated. For symptoms of stagnant Qi and congealed Blood, add S-29 *(Guilai)* and Co-6 *(Qihai)*. For symptoms associated with Cold, add S-36 *(Zusanli)* and B-23 *(Shenshu)*. Electro-acupuncture may also be used, connecting points bilaterally on the lower limb. Use a relatively high frequency current for 10-15 minutes.

Moxibustion
Points: Co-4 *(Guanyuan)*, Co-2 *(Qugu)*, M-CA-18 *(Zigong)*
Method: Warm with moxa stick for 10-20 minutes.

Ear acupuncture
Points: Ovaries, Neurogate, Endocrine, Allergy
Method: Use relatively strong stimulation until the pain is alleviated.

Cutaneous acupuncture
For pain associated with Cold, use the following principal points: B-23 *(Shenshu)*, B-20 *(Pishu)*, Co-4 *(Guanyuan)*, Sp-10 *(Xuehai)*, Co-12 *(Zhongwan)*, K-6 *(Zhaohai)*, Sp-1 *(Yinbai)*, Li-1 *(Dadun)*, Gv-4 *(Mingmen)* and the vertebral points M-BW-35 *(Jiaji)* from the 11th thoracic to the 4th sacral vertebra

Supplementary points: Co-6 *(Qihai)*, Sp-15 *(Daheng)*, S-25 *(Tianshu)*, S-29 *(Guilai)*, Co-3 *(Zhongji)*, Li-3 *(Taichong)*, Sp-3 *(Taibai)*

For pain associated with stagnant Qi and congealed Blood, use these points: Sp-6 *(Sanyinjiao)*, Co-6 *(Qihai)*, LI-4 *(Hegu)*, GB-29 *(Juliao)*, M-BW-24 *(Yaoyan)*, B-18 *(Ganshu)*, Sp-8 *(Diji)*, Co-2 *(Qugu)*, B-31 to 34 *(Shangliao, Ciliao, Zhongliao, Xialiao)* and the vertebral points M-BW-35 *(Jiaji)* from the 11th thoracic to the 4th sacral vertebra

Method: Treat once daily. Use moderate stimulation prior to onset of pain and strong stimulation when pain occurs.

Other prescriptions
1. Difficult menstruation: Co-4 *(Guanyuan)*, Co-3 *(Zhongji)*, S-27 *(Daju)*, S-28 *(Shuidao)*, Sp-10 *(Xuehai)*, Sp-6 *(Sanyinjiao)*. Use a moxa stick or moderate stimulation while retaining the needle. (Source: CAM)
2. Difficult menstruation: Sp-6 *(Sanyinjiao)*, S-36 *(Zusanli)*, Co-4 *(Guanyuan)*, Gv-12 *(Shenzhu)*, B-23 *(Shenshu)*, B-24 *(Qihaishu)*, B-25 *(Dachangshu)*, B-31 *(Shangliao)*, GB-1 *(Tongziliao)*, GB-6 *(Xuanli)*. Use strong stimulation. (Source: NAM)
3. For dizziness and lower abdominal pain accompanying menstruation, use moxa at S-44 *(Neiting)*. (Source: PDM)

Remarks
• The patient should keep warm during the menstrual period and avoid eating raw or cold foods.
• The causes of menstrual pain are numerous. The physician must therefore carefully determine the underlying cause and treat accordingly.
• Acupuncture therapy is quite effective in alleviating the pain associated with this condition.

ABNORMAL UTERINE BLEEDING

In traditional medicine, abnormal uterine bleeding is a condition wherein the Penetrating and Conception channels fail to regulate and retain the Blood in the uterus.

The Liver stores the Blood, the Penetrating channel is the 'sea of Blood', and the Conception channel controls the Blood in the uterus. If the Spleen Qi is Deficient, the Blood is not properly controlled in the vessels. If Heat lodges in the Liver channel, the Blood is not stored. In both cases, the functions of the Penetrating and Conception channels become disrupted and abnormal bleeding results.

Symptoms associated with Deficient Spleen Qi include lassitude, pallid complexion and light red menstrual blood. Symptoms associated with Heat in the Blood include irritability, dizziness and dark red, foul smelling menstrual blood.

Treatment is directed toward regulating the Liver and Spleen so as to retain the Blood and nourish the base of the body's vital functions.

Moxibustion
Principal points: Co-7 *(Yinjiao)*, Sp-6 *(Sanyinjiao)*, B-20 *(Pishu)*, B-18 *(Ganshu)*, Sp-1 *(Yinbai)*
Supplementary points: Gv-4 *(Mingmen)*, Co-4 *(Guanyuan)*, Sp-10 *(Xuehai)*, Li-1 *(Dadun)*, Gv-20 *(Baihui)*
Method: Select 1-3 principal points each session and burn 5-7 small 'grain of rice' sized moxa cones at each point. For Deficient Spleen Qi, burn moxa at Gv-4 *(Mingmen)* and Co-4 *(Guanyuan)*. For Heat in the Blood, add Sp-10 *(Xuehai)* and Li-1 *(Dadun)*. If the quantity of discharge is substantial, add Gv-20 *(Baihui)*.
Discussion of points: Stimulating B-18 *(Ganshu)* and B-20 *(Pishu)*, the Associated points of the Liver and Spleen channels respectively, regulates those Organs. Warming Co-7 *(Yinjiao)* regulates the Penetrating and Conception channels, Sp-1 *(Yinbai)* helps the Spleen control the Blood, and Sp-6 *(Sanyinjiao)* regulates the Blood itself. When the Qi is Deficient, burning moxa at Co-4 *(Guanyuan)* and Gv-4 *(Mingmen)* warms the Kidney Yang. For Heat in the Blood, applying moxa at Sp-10 *(Xuehai)* and Li-1 *(Dadun)* helps to cool the Blood. Excessive discharge indicates that the Qi is weak and sinking. Warming Gv-20 *(Baihui)* serves to raise the Yang (Qi).

Ear acupuncture
Points: Uterus, Subcortex, Endocrine, Ovaries
Method: Retain needles for 1-2 hours with periodic manipulation.

Cutaneous acupuncture
Principal points: Sp-10 *(Xuehai)*, B-17 *(Geshu)*, B-20 *(Pishu)*, Sp-6 *(Sanyinjiao)*, Sp-3 *(Taibai)*,

B-18 *(Ganshu)*, Sp-1 *(Yinbai)*, B-15 *(Xinshu)*, Gv-20 *(Baihui)*, Co-4 *(Guanyuan)*, B-31 to 34 *(Shangliao, Ciliao, Zhongliao, Xialiao)*, and the vertebral points M-BW-35 *(Jiaji)* from the 1st thoracic to the 4th sacral vertebra

Supplementary points: B-23 *(Shenshu)*, Sp-4 *(Gongsun)*, P-6 *(Neiguan)*, Co-6 *(Qihai)*, B-22 *(Sanjiaoshu)*, Li-1 *(Dadun)*

Method: Use the points above in rotation, with strong stimulation. Treat once or twice daily when the discharge occurs.

Foot acupuncture
Points: #20, #26, #30
Method: Retain needles for 1-2 hours with periodic manipulation.

Head acupuncture
Points: Reproduction area, bilaterally
Method: Retain needles for 1-2 hours with periodic manipulation.

Other prescriptions
1. S-36 *(Zusanli)*, Sp-6 *(Sanjinjiao)*, Co-4 *(Guanyuan)*, Co-3 *(Zhongji)*, K-3 *(Taixi)*, L-6 *(Kongzui)*. (Source: HCNMT)
2. B-31 to 34 *(Baliao)*, S-36 *(Zusanli)*, Sp-6 *(Sanyinjiao)*, Sp-10 *(Xuehai)*, Sp-9 *(Yinlingquan)*, B-23 *(Shenshu)*, Co-4 *(Guanyuan)*. (Source: HCNMT)
3. Co-4 *(Guanyuan)*, Sp-6 *(Sanyinjiao)*, Co-3 *(Zhongji)*, Sp-10 *(Xuehai)*, M-CA-18 *(Zigong)*. (Source: HCNMT)
4. Use three small cones of moxa burned directly on M-CA-18 *(Zigong)*, Sp-6 *(Sanyinjiao)*, and Sp-1 *(Yinbai)*. If there is spotting one day and a half after the bleeding stops, burn fifty cones of moxa on Co-4 *(Guanyuan)*, Co-6 *(Qihai)* and Sp-6 *(Sanyinjiao)*. (Source: CAM)
5. Co-6 *(Qihai)*, Li-1 *(Dadun)*, K-10 *(Yingu)*, Co-4 *(Guanyuan)*, Li-3 *(Taichong)*, K-2 *(Rangu)*, Sp-6 *(Sanyinjiao)*, Co-3 *(Zhongji)*, Sp-2 *(Dadu)*, S-12 *(Quepen)*, S-10 *(Shuitu)*, H-1 *(Jiquan)*, P-3 *(Quze)*, B-54 *(Weizhong)*. (Source: NAM)
6. Uterine bleeding: Co-6 *(Qihai)*, Li-1 *(Dadun)*, K-10 *(Yingu)*, Li-3 *(Taichong)*, K-2 *(Rangu)*, Sp-6 *(Sanyinjiao)*, Co-3 *(Zhongji)*. (Source: CDR)
7. Uterine bleeding: Co-3 *(Zhongji)*, M-CA-18 *(Zigong)*. (Source: GCAM)
8. Continuous uterine bleeding: Use moxa on B-17 *(Geshu)*, B-18 *(Ganshu)*, B-23 *(Shenshu)*, Gv-4 *(Mingmen)*, Co-6 *(Qihai)*, Co-3 *(Zhongji)*, P-5 *(Jianshi)*, Sp-10 *(Xuehai)*, K-7 *(Fuliu)*, Li-2 *(Xingjian)*. (Source: IACC).

Remarks
- Acupuncture therapy has proven effective in the treatment of abnormal uterine bleeding.
- When the bleeding is brought under control, it is important that the physician determine and treat the underlying cause.

PROLAPSE OF UTERUS

In Chinese medicine this condition is attributed to weak or sunken Qi of the Middle Burner, such that the Penetrating and Conception channels cannot retain the uterus in place. Alternatively, Damp Heat moves into the Lower Burner and causes the uterus to fall.

Symptoms associated with weakened Qi include pallid complexion, sensitivity to cold, lassitude, palpitations and frequent micturition. Symptoms associated with Damp Heat include irritability, bitter taste, depressed feeling in the chest, and Stomach blockage.

Treatment is directed toward strengthening the Qi so as to raise the uterus.

Needling
Principal points: Gv-20 *(Baihui)*, S-30 *(Qichong)*, GB-28 *(Weidao)*, Sp-6 *(Sanyinjiao)*
Supplementary points: Co-6 *(Qihai)*, Sp-9 *(Yinlingquan)*, Li-3 *(Taichong)*, Li-8 *(Ququan)*

Method: Insert needle at GB-28 *(Weidao)* in a medial, inferior direction using a slanted insertion, to a depth of 1.5-3 units. Insert needle at S-30 *(Qichong)* in an upward direction using a slanted insertion, to a depth of 1.5-3 units. Retain needles for 15-20 minutes with periodic, strong manipulation. Treat once daily. Ten treatments constitute one course. For symptoms of weakened Qi, add Co-6 *(Qihai)*. For symptoms associated with Damp Heat, add Sp-9 *(Yinlingquan)*, Li-3 *(Taichong)* and Li-8 *(Ququan)*. Electro-acupuncture may be used at GB-28 *(Weidao)*, applying relatively strong current in short bursts of stimulation.

Discussion of points: GB-28 *(Weidao)* is the point of intersection of the Girdle channel on the Gall Bladder channel. The needle here should be inserted into the broad uterine ligament. S-30 *(Qichong)* is located over the fallopian ligament and is the point of intersection of the Penetrating channel on the Stomach channel. When the needle is inserted upward at this point, it enters the broad uterine ligament. Gv-20 *(Baihui)* is the point of intersection of the Bladder channel on the Governing channel. Sp-6 *(Sanyinjiao)* is the point of intersection of the three Leg Yin channels. Needling this point strengthens the Spleen. Co-6 *(Qihai)* regulates and strengthens the Source Qi. Li-3 *(Taichong)* and Li-8 *(Ququan)* cool the Heat. Sp-9 *(Yinlingquan)* drains the Damp Excess downward.

Moxibustion
Points: Co-6 *(Qihai)*, Sp-6 *(Sanyinjiao)*
Method: Warm with moxa stick for 10-15 minutes.

Ear acupuncture
Points: Uterus, Kidney, Subcortex
Method: Use intermittent, strong stimulation. Treat once daily. Ten treatments constitute one course.

Injection therapy
Principal points: B-20 *(Pishu)*, B-18 *(Ganshu)*, N-CA-4 *(Tituoxue)*, M-CA-16 *(Weibao)*
Supplementary points: Co-17 *(Shanzhong)*, M-CA-15 *(Qimen)*, Sp-6 *(Sanyinjiao)*
Method: Inject 5% *Angelica sinesis (danggui)* solution into a few points, chosen in rotation. Treat once every other day, alternating the side of the body injected. Insert the needle 0.8-1 unit before injecting medicine. Ten treatments constitute one course.

Embedding thread
Points: Join B-21 *(Weishu)* to B-20 *(Pishu)*, Co-2 *(Qugu)* to K-11 *(Henggu)*, Co-3 *(Zhongji)* to Co-4 *(Guanyuan)*, Co-12 *(Zhongwan)* to Co-13 *(Shangwan)*, M-CA-16 *(Weibao)*
Method: Embed sheep-gut thread at the points above. Allow 20-30 days between treatments.

Other prescriptions
1. Needle M-CA-16 *(Weibao)* inserting the needle in the muscle tissue 2-3 units towards the inguinal canal. The needle sensation should reach the lower abdomen and perineum. Supplementary points: M-CA-18 *(Zigong)* and Sp-6 *(Sanyinjiao)*. (Souce: HNMT)
2. Prolapsed uterus: Li-8 *(Ququan)*, K-6 *(Zhaohai)*, Li-1 *(Dadun)*. (Source: CDR)
3. Postpartum prolpased uterus:Burn 27cones of moxa on a crease beneath the navel, and 7 cones of moxa on K-6 *(Zhaohai)*. (Source: BPW)
4. Prolapsed uterus with itching and pain: Li-8 *(Ququan)* and H-8 *(Shaofu)*. (Source: PDM)

Remarks
• Before acupuncture therapy begins, the prolapsed uterus must be pushed back into the vagina and the buttocks propped up.
• After acupuncture therapy, the patient should lie in a fetal position for 20 minutes.
• Acupuncture therapy is effective in the treatment of mild cases of prolapsed uterus.

LEUKORRHEA

In traditional medicine, this condition is attributed either to a depletion of Qi and Blood, or Dampness and Heat moving into the Lower Burner where they disrupt the Girdle, Penetrating and Conception channels.

Symptoms associated with depleted Qi and Blood include a white, thin discharge, fatigue in the limbs and dizziness. Symptoms associated with Dampness and Heat include a yellow or red discharge, palpitations, and dryness in the mouth.

Treatment is directed toward regulating the Girdle, Penetrating and Conception channels, as well as selecting points for particular symptoms.

Needling
Principal points: GB-26 *(Daimai)*, Sp-6 *(Sanyinjiao)*, Co-6 *(Qihai)*
Supplementary points: Li-2 *(Xingjian)*, Sp-9 *(Yinlingquan)*, Co-4 *(Guanyuan)*, S-36 *(Zusanli)*

Method: Use moderate stimulation, retaining needles up to 15 minutes if desired. Treat once every other day. Ten treatments constitute one course. For symptoms associated with depleted Qi and Blood, add Co-4 *(Guanyuan)* and S-36 *(Zusanli)*. For Dampness and Heat moving into the Lower Burner, add Li-2 *(Xingjian)*, Sp-9 *(Yinlingquan)*. Electro-acupuncture may also be used, connecting one point on the trunk with another on the lower limb. Apply moderate frequency current for 5-10 minutes.

Discussion of points: Needling Co-6 *(Qihai)* strengthens the Qi so as to retain the fluids. GB-26 *(Daimai)* helps to eliminate Dampness, and thereby alleviates the discharge. Sp-6 *(Sanyinjiao)* strengthens and regulates the Qi in the three Leg Yin channels. Li-2 *(Xingjian)* drains the Liver Fire. Sp-9 *(Yinlingquan)* drains Dampness and cools the Heat. Co-4 *(Guanyuan)* strengthens the Source Qi. S-36 *(Zusanli)* regulates the Stomach Qi.

Moxibustion
Points: Gv-4 *(Mingmen)*, Co-8 *(Shenque)*, Co-3 *(Zhongji)*
Method: Warm each point with moxa stick for 5 minutes every other day. Ten to fifteen treatments constitute one course.

Ear acupuncture
Points: Uterus, Bladder
Method: Moderate stimulation on alternating days, 10 treatments constitute a course.

Other prescriptions
1. Co-4 *(Guanyuan)* and Sp-6 *(Sanyinjiao)*; or Co-6 *(Qihai)*, S-29 *(Guilai)*, K-7 *(Fuliu)*; or M-CA-18 *(Zigong)* and Co-3 *(Zhongji)*. Rotate point groups with 10 days constituting one course of treatment. Use moderate stimulation. (Source: HCNMT)

2. Lumps in the abdomen: Co-4 *(Guanyuan)*. Discharge: Co-6 *(Qihai)*, B-27 *(Xiaochangshu)*, Co-7 *(Yinjiao)*. Discharge with irregular periods: B-33 *(Zhongliao)*. Red and white discharge: GB-26 *(Daimai)*, Co-2 *(Qugu)*. (Source: CNLAM)

3. Red and white discharge: Co-6 *(Qihai)*, Co-3 *(Zhongji)*, B-30 *(Baihuanshu)*, B-23 *(Shenshu)*, Sp-6 *(Sanyinjiao)*, GB-35 *(Yangjiao)*. (Source: CDR)

4. Red and white discharge: B-23 *(Shenshu)*, Co-6 *(Qihai)*, Sp-6 *(Sanyinjiao)*, B-30 *(Baihuanshu)*, Co-3 *(Zhongji)*, GB-35 *(Yangjiao)*. (Source: GCAM)

5. Red and white discharge: Burn 7 cones of moxa on Gv-4 *(Mingmen)*, Co-8 *(Qizhong)*, and Co-3 *(Zhongji)*. (Source: IACC)

Remarks
• Acupuncture is definitely effective in the treatment of leukorrhea.

675

● If there is a red or yellow discharge, a thorough gynecological examination should be conducted promptly.

MORNING SICKNESS

According to traditional medicine, when a woman becomes pregnant the Blood in the uterus which no longer passes from the body during menstruation may become 'turbid' and join with Fire in the Stomach and Liver, rebelling upward. Alternatively, Phlegm and Dampness may obstruct the Stomach such that the Qi of that Organ does not properly descend, causing Stomach upset.

Symptoms associated with Fire in the Liver and Stomach rebelling upward include pain in the flanks, depressed feeling in the chest, belching and sighing in discomfort. Phlegm and Dampness obstructing the Stomach is evidenced by a feeling of fullness in the chest and obstruction in the stomach. Food seems tasteless, the fur on the tongue is white and greasy, and the patient may experience palpitations and shortness of breath.

Treatment is directed toward calming the Stomach and moving the Qi.

Needling
Principal points: Co-12 *(Zhongwan)*, P-6 *(Neiguan)*, Sp-4 *(Gongsun)*
Supplementary points: Li-3 *(Taichong)*, S-44 *(Neiting)*, S-40 *(Fenglong)*

Method: Needle the principal points using mild stimulation. Treat once daily, 5-10 treatments constituting one course. For symptoms associated with Fire in the Liver and Stomach, add Li-3 *(Taichong)* and S-44 *(Neiting)*. For Phlegm and Dampness obstructing the Stomach, add S-40 *(Fenglong)*.

Ear acupuncture
Points: Liver, Stomach, Neurogate, Sympathetic
Method: Treat once daily, 5-10 treatments constituting one course.

Cutaneous acupuncture
Principal points: S-34 *(Liangqiu)*, S-36 *(Zusanli)*, P-6 *(Neiguan)*, Co-12 *(Zhongwan)*, Li-3 *(Taichong)*, Sp-4 *(Gongsun)*, B-20 *(Pishu)*, M-HN-3 *(Yintang)*, M-HN-9 *(Taiyang)* and the vertebral points M-BW-35 *(Jiaji)* from the 5th to the 9th thoracic vertebra and from the 1st lumbar to the 4th sacral vertebra
Supplementary points: B-18 *(Ganshu)*, S-44 *(Neiting)*, Co-17 *(Shanzhong)*, Co-13 *(Shangwan)*, B-13 *(Feishu)*
Method: Treat once daily using moderate to strong stimulation, 5-10 treatments constituting one course.

Other prescriptions
1. Severe morning sickness: P-6 *(Neiguan)* joined to TB-5 *(Waiguan)*, moderate stimulation. If appetite is poor, add S-36 *(Zusanli)*. Needle daily. (Source: HNMT)

2. S-36 *(Zusanli)*, P-6 *(Neiguan)*, P-5 *(Jianshi)*, P-7 *(Daling)*, Sp-6 *(Sanyinjiao)*, L-5 *(Chize)*, B-19 *(Danshu)*. During the first five months, Co-12 *(Zhongwan)*, K-21 *(Youmen)*, and Co-11 *(Jianli)* can be added. (Source: NAM)

3. GB-20 *(Fengchi)*, B-18 *(Ganshu)*, B-25 *(Dachangshu)*, B-32 *(Ciliao)*, Co-17 *(Shanzhong)*, S-19 *(Burong)*, K-15 *(Zhongzhu)*, B-10 *(Tianzhu)*, B-19 *(Danshu)*, B-27 *(Xiaochangshu)*, B-33 *(Zhongliao)*, Co-16 *(Zhongting)*, S-20 *(Chengman)*, GB-26 *(Daimai)*. (Source: CAM)

MALPOSITION OF THE FETUS

Treatment of this condition is directed toward regulating the Kidney Qi.

Moxibustion

Point: B-67 *(Zhiyin)*
Method: Warm this point with moxa stick for about 30 minutes daily until the fetus is correctly positioned. During treatment, ask the patient to loosen her clothes at the waist.

An alternative method is to first needle the point with moderate stimulation, then apply moxibustion as described above.

Remarks

• There are many causes of malpositioned fetus, among them deformed uterus, contracted pelvis, tumor, or problems within the fetus itself. The physician should carefully determine the underylying cause and take appropriate measures.

INDUCTION OF LABOR

Treatment is directed toward activating the Blood and Qi so as to strengthen and move the uterus.

Needling

Points: B-31 *(Shangliao)*, B-32 *(Ciliao)*, LI-4 *(Hegu)*, Sp-6 *(Sanyinjiao)*

Method: Use moderate stimulation with continuous needle manipulation for 15-30 minutes. Medium frequency, strong current electro-acupuncture may be used as a substitute for manual manipulation of the needles.

Ear acupuncture

Points: Uterus, Endocrine

Other prescriptions

1. Induction of labor or abortion: Prior to labor, needle Co-4 *(Guanyuan)*, B-32 *(Ciliao)*, LI-4 *(Hegu)*, S-36 *(Zusanli)*, Sp-6 *(Sanyinjiao)*. During labor, needle GB-21 *(Jianjing)*, LI-4 *(Hegu)*, Sp-6 *(Sanyinjaio)*, Li-3 *(Taichong)*, B-60 *(Kunlun)*, B-67 *(Zhiyin)*. (Source: HAM)

2. Inducing labor when the cervix dilates slowly and/or contractions are weak: Use either of the combinations LI-4 *(Hegu)* and S-36 *(Zusanli)*, or Sp-6 *(Sanyinjiao)* and LI-4 *(Hegu)*. After obtaining Qi, stimulate each point strongly for one minute. (Source: HCNMT)

3. Sp-6 *(Sanyinjiao)*, LI-4 *(Hegu)*, Li-3 *(Taichong)*, B-60 *(Kunlun)*, B-67 *(Zhiyin)*. Use strong stimulation. (Source: NAM)

4. Difficult labor: Sp-12 *(Chongmen)*, Li-4 *(Zhongfeng)*, S-30 *(Qichong)*, LI-4 *(Hegu)*, Sp-6 *(Sanyinjiao)*, GB-21 *(Jianjing)*. (Source: PUB)

5. Difficult labor: Use moxa on LI-4 *(Hegu)* and Sp-6 *(Sanyinjiao)*; three cones of moxa on B-67 *(Zhiyin)*. (Source: IACC)

Remarks

• Acupuncture therapy is definitely effective in inducing labor when uterine contractions are slow and weak.

• Body and ear acupuncture may be used simultaneously.

• Because of the many factors which may contribute to causing a difficult delivery, it should be remembered that acupuncture in many cases serves only as a supplementary method of treatment, hastening delivery by strengthening uterine contractions.

INSUFFICIENT LACTATION

In Chinese medicine, a mother's milk is produced by the Qi and Blood in the Penetrating and Conception channels. If, after delivery, lactation is insufficient or suppressed, it is usually because the

Qi and Blood in these channels are Deficient. Alternatively, emotional depression which is associated with the Liver may constrict the vessels and prevent milk from flowing.

Symptoms associated with Deficient Qi and Blood include general weakness in the body, but no distension or pain in the breasts. Depressed Liver Qi, on the other hand, is evidenced by distension and pain in the breasts but otherwise a healthy body.

Treatment is directed toward moving and regulating the Qi and Blood.

Needling
Principal points: Co-17 *(Shanzhong)*, S-18 *(Rugen)*, SI-1 *(Shaoze)*
Supplementary points: B-18 *(Ganshu)*, B-20 *(Pishu)*, S-36 *(Zusanli)*

Method: Needle Co-17 *(Shanzhong)* with a tranverse insertion toward each breast, and S-18 *(Rugen)*, bilaterally, with a transverse insertion toward the breast so that the needle sensation extends in that direction. Use moderate to strong stimulation. Treat once daily, 10 treatments constituting one course. For symptoms of Deficient Qi and Blood, add B-20 *(Pishu)* and S-36 *(Zusanli)*. For symptoms associated with depressed Liver Qi, add B-18 *(Ganshu)*.

Discussion of points: Co-17 *(Shanzhong)* is the Meeting point of the Qi and helps spread the Qi and Blood, thereby inducing lactation. S-18 *(Rugen)* is located at the base of the breast. Stimulating this point facilitates circulation of Qi and Blood through the Stomach channel which crosses the breasts. Needling SI-1 *(Shaoze)* has proved effective in increasing lactation. Needling B-20 *(Pishu)* and S-36 *(Zusanli)* strengthens the Spleen and Stomach so as to produce Blood. B-18 *(Ganshu)* is stimulated to spread the Liver Qi and regulate the Blood.

Moxibustion
Points: Co-17 *(Shanzhong)*, S-18 *(Rugen)*
Method: Warm with moxa stick for 10-20 minutes.

Cutaneous acupuncture
Principal points: B-18 *(Ganshu)*, B-21 *(Weishu)*, Co-17 *(Shanzhong)*, SI-1 *(Shaoze)*, Co-12 *(Zhongwan)*, S-36 *(Zusanli)*, SI-11 *(Tianzong)*, S-18 *(Rugen)*, M-BW-35 *(Jiaji)* from the 5th to the 9th thoracic vertebra and the 1st to the 5th lumbar vertebra, as well as tapping lightly around the perimeter of the breasts
Supplementary points: LI-4 *(Hegu)*, B-20 *(Pishu)*, B-15 *(Xinshu)*, S-42 *(Chongyang)*, Sp-4 *(Gongsun)*
Method: Tap points with moderate stimulation. Treat once daily, 10 treatments constituting one course.

Other prescriptions
1. Abnormal lactation: S-18 *(Rugen)*, SI-15 *(Jianzhongshu)*, B-36 *(Fufen)*, B-37 *(Pohu)*, L-1 *(Zhongfu)*, B-18 *(Ganshu)*, B-15 *(Xinshu)*, H-3 *(Shaohai)*, H-5 *(Tongli)*. (Source: NAM)
2. Women without milk: SI-1 *(Shaoze)*, LI-4 *(Hegu)*, Co-17 *(Shanzhong)*. (Source: GCAM)
3. Lack of milk: Burn moxa on Co-17 *(Shanzhong)* and SI-1 *(Shaoze)*. (Source: GOA)

Remarks
- Acupuncture therapy should be combined with nutritional supplements.
- Acupuncture is relatively effective in the treatment of this condition.

ARTIFICIAL ABORTION

In traditional medicine, treatment is directed toward moving the Qi and Blood so as to induce abortion.

Needling

Prescription #1
   Principal points: LI-4 *(Hegu)*, Sp-6 *(Sanyinjiao)*
   Supplementary points: Gv-1 *(Changqiang)*, Sp-9 *(Yinlingquan)*

Method: Needle LI-4 *(Hegu)* with mild stimulation. Needle Sp-6 *(Sanyinjiao)* with strong stimulation, directing the needle upward so that the sensation extends to the lower abdomen. Use slanted insertion at Gv-1 *(Changqiang)* to a depth of approximately 3 units. Direct the needle upward at this point so that the sensation extends to the lumbosacral region. The needle at Sp-9 *(Yinlingquan)* should also be directed upward so that the sensation reaches the inguinal canal.
   The two principal and two supplementary points should be used in rotation. Treat once daily for 2-3 consecutive days.

Prescription #2
   Principal points: LI-4 *(Hegu)*, Sp-6 *(Sanyinjiao)*
   Supplementary point: B-67 *(Zhiyin)*

Method: Needle LI-4 *(Hegu)* and Sp-6 *(Sanyinjiao)* with strong stimulation for 3-5 minutes, retaining needles with periodic manipulation for 20 minutes thereafter. Alternatively, medium frequency electro-acupuncture may be applied at these points for 20 minutes, twice a day.

Remarks
   • Abortion is considered safest before the 3rd month of pregnancy.

Chapter 8

Diseases of the Eyes, Ears, Nose and Throat

MYOPIA

Treatment of this condition is directed toward regulating the Qi in the channels around the eyes.

Needling
Points: GB-20 *(Fengchi)*, LI-4 *(Hegu)*, B-1 *(Jingming)*, S-1 *(Chengqi)*

Method: Needles placed in the vicinity of the eye should be inserted slowly and with a slight rotating motion, so that the needle sensation is perceived in the eyeball itself. At other points, use moderate stimulation. For GB-20 *(Fengchi)*, best results are obtained if the needle sensation extends as far as the eye region.

Other prescriptions
1. Principal points: S-1 *(Chengqi)*, N-HN-2 *(Xiajingming)*. Supplementary points: S-36 *(Zusanli)*, S-2 *(Sibai)*, LI-4 *(Hegu)*. (Source: HCNMT)
2. M-HN-5 *(Touguangming)* with mild stimulation, retaining the needle for 15 minutes. (Source: HCTM)
3. B-23 *(Shenshu)*, LI-6 *(Pianli)*, Gv-19 *(Houding)*, B-2 *(Zanzhu)*, B-60 *(Kunlun)* for blindness. SI-6 *(Yanglao)*, LI-4 *(Hegu)*, B-4 *(Quchai)*, GB-20 *(Fengchi)*, B-5 *(Wuchu)* for blurred vision. K-5 *(Shuiquan)* for myopia in women. (Source: CNLAM)

Remarks
- Acupuncture therapy is definitely effective in treating non-congenital myopia in the early stages.

COLOR BLINDNESS

Traditional medicine refers to color blindness as the 'see red as white' condition. It is attributed to prenatal malnutrition.
Treatment is directed toward spreading and regulating the Qi in the channels.

Needling
Points: GB-20 *(Fengchi)*, LI-3 *(Sanjian)*, B-2 *(Zanzhu)*, N-HN-6 *(Waiming)*

Method: Insert the needle at N-HN-6 *(Waiming)* slowly, with a slight rotating motion. Use moderate stimulation at other points. At GB-20 *(Fengchi)*, best results are obtained if the needle sensation extends as far as the eye region. Retain needles for 10-20 minutes. Treat on alternating days, 15-20 treatments constituting one course.

Remarks
- This condition has no specific method of cure. The effectiveness of acupuncture therapy is difficult to establish at this time.

GLAUCOMA

Chinese medicine attributes glaucoma to a depletion of the Kidney Yin which causes Wind and Fire in the Liver and Gall Bladder to ascend, disrupting the Qi in the channels.

Treatment is directed toward dispersing Wind to clear the vision, and nourishing the Yin to suppress Fire.

Needling
Principal points: GB-20 *(Fengchi)*, B-2 *(Zanzhu)*, GB-1 *(Tongziliao)*, LI-4 *(Hegu)*, Li-3 *(Taichong)*, K-3 *(Taixi)*, Sp-6 *(Sanyinjiao)*, B-18 *(Ganshu)*
Supplementary points: B-63 *(Jinmen)*, B-62 *(Shenmai)*, Li-2 *(Xingjian)*, S-36 *(Zusanli)*

Method: First needle the principal points with moderate to strong stimulation, retaining needles 15-20 minutes with periodic manipulation. Treat once daily or on alternating days. For acute cases, add B-63 *(Jinmen)*, B-62 *(Shenmai)* and Li-2 *(Xingjian)*. For chronic cases, use S-36 *(Zusanli)*.

Discussion of points: B-2 *(Zanzhu)*, GB-1 *(Tongziliao)* and GB-20 *(Fengchi)* are selected as local points near the eyes. LI-4 *(Hegu)* is the Source point of the Large Intestine channel and is needled to disperse the Wind so as to clear the vision. Needling Li-3 *(Taichong)* and B-18 *(Ganshu)* neutralizes the Fire in the Gall Bladder and Liver. Sp-6 *(Sanyinjiao)* and K-3 *(Taixi)* help nourish the Yin to suppress Fire. Li-2 *(Xingjian)* is added to drain the Liver Fire in acute cases. B-63 *(Jinmen)* and B-62 *(Shenmai)* assist in draining the Fire from the region of the eyes.

Ear acupuncture
Principal points: Allergy, Liver, Eye, Lower Blood Pressure Groove
Supplementary points: Vision #1, Vision #2
Method: First needle the principal points. If the result is unsatisfactory, add the supplementary points. Prick the Lower Blood Pressure Groove to let a few drops of blood. Treat once daily or on alternating days.

Cutaneous acupuncture
This method is suitable for chronic glaucoma only. Tap with firmness along the Bladder channel on the back for several minutes daily or on alternating days. Ten treatments constitute one course.

Other prescriptions
1. Principal points: M-HN-8 *(Qiuhou)*, GB-20 *(Fengchi)*. Supplementary points: B-1 *(Jingming)*, M-HN-9 *(Taiyang)*, GB-8 *(Shuaigu)*, LI-11 *(Quchi)*. For acute cases, needle once or twice a day. (Source: HNMT)
2. GB-20 *(Fengchi)*, GB-6 *(Xuanli)*, B-10 *(Tianzhu)*, GB-14 *(Yangbai)*, TB-16 *(Tianyou)*, GB-16 *(Muchuang)*, S-2 *(Sibai)*. (Source: NAM)
3. Internal obstruction of green Wind with blindness use B-8 *(Luoque)*. (Source: CNLAM)

Remarks
- Acupuncture can alleviate the headache, vomiting and other symptoms associated with this condition. It is definitely effective in the treatment of glaucoma in its early stages. However, if allowed to progress to more severe stages, other methods must be considered in addition to acupuncture.

CONJUNCTIVITIS

Traditional medicine attributes conjunctivitis to Wind and Heat. If these Excesses are not cleansed from the body, an acute condition will become chronic. Overindulgence in alcohol, overuse of the eyes, exposure to wind, poor lighting, and inadequate sleep may all contribute to making the conjunctivitis chronic.

Treatment is directed toward dispersing and draining the Wind and Heat.

Needling

Principal points: GB-20 *(Fengchi)*, M-HN-9 *(Taiyang)*, LI-4 *(Hegu)*
Supplementary points: B-1 *(Jingming)*, GB-8 *(Shuaigu)*

Method: First needle GB-20 *(Fengchi)* until the patient feels a rather strong sensation of soreness and heaviness in the vicinity of the point, then withdraw the needle. M-HN-9 *(Taiyang)* may either be pricked to let a few drops of blood, or joined to GB-8 *(Shuaigu)* with a transverse insertion of the needle. Use mild stimulation at LI-4 *(Hegu)* and B-1 *(Jingming)*. Retain needles for 10-15 minutes. Treat once daily.

Ear acupuncture

1st Prescription
Points: Liver, Eye, Vision #2
Method: Use moderate to strong stimulation. Treat once daily.

2nd prescription
Points: Temple, Ear Apex, Lower Blood Pressure Groove and the posterior auricular veins
Method: Select one point, bilaterally, and prick to let 2-3 drops of blood. Treat once daily.

Piercing method

For piercing, select a point of tenderness between the shoulder blades, a point .5 unit beside Gv-14 *(Dazhui)*, or a point along the frontal branch of the superficial temporal artery between the eyebrows or on the upper eyelid.

Barefoot doctor acupuncture
Points: Barefoot Doctor point, Tip of Tragus
Method: Treat once daily.

Other prescriptions

1. GB-20 *(Fengchi)*, B-2 *(Zanzhu)*, B-1 *(Jingming)*, M-HN-9 *(Taiyang)*, LI-4 *(Hegu)*, GB-37 *(Guangming)*. Use moderate stimulation. (Source: CAM)

2. TB-23 *(Sizhukong)*, GB-1 *(Tongziliao)*, GB-14 *(Yangbai)*, B-1 *(Jingming)*, S-2 *(Sibai)*, P-7 *(Daling)*, LI-4 *(Hegu)*, LI-20 *(Yingxiang)*, LI-5 *(Yangxi)*, GB-42 *(Diwuhui)*, GB-4 *(Hanyan)*, B-10 *(Tianzhu)*, GB-20 *(Fengchi)*, Gv-14 *(Dazhui)*, Gv-12 *(Shenzhu)*, B-18 *(Ganshu)*, B-20 *(Pishu)*. (Source: NAM)

3. Red eyes: B-60 *(Kunlun)*, K-3 *(Taixi)*, LI-5 *(Yangxi)*, P-7 *(Daling)*, B-1 *(Jingming)*, SI-3 *(Houxi)*, GB-1 *(Tongziliao)*, GB-16 *(Muchuang)*. Red and painful eyes: B-2 *(Zanzhu)*, TB-2 *(Yemen)*. Red, painful, and swollen eyes: B-62 *(Shenmai)*, Li-3 *(Taichong)*, Li-8 *(Ququan)*, LI-5 *(Yangxi)*. Red and painful canthi: GB-6 *(Xuanli)*. Red and painful inner canthus: GB-20 *(Fengchi)*, B-18 *(Ganshu)*, Gv-23 *(Shangxing)*. Red outer canthus, dizziness: GB-43 *(Xiaxi)*. (Source: CNLAM)

4. Eyes suddenly becoming red, swollen, and painful: Gv-24 *(Shenting)*, Gv-23 *(Shangxing)*, Gv-22 *(Xinhui)*, Gv-21 *(Qianding)*, prick Gv-20 *(Baihui)*, GB-37 *(Guangming)*, GB-42 *(Diwuhui)*. (Source: OM)

5. Eyes suddenly becoming red, swollen, and painful: Prick M-HN-9 *(Taiyang)*, apply moxa on

M-UE-15 *(Dagukong)* and M-UE-17 *(Xiaogukong).* (Source: JDC)

6. Red, swollen, and painful eyes with diminishing vision: Apply moxa on LI-4 *(Hegu),* LI-2 *(Erjian),* B-18 *(Ganshu),* and S-36 *(Zusanli).* (Source: PDM)

Remarks
- During acupuncture treatment for acute conjunctivitis, the eyes can be bathed with a cold saline solution.

ELECTRIC OPTHALMIA

Treatment of this condition is directed toward dispersing the Wind and Heat.

Needling
Principal points: LI-4 *(Hegu),* GB-20 *(Fengchi),* M-HN-9 *(Taiyang)*
Supplementary points: B-1 *(Jingming),* B-2 *(Zanzhu),* S-2 *(Sibai),* GB-37 *(Guangming)*

Method: First needle principal points with moderate to strong stimulation, retaining needles for 30 minutes with periodic manipulation. Add supplementary points as needed.

Barefoot doctor acupuncture
Points: Barefoot Doctor point, Tip of Tragus

Ear acupuncture
Points: Eye, Liver, Vision #1, Vision #2, Subcortex
Method: Use moderate to strong stimulation, retaining needles for 20-30 minutes.

OPTIC NEURITIS OR ATROPHY

In traditional medicine the pattern which corresponds to optic neuritis ('sudden blindness') is attributed to depleted Yin of the Liver and Kidneys which causes the Yang Excess, Wind, to ascend recklessly. Optic atrophy ('green blindness'), on the other hand, is said to be caused by the exhaustion of Qi and Blood which denies nourishment to the eyes.

Treatment is directed toward nourishing and strengthening the Liver and Kidneys.

Needling
Principal points: GB-20 *(Fengchi),* M-HN-8 *(Qiuhou),* B-1 *(Jingming),* LI-4 *(Hegu)*
Supplementary points: S-1 *(Chengqi),* B-18 *(Ganshu),* B-23 *(Shenshu),* S-36 *(Zusanli),* GB-37 *(Guangming)*

Method: At points near the eye, insert needles slowly and with slight rotation so as to cause the needle sensation to expand into the eyeball. At other points, use moderate stimulation. Retain needles for 10-15 minutes. Treat once every other day, 15-20 treatments constituting one course.

Ear acupuncture
Points: Eye, Liver, Vision #1, Vision #2, Subcortex
Method: Use moderate stimulation, retaining needles 10-15 minutes. Treat once daily or on alternating days, 15-20 treatments constituting one course.

Other prescriptions
1. Optic neuritis: Principal points—M-HN-8 *(Qiuhou),* B-1 *(Jingming),* S-1 *(Chengqi),* N-HN-34 *(Xinzanzhu).* Supplementary points—GB-20 *(Fengchi),* M-HN-9 *(Taiyang),* LI-4 *(Hegu).* Use moderate stimulation. (Source: HCNMT)

2. Atrophy of optic nerve: Principal points—B-1 *(Jingming)*, M-HN-8 *(Qiuhou)*. Supplementary points—N-HN-1 *(Shangjingming)*, GB-20 *(Fengchi)*, M-HN-13 *(Yiming)*. Use mild stimulation. (Source: HCNMT)

3. Atrophy of optic nerve: Principal points—N-HN-1 *(Shangjingming)*, M-HN-8 *(Qiuhou)*. Supplementary points—M-HN-9 *(Taiyang)*, GB-20 *(Fengchi)*, LI-4 *(Hegu)*, GB-37 *(Guangming)*. Electro-acupuncture may be used. Frequency should be set at 200-250 pulses per minute for 15-20 minutes. Treat on alternating days, 7 treatments constituting one course. One week should separate each course. (Source: SCM)

4. Green blindness: LI-1 *(Shangyang)*, S-3 *(Juliao)*, GB-3 *(Shangguan)*, GB-1 *(Tongziliao)*, B-8 *(Luoque)*, B-6 *(Chengguang)*. (Source: CNLAM)

5. Green blindness: Apply 7 cones of moxa on B-18 *(Ganshu)*, B-19 *(Danshu)*, B-23 *(Shenshu)*, and SI-6 *(Yanglao)*; 5 cones of moxa on LI-1 *(Shangyang)*, GB-37 *(Guangming)*. (Source: IACC)

6. Sudden blindness: Needle B-2 *(Zanzhu)*, Gv-24 *(Shenting)*, Gv-23 *(Shangxing)*, Gv-22 *(Xinhui)*, Gv-21 *(Qianding)*, and Gv-20 *(Baihui)*. Prick B-54 *(Weizhong)*. (Source: CDP)

Remarks

• Acupuncture prescriptions for optic atrophy and optic neuritis are largely interchangeable.

STRABISMUS

Treatment of this condition is directed toward regulating the muscles of the eyes.

Needling

Points: For internal strabismus, use GB-20 *(Fengchi)*, LI-4 *(Hegu)* and M-HN-8 *(Qiuhou)*. For external strabismus, use GB-20 *(Fengchi)*, LI-4 *(Hegu)* and N-HN-3 *(Jianming)*.

Method: At points near the eyes, insert needles slowly and with slight rotation. Very mild electro-acupuncture stimulation may be used for a short time. For points on the limbs, use moderate stimulation, retaining needles for 10-15 minutes. Treat once every other day, 15-20 treatments constituting one course.

Barefoot doctor acupuncture

Points: Barefoot Doctor point, Tip of Tragus
Method: Treat once every other day, 15-20 treatments constituting one course.

Other prescriptions

1. External strabismus: B-1 *(Jingming)*, S-2 *(Sibai)* joined to N-HN-2 *(Xiajingming)*. (Source: HCNMT)

2. Internal strabismus: M-HN-8 *(Qiuhou)*, M-HN-9 *(Taiyang)*. Supplementary points: TB-3 *(Zhongzhu)*, LI-4 *(Hegu)*. Treat daily. (Source: HCNMT)

Remarks

• Acupuncture therapy is only a supplementary method for the treatment of this condition. For paralytic strabismus, further examination will be necessary to determine the proper therapy. For concomitant strabismus, acupuncture may be combined with corrective glasses.

AURAL VERTIGO (Meniere's Disease)

Traditional medicine attributes aural vertigo to Phlegm and Dampness obstructing the Middle Burner and suppressing the 'cleansing' Yang Qi (i.e., the Qi of respiration which is said to rise to the eyes, ears, nose and mouth so as to maintain clarity in the senses).

Alternatively, this condition may arise from depletion of Kidney Yin which causes the Liver Yang, in the form of Wind, to ascend.

Symptoms associated with Phlegm and Dampness include nausea and vomiting. Vertigo induced by depleted Kidney Yin and ascendant Liver Yang is evidenced by dizziness, headache, blurred vision and tinnitus.

Treatment is directed toward clearing and draining the Wind, while spreading and regulating the Qi in the channels.

Needling

Principal points: GB-20 *(Fengchi)*, Li-3 *(Taichong)*, TB-17 *(Yifeng)*, SI-19 *(Tinggong)*, P-6 *(Neiguan)*

Supplementary points: S-36 *(Zusanli)*, Co-12 *(Zhongwan)*, K-3 *(Taixi)*, N-HN-54 *(Anmian)*

Method: Needle principal points continuously for 10-30 minutes with moderate to strong stimulation. Treat once daily, 5-7 treatments constituting one course. For symptoms of Phlegm and Dampness, add S-36 *(Zusanli)* and Co-12 *(Zhongwan)*, For symptoms of depleted Kidney Yin and ascendant Liver Yang, add K-3 *(Taixi)* and N-HN-54 *(Anmian)*. Electro-acupuncture may be used at points in the vicinity of the ear. Use relatively high frequency and moderate strength current.

Discussion of points: Needling GB-20 *(Fengchi)* and Li-3 *(Taichong)* extinguishes the Wind, while needling TB-17 *(Yifeng)* and SI-19 *(Tinggong)* restores circulation of the Qi in the channels surrounding the ear. Stimulating P-6 *(Neiguan)* calms the Stomach and alleviates vomiting. S-36 *(Zusanli)* and Co-12 *(Zhongwan)* strengthen the Spleen and Stomach so as to disperse the Phlegm. K-3 *(Taixi)* nourishes the Kidneys, and N-HN-54 *(Anmian)* calms the Spirit.

Ear acupuncture

Points: Forehead, Heart, Sympathetic, Neurogate, Kidney, Endocrine, Adrenal, Occiput

Method: Select 2-4 points each session. Use moderate to strong stimulation, retaining needles for 15-20 minutes with periodic manipulation. Treat once daily, 5-7 treatments constituting one course. Intradermal needles may be used. Alternatively, vitamin B1 may be injected daily into the ear points. Select 2-3 points each session. Ten to fifteen treatments constitute one course.

Head acupuncture

Points: Vertigo and Hearing area, bilaterally

Method: Treat once daily, 5-10 treatments constituting one course.

Cutaneous acupuncture

Principal points: B-18 *(Ganshu)*, Gv-20 *(Baihui)*, B-67 *(Zhiyin)*, M-HN-9 *(Taiyang)*, Co-6 *(Qihai)*, Co-4 *(Guanyuan)*, S-36 *(Zusanli)*, Li-1 *(Dadun)*, TB-17 *(Yifeng)*, M-HN-3 *(Yintang)* and the vertebral points M-BW-35 *(Jiaji)* from the 5th to the 4th sacral vertebra

Supplementary points: B-23 *(Shenshu)*, H-7 *(Shenmen)*, LI-4 *(Hegu)*, Gv-23 *(Shangxing)*, S-34 *(Liangqiu)*, Gv-16 *(Fengfu)*, B-14 *(Jueyinshu)*

Method: Tap once or twice daily with moderate stimulation. Five to ten treatments constitute one course.

Injection therapy

Points: TB-17 *(Yifeng)*, SI-19 *(Tinggong)*

Method: Inject a compound of vitamins B3 and B12 into one of the two points. Treat once every other day, rotating the points.

Other prescriptions

1. Group 1: LI-4 *(Hegu)*, Li-3 *(Taichong)*, M-HN-13 *(Yiming)*. Group 2: P-6 *(Neiguan)*, GB-20 *(Fengchi)*, TB-9 *(Sidu)*. Rotate groups daily. Use strong stimulation. (Source: HNMT)

2. GB-20 *(Fengchi)*, B-23 *(Shenshu)*, LI-4 *(Hegu)*, S-40 *(Fenglong)*, S-41 *(Jiexi)*, B-62 *(Shenmai)*. (Source: HAM)

3. Head spinning: GB-16 *(Muchuang)*, B-8 *(Luoque)*, Gv-20 *(Baihui)*, B-62 *(Shenmai)*, B-67 *(Zhiyin)*. (Source: CDR)

4. Head spinning and ringing in the ears: B-8 *(Luoque)*. Dizziness: B-58 *(Feiyang)*, B-13 *(Feishu)*. Dizziness with headache: SI-7 *(Zhizheng)*, B-22 *(Sanjiaoshu)*. (Source: CNLAM)

5. Dizziness: Gv-24 *(Shenting)*, Gv-23 *(Shangxing)*, Gv-22 *(Xinhui)*, Gv-21 *(Qianding)*, Gv-19 *(Houding)*, GB-19 *(Naokong)*, GB-20 *(Fengchi)*, SI-5 *(Yanggu)*, Sp-2 *(Dadu)*, B-67 *(Zhiyin)*, B-63 *(Jinmen)*, B-62 *(Shenmai)*, S-36 *(Zusanli)*. (Source: OM)

6. Dizziness: Apply moxa on H-5 *(Tongli)* and S-41 *(Jiexi)*. (Source: IACC)

Remarks
- During an attack, reduce water and salt intake.
- Acupuncture therapy is definitely effective in treating this condition.

DEAF-MUTISM

Treatment of this condition in traditional medicine is directed toward restoring the circulation of Qi through the channels which are connected with the ears and tongue.

Needling
Principal points: TB-21 *(Ermen)*, SI-19 *(Tinggong)*, GB-2 *(Tinghui)*, TB-17 *(Yifeng)*, Gv-15 *(Yamen)*, Co-23 *(Lianquan)*
Supplementary points: LI-4 *(Hegu)*, TB-3 *(Zhongzhu)*, TB-5 *(Waiguan)*

Method: Select 1-2 points from among those in the vicinity of the ear. Before needling, ask the patient to open his or her mouth. Insert needles about 1.5-2 units deep. Treat once daily, 10 treatments constituting one course. Allow one week rest, then resume treatment. If hearing ability begins to improve, add Gv-15 *(Yamen)* and Co-23 *(Lianquan)*. Electro-acupuncture may also be applied at the points in the vicinity of the ear. Use a low frequency, medium strength current for a short time only.

Discussion of points: The first four principal points are all situated in the vicinity of the ear. Thus, stimulation of these points helps restore circulation of the Qi in the channels connected with the ear. Gv-15 *(Yamen)* is useful in the treatment of mutism, and Co-23 *(Lianquan)* restores functioning to the tongue. The Triple Burner channel enters the ear. TB-3 *(Zhongzhu)* and TB-5 *(Waiguan)*, situated on this channel, are helpful in the treatment of ear diseases. Likewise, the Large Intestine channel enters the ear and connects with other channels there. LI-4 *(Hegu)*, on the Large Intestine channel, is therefore an effective supplementary point in the treatment of this condition.

Embedding needles
Points: TB-18 *(Qimai)*, TB-17 *(Yifeng)*, M-HN-13 *(Yiming)*, SI-19 *(Tinggong)*
Method: Select 1-2 points for treatment once each day. Embed intradermal needles for 24 hours in points located behind the ear, and for 12 hours in those in front of the ear.

Injection therapy
Points: SI-19 *(Tinggong)*, GB-12 *(Wangu);* or GB-2 *(Tinghui)*, TB-18 *(Qimai);* or TB-21 *(Ermen)*, TB-17 *(Yifeng)*
Method: Select one point grouping each day, in rotation. Inject the following medicine into each of the points at a depth of about 1-2 units: vitamin B12 or anisodamine.

Other prescriptions

[These prescriptions are derived from the Peoples Liberation Army hospitals.]

1. Congenital deafness (total or unilateral): Principal points—TB-21 *(Ermen)*, TB-17 *(Yifeng)*, Gv-15 *(Yamen)*, TB-3 *(Zhongzhu)*, TB-5 *(Waiguan)*. Supplementary points—M-HN-13 *(Yiming)*,

LI-11 *(Quchi)*, Gv-20 *(Baihui)*, Gv-26 *(Renzhong)*, and 3 vertebral points lateral to the spinous processes of the 4th cervical, 2nd thoracic and 2nd lumbar vertebrae.

Method: Treat daily. The points around the ear are stimulated first mildly, then strongly. Insert needle at TB-21 *(Ermen)* with transverse insertion, anteriorly and downward 2-3 units. TB-3 *(Zhongzhu)* and TB-5 *(Waiguan)* are used in rotation. If the supplementary points are used, select 1-2 for each treatment, with moderate stimulation.

2. Trauma-induced deafness (total or unilateral deafness or loss of hearing): Group 1—TB-21 *(Ermen)*, Gv-15 *(Yamen)*, TB-3 *(Zhongzhu)*. Group 2—S-7 *(Xiaguan)*, TB-17 *(Yifeng)*, Co-23 *(Lianquan)*.

Method: Rotate the two groups. Insert needle at TB-21 *(Ermen)* with transverse insertion, anteriorly and downwards 2-3 units. S-7 *(Xiaguan)* is joined posteriorly to SI-19 *(Tinggong)*.

3. Trauma-induced tinnitus: TB-21 *(Ermen)*, TB-17 *(Yifeng)*, Gv-15 *(Yamen)*, TB-3 *(Zhongzhu)*, Gv-14 *(Dazhui)*, P-9 *(Zhongchong)*, LI-11 *(Quchi)*, H-7 *(Shenmen)*, B-23 *(Shenshu)*, S-36 *(Zusanli)*.

Method: Needle daily. Use only 2 of the last 7 points above during any one treatment.

4. Drug-induced deafness: TB-21 *(Ermen)*, M-HN-13 *(Yiming)*, TB-3 *(Zhongzhu)*, TB-5 *(Waiguan)*, GB-2 *(Tinghui)*, TB-18 *(Qimai)*, Gv-15 *(Yamen)*, N-LE-17 *(Lingxia)*, TB-9 *(Sidu)*.

Method: Insert at TB-21 *(Ermen)* as described above. GB-2 *(Tinghui)* is joined to SI-19 *(Tinggong)*. The other points are used in rotation. Moderate stimulation.

5. Drug-induced tinnitus: M-HN-13 *(Yiming)*, TB-20 *(Jiaosun)*, H-7 *(Shenmen)*, Gv-14 *(Dazhui)*.

Method: Join M-HN-13 *(Yiming)* to TB-17 *(Yifeng)*. Use mild stimulation.

6. Drug-induced dizziness: Gv-15 *(Yamen)*, M-HN-13 *(Yiming)*, LI-4 *(Hegu)*, GB-20 *(Fengchi)*, Gv-20 *(Baihui)*, TB-9 *(Sidu)*.

Method: Rotate two groups of points. Use mild stimulation.

7. Deafness from otitis media (deafness, mutism, hearing loss): TB-21 *(Ermen)*, TB-17 *(Yifeng)*, TB-3 *(Zhongzhu)*, TB-5 *(Waiguan)*, Gv-15 *(Yamen)*.

Method: Insert at TB-21 *(Ermen)* as described above. Points on the upper extremities are used in rotation. Gv-15 *(Yamen)* is only used in cases of mutism.

8. Tinnitus from otitis media: TB-21 *(Ermen)*, Gv-15 *(Yamen)*, TB-3 *(Zhongzhu)*, M-HN-13 *(Yiming)*, LI-11 *(Quchi)*, Gv-14 *(Dazhui)*, S-36 *(Zusanli)*.

Method: Insert at TB-21 *(Ermen)* as described above. Use 2 of the other points each treatment. Mild stimulation. If the tympanic membrane is retracted, add S-7 *(Xiaguan)*. If there is suppurative inflammation, needle and moxi TB-17 *(Yifeng)*.

9. Deafness, mutism after infectious disease: TB-21 *(Ermen)*, S-7 *(Xiaguan)*.

Method: Insert at TB-21 *(Ermen)* as described above. Use moderate stimulation.

10. Hearing loss after infectious disease: TB-21 *(Ermen)*, TB-17 *(Yifeng)*, TB-3 *(Zhongzhu)*, TB-5 *(Waiguan)*.

Method: Insert at TB-21 *(Ermen)* as described above. Upper extremity points are used in rotation. Mild stimulation.

11. Tinnitus after infectious disease: S-7 *(Xiaguan)*, GB-20 *(Fengchi)*, TB-20 *(Jiaosun)*, Gv-20 *(Baihui)*, M-HN-13 *(Yiming)*, TB-18 *(Qimai)*, SI-19 *(Tinggong)*, H-7 *(Shenmen)*, S-36 *(Zusanli)*, Gv-20 *(Baihui)*.

Method: Insert at TB-21 *(Ermen)* as described above.

Remarks
- When needling Gv-15 *(Yamen)*, extreme caution must be observed regarding both the direction and depth of needle insertion.
- After hearing ability has been restored, further speech therapy is necessary.

TINNITUS, DEAFNESS

In traditional medicine, these disorders are primarily attributed to two causes. Fire in the Liver and Gall Blader can generate Phlegm and ascend, disrupting the functions in the head. Or, Deficient Kidneys may cause the Yang to rise to the head. The former is a condition of Excess, the latter a condition of Deficiency.

Symptoms associated with Fire in the Liver and Gall Bladder include dizziness, fever, insomnia, soreness in the waist and weakness in the knees.

Treatment is directed toward nourishing the Yin and restraining the Yang.

Needling
Principal points: TB-17 *(Yifeng)*, GB-20 *(Fengchi)*, TB-3 *(Zhongzhu)*
Supplementary points: Li-2 *(Xingjian)*, S-40 *(Fenglong)*, K-3 *(Taixi)*, B-23 *(Shenshu)*

Method: Needle the principal points with moderate stimulation once every other day. Ten to fifteen treatments constitute one course. For symptoms of Fire in the Liver and Gall Bladder, add Li-2 *(Xingjian)* and S-40 *(Fenglong)*. For symptoms associated with Deficient Kidneys, add B-23 *(Shenshu)* and K-3 *(Taixi)*.

Injection therapy
Points: TB-17 *(Yifeng)* or GB-20 *(Fengchi)*
Method: Inject vitamin B1, vitamin B12, anisodamine or procaine hydrochloride at one of the points. For tinnitus due to old age, inject procaine hydrochloride. Rotate the points. Treat once every 3 days. Ten treatments constitute one course. An allergy test should be given prior to injecting procaine hydrochloride.

Ear acupuncture
Points: Ear, Inner Ear, Neurogate, Kidney, Endocrine, Occiput
Method: Treat once daily with moderate stimulation. Ten to fifteen treatments constitute one course.

Other prescriptions
1. For tinnitus and deafness: GB-3 *(Shangguan)*, S-7 *(Xiaguan)*, S-2 *(Sibai)*, Gv-20 *(Baihui)*, Gv-22 *(Xinhui)*, TB-17 *(Yifeng)*, TB-21 *(Ermen)*, GB-4 *(Hanyan)*, SI-16 *(Tianchuang)*, LI-5 *(Yangxi)*, TB-1 *(Guanchong)*, TB-2 *(Yemen)*, TB-3 *(Zhongzhu)*. (Source: TDP)
2. Sound of cicada in the ears: SI-17 *(Tianrong)*, GB-2 *(Tinghui)*, SI-19 *(Tinggong)*, TB-3 *(Zhongzhu)*. Ringing in the ears: SI-4 *(Wangu)*, SI-5 *(Yanggu)*, SI-9 *(Jianzhen)*, GB-11 *(Qiaoyin)*, GB-43 *(Xiaxi)*, LI-1 *(Shangyang)*, LI-5 *(Yangxi)*, B-8 *(Luoque)*, SI-2 *(Qiangu)*. (Source: CNLAM)
3. Ringing in the ears: Gv-20 *(Baihui)*, GB-2 *(Tinghui)*, SI-19 *(Tinggong)*, TB-21 *(Ermen)*, B-8 *(Luoque)*, LI-5 *(Yangxi)*, SI-5 *(Yanggu)*, SI-3 *(Houxi)*, SI-4 *(Wangu)*, TB-3 *(Zhongzhu)*. Indistinct hearing: TB-21 *(Ermen)*, TB-17 *(Yifeng)*, GB-20 *(Fengchi)*, GB-43 *(Xiaxi)*, GB-2 *(Tinghui)*, SI-19 *(Tinggong)*. (Source: CDR)
4. Deafness: 14 cones of moxa on Gv-23 *(Shangxing)*; 7 cones of moxa on TB-17 *(Yifeng)*. SI-19 *(Tinggong)*, B-23 *(Shenshu)*, TB-5 *(Waiguan)*, LI-6 *(Pianli)*, LI-4 *(Hegu)*. (Source: IACC)

Remarks
- Acupuncture therapy is definitely effective in the treatment of neural deafness and tinnitus.

RHINITIS

According to traditional medicine, treatment of rhinitis is directed toward dispersing the Excesses so as to clear the nasal cavity.

Needling
Points: M-HN-3 *(Yintang)*, LI-4 *(Hegu)*, LI-20 *(Yingxiang)*, M-HN-14 *(Bitong)*

Method: Use points in rotation, applying moderate to strong stimulation. Treat once every other day.

Discussion of points: M-HN-3 *(Yintang)*, LI-20 *(Yingxiang)* and M-HN-14 *(Bitong)* are all local points in the vicinity of the nose. Needling these points will clear the nasal cavity. Stimulating LI-4 *(Hegu)* disperses the Wind and Exterior condition. Furthermore, inasmuch as this point is situted on the Large Intestine channel which enters the nose, needling this point contributes to opening the nasal passages.

Injection therapy
Points: Same points as needling method above
Method: Inject vitamin B complex into one of the points.

Ear acupuncture
Points: Inner Nose, Adrenal, Endocrine
Method: First, try to find the specific site of tenderness in the vicinity of each of these points. Use moderate to strong stimulation, retaining needles for one hour. Alternatively, intradermal needles may be embedded at the points for one week.

Other prescriptions
1. Chronic rhinitis: GB-20 *(Fengchi)*, Gv-23 *(Shangxing)*, M-HN-3 *(Yintang)*, LI-20 *(Yingxiang)*, LI-4 *(Hegu)*. (Source: HAM)
2. GB-20 *(Fengchi)*, B-10 *(Tianzhu)*, Gv-23 *(Shangxing)*, LI-20 *(Yingxiang)*, LI-4 *(Hegu)*. Use moderate stimulation. Moxa can also be applied on Gv-23 *(Shangxing)*. (Source: CAM)
3. GB-20 *(Fengchi)*, B-10 *(Tianzhu)*, Gv-14 *(Dazhui)*, Gv-16 *(Fengfu)*, B-12 *(Fengmen)*, LI-19 *(Heliao)*, LI-20 *(Yingxiang)*, LI-4 *(Hegu)*, Gv-20 *(Baihui)*, P-8 *(Laogong)*, SI-2 *(Qiangu)*. (Source: NAM)
4. Loss of smell: Tip of nose, B-13 *(Feishu)*, LI-20 *(Yingxiang)*. Inject 5% *Angelica sinesis* fluid every other day. Alternate sides. (Source: SCM)

Remarks
• Acupuncture is definitely effective in treating rhinitis, whether acute or chronic.

CHRONIC SINUSITIS

Traditional medicine attributes this condition to Wind and Cold which attack the Lungs and disrupt the 'cleansing' function of that Organ. Alternatively, this condition may arise from Heat in the Lungs, or Fire in the Liver and Gall Bladder, which ascends to the Head.

Treatment is directed toward clearing the Lungs and nasal cavities.

Needling
Principal points: LI-20 *(Yingxiang)*, B-2 *(Zanzhu)*, B-7 *(Tongtian)*

Supplementary points: GB-30 *(Fengchi)*, LI-4 *(Hegu)*, Li-2 *(Xingjian)*, L-7 *(Lieque)*

Method: Use moderate to strong stimulation. Treat once every other day, 10-15 treatments constituting one course. For symptoms associated with Heat in the Lungs (coughing with sputum), add L-7 *(Lieque)* and LI-4 *(Hegu)*. For Fire in the Liver and Gall Bladder, add GB-20 *(Fengchi)* and Li-2 *(Xingjian)*.

Discussion of points: LI-20 *(Yingxiang)*, situated beside the nose, is effective in clearing the nasal cavities. B-2 *(Zanzhu)*, on the Bladder channel, is connected with the nose and cheeks, and may be used to clear the nasal cavities and alleviate sinus headache. B-7 *(Tongtian)*, also on the Bladder channel, may be needled to clear a stuffy nose (i.e., draining an Exterior symptom). GB-20 *(Fengchi)*, on the Gall Bladder channel, drains Fire from the Gall Bladder. Li-2 *(Xingjian)*, on the Liver channel, spreads the Liver Qi.

Ear acupuncture
Points: External Nose, Inner Nose, Adrenal, Endocrine, Forehead
Method: Use moderate to strong stimulation, treating once every other day. Retain needles for 10-15 minutes. Ten to fifteen treatments constitute one course.

Piercing lymph nodes
Inject Ringer's solution into one of the submaxillary cervical lymph nodes.

Other prescriptions
1. LI-20 *(Yingxiang)*, LI-4 *(Hegu)*, GB-20 *(Fengchi)*. Treat daily with moderate stimulation. (Source: HCNMT)
2. GB-20 *(Fengchi)*, SI-15 *(Jianzhongshu)*, Gv-23 *(Shangxing)*, LI-20 *(Yingxiang)*, LI-10 *(Shousanli)*, LI-4 *(Hegu)*, B-17 *(Geshu)*. Burn 5-7 cones of moxa on Gv-23 *(Shangxing)*. (Source: CAM)
3. Gv-23 *(Shangxing)*, B-4 *(Quchai)*, M-HN-3 *(Yintang)*, B-12 *(Fengmen)*, LI-4 *(Hegu)*. (Source: IACC)
4. Gv-23 *(Shangxing)* and Gv-16 *(Fengfu)*. If ineffective add LI-19 *(Heliao)*, GB-20 *(Fengchi)*, Gv-26 *(Renzhong)*, M-HN-30 *(Bailao)*, B-12 *(Fengmen)*. (Source: GCAM)

Remarks
• Acupuncture therapy can improve the symptoms associated with this condition.

ACUTE TONSILLITIS

Traditional medicine attributes tonsillitis to a collection of Heat in the Lungs and Stomach, complicated by an attack of Wind.
Treatment is directed toward dispersing the Heat.

Needling
Principal points: SI-17 *(Tianrong)*, L-11 *(Shaoshang)*
Supplementary points: LI-4 *(Hegu)*, LI-11 *(Quchi)*

Method: Treat once daily, using moderate to strong stimulation. When needling SI-17 *(Tianrong)*, the needle sensation should extend to the pharynx. Prick L-11 *(Shaoshang)* to let a few drops of blood. For high fever, add LI-4 *(Hegu)* and LI-11 *(Quchi)*.

Discussion of points: The tonsils are beneath point SI-17 *(Tianrong)*. Needling this point disperses the Qi and Blood which has collected there. Pricking L-11 *(Shaoshang)* disperses Wind and Heat along the Lung channel. LI-4 *(Hegu)* and LI-11 *(Quchi)* drain the Heat of a fever.

690

Ear acupuncture

Prescription#1
Points: Throat, Tonsils
Method: Use moderate to strong stimulation with continuous manipulation of the needles for 2-3 minutes. Thereafter, retain needles for one hour. Treat once daily.

Prescription#2
Points: Helix #1, #2, and #3 as well as the posterior auricular veins
Method: Select a couple of the points and prick to let 2-5 drops of blood.

Foot acupuncture
Points: #1, #3, #45

Barefoot doctor acupuncture
Points: Barefoot Doctor point, Cervical #7

Piercing the lymph nodes
Inject Ringer's solution into one of the submaxillary lymph nodes. Treat once daily, 3 treatments constituting a course.

Injection therapy
Point: LI-4 *(Hegu)*
Method: Inject .5-1% procaine into this point, once daily.

Other prescriptions
1. LI-4 *(Hegu)*, S-44 *(Neiting)*, LI-11 *(Quchi)*. Treat daily with strong stimulation. (Source: HCNMT)

2. GB-20 *(Fengchi)*, B-10 *(Tianzhu)*, B-11 *(Dazhu)*, L-5 *(Chize)*, L-11 *(Shaoshang)*, LI-1 *(Shangyang)*. Daily with strong stimulation. (Source: CAM)

3. GB-20 *(Fengchi)*, B-10 *(Tianzhu)*, S-9 *(Renying)*, LI-17 *(Tianding)*, SI-16 *(Tianchuang)*, S-6 *(Jiache)*, B-11 *(Dazhu)*, B-12 *(Fengmen)*, SI-15 *(Jianzhongshu)*, GB-21 *(Jianjing)*, LI-4 *(Hegu)*, LI-11 *(Quchi)*, TB-17 *(Yifeng)*, TB-3 *(Zhongzhu)*, TB-1 *(Guanchong)*, LI-3 *(Sanjian)*, L-11 *(Shaoshang)*. (Source: NAM)

4. Throat blockage with inability to talk: LI-10 *(Shousanli)*, LI-7 *(Wenliu)*, LI-11 *(Quchi)*, TB-3 *(Zhongzhu)*, S-40 *(Fenglong)*. Throat blockage: H-7 *(Shenmen)*, LI-4 *(Hegu)*, GB-20 *(Fengchi)*. Throat blockage with Cold and Hot obstruction: SI-17 *(Tianrong)*, S-12 *(Quepen)*, B-11 *(Dazhu)*, B-17 *(Geshu)*, L-2 *(Yunmen)*, L-5 *(Chize)*, LI-2 *(Erjian)*, S-45 *(Lidui)*, K-1 *(Yongquan)*, K-2 *(Rangu)*. (Source: CNLAM)

5. Throat blockage; LI-4 *(Hegu)*, K-1 *(Yongquan)*, Co-22 *(Tiantu)*, S-40 *(Fenglong)*. (Source: GOA)

6. Throat blockage: B-10 *(Tianzhu)*, Co-23 *(Lianquan)*, Co-22 *(Tiantu)*, SI-5 *(Yanggu)*, LI-4 *(Hegu)*, SI-3 *(Houxi)*, LI-3 *(Sanjian)*, L-11 *(Shaoshang)*, TB-1 *(Guanchong)*, S-36 *(Zusanli)*, S-40 *(Fenglong)*, Sp-6 *(Sanyinjiao)*, Li-2 *(Xingjian)*. (Source: IACC)

7. Bilateral tonsillitis: L-11 *(Shaoshang)*, M-HN-20 *(Jinjin)*. Unilateral tonsillitis: L-11 *(Shaoshang)*, L-4 *(Hegu)*, M-HN-37 *(Haiquan)*. (Source: GCAM)

Remarks
• Relatively good results are obtained from the use of either the ear acupuncture or needling methods.

TOOTHACHE

Traditional medicine attributes toothache to either Fire in the Stomach, or Deficient Kidneys. The first is called Excessive pain, the second, Deficient pain.

Therapy

Treatment is directed toward spreading Qi through the channels near the affected area.

Needling
Principal points: LI-4 *(Hegu)*, S-6 *(Jiache)*, S-7 *(Xiaguan)*
Supplementary points: S-44 *(Neiting)*, K-3 *(Taixi)*

Method: First, needle the principal points with moderate to strong stimulation. Thereafter, retain needles for 10 minutes with periodic manipulation. Treat once daily. For symptoms associated with Fire in the Stomach (hallitosis, constipation), add S-44 *(Neiting)*. For symptoms associated with Deficient Kidneys (lassitude, loose teeth), add K-3 *(Taixi)*.

Discussion of points: Needling S-6 *(Jiache)* and S-7 *(Xiaguan)* spreads the Qi through the channels where it has collected around the teeth. LI-4 *(Hegu)* is situated on the Large Intestine channel, a branch of which penetrates beneath the teeth. Needling this point also spreads the Qi through the affected region. S-44 *(Neiting)* drains the collected Heat in the Stomach channel. K-3 *(Taixi)* strengthens the Kidneys.

Ear acupuncture
Points: Maxilla, Mandible, Tragus Apex
Method: Use moderate to strong stimulation, retaining needles for one hour.

Hand acupuncture
Point: Toothache

Foot acupuncture
Points: #14, #45

Head acupuncture
Points: Middle 2/5 of the Sensory area

Barefoot doctor acupuncture
Points: Barefoot Doctor point, Posterior *Hegu*, Tip of Tragus

Other prescriptions
1. Principal points: N-UE-1 *(Yatongzue)*, LI-4 *(Hegu)*. Supplementary points: S-7 *(Xiaguan)*, S-6 *(Jiache)*. Use strong stimulation. (Source: HCNMT)
2. Principal points: S-7 *(Xiaguan)*, LI-4 *(Hegu)*. Supplementary points: GB-20 *(Fengchi)*, B-11 *(Dazhu)*. (Source: CAM)
3. S-6 *(Jiache)*, SI-17 *(Tianrong)*, LI-4 *(Hegu)*. Continuously manipulate needles. (Source: NAM)
4. Toothache with chills: S-5 *(Daying)*, SI-18 *(Quanliao)*, GB-2 *(Tinghui)*, LI-11 *(Quchi)*, LI-1 *(Shangyang)*. Jaw pain: TB-17 *(Yifeng)*. Toothache with closed jaw: GB-3 *(Shangguan)*. (Source: CNLAM)
5. Toothache: LI-4 *(Hegu)*, S-44 *(Neiting)*, GB-10 *(Fubai)*, GB-14 *(Yangbai)*, LI-3 *(Sanjian)*. (Source: GOA)
6. Toothache: 3 cones of moxa on Co-24 *(Chengjiang)* and S-6 *(Jiache)*. 7 cones of moxa on LI-15 *(Jianyu)*, L-7 *(Lieque)*, L-9 *(Taiyuan)*, L-10 *(Yuji)*, SI-5 *(Yanggu)* for upper teeth; LI-4 *(Hegu)*, LI-3 *(Sanjian)* for lower teeth; S-36 *(Zusanli)* for upper teeth; K-3 *(Taixi)*, S-44 *(Neiting)* for upper teeth. (Source: IACC)

Remarks
- Acupuncture therapy is effective in alleviating the pain of toothache. However, the source of the pain must be determined and treated by other means.

Appendix I

Table of Abbreviations

ATDP	*Appendix to Thousand Ducat Prescriptions**
BBQS	*Book of Bian Que's Secrets**
BDH	*Barefoot Doctors' Handbook*
BPW	*Complete Collection of Beneficial Prescriptions for Women**
CAM	*Chinese Acupuncture and Moxibustion*
CBCA	*Complete Book of Carbuncles and Abscesses**
CBZJ	*Complete Book of Zhang Jingyue**
CCAM	*Complete Collection of Acupuncture and Moxibustion**
CCMHCD	*Clinical Chinese Medical Handbook for Common Diseases*
CDP	*Confucians' Duties to Their Parents*
CDR	*Classic of Divine Resonance**
CNLAM	*Classic of Nourishing Life with Acupuncture and Moxibustion**
COAM	*Compilation of Acupuncture and Moxibustion**
ECAM	*Essentials of Chinese Acupuncture and Moxibustion*
FCAM	"Fujian Traditional Chinese Medicine" (journal)
GCAM	*Great Compendium of Acupuncture and Moxibustion**
GOA	*Gatherings from Outstanding Acupuncturists**
GS	*Guidelines for Surgery**
HAM	*Handbook of Acupuncture and Moxibustion*
HCNMT	*Handbook for Common New Medical Therapies*
HCTM	Hebei College of Traditional Medicine [not a publication]
HIM	*Handbook of Internal Medicine*
HNMT	*Handbook of New Medical Therapies*
IACC	*Illustrated Appendices to the Classic of Categories**
ICAP	*Illustrated Classic of Acupuncture Points as Found on the Bronze Model**
JCM	"Jiangsu Traditional Chinese Medicine" (journal)
JDC	*Bian Que's Divine Resonance Acupuncture and Moxibustion Jade Dragon Classic**
JTM	"Journal of Traditional Chinese Medicine" (journal)
MQK	*Meaning of Qian and Kun**
MSAM	*Meeting the Source of Acupuncture and Moxibustion**
NAM	*New Acupuncture and Moxibustion*
NCM	"New Traditional Chinese Medicine" (journal)
NFO	*Necessities of a Frontier Official**
NOCM	*New Outline of Chinese Medicine*
NPA	*Necessities for Practicing Acupuncture**

OHS	*Ode of a Hundred Syndromes**
OM	*Outline of Medicine**
OSM	*Ode to the Standard of Mystery**
OXH	*Ode of Xi Hong**
PDM	*Principles of Divine Moxibustion**
PUB	*Prescriptions for Universal Benefit**
RAT	*Rapid Acupuncture Therapy*
SCCM	*Secrets of the Cinnabar Creek Master**
SCM	Shenyang College of Medicine [not a publication]
SGC	*Song of the Glorious Jade**
SJD	*Song of the Jade Dragon**
SJTM	"Shanghai Journal of Traditional Chinese Medicine" (journal)
SPDM	*Song of Points for Miscellaneous Diseases**
TAA	*Combined Chinese and Western Medicine in the Treatment of Acute Abdominal Disorders*
TDP	*Thousand Ducat Prescriptions**
TLM	*True Linneage of Medicine**
TMLP	*Treasured Mirror of Life Protection**
TWD	*Ten Works of Dongyuan**

*Written prior to 1911. For full bibliographic information, see Bibliography.

Appendix II

Guide to Pinyin Pronunciation

Consonants

b-	like *b-* in *obstinate*
c-	like *-ts* in *its*
ch-	like *ch-* in *chair* but with the tongue on the palate
d-	as in English but not as voiced
f-	as in English
g-	as in English but not as voiced
h-	between the *h-* in *how* and the *ch-* in *chutzpah*
j-	as in English but with the tip of the tongue on the lower teeth
k-	as in English but more strongly aspirated
l-	as in English
m-	as in English
n-	as in English
p-	as in English but more strongly aspirated
q-	like *ch-* in *chair* but with the tip of the tongue on the lower teeth
r-	something like *r-* in *raid* but with the tongue on the palate
s-	as in English
sh-	as in English but with the tongue on the palate
t-	as in English but more strongly aspirated
w-	as in English but softer
x-	something like *sh-* in *she* but with the tip of the tongue on the lower teeth
y-	as in English but softer
z-	like *-ds* in *pads*
zh-	like *j-* in *jar* but with the tongue on the palate

Vowels, Diphthongs and Finals*

a or *-a*	like *-a* in *father*
-ai	like *-ye* in *rye*
-an	like *-ohn* in *John*
-ang	something like *-ang* in the German *angst;* *ng* has both a nasalizing and gutteralizing action on the vowel
-ao	like *-ow* in *cow* but less fused

697

-e	like *-a* in *sofa*
-ei	like *-ay* in *bay*
-en	like *-un* in *fun*
-eng	like *-ung* in *lung*
er or *-er*	like *-ar* in *far*
-i	after *c-*, *ch-*, *s-*, *sh-*, *z-*, *sh-* something like the *-urr* in *burr* but shorter and with the tongue on the palate; after any other letter, like *-e* in *be*
-in	like *-een* in *sheen*
-ing	like *-ing* in *ring*
-iu	like *yo* in *yo-yo*
-o	like *-au* in *maudlin*
-ong	like *-ung* in *hung*
-ou	like *-ow* in *mow* but less fused
-u or *-ü*	after *j-*, *q-*, *x-*, *y-*, *l-*, or *n-* something like *-ew* in *knew* but with lips more pursed; after any other letter, like *-oo* in *boo*
-ua	like *-ua* in *Guam*
-uai	like *-ui* in *quiet*
-uan	like *-uan* in *quantity*
-uang	similar to *-uan* above but with a gutteral ending
-ui	like *-uay* in *quay* but slightly shorter
-un or *-ün*	after *j-*, *q-*, *x-*, *y-*, *l-*, or *n-* something like the *-une* in *June* but with lips more pursed; after any other letter, between the *-one* of *done* and the *-win* of *twin*
-uo	something like the *wa-* in *war*

*Diphthongs that are pronounced as expected from the respective vowels are not further discussed.

Appendix III

Table of Chinese Dynasties

Shang	16th cent. B.C. - 1066 B.C.
Zhou	1066 B.C. - 221 B.C.
Warring States	403 B.C. - 221 B.C.
Qin	221 B.C. - 206 B.C.
Western (Former) Han	206 B.C. - 23 A.D.
Eastern (Later) Han	25 A.D. - 220 A.D.
Three Kingdoms	220 A.D. - 280 A.D.
Jin	265 A.D. - 420 A.D.
North and South Kingdoms	420 A.D. - 581 A.D.
Liang	502 A.D. - 557 A.D.
Sui	581 A.D. - 618 A.D.
Tang	618 A.D. - 907 A.D.
Five Dynasties	907 A.D. - 960 A.D.
Song	960 A.D. - 1279 A.D.
Southern Song	1127 A.D. - 1279 A.D.
Jin (Tartar)	1115 A.D. - 1234 A.D.
Yuan (Mongol)	1279 A.D. - 1368 A.D.
Ming	1368 A.D. - 1644 A.D.
Qing (Manchu)	1644 A.D. - 1911 A.D.

Appendix IV

Cross Index of Acupuncture Points (Pinyin)

*=alternate name
°=point is not discussed in this text

A

Anmian   N-HN-54
Anmian #1   N-HN-22(a)
Anmian #2   N-HN-22(b)
Anmian #3   N-BW-21
Anmian #4   N-LE-50

B

Bafeng   M-LE-8
Bahua   M-BW-3
Baichongwu   M-LE-34
Baihuanshu   B-30
Baihui   Gv-20
Bailao   M-HN-30
Bailiao   B-31-34
Baizhongfeng   M-BW-2
Banmen   M-UE-13
Baohuang   B-48
Baxie   M-UE-22
Bazhuixia   M-BW-11
Benshen   GB-13
Biantao   M-HN-26
Bichuan*   M-HN-14
Biguan   S-31
Bijian*   Gv-25
Bikong   N-BW-34
Biliu   M-HN-16
Binao   LI-14
Bingfeng   SI-12
Bitong   M-HN-14
Bizhong   M-UE-30
Bulang   K-22
Burong   S-19

C

Changfeng   M-BW-18
Changqiang   Gv-1
Changyi   M-CA-17
Chengfu   B-50
Chenggu   M-LE-36
Chengguang   B-6
Chengjian   N-LE-12
Chengjiang   Co-24
Chengjin   B-56
Chengling   GB-18
Chengman   S-20
Chengming   M-LE-20
Chengqi   S-1
Chengshan   B-57
Chiqian   N-HN-17
Chirao   M-UE-36
Chixia   N-HN-40
Chixue   M-CA-1
Chize   L-5
Chonggu   M-HN-31
Chongjian   N-CA-5
Chongmen   Sp-12
Chongyang   S-42
Chuangxinmen   N-CA-9
Chuanxi*   M-BW-1
Chuqixue   N-LE-48
Ciliao   B-32
Cunping   M-UE-34

D

Dabao   Sp-21
Dachangshu   B-25

Dadu   Sp-2
Dadun   Li-1
Dagukong   M-UE-15
Dahe   K-12
Daheng   Sp-15
Daimai   GB-26
Daju   S-27
Daling   P-7
Dalun   M-LE-32
Damen   M-HN-40
Dannangxue   M-LE-23
Danshu   B-19
Dazhu   B-11
Dayan   N-BW-32
Daying   S-5
Dazhong   K-4
Dazhui   Gv-14
Dianxian   M-BW-36
Dicang   S-4
Dihe   M-HN-19
Diji   Sp-8
Dijian #1   N-HN-50(a)
Dijian #2   N-HN-50(b)
Dijian   N-LE-15
Dingchuan   M-BW-1
   (N-BW-4)*
Dingshen   N-HN-32
Dingshu   M-UE-28
Diwei   N-BW-28
Diweishu   N-BW-29
Diwuhui   GB-42
Dongfeng*   M-HN-26
Dubi   S-35 or M-LE-16

Duiduan Gv-27
Dushu B-16

E

Eni M-CA-21
Erbai M-UE-29
Erbeijingmaisantiao
   M-HN-12
Erjian (hand) LI-2
Erjian (ear) M-HN-10
Erliban N-LE-59
Ermen TB-21
Ershanmen° M-UE-19 (see
   Neumen N-UE-2)
Erzhuixia M-BW-5
Ezhong M-HN-2

F

Feichang* N-LE-44
Feirexue N-BW-20
Feishu B-13
Feiyang B-58
Fengchi GB-20
Fengfu Gv-16
Fengguan M-UE-4
Fenglong S-40
Fengmen B-12
Fengshi GB-31
Fengyan M-HN-28
Fengyan M-UE-7
Fuqi Sp-16
Fubai GB-10
Fufen B-36
Fujie Sp-14
Fuliu K-7
Fushe Sp-13
Futonggu* K-20
Futu (leg) S-32
Futu (neck) LI-18
Fuyamen N-HN-46
Fuyang B-59
Fuxi B-52
Fuxing* N-LE-34

G

Gangmensixue N-BW-39
Ganrexue N-BW-8
Ganshi N-CA-8
Ganshu B-18
Ganyandian N-LE-14
Gaohuang(shu) B-38
Gaoweishu N-BW-27
Geguan B-41
Genjin N-LE-9

Genping N-LE-3
Geshu B-17
Gongsun Sp-4
Gongzhong N-UE-9
Guanchong TB-1
Guangcai N-HN-33
Guangming GB-37
Guanmen S-22
Guantu M-LE-30
Guanyuan Co-4
Guanyuanshu B-26
Guilai S-29
Gunei* N-LE-31

H

Haiquan M-HN-37
Hanyan GB-4
Heding M-LE-27
Hegu LI-4
Heliao (ear) TB-22
Heliao (neck) LI-19
Henggu K-11
Hengwen° M-CA-9 (See
   Tongbian N-CA-11)
Heyang B-55
Hongyin M-HN-23
Houcong N-HN-16
Houding Gv-19
Houqimen° M-BW-22
Houtinggong N-HN-13
Houtinghui* N-HN-15
Houtingxue N-HN-14
Houxi SI-3
Houxuehai N-LE-30
Houyangguan N-LE-32
Houye° M-UE-44
Huagai Co-20
Huangmen B-46
Huangshu K-16
Huantiao GB-30
Huanmen M-BW-6
Huanzhong M-BW-34
Huanyue N-BW-37
Huaroumen S-24
Huatuojiaji* M-BW-35
Hubain N-UE-15
Huiyang B-35
Huiyin Co-1
Huizong TB-7
Hunmen B-42
Huxi N-HN-52

J

Jiabi° M-HN-15

Jiache S-6
Jiachengjiang M-HN-18
Jiaji M-BW-35
Jiali* N-HN-29
Jianei N-HN-29
Jianjing GB-21
Jiankua N-LE-55
Jianli Co-11
Jianliao TB-14
Jianming N-HN-3
Jianming #1 N-HN-3(a)
Jianming #2 H-HN-3(b)
Jianming #3 H-HN-3(c)
Jianming #4 N-HN-3(d)
Jianming #5 N-BW-12
Jainming N-UE-13
Jianneiling M-UE-48
Jianqian* M-UE-48
Jianshi P-5
Jianshu° M-UE-42 (See
   Zhitan #1 N-UE-29)
Jiantongdian N-BW-9
Jianwaishu SI-14
Jianweidian* M-LE-13
Jianxi N-LE-18
Jianyang* N-HN-3
Jianyu LI-15
Jianyuxia* N-UE-14
Jianzhen SI-9
Jianzhongshu SI-15
Jiaoling N-LE-24
Jiaosun TB-20
Jiaoyi M-LE-21
Niaxin K-8
Jiegu M-BW-15
Jiehexue N-BW-6
Jiejian N-LE31
Jiexi S-41
Jifeng M-BW-38
Jijupikuai* M-BW-19
Jimai Li-12
Jimen Sp-11
Jingbi M-HN-41
Jinggu B-64
Jingling° M-UE-26 (See
   Yaotong #2 N-UE-19(b))
Jingmen GB-25
Jingming B-1
Jingqu L-8
Jingxia* N-HN-2
Jingxia N-LE-5
Jingzhong M-CA-11
Jingzhong N-HN-28
Jinjin M-HN-20

Jinmen B-63
Jinsuo Gv-8
Jiquan H-1
Jisanxue M-BW-37
Jisibian M-CA-8
Jiudianfeng° M-UE-5
Jiuneifan N-LE-11
Jiuqi M-BW-28
Jiuwaifan #1 N-LE-10(a)
Jiuwaifan #2 N-LE-10(b)
Jiuwei Co-15
Jixia N-LE-20
Jixin* N-CA-1
Jizhong Gv-6
Jubi N-UE-10
Juegu* GB-39
Juejin #1 N-BW-30(a)
Juejin #2 N-BW-30(b)
Juejin #3 N-BW-30(c)
Juejin #4 N-BW-30(d)
Jueyinshu B-14
Jueyun M-CA-13
Jugu LI-16
Juguxia N-BW-19
Jujue° M-BW-4
Juliao (face) S-3
Juliao (hip) GB-29
Juquan M-HN-36
Juque Co-14
Juqueshu M-BW-7

K

Keliao* M-HN-18
Kongzui L-6
Kuangu M-LE-28
Kuanjiu N-LE-56
Kufang S-14
Kuiyangxue N-BW-13
Kunlun B-60

L

Lanweixue M-LE-13
Laogong P-8
Liangmen S-21
Liangqiu S-34
Liangyan° M-BW-8
Lianquan Co-23
Liaoliao M-LE-31
Libian N-BW-33
Lidui S-45
Lieque L-7
Ligou Li-5
Lijimingandian N-LE-51
Lineiting M-LE-1

Lingbao M-LE-40
Lingdao H-4
Linghou M-LE-24
Linghouxia M-LE-25
Lingtai Gv-10
Lingxia N-LE-17
Lingxia N-LE-60
Lingxu K-24
Liniao* N-CA-3
Linqi (foot) GB-41
Linqi (head) GB-15
Lishang N-LE-8
Liuhua M-BW-3
Liujingzhuipang N-BW-1
Liwai N-LE-7
Lizhong* N-BW-19
Longhan M-CA-3
Longmen M-CA-24
Longxue* N-HN-8
Longzhong* N-LE-16
Lougu Sp-7
Luodi* N-LE-9
Luojing M-HN-27
Luolingwu N-UE-3
Luoque B-8
Luoshang N-UE-6
Luozhen M-UE-24
Luxi TB-19

M

Maibu N-LE-23
Maigen N-BW-31
Meichong B-3
Meihua M-CA-5
Meitou* B-2
Meixiao* TB-23
Meizhong* M-HN-6
Mingmen Gv-4
Mingyan M-UE-8
Muchuang GB-16
Muming M-HN-32
Muzhihenglisanmao°
  M-LE-7
Muzhijian M-UE-2
Muzhijiehengwen M-UE-6
Muzhilihengwen M-LE-2

N

Naohu Gv-17
Naohui TB-13
Naokong GB-19
Naoqing N-LE-4
Naoshang N-UE-14
Naoshu SI-10

Neiguan P-6
Neihegu N-UE-17
Neihuaijian M-LE-17
Neijingming M-HN-33
Neikunlun* N-LE-12
Neiming* N-HN-1
Neiting S-44
Neiyangchi M-UE-12
Neiyingxiang M-HN-35
Niushangxue N-UE-8
Nuemen N-UE-2
Nuxi M-LE-9

P

Panggu N-LE-2
Pangguangshu B-28
Panglaogong M-UE-11
Panglianquan M-HN-24
Pangqiang N-BW-18
Pianli LI-6
Pigen M-BW-16
Pinxueling M-BW-32
Pirexue N-BW-10
Pishu B-20
Pohu B-37
Pushen B-61

Q

Qiabinzhong N-LE-42
Qiahoushangji N-BW-36
Qiading Gv-21
Qianfengshi° N-LE-22
Qiangjian Gv-18
Qiangkua N-LE-57
Qiangu SI-2
Qiangyin N-HN-25
Qianhouyinzhu M-LE-3
Qianjin N-LE-35
Qianzheng N-HN-20
Qiaoyin (foot) GB-44
Qiaoyin (head) GB-11
Qibiansixue M-CA-8
Qichong S-30
Qichuan M-BW-9
Qiduan M-LE-6
Qihai Co-6
Qihaishu B-24
Qihu S-13
Qijingzhuipang N-BW-3
Qimai TB-18
Qimen Li-14
Qimen M-CA-15
Qinglengyuan TB-11
Qingling H-2

Qishe S-11
Qiuhou M-HN-8
Qiuxu GB-40
Qixue K-13
Qiying N-HN-43
Qizhong Co-8
Qizhong M-CA-10
Quanjian M-UE-21
Quanliao SI-18
Quanshengzu M-LE-10
Qubin GB-7
Quchai B-4
Quchi LI-11
Quepen S-12
Qugu Co-2
Ququan Li-8
Quyangwei° M-UE-37
Quyuan SI-13
Quze P-3

R

Rangu K-2
Renying S-9
Renzhong Gv-26
Riyue GB-24
Ronghou N-HN-24
Rugen S-18
Ruzhong S-17

S

Sanchi M-UE-8
Sanjian LI-3
*Sanjiaoji** N-UE-14
Sanjiaojiu M-CA-23
Sanjiaoshu B-22
Sanliwai N-UE-20
Sanshang M-UE-14
Sanxiao M-HN-17
Sanyangluo TB-8
Sanyinjiao Sp-6
Shangbafeng M-LE-41
Shangbaxie M-UW-50
*Shangchengqi** N-HN-4
Shangen M-HN-4
Shangergen N-HN-12
Shangfengshi N-LE-34
Shangquan GB-3
*Shangheyang** N-LE-25
Shanghouxi N-UE-4
*Shangjiexi** N-LE-4
Shangjingming N-HN-1
Shangjuxu S-37
Shanglian LI-9
Shanglianquan M-HN-21

Shangliao B-31
Shanglong N-HN-37
Shangming N-HN-4
Shangqiu Sp-5
Shangqu K-17
Shangquan N-LE-52
Shangquchi N-UE-22
Shangtianzhu N-HN-44
Shangwan Co-13
Shangxi N-LE-13
Shangxing Gv-23
Shangxuehai N-LE-54
Shangyang LI-1
Shangyangquan N-LE-33
*Shangyilong** N-HN-15
*Shanyingxiang** M-HN-14
Shanzhong Co-17
Shaochong H-9
Shaofu H-8
Shaohai H-3
Shaoshang L-11
Shaoyangwei M-LE-19
Shaoze SI-1
Shencang K-25
Shendao Gv-11
Shenfeng K-23
Shenji N-BW-15
*Shenjue** Co-8
Shenmai B-62
Shenmen H-7
Shenque Co-8
Shenrexue N-BW-11
Shenshu B-23
Shentang B-39
Shenting Gv-24
Shenxi M-LE-29
Shenxin N-BW-23
Shenzhou N-UE-24
Shezhu M-HN-38
Shicang M-CA-6
Shidou Sp-17
Shiguan K-18
Shiguan M-CA-7
Shimen Co-5
Shimian M-LE-5
*Shiming** N-HN-3
Shiqizhuixia M-BW-25
Shiwang M-UE-49
Shixuan M-UE-1
Shoujinmen M-UE-27
Shousanli LI-10
Shouzhongping M-UE-10
Shuaigu GB-8
Shubian M-BW-13

Shufu K-27
Shugu B-65
Shuidao S-28
Shuifen Co-9
*Shuigou** Gv-26
Shuiquan K-5
Shuishang N-CA-1
Shuitu S-10
Shuxi N-CA-6
Sibai S-2
Sidu TB-9
Sifeng M-UE-9
Sili N-LE-37
Silian M-LE-38
Siman K-14
Siqiang N-LE-19
Sishencong M-HN-1
Sizhong N-HN-30
Sizhukong TB-23
Suliao Gv-25

T

Taibai Sp-3
Taichong Li-3
Taijian N-UE-11
Taixi K-3
Taiyang M-HN-9
Taiyi S-23
Taiyingiao M-LE-11
Taiyuan L-9
Tanchuan M-CA-2
Tanfu N-LE-39
Tankang N-LE-41
Tanli N-LE-40
Taodao Gv-13
Tianchi P-1
Tianchong GB-9
Tianchuang SI-16
Tianding LI-17
Tianfu L-3
Tianjing TB-10
Tianliao TB-15
Tianling M-UE-41
Tianquan P-2
Tianrong SI-17
Tianshu S-25
Tianting N-HN-19
Tiantu Co-22
Tianxi Sp-18
Tianyou TB-16
Tianzhu B-10
Tianzong SI11
Tiaokou S-38
Tiaoyue N-BW-16

703

Tigangjixue N-CA-16
Tingcong N-HN-10
Tinggong SI-19
Tinghui GB-2
Tingling N-HN-9
Tinglongjian N-HN-38
Tingmin N-HN-11
Tingtou M-CA-19
Tingxiang N-HN-36
Tingxue N-HN-8
Tituo(xue) N-CA-4
Tiwei N-CA-10
Tongbian N-CA-11
Tongerdao N-HN-41
Tonggu (abdomen) K-20
Tonggu (foot) B-66
Tongli H-5
Tongling N-UE-18
Tongming N-HN-35
Tongtian B-7
Tongziliao GB-1
Touguangming M-HN-5
Tounie N-HN-31
Touqiaoyin GB-11
Touwei S-8
Tunzhong M-BW-33

W

Waidingchuan N-BW-5
Waierdaokou N-HN-42
Waiguan TB-5
Waihuaijian M-LE-22
Waijingming* N-HN-6
Waijinjin M-HN-22
Wailaogong° M-UE-23 (see *Yaotong #1* N-UE-19(a))
Wailing S-26
Waiming N-HN-6
Waiqiu GB-36
Waisiman M-CA-12
Waiyinlian N-LE-58
Waiyuye M-HN-22
Waizhili N-LE-27
Wangu (head) GB-12
Wangu (wrist) SI-4
Wanli N-LE-6
Weibao M-CA-16
Weicang B-45
Weidao GB-28
Weigupang N-BW-35
Weile N-CA-2
Weiling° M-UE-25 (see *Yaotong #3* N-UE-19(c))
Weirexue N-BW-7

Weishang N-LE-25
Weishangxue N-CA-18
Weishu B-21
Weishu N-BW-14
Weixia N-LE-44
Weiyang B-53
Weizhong B-54
Wenliu LI-7
Wuchu B-5
Wuhu M-UE-45
Wuli (arm) LI-13
Wuli (thigh) Li-10
Wuling M-LE-39
Wushu GB-27
Wuyi S-15

X

Xiyan S-35
Xinzhongji N-CA-13
Xuanzhong GB-39
Xuechou M-BW-17
Xuefu M-BW-19
Xuehai Sp-10
Xueyadian N-BW-2

Y

Yamen Gv-15
Yaming N-HN-39
Yanchi N-HN-21
Yangbai GB-14
Yangchi TB-4
Yangfu GB-38
Yanggang B-43
Yanggu SI-5
Yangjiao GB-35
Yangkang N-LE-46
Yanglao SI-6
Yanglingquan GB-34
Yangwei #1 N-LE-39
Yangwei #2 N-LE-40
Yangwei #3 N-LE-41
Yangxi LI-5
Yankou M-HN-34
Yaogen M-BW-27
Yaoqi M-BW-29
Yaoshu Gv-2
Yaotong #1 N-UE-19(a)
Yaotong #2 N-UE-19(b)
Yaotong #3 N-UE-19(c)
Yaoyan M-BW-24
Yaoyangguan Gv-3
Yaoyi M-BW-23

Yatong N-UE-1
Yaxue M-HN-25
Yeling M-UE-40
Yemen TB-2
Yeniao N-CA-14
Yifeng TB-17
Yijing M-CA-14
Yilong N-HN-15
Yiming M-HN-13
Yimingxia N-HN-18
Yinbai Sp-1
Yinbao Li-9
Yinbian N-CA-17
Yindu K-19
Yingchuang S-16
Yingshang N-UE-12
Yingu K-10
Yingxia N-UE-7
Yingxiang LI-20
Yiniao N-LE-49
Yinjiao (abdomen) Co-7
Yinjiao (mouth) Gv-28
Yinkang N-LE-29
Yinkou M-BW-10
Yinlian Li-11
Yinlingquan Sp-9
Yinmen B-51
Yinshang N-LE-28
Yinshi S-33
Yintang M-HN-3
Yinwei #1 M-LE-37(a)
Yinwei #2 M-LE-37(b)
Yinwei #3 M-LE-37(c)
Yinxi H-6
Yinxia N-LE-45
Yishanmen M-UE-18
Yishe B-44
Yishu M-BW-12
Yixi B-40
Yongquan K-1
Youmen K-21
Youyi M-CA-4
Yuanye GB-22
Yuji L-10
Yunmen L-2
Yuqian° M-UE-43
Yutang Co-18
Yutain M-BW-31
Yuwei M-HN-7
Yuxia* N-HN-4
Yuyao M-HN-6
Yuye M-HN-20
Yuzhen B-9
Yuzhong K-26

Bibliography

BIBLIOGRAPHY A: CHINESE PUBLICATIONS PRE-1911

Bian Que's Divine Resonance Acupuncture and Moxibustion Jade Dragon Classic (Bian Que Shenying Zhenjiu Yulong Jing), Wang Guorui, Yuan, 1329.
扁鹊神应针灸玉龙经

Book of Bian Que's Secrets (Bian Que Xin Shu), Dou Cai, Song, 1146.
扁鹊心书

Classic of Categories (Lei Jing), Zhang Jiebin, Ming, 1624.
类经

Classic of Difficulties (Nan Jing), author unknown, Han. Commentaries collected by Wang Jiusi (Ming), Hua Shou (Ming), Xu Lingtai (Qing).
难经

Classic of Divine Resonance (Shenying Jing), Chen Hui, Ming, 1425.
神应经

Classic of Nourishing Life with Acupuncture and Moxibustion (Zhenjiu Zisheng Jing), Wang Weiyi, Song, 1220.
针灸资生经

Classic of the Pulse (Mai Jing), Wang Shuhe, Jin, c. 300.
脉经

Compilation of Acupuncture and Moxibustion (Zhenjiu Jicheng), Liao Runhong, Qing.
针灸集成

Complete Acupuncture and Moxibustion Book of Yang Jingzhai (Yang Jingzhai Zhenjiu Quanshu), Chen Xin, Ming.
楊敬斋针灸全书

Complete Book of Carbuncles and Abscesses (Chuang Yang Quanshu), also known as *Dou's Complete Book of External Medicine (Doushi Waike Quanshu),* Dou Menglin, Ming, 1569.
疮疡全书 , also known as 窦氏外科全书

707

Complete Book of Zhang Jingyue [Jiebin] (Jingyue Quanshu), Zhang Jiebin, Ming, 1624.
景岳全书

Complete Collection of Acupuncture and Moxibustion (Zhenjiu Daquan), Xu Feng, Ming, c. 1439.
针灸大全

Complete Collection of Beneficial Prescriptions for Women (Furen Da Quan Liangfang), Chen Ziming, Song, c. 1237.
妇人大全良方

Concise Prescriptons from the Golden Casket (Jingui Yaolue Fang Lun), Zhang Zhongjing, Han, c. 220.
金匮要略方论

Confucians' Duties to Their Parents (Rumen Shiqin), Zhang Congzheng, Jin Tartar, 1228.
儒门事亲

Continuation of Notes on the "Simple Questions" (Xu Suwen Chao), Wang Ji, Ming.
续素问钞

Discussion of Cold-Induced Disorders (Shanghan Lun), Zhang Zhongjing, Han, c. 220.
伤寒论

Discussion of the Origins of Symptoms of Disease (Zhubing Yuanhou Lun), Chao Yuanfang, Sui, 610.
诸病源候论

Elucidation of the Fourteen Channels (Shisi Jing Fahui), Hua Shou, Yuan, 1341.
十四经发挥

Emergency Moxibustion Methods (Beiji Jiufa), Wenren Qinian, Song, 1226.
备急灸法

Emergency Prescriptions to Keep Up One's Sleeve (Zhouhou Beiji Fang), originally by Ge Hong (Jin), c. 340. Edited by Tao Hongjing (Liang).
肘后备急方

Extensive Treasures to Protect Life (Weisheng Hongbao), Luo Tianyi, Yuan, 1343.
卫生鸿宝

Gatherings from Outstanding Acupuncturists (Zhenjiu Juying), Gao Wu, Ming, 1537.
针灸聚英

Great Compendium of Acupuncture and Moxibustion (Zhenjiu Dacheng), Yang Jizhou, Ming, 1601.
针灸大成

Guide to the Classics of Acupuncture (Zhenjing Zhinan), Dou Hanqing, Jin-Yuan, 1241.
针经指南

Illustrated Appendices to the Classic of Categories (Lei Jing Tu Yi), Zhang Jiebin, Ming, 1624.
类经图翼

Illustrated Classic of Acupuncture Points on the Bronze Model (Tongren Zhenjiu Shuxue Tu Jing), Wang Weiyi, Song, 1026.
铜人针灸俞穴图经

Illustrated Studies of the Channels (Jingmai Tukao), Chen Huichou, Qing.
经脉图考

Inner Classic (Nei Jing), (see *Yellow Emperor's Inner Classic* below).
内经

Introduction to Medicine (Yixue Rumen), Li Ting, Ming, 1575.
医学入门

Meaning of the "Classic of Difficulties" (Nan Jing Benyi), Huo Shou, Yuan, 1361.
难经本义

Meaning of Qian and Kun (Qian Kun Shengyi), author and date unknown.
乾坤生意

Meeting the Source of Acupuncture and Moxibustion (Zhenjiu Fengyuan), Li Xuechuan, Qing.
针灸逢源

Methods of Acupuncture and Moxibustion from the Golden Mirror of Medicine (Yizong Jinjian Cijiu Xinfa), Wu Qian, Qing, 1742.
医宗金鉴刺灸心法

Necessities of a Frontier Official (Waitai Biyao), Wang Tao, Tang, 952.
外台必要

Necessities of Practicing Acupuncture (Xing Zhen Zhiyao), found in the *Great Compendium of Acupuncture and Moxibustion,* (see above).
行针指要

New Edition of the Pharmacopeia (Bencao Congxin), Wu Yiluo, Qing, 1757.
本草从新

Ode of a Hundred Syndromes (Bai Zheng Fu), Gao Wu, Ming, 1529.
百症赋

Ode of the Essentials of Understanding (Tongxuan Zhiyao Fu), found in the *Great Compendium of Acupuncture and Moxibustion,* (see above).
通玄指要赋

Ode of the Golden Needle (Jinzhen Fu), found in the *Complete Collection of Acupuncture and Moxibustion,* (see above).
金针赋

Ode of the Standard of Mystery (Biao You Fu), Dou Hanqing, Jin Tartar, c. 1235.
标幽赋

Ode of the Subtleties of Flow (Liuzhu Zhiwei Fu), He Ruoyu, Jin Tartar, found in the *Great Compendium of Acupuncture and Moxibustion,* (see above).
流注指微赋

709

Ode of Xi Hong (Xi Hong Fu), found in *Gatherings from Outstanding Acupuncturists*, (see above).
席弘赋

Outline of Medicine (Yixue Gangmu), Lou Ying, Ming, 1565.
医学纲目

Pouch of Precious Pearls (Zhenzhu Nang), Zhang Yuansu, Jin Tatar.
珍珠囊

Prescriptions of Universal Benefit (Puji Fang), Zhu Xiao, Ming, 1406.
普济方

Principles of Divine Moxibustion (Shenjiu Jing Lun), Wu Yancheng, Qing.
神灸经论

Questions and Answers About Acupuncture and Moxibustion (Zhenjiu Wendui), Wang Ji, Ming, 1532.
针灸问对

Research on Points Along Channels (Xunjing Kao Xue Pian), author probably Yan Zhenshi, Ming, c. 1575.
循经考穴编

Sagelike Prescriptions from the Taiping Era (Taiping Shenghui Fang), Wang Huaiyin, Song, 992.
太平圣惠方

Secrets of the Cinnabar Creek Master (Danxi Xinfa), Zhu Zhenxiang, Yuan, 1347.
丹溪心法

Selected Materials Beneficial to Life (Jisheng Bacui), Du Sijing, Yuan, 1315.
济生拔粹

Simple Question (Su Wen), one of two parts of the *Yellow Emporer's Inner Classic*, (see below).
素问

Six Collections of Acupuncture Prescriptions (Zhenfang Liu Ji), Wu Kun, Ming.
针方六集

Song of the Glorious Jade (Shengyu Ge), found in the *Great Compendium of Acupuncture and Moxibustion*, (see above).
胜玉歌

Song of the Jade Dragon (Yulong Ge), found in *Gatherings from Outstanding Acupuncturists*, (see below).
玉龙歌

Song of Points for Miscellaneous Diseases (Zabing Xuewei Ge), found in *Gatherings from Outstanding Acupuncturists*, (see below).
杂病穴位歌

Spiritual Axis (Ling Shu), one of two parts of the *Yellow Emperor's Inner Classic*, (see below).
灵枢

Studies of the Eight Miscellaneous Channels (Qijing Bamai Kao), Li Shizhen, Ming, 1578.
奇经八脉考

Supplement to the Thousand Ducat Prescriptions (Qianjin Yi Fang), Sun Simiao, Tang, 659.
千金翼方

Systematic Classic of Acupuncture and Moxibustion (Zhenjiu Jiayi Jing), Huangfu Mi, Jin, 282.
针灸甲乙经

Ten Works of Dongyuan (Dongyuan Shi Shu), author unknown, early Ming.
東垣十书

Therapeutic Importance of the Acupuncture Points from the Bright Hall (Mingtang Kongxue Zhenjiu Zhiyao), author unknown, probably Han, c. 100. (Only extant fragments in *Systematic Classic of Acupuncture and Moxibustion.)*
明堂孔穴针灸治要

Thousand Ducat Prescriptions (Qianjin Yao Fang), Sun Simiao, Tang, 652.
千金要方

Treasured Mirror of Life Protection (Wei Sheng Baojian), Luo Tianyi, Yuan.
卫生宝鉴

True Linneage of Medicine (Yixue Zhengchuan), Yu Tianmin, Ming, 1515.
医学正传

Warp and Woof of Febrile Diseases (Wenre Jingwei), Wang Mengying, Qing.
温热经纬

Yellow Emperor's Inner Classic (Huang Di Nei Jing), authors unknown, for the most part compiled around 100 B.C. Present edition contains two books, the *Simple Questions* and the *Spiritual Axis.* Commentaries compiled by Zhang Jiebin (Ming), Ma Shi (Ming), and Zhang Zhicong (Qing).
黄帝内经

Yellow Emperor's Inner Classic: Categorization of the Bright Hall (Huang Di Nei Jing Mingtang Leicheng), author unknown. Commentary by Yang Shangshan, Sui, c. 610.
黄帝内经明堂类成

Yellow Emperor's Inner Classic: Great Simplicity (Huang Di Nei Jing Tai Su), author unknown. Commentary by Yang Shangshan, Sui, c. 610.
黄帝内经太素

BIBLIOGRAPHY B: PUBLICATIONS POST-1911

Acupuncture and Moxibustion (Zhenjiu Xue), Jiangsu Provincial School of Traditional Medicine.
针灸学

Acupuncture Point Chart (Zhenjiu Xuewei Gua Tu), Health Group of the Support Services for the Guangzhou Section of the People's Liberation Army and the Revolutionary Committee of the Guangzhou Arts Academy.
针灸穴位挂图

Acupuncture Point Loop-tying Therapy for the Sequelae of Infantile Paralysis (Xiaoer Mabizheng Houyizheng Xuewei Ciji Jiezha Liofa), People's Liberation Army Hospital #208.
小儿麻痹症后遗症穴位

'Beard of Wheat' Needle Therapy (Mang Zhen Liao Fa), Beijing City Acupuncture Clinic.
芒针疗法

Barefoot Doctors' Handbook (Chijiao Yisheng Shouce), Shanghai College of Traditional Medicine.
赤脚医生手册

Chart and Explanation of Off-Channel Miscellaneous Points (Zhenjiu Jingwai Qixue Tupu), Hao Jinkai.
针灸经外奇穴图谱

Chinese Acupuncture and Moxibustion (Zhongguo Zhenjiu Xue), Cheng Danan.
中国针灸学

Clinical Chinese Medical Handbook for Common Diseases (Changjianbing Zhongyi Linchuang Zhiliao Shouce), Jiangsu College of New Medicine.
常见病中医临床治疗手册

Combined Chinese and Western Medicine in the Treatment of Acute Abdominal Disorders (Zhongxiyi Jiehe Zhiliao Jifuzheng), Tianjin City Nankai Hospital.
中西医结合治疗急腹症

Complete Book to Popularize Medicine and Hygiene (Yixue Weisheng Puji Quan Shu), Shanghai Number 1 Hospital.
医学卫生普及全书

Cupping Therapy (Bahuo Liaofa), Huo Kangguo and Zhang Yongzeng.
拔罐疗法

Ear Acupuncture Therapy (Erzhen Liaofa), Zoological Institute of the Academia Sinica.
耳针疗法

Educational Materials for Colleges of Traditional Medicine by the Beijing College of Traditional Medicine.

Educational Materials of the Shanghai College of Traditional Medicine.

Essentials of Chinese Acupuncture and Moxibustion (Zhongguo Zhenjiuxue Gaiyao), Nanjing College of Traditional Medicine.
中国针灸学概要

Explanatory Charts for Clinical Location of Acupuncture Points (Zhenjiu Linchuang Quxue Tujie), Beijing College of Traditional Medicine.
针灸临床取穴图解

Handbook for Rural Physicians (Nongcun Yisheng Shouce), Hubei Medical School.
农村医生手册

Handbook of Acupuncture and Moxibustion (Zhenjiuxue Shouce), Wang Xuetai.
针灸学手册

Handbook of Common New Medical Therapies (Changyong Xinyi Liaofa Shouce), Health Group

712

of the Support Services for the Guangzhou Section of the People's Liberation Army.

常用新医疗法手册

Handbook of Internal Medicine (Neike Shouce), Shanghai Number 2 Medical School.

内科手册

Handbook of New Medical Therapies (Xinyi Liaofa Shouce), Health Group of the Support Services for the Shenyang Section of the People's Liberation Army.

新医疗法手册

Illustrated Reference for Acupuncture Channel Points (Zhenjiu Jingxue Tukao), Huang Zhuzhai.

针灸经穴图考

New Acupuncture and Moxibustion (Xin Zhenjiu Xue), Zhu Lian.

新针灸学

New Outline of Chinese Medicine (Xinpian Zhongyixue Gaiyao), Health Group of the Support Services for the Guanzhou Section of the People's Liberation Army.

新编中医学概要

Practical Internal Medicine (Shiyong Neike Xue), Shanghai Number 1 Medical School.

实用内科学

Rapid Acupuncture Therapy (Kuaisu Zhenci Liaofa), People's Liberation Army Air Force, Shenyang Hospital.

快速针刺疗法

Seven-Star Needle Therapy (Qixingzhen Liaofa), Wu Yiqing.

七星针疗法

Various Journals of Traditional Chinese Medicine.

TRANSLATORS' BIBLIOGRAPHY

Academy of Traditional Medicine and the Guangdong College of Traditional Medicine, editors, *Dictionary of Traditional Chinese Medical Terms and Nomenclature (Zhongyi Mingci Shuyu Cidian)*, Hong Kong: Commercial Press, 1975.
中医名词术语词典

Academy of Traditional Medicine, Guangzhou College of Traditional Medicine, et al., *Concise Dictionary of Traditional Chinese Medicine (Jianming Zhongyi Cidian)*, Hong Kong: Joint Publishing Co., 1979.
简明中医词典

Capital Hospital, *Classified Nomenclature of Diseases and Operations (Jibing Fenlei Ji Shoushu Fenlei Mingchen)*, Beijing: Peoples Health Publishing Company, 1980.
疾病分类及手术分类

Chen Biliu and Zheng Zhuoren, *Vernacular Explanation of the "Spiritual Axis" (Ling Shu Jing Baihua Jie)*, Beijing: People's Health Publishing Company, 1974.
灵枢经白话解

Chen Xinqian, et al., *New Edition of Pharmcology (Xin Bian Yaowu Xue)*, Beijing: People's Health Publishing Company, 1974.
新编药物学

Davies D.V. and Coupland, R.E., *Gray's Anatomy: Descriptive and Applied*, 34th Edition, London: Longmans, Green, and Co., Ltd., 1967.

Jia Dedao, *Brief History of Chinese Medicine (Zhongguo Yixue Shilue)*, Taiyuan: Shanxi People's Publishing Company, 1979.
中国医学史略

Jiangsu College of New Medicine, *Great Dictionary of Chinese Medicinal Substances (Zhongyao Da Cidian)*, Shanghai: Shanghai Science and Technology Publishing Co., 1977.
中药大词典

Lu Gwei Djen and Needham, Joseph, *Celestial Lancets*, Cambridge: Cambridge University Press, 1980.

W.B. Saunders Co., editor, *Dorlund's Illustrated Medical Dictionary*, translated into Chinese by the Modern Medical Society, Taibei: College Publishing Co., 1970.

Zhou Fengwu, Wang Wanjie, Xu Guoqian, *Vernacular Explanation of the Yellow Emperor's Inner Classic: Simple Questions (Huangdi Nei Jing Su Wen Baihua Jie)*, Beijing: People's Health Publishing Company, 1958.
黄帝内经素问白话解

717

NEW POINTS

BAREFOOT DOCTOR POINTS

EAR POINTS

Point Index

POINT CLUSTERS

General Index

Gastroenteritis
  acute, 246
  chronic, 289
Gatherings from Outstanding Acupuncturists, 64
  amenorrhea, 670
  back strain, 655
  Blockage, throat, 691
  carbuncles, 637
  cough, 592-93
  drowning, 568
  infantile convulsions, 578
  milk, lack of, 678
  needling methods, 517-18
  pain, low back, 656
  pain, rib, 643
  toothache, 692
  urinary dysfunction, 586
Girdle channel, 70,
Glaucoma, 149, 293, 681
Goiter, 165, 601-3
Golden Mirror of Medicine
  moxibustion, 439
  number of points in, 120
  organ, 'irritated', 628
Governing channel, 46, 67-68, 329-31
Great Compendium of Acupuncture and Moxibustion,
  46, 64, 120, 410, 411
  abdomen, distended, 278
  abdomen, fullness in, 276
  amenorrhea, 188, 670
  apoplexy, 158
  asthma, 179,595
  carbuncles, 637
  chest pain, 246, 250
  constipation, 181
  cough, chronic, 593
  coughing red sputum, 588
  diarrhea, 293
  discharge, red and white, 675
  draining methods, 522
  dysentery, 578
  dysmenorrhea, 279
  edema, 295
  eye membranes, 472
  eye pain, 275
  eye tics, 143
  fainting, 275
  face, swollen, 154
  feet, numb, 613
  hand, burning sensation in, 243
  headache, 158, 626
  heat exhaustion, 570
  hematuria, 250
  hemorrhoids, 645
  hyperextension, 167, 659
  incontinence, 276
  indigestion, 273
  indigestion, infantile, 632
  intestinal abscess, 640
  jaundice, 239
  jaw, locked, 156
  kyhosis, 168
  labor, difficult, 288
  Leg Qi, 289
  low back strain, 655
  madness, 249, 630

Great Compendium of Acupuncture . . . (continued)
  mental instability, 178
  mastitis, 638
  menstruation, irregular, 669
  milk, insufficient, 177, 241, 678
  mouth awry, 610
  needling methods, 518-19, 520-21
  nosebleed, 206
  pain, arm, 607
  pain, back, 280
  pain, elbow, 659
  pain, low back, 266, 280, 656
  pain, low back and legs, 612
  pain, rib, 236-279
  pain, shoulder, 658
  paralysis, 622
  rash, 635
  rectum, prolapsed, 645
  scrofula, 590
  seizures, 624
  sinusitis, 690
  strengthening methods, 522, 523
  sweating, insufficient, 233
  throat, dry, 244
  throat, swollen, 238, 246
  testicle, distended, 185
  tidal fevers, 142, 238, 241, 585
  tonsillitis, 691
  urination, difficult, 653
  uterine bleeding, 252, 290, 293, 673
  uterine, prolapsed, 291
  vomiting, 183
  vomiting blood, 231
  wet dreams, 651
  wheezing, 282
Great needle acupuncture, 428-29
Guide to the Classics of Acupuncture, 514-16, 519
Guidelines of Surgery
  carbuncles, 637
Gynecological diseases, 70, 75

H

Hand
  acupuncture, 501-5
  burning sensation in, 243
  numb, 662-63
Handbook of Acupuncture and Moxibustion
  amenorrhea, 670
  infantile paralysis, 583
  labor, induction of, 677
  neurodermatitis, 655
  rhinitis, 689
  vertigo, aural, 685
Handbook of Common New Medical Therapies
  arthritis, 607
  cerebrovacular accident, 622
  goiter, 602
  hyperthyroid, 604
  impotence, 652
  intestinal obstruction, 641
  leukorrhea, 675
  mastitis, 638
  menstrual disorders, 669
  morning sickness, 676
  multiple neuritis, 614
  myopia, 680

733

Handbook of Common New . . . Therapies (continued)
  neurasthenia, 627
  optic nerve atrophy, 684
  optic nerve neuritis, 683
  prostatitis, 650
  psychosis, 630
  renal colic, 649
  roundworm in the biliary tract, 643
  seizures, 624, 629
  shoulder problems, 658
  sinusitis, 690
  strabismus, 684
  tonsillitis, 691
  toothache, 692
  trigeminal neuralgia, 609
  urinary retention, 653
  urinary tract infection, 648
  uterine bleeding, abnormal, 670
  uterus, prolapsed, 674
Handbook of Internal Medicine
  drowning, 568
  heat exhaustion, 570
  pertussis, 576
Handbook of New Medical Therapies
  asthma, 594
  bronchitis, 592
  glaucoma, 681
  hepatitis, 579
  shock, 571
  vertigo, aural, 685
Half exterior/half interior, 20, 25
He Ruoyu, 514
Head acupuncture, 497-501
Head wind, 626
Headache
  frontal, 147, 172
  lateral, 172
  migraine, 143, 148, 278
  occipital, 285
  symptom, 25, 48, 55, 59, 60, 85
  treatment, 141, 142, 143, 144, 145, 152, 158, 159, 235, 237, 279, 283, 624-26
  vertex, 172
Hearing, impaired, 628, 687
Heart, traditional, 12-13, 401-2, 628
  Blood, Deficient, 13, 26
  channel, Arm Lesser Yin, 51-52, 307
  Fire, 13, 24, 40, 627
  Qi, Deficient, 13
  stuffy, 251
  Yang, Deficient, 13, 595
  Yin, Deficient, 13, 26
Heart blockage, 177, 606
Heart disease (see Rheumatic heart disease)
Heat (one of Six Excesses)/other see Hot, 17, 24, 26, 27, 29, 95, 402
Heat blockage, 606
Heat
  Deficient, 22, 24
  Excessive, 22, 24, 30, 568
  and Dampness (see Damp heat)
Heat exhaustion, 158, 257, 280, 568-70
Heaviness, feeling of, 51, 68, 88
Hebei College of Traditional Medicine
  myopia, 680
Hematuria, 250

Hemiplegia, 228, 247, 276, 621
Hemoptysis, 98, 225, 243, 245, 248, 588
Hemorrhage, upper digestive tract, 289
Hemorrhoids, 68, 281, 644-45
Hepatitis, 181, 203, 205, 292, 578-80
Hernia
  symptom, 60, 72, 93
  treatment, 190, 291
Herpes zoster, 618
Hiccoughs (also see Diaphragm, spasm of), 174, 557, 619
Hoarseness, 556
Hot (one of Eight Parameters), 20-21, 90, 93, 509
  Exterior, 19
  false, 21
  Interior, 20
Hot needle acupuncture, 430-31
Hua Tuo lining the spine points (see M-BW-35 *(Jiaji)* in Point Index), 217
Hunger, 51
Hyperextension (of spine), 167, 639
Hypersomnia, 252, 629
Hypertension, 144, 165, 168, 596-99
Hyperthyroid, 249, 603-4
Hypotension, 153, 165, 250
Hysteria, 158, 251, 628-29

I

Illustrated Appendices to the Classic of Categories, 64, 121
  asthma, 595
  blindness, green, 684
  Blockage, throat, 691
  cough, 593
  deafness, 688
  discharge, red and white, 675
  dizziness, 686
  enuresis, 633
  hemorrhoids, 645
  impotence, 652
  labor, induction of, 677
  low back strain, 654
  mastitis, 638
  menstruation, irregular, 669
  number of points in, 120
  pain, back, 656
  paraplegia, 616
  rectum, prolapsed, 646
  roundworm, chest pain from, 643
  scrofula, 590
  sinusitis, 690
  tidal fevers, 584
  toothache, 692
  urinary dysfunction, 586
  uterine bleeding, 675
  wet dreams, 651
  wheezing, 595
  worm, poisonous, 587
Illustrated Classic of Acupuncture Points as Found on the Bronze Model, 46
  number of points in, 120
  roundworm, chest pain from, 643
Illustrated Studies of the Channels, 46
Impotence
  symptom, 14, 55, 70, 95, 651
  treatment, 185, 188, 557, 651-52